NATUROPATHIC ONCOLOGY

An Encyclopedic Guide for Patients and Physicians

Dr. Neil McKinney, BSc, ND

NATUROPATHIC ONCOLOGY

An Encyclopedic Guide for Patients and Physicians

Dr. Neil McKinney, BSc, ND

LIAISON PRESS

VANCOUVER | CANADA

Naturopathic Oncology – An Encyclopedic Guide for Patients and Physicians
Dr. Neil McKinney, BSc, ND

Published by Liaison Press, Vancouver, BC, Canada
www.liaisonpress.com
ISBN-10: 1-894953-73-8
ISBN-13: 978-1-894953-73-3
First printing: November 2010
© 2010 Neil McKinney
All rights reserved.

This book is dedicated to the memory of John McKinney.
My twin, my true friend, my brother.
A man of peace, whose generous heart reached out to help everyone he could.
You're the best!

TABLE OF CONTENTS

PART ONE – A REALLY SIMPLE APPROACH TO CANCER

PART TWO – INTEGRATIVE ONCOLOGY

PART THREE – A DEEPER LOOK AT THE BIOLOGY OF CANCER

PART FOUR – A DEEPER LOOK AT NATUROPATHIC ONCOLOGY

PART SIX – PREVENTING CANCER

PART ONE – A REALLY SIMPLE APPROACH TO CANCER

Preface: How to Use This Book

This third edition on naturopathic oncology is updated with the rewards of clinical practice, study, research and reader feedback from the last several years.

I hope patients will find it easier to navigate, more complete, and of real service. I also hope it will provide inspiration to their integrative physicians and entire health team.

The **Introduction** gives you a narrative of my personal journey through teaching, medical research and study to practicing naturopathic medicine with a focus towards cancer care.

Part One – A really simple look at cancer – introduces the basic concepts and vocabulary of naturopathic cancer care in a very straight-forward way. This is intended for those with no training in science or medicine, who just want to know the bottom line in plain English. Then I introduce the fundamentals of naturopathic cancer care. The core products and protocols I have seen benefit many patients are introduced. Remedies are suggested for most common cancers. These are to be discussed with your doctors, who may have other suggestions.

Part Two – Integrative oncology – shows how naturopathic supports integrate with medical therapies to improve effectiveness and reduce harm. Surgery, radiation, chemotherapy, hormone therapy and immune therapy supports are described in a brief and simple style. Again, all cancer treatments require supervision by an attending physician , and all integrative cancer care requires the oversight of a qualified integrative physician in oncology.

Part Three – A deeper look at the science of cancer – introduces the essential vocabulary and concepts in naturopathic oncology. This gives a deeper insight into how a professional puts together an effective program tailored to each cancer patient. When you understand the biochemistry and biology of cancer, obstacles become opportunities, and strategies emerge to harmonize and heal.

Part Four – A deeper look at the arts and science of naturopathic oncology and integrative oncology – is for those who would like a more detailed scientific and technical explanation of the key concepts of naturopathic oncology in integrative cancer care. More detail is provided on the naturopathic repertoire of remedies. The major components and mechanism of action of many botanicals and nutraceuticals are provided. The biochemical rationale of diets and Complementary and Alternative Medicines (**CAM**) programs are discussed.

Part Five – Integrated treatment of common cancers – Using the more advanced language and knowledge acquired in Parts Three and Four, we re-examine in detail the common cancers – their diagnosis, medical treatment, and integrative care. Naturopathic medicines which target specific growth factors, receptors, hormones, cytokines and signalling pathways are matched to specific types and stages of cancer. Samples of protocols which have given good clinical responses are provided. You will find my best clinical pearls for the treatment of each major class of cancer. This may be the foundation of your personal prescription for healing, under the supervision of a qualified naturopathic physician.

While I give a great deal of detail on products and protocols which can give great results, you need and deserve to have an individualized program, close monitoring, and a trusted advisor in these matters. *Do NOT attempt to treat yourself!*

Do use this book to be informed about your best options, and what to expect them to accomplish. Get expert guidance from a licensed, accountable, health professional team experienced in treating cancer. Cancer is a life-threatening disease in most cases. You do not have the objectivity, experience or knowledge to make critical medical decisions alone. *This is not just a legal disclaimer.* I do not treat myself! *Cancer is unforgiving of delays and poor choices.*

Your cancer care team may offer other options than I have outlined in this book. *This book is not a self-help manual, nor is it a cookbook.* It is a contribution to the field of integrative oncology, not the final word on how you are going to get well.

Every remedy mentioned in this book may cause harm in a particular person or in combination with some other medications. It is your responsibility to seek the professional advice of your personal naturopathic physician or integrative physician to direct the use of any of these agents for any serious disease.

I hold some strong opinions against remedies many patients are taking, and even some my peers encourage. These are based on my simple criterion – either show me conventional scientific studies of merit supporting use of a high-risk agent, or show me reasonably consistent results with traditional and trusted natural remedies among those of my peers who I know to be objective and trustworthy. We verify safety and efficacy with the best available evidence. If I see little value in something purported to treat cancer, I say so. I have seen thousands of patients do many different therapies, so I have clinical experience to report.

I hope readers will realize that we continue to learn and progress. If you find you would like to try some of the therapies from this book, that is OK, but you should be asking your naturopathic doctor what is new and exciting, and what they can add to the mix. Medical doctors hold tumour boards, meetings where cases are discussed and a multi-disciplinary team discuss the latest trends in research and care, and come up with a consensus. This book is intended to be just one of the voices at that table.

Part Six – Preventing cancer – the new edition concludes with a discussion of the most effective treatment for cancer – prevention! Learn what to avoid, what to do, and find resources to reduce risk and maximize vitality.

INTRODUCTION
A Journey to Healing

I was born with the help of a nurse midwife at Vancouver General Hospital. The doctor never did show up. Alternative medicine is the theme of my whole life.

I had an epiphany at age 15 which made me aware that there was something more to healing than drugs or surgery. I had an extraordinary healing of a severe burn by Reiki therapy. It was actually a miracle.

I credit my first encounter with homeopathic medicine in India in 1975 with saving my life from terrible dysentery. I have met others with similar experiences of extraordinary healing by simple, natural means.

I have finally now begun to reach a goal set so long ago, to help people with cancer using the healing power of Nature. Wonderful outcomes, even miracles, continue to occur in my life and in that of my patients. Yes, we do see more healings than cures, and some people have a very hard path despite our walking with them. Still, it is my joy to join them in hope, and offer care with loving kindness.

I can claim some contributions and innovations in the cancer field, some large, some small:

- The synergistic combination of green tea EGCG, curcumin and grapeseed extracts to control the growth and spread of many cancers. Inspired by Boik and many others, this trilogy remains a core therapy.
- The rapid dose-escalation protocol for Iscador mistletoe, which gets to the full dose in 3 weeks instead of the traditional 6 week build-up, and with fewer problems.
- Mitochondrial rescue protocol – a very useful program for difficult cancers.
- Using homeopathic "kickers" in herbal tinctures for cancer.
- Low-glycemic and wholesome meal replacements with greens powders, whey protein isolates and vitamins in smoothies.
- Wart Death escharotic formula.
- Describing apoptosis simply as "the off-switch for bad cells."
- Original integrative protocols to support radiation, chemotherapy, and other standard medical treatments.
- Matching natural medicines to proven growth factors for each type of cancer, recognizing the unique biology of the various forms of cancer.
- Organizing a reference database of scientific research on natural medicines and cancer.
- Mentoring and teaching doctors around the world.

Natural medicines can be integrated into medical cancer therapies with great success. I have created some novel cancer treatment plans and formulas, and have found a network of other reputable doctors and scientists who have reached similar conclusions. There are many whose work parallels mine. Many of the therapies I use are becoming common among my peers in naturopathic medicine and medical oncology. Others are very time-tested classical formulae from Traditional Chinese Medicine TCM, as well as some very modern TCM advances in cancer care. In turn, my medical and naturopathic peers have mentored me and shared their excellent treatment ideas.

There are humane physicians around the world who integrate standard cancer medicine with natural therapies such as diet, detoxification, exercise, emotional support, music, and spiritual practices. These greatly impact quality of life. They may be considered scientifically "unproven," but of course they can still be much sought after by patients. Patients can choose, and do have the right to choose, treatments even if research on them has not yet found a rich sponsor. I think anything alive has value, and so does anything perceived as supporting life.

Natural therapies with plant medicines, living foods and nutritional supplements are rationally directed to immune strengthening, normalizing cell regulation, and encouraging bad cells to recycle themselves. Working with Nature, we can bring the order of biological self-regulation to bear on the chaos that is cancer. Naturally, there's always hope!

Chapter One: What is cancer?

What causes cancer?

Your body is made up of trillions of cells, each a little living organism unto itself. They specialize into many different roles (differentiate), and collect into various tissues and organs. All cells should communicate and cooperate with all the others in a harmonious way, for the good of the whole.

Cancer means cells are:

- growing too fast
- growing out of control, wounding local tissues.
- losing the ability to perform the cellular tasks they should do
- learning to do things and to make cell products they should not be making
- recruiting stem cells and immune cells to support and feed them –in "repair mode," vainly trying to fix the "wound that will not heal," but unable to repair the genetic faults at the root of the malignancy.
- becoming capable of invading into places they shouldn't go, with immune cell and stem cell support
- becoming capable of living in distant parts of the body (metastasis)
- progressively mutating into potentially even more dangerous cells.

Therefore, cancer is parasitic, toxic and destructive. It can disrupt the entire biochemistry and metabolism of the body. It can eat up all the resources, wreck essential organs and ruin life support functions such as blood clotting and the immune system.

The disorganization of whole body systems, organs, tissues and cells begins in the information library of the cell, the genetic material in the cell center (nucleus). The chromosomes from our parents are made up of **DNA** organized into genes. DNA carries the code to make proteins such as enzymes. Enzymes are living catalysts which make all of life's chemical reactions (biochemistry) happen, at body temperature and at the atmospheric pressure we live under. Every scrap of every cell, and every chemical in the body, is assembled by enzymes based on the instructions contained in the DNA.

Cancer begins with **oxidative stress** on the DNA. Oxygen is highly reactive – most things on this Earth can either burn or rust. Inside our bodies we make super-reactive forms of oxygen we call **free radicals of oxygen** or **reactive oxygen species ROS**. We generate a lot of them in the combustion chambers inside cells (mitochondria) where we burn sugars with oxygen for energy. We harness the power of these oxygen bombs for detoxifying any chemical we want out of the body, and use them in our immune system as potent anti-microbial weapons. We have natural defences we call **anti-oxidants** which control oxygen reactions. Most we get from food, some we make for ourselves.

Antioxidants – such as vitamin C, vitamin E, selenium, alpha lipoic acid, beta carotene (provitamin A) and related carotenes and retinoids found in diets loaded with fresh whole fruits and vegetables – can prevent cancer!

Radiation, cancer-causing chemicals, stress hormones and everything else which can cause cancer (carcinogens) produce oxidation of the DNA. This disrupts the information stored in the DNA, making a mutant gene. A mutation results in a wrong enzyme or no functioning enzyme at all.

When several very specific mutations occur, without killing the cell, it can be permanently transformed into a cancer cell (carcinogenesis). It takes a multitude of insults to the cell, and an accumulation of several survival skills before a cell gets to a state of radical growth, yet is so altered it cannot die no matter how damaged or stressed that mad growth makes them..

An example is the loss of normal cell-to-cell communication which tells normal cells to stop growing when they are touching another cell. Cancer cells lose this contact inhibition, and keep on growing, piling up into abnormal lumps of cells we call tumours.

By the time the cancer cell doubles 20 times there will be over a million cancer cells in the tumour. It will be a very small lump, perhaps 1 millimetre in diameter, too small to be causing any significant symptoms, and too small to be seen on diagnostic screening tests. The cells will be burning energy and metabolizing at 30 to 40 times the rate of normal cells of the same type.

At this point tumours may start to run low on oxygen, which we call hypoxia. The cancer must at this point have developed the ability to generate more than normal amounts of chemicals which attract new blood vessels to grow into the lump. If it cannot sustain aggressive in-growth of new blood vessels, it will stop growing rapidly, and in fact may die off completely.

Tumours that grow to a detectable size have mastered getting blood vessels to grow. They also must make new lymphatic vessels grow out to provide drainage of waste fluids. These new vessels are always disorganized, thin-walled and leaky, so the tumour starts to build up fluid pressure. This crushes the weak vessels, lowering oxygen and nutrient supply, in turn triggering another round of new blood vessel growth. No matter how much new blood vessel growth there is to feed new tumour growth, the pressure of more cells and fluid leakage will always create areas of low oxygen.

The low oxygen zones will now start to switch from burning sugars with oxygen to making energy by **fermenting** sugars without oxygen. This is like what yeast and other very primitive cells do for energy. It is 19 times less efficient than getting energy by burning sugars, so the tumour starts to become a bottomless pit into which the life energy starts to drain. Advanced cancer leads to fatigue and weight loss because the tumour is growing very fast but very wastefully.

I once made a long road trip in an old Rambler station wagon with a big V-8 motor equipped with dual Holley carburetors. You could see the gas gauge falling visibly as you drove. We had to stop at pretty much every gas station on the way there and back. The next trip I took was in a Volkswagen Beetle, and I got there and back on one tank of gas. Cancer is like the old Rambler. Their big motors are terribly inefficient.

The low oxygen zones in the tumour become filled with lactic acid, the same waste product you build up in your muscles after strenuous exertion. It makes a person tired, and even achy, but even worse, it actually makes cancer cells grow and spread even faster!

Cancer cells are acidic and low in oxygen, but it is not possible to cure cancer with oxygen therapies or with alkaline pH therapies. Alkaline diets help, but not just because they are alkaline. Oxygen and pH based therapies are red flags for possible quackery!

After just a handful of doublings, the tumour can now be 1 to 2 centimetres in diameter. This is the point at which the cancer is often detected, and a diagnosis is made. Unfortunately it is also the point at which the cancer has often begun to spread.

When a human cell has doubled 50 times, or in other words when its DNA has been copied 50 times, it should recognize it may be full of errors. It stops at a checkpoint before committing to split into two new cells and checks itself for DNA nicks, missing pieces, and other glitches. This process operates rather like the "scan disc" program on your computer. It looks through the "hard drive" in the cell, and if there are too many errors to repair, it will throw the built-in off switch for bad cells. The "apoptosis" program causes it to break up into bits, turn its membranes inside-out and it gets recycled. It is a normal process to remove old or damaged cells for the good of the community of cells in which it lives. Deleted cells are then replaced by fresh new cells created from stem cells. The new cell starts the counter at zero, and has pristine new DNA. If a normal cell gets damaged by radiation or chemicals, it should also throw the apoptosis switch before 50 doublings.

We are replacing cells all the time, whether they are old or damaged, or both. Cancer is when new cells form where not needed as replacements, and arise from mutated cells that have lost control and purpose.

The most abnormal thing about cancer cells is that they have blocked the off-switch for bad cells, called *apoptosis*. These malignant cells will not die, even when highly mutated, damaged and very old. They become very sick, but almost immortal. Once cancer cells pass this threshold, at about a diagnosable size, they have become very difficult to kill. Restoring the off-switch in the cancer cell is the number one goal of cancer therapy.

For years I grew human and animal cells in a cancer research laboratory. Normal cells we got from patients would die off after 50 doublings, which is called the Flickman Limit. I was good at tissue culture, but no one can beat this built-in safety system. However, I also grew cancer cells, and they just go on forever, like the Energizer Bunny of cells. One cell line we used in research was "Hela cells," from the cervical cancer of a woman named Henrietta Lacks – who died in the 1950's. Her cancer cells are alive and well in labs all over the world. They will always grow, as long as someone keeps feeding them.

BEYOND the DNA

While genetics are important in the life of a cell, it is after all only a reliable way of passing down information. A living cell is made of all the products the enzymes make, and they breathe actual life into the cell. The cell must get nutrients and information from its environment. It does this through the cell membrane – its overcoat, studded with sensors and signalling devices called receptors.

Most important in cancer are the hormone and growth factor receptors. These accept only very specific molecules, most of which are the sex hormones estrogen or testosterone, or chemicals from outside the body which are very similar, called **xenohormones** or **xenobiotics**.

Other often important cancer growth factors include insulin-like growth factors IGF-1 and IGF-2 made in the liver, and a protein made during inflammation called cyclooxygenase two – COX-2. There are many growth factors, and all growth factors are bad for cancer. It is already a disease because the cells are growing too fast!

We act to reduce the number of receptors, block the receptors, or cut off the growth factor supply to slow the growth of tumours. If we do not, cancers will develop more and more of the receptors, and even start making their own growth factors, to grow faster and faster.

Outside the cell lies the extracellular matrix ECM, made up of a gelatinous ground substance, connective tissue, blood and lymph vessels, nerves, dormant immune cells, stem cells, and more. The ECM turns out to be a major regulator of cell growth, promoting or blocking cancer development and progression. The single most important regulator in the ECM is vitamin A. It acts on the immune cells and stem cells in the area that are supporting and nurturing their neighbours.

My Chinese medicine training taught me that cancer is associated with "blood stasis." The Chinese knew this over a thousand years ago, and it is easily diagnosed by TCM pulse and tongue assessment. About 150 years ago Western physicians began to notice cancer patients had a very high risk of forming blood clots – depending on the cancer, 7 to 30 times normal risk of clots.

I was taught in TCM college that cancer patients who developed "fire poison" or "heat toxin" are on a slippery slope to doom, and in fact this is very true in practice. Well, this is just **inflammation**. Treated in a timely way, cancer patients recover and live for months or years in good health. I lectured on this to medical oncologists at Grand Rounds at the BC Cancer Agency a few years ago, and they had not realized the importance of controlling inflammation. Now it is in all the medical journals, and is a hot topic. However, they still do not consistently test for it, don't treat it adequately, and the drugs they do use for it are dangerous.

Immune cells are attracted to cancerous tumours, due to stress signals from over-crowding and nutrient depletion. They see damaged cells, and immediately start to try to repair the problems. The entire wound-healing mechanism kicks in, creating growth factors, blood and lymph vessel support, and enzymes to assist **invasion** and movement of the cancer cells. Once cancer starts to invade adjacent tissues, it can begin to severely damage tissue and organ function, as well as that of its neighbours.

The most dangerous thing that this disease called cancer does is **metastasize** or spread into distant sites. It may start as a single cell entering a leaky lymph or blood vessel in the tumour, carrying it in the circulation to somewhere else. It may be by invasion into a vessel or body cavity. It may be by a clump of cells being shed during handling in surgery or even at biopsy for diagnosis.

If the cancer cell is still much like the normal tissue it is supposed to be, we call it "well **differentiated**." It will be very highly adapted to doing a specialized job in a specific place, and is not likely to be able to adapt to life in a new part of the body. If it is de-differentiated, poorly differentiated, or even worse, anaplastic, it is no longer focussed on its assigned task. All it is concentrating on is growing and invading.

If a cancer cell can invade its way out of the blood or lymph vessels it can easily attach to a sticky platelet and be carried off to a new location. If it can move out of the bloodstream, attach in a new organ, and get new blood vessels to feed it, a new metastatic tumour may form. These **mets** in vital organs like the brain, liver, adrenal glands and bones cause the most harm and suffering. Widespread cancer is very difficult to control, much less cure.

However grim your medical prognosis may sound, always remember these wise words of hope:

Cancer is only a word – not a "sentence."

Chapter Two: Introduction to naturopathic cancer care

Oncology is the medical term for cancer care and treatment. Like all of medicine, it is an art and a science, and there are many traditions and styles of practice available to you.

A naturopathic physician's job description has been defined by the US government as "Diagnose, treat and help prevent diseases using a system of practice that is based on the natural healing capacity of individuals. May use physiological, psychological or mechanical methods. May also use natural medicines, prescription or legend drugs, foods, herbs or other natural remedies." For a detailed look at the Canadian description of our training and practices, please see the website of the Canadian Association of Naturopathic Doctors www.cand.ca

Integrative and naturopathic oncology is the application of all the licensed and regulated medical arts to the care of the person with cancer. It is concerned with healing as well as cure, with humane care as well as medications, and with personal empowerment as well as medical interventions. We integrate all effective therapies, be they natural, drug, food, emotional, spiritual or the therapeutic relationship with your partners in health.

Remember the contents of this book are not to be construed as medical advice to any reader. You require professional assistance by a licensed health care provider experienced in integrative cancer care to use any method or product described in this book. This information is only illustrative of some options for cancer care you might discuss with your doctors.

Why bother adding extra costs and complexities to treating cancer? Why should we search the margins of scientific research for novel ideas based on medicines the pharmaceutical and medical industries have long portrayed as unimportant?

The answer is that the number of cancer deaths is rising faster than the growth of population in Canada – 48% in the last 20 years. The incidence of many cancers is on the rise too.

Furthermore, the treatments are always harsh and despite the costs and rigors of oncological medicine, about half of cases diagnosed with cancer will still die from cancer. Some sources say up to 64% still die, when relatively innocent skin cancers are subtracted. So, there is a great need to do far more to prevent, treat, support and cure cancers. I have seen naturopathic cancer strategies make an enormous difference in most cases.

The most cost-effective solution for the cancer epidemic is to put together all the current healing arts and sciences into an integrated plan.

Starting your integration:

1. Get a proper diagnosis, including where it is and is not in your body (staging)

so we know what we are up against, and can be as aggressive as is necessary. Have your medical file including laboratory tests, scans and pathology report, and pertinent medical reports sent to your naturopathic doctor.

2. Use naturopathic medicines at all stages of cancer to restore quality of life, stabilize disease progression, create remission and cure. Start immediately with the prescribed basic core supplement program, most of which will be taken from the **Leading Remedies for Integrative Cancer Care** list. I call this "Interval Care," as it is to be used while awaiting staging or medical therapies, between rounds of medical care, and on a long-term basis after the medical interventions.

3. Integrate naturopathic and traditional Chinese medicine into your medical cancer care. You can reduce harm and substantially increase the chance of a durable remission or cure from conventional surgery, radiation, chemotherapy, hormone therapy and immune therapies. Not all the medicines in the Leading Remedies list are compatible with oncology procedures such as surgery, radiation, chemotherapy, hormone blockade, immune and biological therapies. Keep your naturopathic physician informed of any change in your medications or medical treatment plan.

4. Return for regular follow-ups to keep this program well tuned to your current health needs and medications.

5. Change to whole organic foods and low sugar (low glycemic) diet.

6. Develop a maintenance program to reinforce remission and push for a cure.

7. Do NOT self-treat, including using advice from unlicensed persons, multi-level marketing products, or internet sources. You are the CEO of your own body, and a sovereign person, but you need the expertise of a naturopathic physician skilled in the arts and science of interactions between drugs and natural medicines. To marshal all your resources, anticipate what is going to happen next, and to personalize a program requires an objective person with the experience to make sound judgements. Cancer is unforgiving of mistakes and time wasted!

A philosophy of naturopathic oncology

The body has an innate gift for healing itself. It must be properly nourished, kept clean, and supported to do this job. Naturopathic medicines from all the healing traditions of the world are applied in a manner which respects the nature of the human being. Naturopathy is biologically sound, wholesome, and tailored to the individual patient. We have a physical body which is shaped by a genetic code inherited from people who were well adapted to a hunter-gatherer diet, radically different from the modern diet. They inhabited an unpolluted world, and had a lot less time stress. We also have an emotional life, a discerning mind, and a spiritual dimension. Naturopathic medicine keeps these facts in focus in its healing process.

I believe in the principle of *Vis Medicatrix Naturae* – the healing power of Nature.

I understand we are created in the divine spirit which is manifesting by expressing and experiencing itself in ways that are non-linear, non-local and yet coherent. Life is chaotic, but more brilliantly organized than current medicine paradigms can understand.

Naturopathic Oncology

"The deeper we go into the facets of life, the more mysteries we encounter. Analyzing living systems, we often have to pull them to pieces, decompose complex biological happenings into simple reactions. The smaller and simpler systems we study, the more it will satisfy the rules of physics and chemistry, the more we will understand it, but also the less 'alive' it will be. So when we have broken down living systems to molecules and analyzed their behaviour, we may kid ourselves into believing that we know what life is, forgetting that molecules have no life at all."—Albert Von Szent-Gyorgyi, MD Nobel laureate, discoverer of vitamin C.

Every modern disease can be improved by gentle therapies which feed, harmonize, cleanse and balance the complex biological systems that synergize in great networks that make a whole person. We start with a sound diet of whole, living foods. Food concentrates, vitamins and minerals are important to shift the health rapidly in the face of aggressive disease. In this respect they are used as drugs. Later, as health returns, we can rely on dietetics alone. I cannot fathom doctors who think a few milligrams of this drug or that drug is all important, while the pounds of chemicals we take in as food are ignored as irrelevant.

As a well trained and experienced researcher and scientist, I know science from nonsense. I have won several awards for raising the standards in my profession. I have seen enough scientific and clinical evidence to ethically integrate naturopathic medicine into modern oncology. If a therapy is not "proven" to the highest possible standard, then informed consent is still a reasonable basis to proceed. The safer the therapy and the greater the need, the lower we can set out threshold of what is utilitarian and can be offered in good faith. If it appears to benefit a majority of my patients and those my peers, in a reproducible way, then I think our patients have a right to know. All I ask is that they get better taking it, could become worse on stopping it, and that it be safe.

The American Food and Drug Administration (FDA) suggests that 2 or more randomized controlled clinical trials are needed to qualify as "substantial evidence." This is *more than an iota, but less than a preponderance.*

Evidence for natural medicines in cancer care is now readily found to this level and beyond. It is fine to run an institution such as the venerable BC Cancer Agency as a research-oriented and research-driven collective, with treatment decisions screened by a panel of experts. High standards of evidence are noble. However, the present model of evidence-based medicine EBM is often used too restrictively. It may make an easy cookbook style medicine that serves reimbursement coding and legal tort defence, but translating research into humane medical practice is still an art that requires judgement and skill.

Where the rubber really hits the road in medicine is in the very personal and interactive doctor-patient relationship.

All forms of medicine must ultimately in the end serve the patient's best interests, and have to respect the patient's right to choose or refuse any therapy offered. People do not always choose care based on volumes of scientific research. They and their doctor are actually the only ones who have ever experimented on their particular case.

Sometimes they actually know what is right for themselves, even if science doesn't.

Cancer is close to becoming the leading cause of death for Canadians. It is bound to strike nearly every family of two parents and a child, as nearly one in three of us will develop cancer in our lifetime. Nearly half of all patients diagnosed with cancer still eventually die of the cancer despite the best of medical care. Nearly all patients are being harmed by standard cancer therapies. This provides the rationale for more than two out of three cancer patients seeking out further cancer care from licensed practitioners of complementary and alternative medicine.

Complementary care includes measures to increase the effectiveness of medical therapies such as surgery, chemotherapy and radiation, and reduce their harm. Alternative therapies are intended to extend life and improve quality of life between and beyond medical therapies. Major cancer treatment centers in America and Asia blend drugs and surgery with herbal medicine, homeopathy, traditional Chinese medicine, nutrition and mind-body medicine. The result is improved patient outcomes.

The great weight of scientific evidence is that anti-oxidants, herbs and many other types of natural medicine and healing arts can be integrated into specific procedures of medical oncology to significantly improve responses to therapy while lessening complications. Complementary and alternative medicine is part of the current treatment model at leading oncology hospitals such as Memorial Sloan Kettering in New York, MD Anderson in Houston, Dana-Farber in Boston, Keith Block's Integrative Cancer Care Institute in Chicago, and all the Cancer Treatment Centers of America five hospitals and clinics.

Naturopathic Physicians have a potent armamentarium to tackle many of the problems of the cancer patient, at all stages of disease and at all stages of therapy. In following chapters you will learn how to use naturopathic supports for surgery, radiation and chemotherapy.

Most "spontaneous remissions" from terminal cancer are associated with major changes in diet and psychological patterns. Copying nature, we provide care intended to prolong life and restore meaning and usefulness.

After the standard medical therapies there is still a significant risk of relapse. We offer cancer suppressive natural agents which can arrest further growth and spread. I have found great inspiration from the work of John Boik who assembled world research on natural agents for cancer, and from the naturopathic doctors at Cancer Treatment Centers of America. I can tell you, from twenty-five years of clinical practice, which products and processes work consistently for cancer, and which of them does not.

Every ill person can benefit by gentle therapies which feed, harmonize, cleanse and balance the complex biological systems that synergize to make up the whole person. We start with a sound diet of whole, living foods. We are what we eat. What else could we be made of? In all cases we want to reduce sugar and refined starches, increase clean protein, give good fats, increase fibre, and supply lots of antioxidants. Food concentrates, vitamins and minerals are important to shift the health rapidly in the face of aggressive disease. In this respect they are used as drugs. Later, as health returns, we can rely on dietetics alone – "food shall be our medicine."

Naturopathic Oncology

We use medicinal as well as food plants, in as whole a form as possible, and in complex combinations to take advantage of the natural synergies that exist. Every living thing on this Earth is working with the same issues, the same stresses and problems, and many strategies have evolved in other living beings to regulate growth and restore balance. We can integrate their successes into our biology to correct our health.

We use various gentle medicines which satisfy our commitment to the Hippocratic Oath, to FIRST DO NO HARM. We cannot gain health just by cutting out disease. We respect the subtle and elegant power of the mind, of the immune system, and the homeostatic regulation in the body, and address all of them with medicines which are not necessarily cancer specifics. We are treating the person, not the disease. The Chinese call my approach *Fu Zheng Pai Beng*, which means **support and nourish the patient to fight the disease**.

Healing is about restoring sufficient balance to allow proper relationships in our physical, emotional, and spiritual dimensions. We hope to create enough time and vitality to allow each person to experience the joys of life, personal relationships, and awareness of our interconnections with things greater than ourselves

Curing cancer is not always possible. Achieving clinical stability with good quality of life is usually possible, and significant life extension is also quite common.

Primary Strategies in Naturopathic Oncology

The more of these issues we successfully address, the greater is the likelihood of surviving the cancer with a minimum of harm:

- Improve the terrain (the internal biochemical milieu) to support normal cell division, primarily by improving nutrition. Dr. Block suggests the cancer terrain is set by these factors: oxidative stress, inflammation, insulin-like growth factor IGF-1, blood coagulation parameters, immunity and stress hormones.
- Support differentiation of cells back to their normal function
- Remove promoters – environmental toxins, dietary hazards, and toxic emotional stressors such as fear and despair. Apply physical, dietary and mental hygiene principles to make a safer lifestyle.
- Detoxify from accumulated carcinogens.
- Deal with toxic emotions, address fears and feelings, practice positive attitudes and lifestyle.
- Stop mutation, stabilize the DNA genome and support DNA repair
- Inhibit invasion and metastasis
- Enhance cell-to-cell communication
- Support apoptosis – the off-switch for bad cells – a built-in cellular program for natural removal of cells with unhealthy DNA, or cells that are no longer needed. Resuscitate the burning of sugars by oxygen in the mitochondria, to restore the off-switch in cancer cells.
- Modulate activity of bone marrow derived and local stem cells, recruited to control inflammation, which resist treatment and cause recurrence and spread.

- Control inflammation and its growth factors that speed progression
- Enhance cell-to-cell communication
- Destroy tumours with natural medications – use synergies of non-toxic natural drugs to directly kill cancer.
- Target specific growth factors and their receptors with natural medicines.
- Support balanced immune function, including removal of toxic fungi and parasites, control viral replication, restore the good flora and fauna of the gut.
- Inhibit invasion
- Stop metastasis or spread to distant sites.
- Inhibit blood vessel growth into tumours and cancer cell clusters.
- Reduce side-effects and symptoms of the disease and treatments.
- Detoxification from chemo drugs and other harsh medications after treatment.
- Rejuvenation – restore real health and vitality.
- Prevention of re-occurrence or new cancers or other chronic diseases.

How a naturopathic physician thinks about a cancer case:

My naturopathic physician colleagues at the Cancer Treatment Centers of America have laid out a simple set of issues to explore with every new patient.

What is the exact diagnosis? What is the stage of the disease? What is the natural history of that form of cancer at that stage – the average survival & prognosis? Develop realistic expectations, and then strive to be an uncommon success.

Why this person at this time with this disease? Disease has meaning, it is not random. Find the cause, physically, chemically, emotionally.

What other medical conditions e.g. hypertension, diabetes, cardiovascular, immune, renal or liver complications?

Is the, digestion, absorption and overall nutritional status adequate to fight this disease?

Assess primary care treatment options, as well as adjuncts, complementary care, alternative medicines, palliation, social supports, psychological and self-healing assets. Integrate the best available evidence from systematic medical research, but not to the exclusion of the conscientious application of good judgement and individual clinical experience. Always remember that **the only medical experiment that truly matters is the one you and your physician decide to try on you.**

Set up a method and schedule for monitoring progress. Tumour markers in the blood can guide therapy, subject to expert interpretation. Monitor health parameters such as body weight and lean body mass index BMI, blood albumen, liver enzymes, kidney function, blood chemistry.

After treatment and recovery, detoxify and then start a prevention program.

Diagnosing Cancer

Biopsy and histological evaluation are the only way to confirm cancer. This means a doctor or surgeon gives suspected tumour tissue to a medical doctor certified in the medical specialty of pathology. This expert in the structure and chemistry of living tissue looks at your cells under a microscope, and may perform various biochemical tests on your biopsy tissue.

It is unethical to offer to treat as cancer a case that has not been medically confirmed, nor can one claim a cure until all positive medical test results related to cancer are reversed in a lasting way.

Cytology is a method of looking at loose cells taken off tumours or from around them. Pap smears, washings or brushings during endoscopies, and needle aspiration are alternatives to removing the primary tumour for evaluation.

Diagnosis is supported by physical exam, scans, X-ray imaging, neurological findings, tumour specific scans, tumour markers and other chemicals in the blood such as hormones, tumour antigens and antibodies.

It can be very frustrating for patients to go through test after test, as the doctors determine exactly what the nature of the cancer is, and how advanced it is. "Staging" tests show if it has spread locally or widely. Only when all this is known can the overall treatment plan be made. However, it is my firm conviction that taking steps at the first diagnosis to prevent further growth and spread can be fruitful. It is understood that the program will be fine-tuned later, and all the naturopathic and medical strategies integrated. Still, some basic and generic methods to arrest growth and spread make sense, to ease stress, and reduce the risk of the cancer running wild in the interim.

As strange as it may seem, with all the modern scans and molecular techniques, not all cancers can be definitively diagnosed. About 3 to 5% of cancers show up as metastases from an unknown primary source. Some cancers are just so mutated that one cannot say with certainty what tissue or organ they came from.

Measuring response to therapy

A response to therapy is a good thing, but does not in any way guarantee longer survival, or even longer disease-free survival. For example about 75% of patients get a therapeutic response in cancers of the prostate, head and neck, ovary, chronic leukemias, multiple myeloma, mycosis fungoides and stage 3 to 4 breast cancers, yet it is rare not to have a reoccurrence. Often the recurrent cancer is quite treatment resistant.

Complete response – the disappearance of all evidence of tumour/s, including any metastases, for at least 2 measurement periods separated by at least 4 weeks.

Partial response – a decrease of 50% or more in one or more measureable lesions with no progression of any lesion and no appearance of any new lesions for at least 4 weeks.

Stable disease – a decrease of less than 50% to an increase up to 25% in lesion diameter = no change

Progression – an increase of over 25% in diameter of a lesion or the appearance of any new lesions.

Standards of care

Patients expect every type of physician to provide good care, even if the treatment is unorthodox or experimental.

I do not operate a crusade to convert people to natural medicine, and medical oncologists should not act as if they have all the answers either. We all need to get involved early, act promptly, and respond quickly.

Always act in the patient's best interest. This means putting the patient's welfare ahead of any desire by the practitioner for money, control, power, gratification or any self-serving interest. I define the core professional ethics as "service and sacrifice."

Informed consent must always be obtained, preferably in writing. This basic legal principle means the patient needs to be told what the diagnosis is, what will happen without treatment, what all the treatment options are, and what the consequences of those choices will be. These must be explained in such a way that the patient actually understands them, and is able to give permission to the doctor without feeling pressured or coerced in any way.

It is the patient who knows best what is right for them, and they have" the right to be wrong" – to choose care or a lifestyle different from what we would do or advise them to do.

Tumour regression frequently occurs early in the course of effective treatment. If there is no objective evidence of a reasonable response to treatment in 4 to 6 weeks, then new options must be examined, or a referral made to another practitioner for exploration of other options. Natural therapies may not act as fast as drugs, but they must act by this time frame or be abandoned. Most good outcomes begin with a response within a day or two. I always recommend an objective test such as a CT scan, PET scan, or reliable tumour marker test by 6 weeks to confirm a response. If the cancer growth and spread is not at least stabilized by that time, another therapy should be tried.

Assess every 3 months for the first year, every 6 months in the second year, and annually thereafter. Usually after 5 years cancer free the patient is considered "cured." The odds of reoccurrence fall off sharply by that time. 20 year survival is about 85% of the 5 year levels.

ALTERNATIVE AND COMPLEMENTARY NATUROPATHIC MEDICINE IN CANCER CARE

There are hundreds of excellent naturopathic medicines and procedures which can help in the healing of cancer patients. These are discussed in more detail in Part Four – a deeper look at naturopathic oncology. This simpler introductory section is for the patient who does not need to know all the whys and wherefores, but just wants to know what to ask the doctor about. Consider exploring the following general subjects:

- Nutrition – dietetics and food supplements
- Botanicals – herbs and medicinal plants
- Homeopathic remedies – for body, mind and spirit.

Naturopathic Oncology

- Traditional Chinese Medicine TCM – herbs, acupuncture, qi gong.
- Psychology – mind-body healing – such as Dr. Teresa Clarke's *Remembered Wellness* CD
- Expressive therapies – art, music, journaling
- Intravenous oxidative medicines – vitamin C, glutathione, ozone.
- Vaccines and immune therapies.

You will find the naturopathic repertoire to be so vast as to be overwhelming. You cannot become an instant expert in such a vast field. So, how are you going to get to the right program for your cancer care? Do you need homeopathic medicines, acupuncture, massage, colon therapy, detoxification, intravenous therapy, psychotherapy or expressive therapies? This clearly requires professional guidance from someone familiar with the role of each of these modalities in cancer. Consult a licensed naturopathic physician to boil it all down to something practical. If you want to go on to read the more technical parts of the book – Parts 4 and 5 – you may get some insight into the nuances of what drives certain cancers to grow and spread, and how to mix targeted agents together for synergies, while avoiding medication conflicts. It should be absolutely clear there are many great therapeutic strategies to discuss with your health care team. We do not lack for good ideas, and you do not have the qualifications to decide where to start and when to change your program.

Naturopathic Diet for Cancer

Emphasize fresh fruits and vegetables. Eat an entire rainbow of various plant foods. The very best foods to fight cancer are organic green vegetables and red fruits. Raw foods are alive, energizing and healing. Try salads, veggie dips, smoothies, or chunky style. For an excellent review of what is in these brightly coloured plant foods see the book *"Foods That Fight Cancer"* by Drs. Beliveau and Gingras of McGill University. They have also published a cookbook on this topic. These coloured food compounds are real cancer drugs, but are of course safe.

Many herbicides and pesticides act like our hormones estrogen or testosterone. *Xenobiotics* or *xenohormones* (foreign hormones) such as dioxins and bisphenol act like estrogen. They are fat soluble, and so accumulate in our fatty tissues. That would obviously be a problem in most breast cancers. If you cannot buy all organic or grow your own, thoroughly soak, wash and scrub produce to remove as much of these chemicals as possible.

Home-made juices such as carrot, celery, and cabbage are encouraged. Beet juice should be limited to 2 ounces daily, from one medium beet. Greens such as parsley, beet tops, kale or wheatgrass make excellent additions to fresh juice. Apple juice may be added for taste.

Animal foods can be OK for cancer patients, but the quality is critical. Most integrative medicine doctors will tell you to eat strictly vegetarian if you have cancer, because commercial grade red meat noticeably increases tumour growth rates. I believe this is because the omega 3 to 6 fat ratio in grain or corn silage fed red meats promotes inflammation. Find wild game, or organic meat, <u>pasture grass fed</u>. Grass gives meat lots of anti-inflammatory omega 3 oils. Buffalo (bison) and lamb are typically only grass-fed. Beef can be grass-fed, but costs more to finish on grass. It is also the accumulation of xenohormones which make common grocery and restaurant grade meats dangerous for a cancer patient. You must <u>only eat clean meat grown on clean feed</u>. It must be <u>hormone and drug free</u>. The same goes for poultry and eggs, which need to be fed real grains and food, not some mystery filth pellets of rendered animals and waste products. Wrapping fatty foods like meat and cheese in plastic taints them with plasticizers which are nasty xenobiotics. Ask for meat packaged in butcher paper, and use it at home too. There is not yet a certified organic system in place for animal foods, so the only real system is "buyer beware."

If you find proteins or meat hard to digest, ask your naturopathic doctor if you might benefit from supplementing the stomach hydrochloric acid with betaine hydrochloride. Consider plant-source protease enzymes to augment stomach or pancreatic enzyme deficiency.

Poultry is certainly safer than red meat, and so deserves to be more of a staple food for healing. No-one controls what is meant by "free-range" eggs or "free-range" chickens, and it is more important what they have been eating than how much exercise they got. It is acceptable to feed grain to birds, but we cannot support feeding them "mystery filth pellets" of rendered waste. Clean, hormone and drug free poultry is preferable. Just like the difference between farmed salmon and wild is apparent in the taste, smell and texture of the fish, it is obvious that poultry raised in the traditional ways of our grandparents are superior to agri-business poultry. They will cost more, but are so much more satisfying to eat, and even digest easier. It is well worth the effort and expense.

We are now seeing certified **organic milk and dairy foods**. Cultured and soured organic milk products are very good for you. If you cannot get organic dairy, stick with skim or non-fat products. Many doctors advocate a vegan diet- no eggs or dairy or fish, as well as no meat. The issue with milk and cheese is the potential to form "mucus," which some believe protects cancer cells from the immune system, and the potential to form compounds which promote tumour invasiveness. The invasion factor is only made by rare dangerous bacteria that most people do not harbour in their gut. I don't worry about these issues, and my patients do well eating clean dairy foods.

Fresh wild fish is a terrific form of protein, and easily digested. Most fish do contain some heavy metals and nasty chemicals such as dioxins, flame retardants, and pesticides. However, because of their wonderful nutritional value, they still have a definite net health benefit.

Avoid farmed salmon and trout, which are fed filthy things, and taste like it too.

Avoid tuna, shark, swordfish/marlin and other large predators which accumulate too much mercury. Mercury certainly promotes many cancers, and poisons our innate healing systems.

We can scare ourselves into accepting only a limited and unbalanced diet. The more we study food science the more concerns and confusion we find. An excellent book on this topic is Dr. Steven Bratman's *Health Food Junkies: Orthorexia Nervosa: Overcoming the Obsession with Healthful Eating.* "Orthorexia nervosa" is a term he coined for the neurosis of overly-correct eating. Dr. John Bastyr, ND once gave a brilliant talk on avoiding the worst thing we can swallow at mealtime – *worry* – including the fear of being poisoned and of dietary mistakes, and the guilt of eating what we actually like. Once you make a food choice, enjoy it with gusto!

Our bodies can detoxify a lot, and need a variety of food, so keep your core diet clean, and allow yourself a little wiggle-room to bend some of the rules. The better the food quality is, the more you should eat, and the worse it is, the smaller the portion size and the less often you should be having it. Above all, be thankful for any food you decide to eat, and do not turn it into a poison by worry. Replace worry with concern. Pick the best food available, but once chosen, eat it with a happy heart. Bless it to your needs, and enjoy it with gusto and gratitude.

You can have quality fish, dairy, poultry and even red meat in moderation. If you choose instead to be vegetarian or vegan, remember that adequate quality protein is a key to healthy immune function and the healing of tissues.

I think a lot of **completely raw food and juice plans such as the Gerson diet and the Hallelujah Acres plan are dangerous to the majority of cancer patients** because they are grossly deficient in protein, and often add a high glycemic load.

Some protein requirements may come from fresh nuts. Seeds are excellent, such as fresh sesame seeds, flax seeds, pumpkin seeds, sunflower seeds. Fresh nuts and seeds provide healthful omega 3 oils.

Peas, lentils, beans and other legumes are a good source of protein and fibre. Soybeans are best eaten in fermented forms, such as miso.

Cook with extra virgin-grade olive oil to obtain the healthy **omega 9** oil oleic acid. Organic grapeseed oil, sesame oil, cold-pressed canola, sunflower and coconut may be used. Butter is permitted in small quantities.

Reduce or eliminate inflammation-promoting omega 6 fats: man-made trans-fatty acids and arachidonic acid, such as corn oil, margarine, shortening, and hydrogenated fats.

Pure water, green tea, rooibos (red bush) tea and taheebo (pau d'arco) tea are the preferred beverages.

Sugar Feeds Most Cancers!

Eat a low glycemic diet to reduce the insulin and insulin-like growth factors driving the growth of your cancer.

If insulin, IGF-1, IGFR or IGFBP are listed in the "targets of therapy" in the chapter devoted to the integrative care of your type of cancer, then it is sugar sensitive. Breast, prostate and all GI cancers are sugar sensitive.

Some cancers, surprisingly, are not sensitive to sugar.

A low sugar or low glycemic load diet helps prevent most cancers, improves responses to medical therapies for cancer, and slows the progression of these cancers.

Low glycemic means far less sugar and fast sugar-releasing starches, including wheat, potatoes and bananas. It means more heavy rye bread, real oatmeal porridge, peas and beans, berries and sweet potato.

Glycemic index refers to the rate at which foods turn into blood sugar. Almost all sugars and starches we eat get reprocessed in the liver into glucose. After a meal the surge of glucose or "blood sugar" in the bloodstream causes the pancreas to release insulin. Insulin attaches to cells and pumps nutrition into them – sugars, proteins and fats. One way cancer cells grow too fast is by always having far more insulin than normal cells.

Cancer cells build more receptors on their surface for insulin. This is like putting a turbocharger on a motor. By pumping more fuel in, it is able to run faster than normal. A typical breast cancer cell will have triple the insulin loading docks compared to a non-cancerous breast cell of the same type.

If the insulin spikes up the liver responds by releasing insulin-like growth factors one and two IGF-1, IGF-2 which tell the cell, "Now you have food, grow!" Many cancers will grow faster after a high sugar-load meal. A recent study showed that colon cancer cells that spread into the liver grew at 8 times the normal rate for about 3 hours after a high glycemic meal – with no obvious sugars or dessert included. This is just like throwing gas on a fire!

Like a diabetic, make "food exchanges" to keep the high sugar-releasing foods to smaller portions, less often, and not too many together in a meal or too much in a day. It is all about moderation. Trade a sweet you like for a sweet you don't care as much about.

There are many good websites with food lists, such as **www.lowglycemicdiet.com**. Google or any other internet search engine can give you a hundred lists. There are also a lot of books on this subject in the public library system. My favourite is *The New Glucose Revolution,* 3rd edition, by Dr. Jennie Brand-Miller, MD, or any of her "GI" Revolution books. She does not make the cancer connection in any of her books, but she does a great job of explaining about the glycemic index and the glycemic load, with recipes and menu plans.

Be aware that as you peruse different lists created by various labs over the last 25 or more years, the numbers attributed to a given food may not be consistent. The current contender for the next international standard is referenced to glucose. A glycemic index of 100 is the blood sugar and insulin response seen after ingesting pure glucose, made from corn sugar, given in an amount proportional to your body surface area, as standardized in medical testing for diabetes or glucose tolerance. An old standard was referenced to the impact of eating white bread, with a difference of 40%.compared to the glucose test. The glycemic index value assigned to a food also depends on the variety tested, its ripeness and what the investigator chose as a portion size. The glycemic value is only an estimate of what you will actually consume, and allow us to roughly rank foods. Don't put too fine a point on the exact numbers. Whatever list you are looking at, **the basic concept is eat less of the foods with the higher numbers and more of the foods with the lower numbers.**

Assuming a rating of 100 is referenced to eating a measured amount of glucose from corn sugar, according to your body surface area, as in a diabetes or glucose tolerance medical test, then GI under 60 (plus or minus a few points) is a non-stress food that can be eaten freely. These foods should become a core part of your diet, a staple food. Those rated 65 to 80 will be less healthful, and should be limited. Those over 80 are definitely going to pump up the IGF if taken often in large amounts. Eat them a lot less often and in much smaller portions.

The real core issue is the **glycemic load**, or total sugar intake in a day. If you over-eat a moderate glycemic index food, it will have the same effect as less of a higher index food. It is always all about balance and moderation.

Some fruits to limit: kiwi, banana, mango, pineapple, watermelon, all dried fruit – including dates and raisins.

Fruit canned in juice is OK, but not fruit canned in syrup. Dilute fruit juices by ½, – except for red grape, pomegranate, blueberry, raspberry or unsweetened cranberry juices.

Vegetables to limit: beets (cooked), carrots (cooked), potato, corn, parsnips. Raw grated or juiced carrots are fine, and the same goes for raw or juiced beets, in moderation.

Basmati rice is superior to polished white rice, and brown rice is best. I like to mix in red rice and wild rice.

Grains to limit: anything refined or white, and very soft breads. Very dense breads are better, such as true rye pumpernickel, also called full-korn bread, the kind that looks like a bunch of grain pressed together and is solid as a brick. If it is mostly wheat and is spongy or soft, it will be higher glycemic. The leavening process of bread making alters the starch structure, which breaks up fast into sugars in our digestive tracts. Flat unleavened breads such as wraps, pitas and tortillas have a low glycemic index, while the same amount of that flour puffed up into a baguette or loaf will often be very high glycemic. Choose organic whole grain cereals such as real oatmeal and Red River mixed grains.

Provided the core foods are OK, some treats and sweets are permitted. For example, 70 – 85% cacao chocolate is OK in moderation. We give you a little "wiggle room" to enjoy life. It is all about balance.

Use Stevia as a sugar substitute for adding sweetness. Stevia is good for baking only up to temperatures of about 350° F. Stevia may be toxic in high amounts, and certainly is very, very sweet, so use sparingly.

Use Xylitol sugar-alcohol for higher temperature baking. Other sugar alcohols include Maltitol, Mannitol – note they all end in "-ol." The newest is erythritol, being sold as Organic Zero. Also note that sugar alcohols can provoke diarrhea if eaten in excess. This can sometimes persist long after the intake of sugar-alcohols is stopped. Use moderately.

Blue agave cactus syrup is promoted as a low glycemic substitute for syrups or honey. It is very high in fructose, which can increase insulin resistance and diabetes risk. It is not recommended.

Splenda is the most user-friendly sugar substitute, although not 100% natural. I think it will do you more good than harm. Use moderately.

In addition to a low sugar load diet, we recommend you consider further measures to regulate the insulin-like growth factors such as drinking green tea, eating cooked tomatoes for lycopene, supplementing with flaxseed and vitamin D3 and exercising regularly.

Avoid human growth hormone HGH or supplements which increase these hormones, such as colostrum. Colostrum from cows is a silly idea for a health food anyway.

Low Glycemic Index Summary

Name of Food	GI Value	GI Level
Beans and Legumes (dried, soaked, and boiled; preferably not canned)	from 30 to 51	LOW
Bread: grain should be as unprocessed as possible and with lots of seeds. Sprouted wheat, sourdough rye, stone-ground whole wheat, Pumpernickel. BEST: pitas, wraps, tortillas	from 45 to 59	LOW
Breakfast Cereals Oats (large flake, steel-cut oats, not instant), Oat bran, All Bran (Kellogg's), Muesli with oats and various seeds	from 34 to 58	LOW
Cakes and Muffins, Pancakes Bran muffins, pancakes from pancake mix. Use whole wheat flour or stone-ground flour in moderation. AVOID white flour	from 60 to 67	MED
Cereal Grains Buckwheat, bulgur wheat, quinoa, barley, oats	from 22 to 58	LOW
Cookies and Crackers Digestives cookies (plain), oatmeal cookies (plain), Wasa rye crackers	from 54 to 59	MED
Dairy Products Milk (1% and 2%) Yogurt (low-fat, plain), Yoplait Lite with fruits Cheese (low-fat) , butter (organic, in moderation)	from 20 to 35	LOW
Fruit Berries, apple, grapes, orange, apricots, pears, peaches, plums, cherries, papaya, lemon, avocado, rhubarb. Canned in pear juice is OK, but no light or heavy syrup	from 0 to 57	LOW to MED
Fruits – BEST: Apple, peach, pear, plum, all berries –strawberry, blueberry, raspberry.	From 38 to 42	LOW

Fruits to Avoid Banana, kiwi, mango, pineapple, watermelon, grapefruit, all dried fruit	> 60	HIGH
Fats (Nuts, Oils, Spreads) Cashews, Peanuts, Almonds, almond butter, flax seeds, other nuts (in moderation), olives and olive oil, sesame oil, canola oil, tahini.	10 – 22	LOW
Meat, Seafood, Protein Chicken, turkey, and fish are preferred over any red meat. Buy only lean, organic grass fed meat. Eggs in moderation, soy milk, tofu	0	LOW
Pasta and Noodles (*Al dente* – not overcooked) Spaghetti (linguine, macaroni, fettuccini) noodles (white and whole wheat, protein-enriched), rice vermicelli, Udon noodles, Soba noodles	from 27 to 62	LOW to MED
Rice NO RICE CAKES Brown rice, basmati, wild rice (mixed with basmati), red rice	from 50 to 58	LOW to MED
Sweeteners Splenda, Stevia, Maltitol, Erythritol	from 0 to 19	LOW
Vegetables Almost all vegetables are fine. Cooked carrots, corn and sweet potatoes in moderation and/or combined with low-glycemic foods such as green beans, peas, lentils, beans.	0	LOW to MED
Vegetables to Avoid Beets (cooked), parsnip, potatoes – high if boiled, worse when baked. Always combine with low glycemic foods such as legumes, and high fibre foods to moderate the high glycemic effect of these foods.	from 64 to 101	MED to HIGH

(Source: *The New Glucose Revolution*, Dr. Jennie Brand-Miller, Dr. Thomas M.S. Wolever, Kaye Foster-Powell, Dr. Stephen Colagiuri).

Having a salad prepared with **vinegar** or **lemon juice** with your meal, will help keep your blood glucose under control.

Combining low-glycemic foods with high-glycemic foods also moderates glucose levels. For example, eating beans with corn tortillas, green beans with a baked potato, and peas with carrots.

For more information you may purchase from our clinic the *Glycemic Index Nutrition Package* prepared by our daughter Talia Ripley. This contains recipes, menus, further resource listings, and more.

The bottom line: Eat food your ancestors could have hunted, fished or milked, that has been raised in as simple and natural way as possible. Read *The Schwarzbein Principle* by Dr. Dianna Schwarzbein, MD to see how to shop like a hunter-gatherer in a modern supermarket. www.schwarzbeinprinciple.com

For more on this subject read *Beating Cancer with Nutrition* by Dr. Patrick Quillin,

RD, PhD. Dr. Quillin works for Cancer Treatment Centers of America, and has been a real inspiration to me.

Cancer Myths: Acid / Alkaline balance and Oxygen

I often hear it said that cancer can be cured by alkalizing the tumours, but it just isn't so. The idea that oxygen kills cancer cells is another popular myth. These widely held, but misguided beliefs are a misinterpretation of the work of Otto Warburg, whose research on the biochemistry of sugar metabolism in the 1920's to 1940's won him a Nobel Prize. He found that cancer cells could survive in very low oxygen conditions by switching to a yeast-like fermentation of sugars without oxygen. This causes a build up lactic acid and the cancer becomes quite acidic, i.e. have a low pH. From these bare facts, some mistakenly assume that:

"Cancer is created by acidic and low oxygen conditions" – This is putting the cart before the horse. Cancers certainly do occur in alkaline persons, and in well oxygenated tissues, such as the lungs. Only quite advanced cancers become acidic, never at the start. Cancer cells have several metabolic sources of acid, independent of Warburg's famous fermentation. Oxygen levels fluctuate, from very low to very high, but even in a well oxygenated tumour, fermentation of sugars without oxygen continues vigorously, and this makes lots of lactic acid. So acid is not linked to oxygen, and it turns out neither really control tumour growth.

"Cancer can be cured by oxygen therapies" – It does not work. They love oxygen, and can die without it. They can be stressed to death by free radicals of oxygen, and hydrogen peroxide – but not by oxygen drops, hyperbaric oxygen, oxygen in steam cabinets, and so forth. This is a bait-and-switch illusion. To begin with, oxygen in drops or powders does not have a significant dose of oxygen to make any real change. Even if they were pure liquid oxygen, it is a tiny fraction of what you already breathe every minute. Hyperbaric oxygen makes blood vessels grow into tumours, completely cancelling any other benefit. If oxygen or ozone could be taken up by our skin we could all go around with plastic bags over our heads. I think only a few creatures such as frogs and newts can actually breathe through their skin. Toe of frog and eye of newt, anyone?

"Alkalizing a tumour will cure cancer" – it is not possible to alkalize a tumour significantly, but if it were possible, it would not help. Tumour acidification is the result of several defects in energy metabolism, including the fermentation of sugars to acids. Alkalizing a cancer cell does not correct the central failure of these cells –their inability to throw a built-in off-switch for bad cells that are old and mutated

The truth is:

An acid-ash diet turns out to be one high in pro-inflammatory omega 6 from meats and grains such as corn. Grass fed meats –free of hormones, drugs, herbicides and pesticides – and also nuts and seeds, gave our ancestors more anti-inflammatory omega 3 fats. This alone is why acidic foods need to be curtailed: inflammation gets immune cells to help cancer grow and spread. Grain-based diets also increase insulin-like growth factors.

An alkaline-ash diet is mostly vegetables, fruits, and legumes. Plant foods provide many potent cancer-fighters such as indoles, sulphoranes, polyphenols, ellagic acid, vitamins and minerals. These completely explain the excellent responses seen in scientific studies on cancer patients who simply adopt a wholesome and whole foods diet, and increase physical fitness with moderate exercise.

Monitoring your urine and saliva pH is unnecessary, and potions to alkalize are pointless. Your blood is so heavily buffered against any deviation in the acid/alkaline pH balance that it takes extreme measures to shift it. If it does go even slightly off normal pH, a person becomes severely ill. Breathing and kidney functions are immediately altered to compensate. But even if you miraculously survived this and only alkalized the tumour, it would have absolutely no effect. Similarly the Simoncini IV-bicarbonate therapy has shown no efficacy.

[See *Early and late apoptosis events in human transformed and non-transformed colonocytes are independent on intracellular acidification*, Wenzel U, Daniel H. **Cellular Physiology and Biochemistry**. 2004; 14 (1-2): 65-76.]

Eat lots of fruits, vegetables, peas and beans. Moderate and watch the qualities of the animal foods and grains. You will become very slightly more alkaline on a proper diet and lifestyle regime, but that is only a sidebar to the real goal of getting control over the cancer. Genuine metabolic rebalancing during cancer requires the scientific expertise of a naturopathic physician trained in integrative oncology.

Leading Remedies for Integrative Cancer Care

The following natural medicines are my primary tools to arrest the growth and spread of most cancers. Several of these agents are usually clustered into a rational program I would call a protocol. Various protocols I have developed out of this set of remedies have been sufficient to shrink away tumours, produce good remissions, and even cure some cases. At least they may improve quality of life and slow the progress of the disease. Most of my patients become stable or better.

This section describes some of the most potent cancer therapies I know, but it is only the tip of the iceberg. This book is not intended to show you the entire naturopathic repertoire. Naturopathic physicians and their networks of healing practitioners will tailor a program to fit the person, and will select homeopathic remedies, perform acupuncture, prescribe detoxification regimes, exercise programs and more. We are a gold-mine of good ideas, and the items mentioned here are only nuggets to pique your interest.

I prescribe professional brands including the **Vital Victoria** label prepared to my specifications by a local compounding pharmacist. I am not prescribing these to any reader of this book. I can only be responsible for their application in patients I have actually examined, interviewed, and where I have reviewed their medical records, labs and imaging. Unless I know your case and all your medications, I cannot help you.

Your health care providers will have their own knowledge and experience to contribute, and their own protocols. They may prefer other products or doses. You may receive other recommendations depending on your general health, the type of cancer you are experiencing, and your medications. In every case, your physicians have the final word regarding your care. The following are merely reasonable suggestions worthy of consideration by you and your health care team. All are to be taken with some food, unless otherwise indicated.

Eat whole fresh organic foods, typically with emphasis on low glycemic load.

Green tea EGCG 95% polyphenol concentrate (low caffeine) – a 700 mg capsule 3 times a day This is equal to dozens of cups of green tea as it is normally brewed. You could not possibly drink enough tea to get this amount of medicine, so you must get it as a concentrate in a pill. EGCG stops cancer in many different ways.

Vitamin E – 400 IU once daily with food when on EGCG therapy to prevent kidney and liver harm from high-dose tea polyphenols. Use only mixed tocopherols with gamma vitamin E, such as Vitazan E-10.

Can-Arrest – bromelain, boswellia, curcumin and quercetin – 2 capsules 3 times a day to control inflammation and its many growth factors. From Vitazan, a professional label sold only through doctors. Curcumin and quercitin may be given separately. I use Thorne Research brand Meriva SR slow release phytosome curcumin, often at 1 capsule 3 times daily. Brand Albi Curcumin 7X is a large softgel, taken twice daily in most cases. Quercitin is usually dosed at 2 of 500 mg capsules 2 to 3 times daily.

Jingli Neixao is a Chinese herbal formula made by my pharmacist. Take 2 capsules 3 times a day to strengthen the organs and general vitality, including the immune system. This has been used in a number of Chinese hospitals, and is a tremendous tonic and healer.

Vitamin C – 1 level tablespoonful in water, taken in 3 or more portions daily – start with 1 tsp, then increase daily to 1 ½, 2, 2 ½ and finally 3tsp or 1 tbsp = 12 grams, or to bowel tolerance – which means until you get a little diarrhea. Once you are at your top dose, you must never come off it suddenly – reduce it at the same rate as you increased it or you risk rebound scurvy. In advanced cases we may add intravenous vitamin C therapy.

Vital Victoria multivitamin & minerals – 1 capsule per day. Custom made for my cancer patients needs. The B-vitamins are particularly important in regulating cancer's abnormal energy production.

Benfotiamine – a fat-soluble form of vitamin B1 (thiamine), 160 mg twice daily to regulate energy metabolism and the shut-off switch for bad cells.

Modified Citrus Pectin MCP – 4 caps or 1 tsp. twice daily. Halts cancer spread, inhibits growth. Professional products are standardized by size of the pectin fragments, to maximize effectiveness.

Iscador or Helixor mistletoe – 1 ampoule by injection just under the skin about 3 times per week. Mistletoe makes the immune system stop supporting the tumour growth, and turn into attack mode. Huge impact on quality of life is expected. Mistletoe will usually stabilize advanced cancers. Over 50% of advanced cancer cases get a strongly positive response, with real life extension.

Indole-3-carbinol – 200 mg capsules 3 times daily for detoxifying and reducing growth stimulating hormones, as well as controlling various growth factors. Found in all the cabbage and mustard family food plants.

Coenzyme Q-10 – 100 mg, 3 times daily to promote repair and restoration of normal energy metabolism.

R+alpha lipoic acid – time release – 150 to 300 mg 3 times daily to rescue mitochondria and turn on the off-switch for bad cells, killing the tumours. Helps detoxify from chemicals and heavy metals too.

Grapeseed extract OPCs – 200 to 400 mg 3 times daily – antioxidant, cancer killer, normalizes blood vessels and prevents unwanted hormone production.

Reishi mushroom extract – 1 to 2 capsules 3 times daily with food. Only the hot water extracts balance immune responses and heal cancer.

Ellagic acid –as found in 8 ounces of unsweetened pomegranate, grape or berry juices – cranberry, raspberry, blueberry, blackberry. These are very powerful anti-cancer foods.

Melatonin – 3 to 20 mg at bedtime only – 8 pm to 12 midnight. The usual dose of this pineal gland hormone is 10 to 20 mg for cancer. Gradually increase by 3 mg per night, and drop the dose down if you get nightmares or feel groggy in the morning. Antioxidant and hormone regulator. Melatonin extends lifespan significantly.

Artemisinin –wormwood extract burns iron out of cancer cells. Take daily for one week, then take a week break. Repeat as needed, under close medical supervision of your blood counts, iron status and liver health.

Selenomethionine – 200 mcg capsule 1 to 2 times daily with food. A non-toxic organic from of the mineral selenium, which assists in repairing DNA damage, and supports thyroid hormone activation.

Milk thistle extract – 2 capsules or 1 dropper-full tincture 3 times daily restricts the growth factor active in 85% of cancers. Also heals the liver and strongly detoxifies.

Vitamin A – 1000 to 10,000 IU capsule 1 to 2 times daily at meals. Controls and normalizes cell growth.

Vitamin D3 – 2000 to 3,000 IU daily, after a larger loading dose. Some protocols go as high as 500,000 IU in a single dose and 50,000 IU once monthly. Strongly prevents cancer. Cancer cells actually try to deactivate it and prevent its manufacture. Foil them by taking this potent cell growth regulator.

Hoxsey herbal tincture – 1 dropper-full (20-25 drops) 3 to 4 times daily – usually I will add a personalized homeopathic remedy to the tincture. Balances cell charge, hormones and liver function.

Low dose naltrexone LDN – a small nightly dose of this drug calms and slows cancers.

Remembered Wellness CD for relaxation, visualization exercises and stress management.

Psychotherapy can unleash the tremendous pharmacy in our brains, and the healing power of the mind and body. I regularly refer patients for counselling, neuro-linguistic programming NLP, Time-line therapy, expressive therapies (art, music).

Reiki universal healing energy treatments for healing spirit and body. I am most enthusiastic about the Usui method, a traditional Japanese healing art. People make dramatic shifts both physically and emotionally. It is deliciously relaxing, rejuvenating and healing.

Natural medicines which can be very useful for better nutrition, to alleviate side-effects, to restore real health, and create healing conditions:

Vitazan milk thistle combination – 2 capsules 3 times daily is a true life-saver in liver failure, and a great detoxifier. Globe artichoke, dandelion root, curcumin and alpha lipoic acid make it work beautifully.

L-carnitine or **acetyl-L-carnitine** 1,000 mg 2 to 3 times daily restores energy to heal the gut, and chemo brain.

Vitazan psyllium husks with acidophilus probiotics to detoxify, and to create healing short-chain fats.

Seal oil omega 3 – EPA, DHA and DPA – 2 capsules 2 times daily. Anti-inflammatory and blood mover so it reduces pain and risk of clots. Supports the brain, heals leaky gut syndrome, and stops wasting.

Ashwagandha herb 2 capsules 3 times daily helps manage stress. We may also use theanine, rhodiola or ginseng.

Greens First – 1 scoop 2 times daily. *Doctors Choice* brand tastes great and delivers the nutrition of several servings of vegetables.

Red Alert – 1 scoop daily as a super food concentrate equal to several servings of fruit and vegetables.

Dream Protein whey – 1 scoop 2 times daily for albumen protein, strengthens weal patients and speeds healing.

Smoothies: note that all capsules can be opened and made into a blender drink with fruit, milk, yoghurt or whatever is appealing, adding the Dream Protein powder, some Greens First , Red Alert and vitamin C powder. We may add a multivitamin to make a natural meal substitute that is far superior to Boost or Ensure.

We find blueberry, grape and pomegranate juices to be excellent to mask any odd flavours and odours.

UltraClear defined food diet. This is a potent tool for detoxification.

If you are nauseated take 2 ginger caps or hot grated ginger tea 1/2 hour before eating or taking any medications.

A SAMPLE BASIC CANCER PROGRAM

One successful protocol is based on what I call **Mitochondria Rescue** – using natural agents which wake up dormant mitochondria to restore the off-switch in cancer cells:

- The most important part is natural inhibitors of pyruvate dehydrogenase kinase: Alpha lipoic acid (R+ form) 150 to 300 mg 3 times daily, best in time-release form.
- Gamma vitamin E in mixed tocopherols – 800 IU daily.
- Coenzyme Q-10 – 100 mg 3 times daily – absorbs best when taken with fats or oils
- Quercetin (with bromelain or bioperine for absorption) – 2 capsules 2 to 3

times daily
- Grapeseed extract (oligomeric proanthocyanidins) – 100 to 400 mg 3 times daily. I prefer *NASOBIH NutraCaps* with added resveratrol.
- *Ganoderma lucidum* (Reishi) mushroom extract – 500 to 1,000 mg 3 times daily
- Indole-3-carbinol 200 mg 2 to 3 times daily
- Ellagic acid – can be as 8 ounces of unsweetened pomegranate, grape or berry juices
- B-vitamins riboflavin (B2) and niacin (B3) as nicotinamide – 50 to 100 mg 2 to 3 times daily.
- B1 or thiamine, especially as benfotiamine 80 to 160 mg 2 times daily.

This program has produced good responses in many advanced cases and tough cancers, including rapid tumour shrinkage. It is based on biochemical principles from animal and cell studies, correlated with results from limited human cancer trials. It is my own innovation. It is completely new and unproven by scientific trials, so I am not advising readers to try this on their own. As with any treatment, I have seen cases which do not respond to this approach.

On this foundation one can develop a complete program of diet, supplements, exercise, mind-body healing, stress management, self-expression, detoxification and all the elements that create real healing conditions.

ANOTHER SAMPLE CORE PROTOCOL FOR A VARIETY OF CANCERS

The core group of therapies I advised in the first edition *Naturally There's Hope*, in adequate doses and with supporting agents:
- Curcumin – as in *CanArrest* – with bromelain for absorption, or *Curcumin 7X* based on lecithin.
- Green tea EGCG – with vitamin E to prevent toxicity
- Grapeseed extract OPCs – I prefer the NASOBIH *NutraCaps* with added resveratrol.

This is still a good combination, and I might commonly add the following to make a basic protocol:
- Indole-3-carbinol
- Modified citrus pectin
- Jingli Neixao
- Whole foods, clean protein, low glycemic load diet.
- Reiki healing

The following brief suggestions for specific cancers may supplant or augment the core protocols mentioned earlier. In all cases they serve only as highlights of therapies of special interest. To learn more about these natural medicines see the more detailed chapters on botanicals, nutrition, and other naturopathic therapies.

Parts Four and Five of this book will provide a more detailed look at all the natural agents shown to be effective for a given type of cancer, and which molecular targets and tumour growth factors they address. To really understand that section you will need to learn more technical language, the scientific logic behind targeted therapies, and the algorithms for treatment that allow for individual differences. Sample foundation protocols which have given good clinical responses will be posted there.

KEY COMPOUNDS FOR INTEGRATIVE CARE OF SPECIFIC TYPES OF CANCER

Assuming you have a base program in mind, such as one of the core protocols outlined above, you can use these lists to add **important items for discussion with your health care team**. Listed are agents that target critical growth factors and exploit weakness in these cancers. If you want more detail on why these are used, and some secondary remedies, see Part Five. For those of you who are inclined to say, "Doc, just tell me what to take," here are the most used substances in naturopathic oncology.

Bladder	Leukemia	Ovary
Brain	Liver & Gallbladder	Pancreas
Breast	Lung	Prostate
Cervical (+Vulva)	Lymphoma	Sarcoma
Colorectal	Melanoma	Skin
Esophagus	Multiple Myeloma	Stomach
Kidney	Nasopharyngeal, head & neck	Thyroid
Uterus		

BLADDER CANCER

- milk thistle extract
- high-dose vitamin C
- carotenes
- green tea EGCG. concentrate with vitamin E
- grapeseed extract OPCs
- hyperthermia.
- GLA oils such as evening primrose.
- MSM – methylsulfonylmethane
- indole-3-carbinol and sulforaphanes from cruciferous vegetables, i.e. broccoli or broccoli sprouts.
- TCM – Ping Xiao Pian, Anti-cancerlin

BRAIN & NERVE CANCERS

- grapeseed extract OPCs
- co-enzyme Q-10
- B-vitamin complex
- acetyl-L-carnitine
- alkylglycerols from shark liver oil
- omega 3 oils
- vitamin E – gamma and mixed tocopherols
- boswellia – especially to control tumour swelling (edema)
- CanArrest
- green tea EGCG concentrate with vitamin E
- reishi mushroom extract
- milk thistle extract
- artemisinin and artemether from wormwood
- detox from fat-soluble pesticides and solvents. I use homeopathic and botanical medicine, along with a defined diet; elimination diet, brown rice diet or modified fast. Foods to increase include beets, cilantro leaf, fish, walnuts, almonds, and of course, pure water

BREAST CANCER

- Can-Arrest – for curcumin and quercetin
- flaxseed – fresh-ground and organic
- green tea EGCG concentrate with vitamin E
- indole-3-carbinol
- melatonin
- grapeseed extract OPCs
- resveratrol
- co-enzyme Q-10
- R+ alpha lipoic acid
- reishi mushroom extract
- milk thistle extract
- Ping Xiao Pian or Jingli Neixao
- artemisinin
- vitamin D3
- exercise, relaxation, expressive arts
- mistletoe injections – Iscador M for pre-menopausal, and Iscador P for post-menopausal.
- Naturopathic physicians have solutions for lymphedema and all other aspects of your care.

CARCINOID (GI NEUROENDOCRINE) TUMOUR

- R+ alpha lipoic acid
- curcumin
- green tea EGCG extract
- grapeseed extract OPCs
- rhodiola
- plant source digestive enzymes
- milk thistle extract
- vitamin D3
- nattokinase
- ginkgo biloba extract
- artemisinin and lactoferrin

CERVICAL CANCER

- folic acid or folate B-vitamin
- vitamin A
- vitamin C
- mistletoe
- sterols and sterolins
- reishi mushroom extract or Immune Assist mushroom formula
- quercetin
- grapeseed extract
- green tea EGCG concentrate
- melatonin
- Engystol
- zinc citrate
- indole-3-carbinol

COLORECTAL CANCER

- CanArrest for curcumin and quercetin
- indole-3-carbinol
- calcium-D-glucarate
- grapeseed extract
- resveratrol
- green tea EGCG concentrate with vitamin E
- R+ alpha lipoic acid
- omega 3 marine oils
- probiotic friendly bacteria
- milk thistle extract
- aloe vera gel
- retinol form of vitamin A.

Naturopathic Oncology

ESOPHAGUS CANCER

- green tea EGCG & vitamin E
- grapeseed extract
- CanArrest
- milk thistle extract
- R+ alpha lipoic acid
- Liu Wei Di Huang Wan
- zinc citrate
- vitamin A

KIDNEY CANCER

- CanArrest – for quercetin
- green tea EGCG
- indole-3-carbinol
- grapeseed extract
- milk thistle extract
- co-enzyme Q-10
- R+ alpha lipoic acid with the full mitochondrial rescue protocol
- niacinamide
- reishi mushroom extract
- vitamin C
- melatonin
- mistletoe injections

LEUKEMIA

- curcumin, quercetin, boswellia = CanArrest
- green tea EGCG plus vitamin E
- grapeseed extract OPCs
- resveratrol
- omega 3 DHA
- milk thistle extract
- reishi extract
- vitamin A
- vitamin D3
- vitamin K2
- indole-3-carbinol
- Bu Zhong Yi Qi Wan.
- beta carotene
- astragalus
- holy basil
- selenomethionine

LIVER & GALLBLADDER CANCER

- Iscador mistletoe
- CanArrest for curcumin and quercetin
- green tea EGCG concentrate with vitamin E
- vitamin C
- R+ alpha lipoic acid
- astragalus
- milk thistle extract
- melatonin
- Xiao Chai Hu Tang or Sho-saiko-to (Honso H09)
- reishi extract or *Immune Assist* mushroom complex
- Hoxsey herbal tonic

LUNG CANCER

- grapeseed extract
- co-enzyme Q-10
- CanArrest – for curcumin and quercetin
- green tea EGCG
- R+ alpha lipoic acid
- L-carnitine
- milk thistle extract
- astragalus
- vitamin E
- resveratrol
- ellagic acid from pomegranate
- reishi extract
- alkylglycerols
- indole-3-carbinol
- artemisinin and lactoferrin
- mistletoe injections

LYMPHOMA

- Can-Arrest
- green tea EGCG plus vitamin E
- grapeseed extract OPCs
- vitamin D3
- indole-3-carbinol
- R+ alpha lipoic acid
- Jingli Neixao
- beta carotene
- reishi extract

Naturopathic Oncology

- R+ alpha lipoic acid
- pomegranate and grape juice
- omega 3 EPA and DHA

MELANOMA

- modified citrus pectin
- bromelain
- green tea EGCG plus vitamin E
- milk thistle extract
- co-enzyme Q-10
- sterols and sterolins
- Bu Zhong Yi Qi Wan
- reishi mushroom extract
- vitamin C
- vitamin D3
- melatonin
- astragalus
- P type mistletoe
- vitamin K3
- Chaga mushroom betulinic acid extract, or mushroom beta-glucan extracts
- CanArrest for boswellia, curcumin and quercetin

MULTIPLE MYELOMA

- DHA omega 3 marine oil
- green tea EGCG concentrate with vitamin E
- milk thistle extract
- reishi mushroom extract
- curcumin with bromelain
- indole-3-carbinol
- vitamin D3
- vitamin K2
- R+ alpha lipoic acid
- MCHA calcium complex
- Helixor A type mistletoe injections

MYELODYSPLATIC SYNDROME

- green tea EGCG plus vitamin E
- curcumin, quercetin, boswellia , bromelain = CanArrest
- vitamin D3
- pomegranate, bilberry and grapeseed anthocyanidins and proanthocyanidins, resveratrol, ellagic acid.

- melatonin
- reishi mushroom extract
- genestein from soy
- EPA marine oils
- alkylglycerols from shark liver oil

NASOPHARYNGEAL, HEAD and NECK CANCER

- CanArrest
- green tea EGCG concentrate with vitamin E
- Jingli Neixao
- indole-3-carbinol
- milk thistle extract
- Engystol
- vitamin A
- vitamin C
- plant sterols and sterolins
- R+ alpha lipoic acid
- P type mistletoe injections

OVARIAN CANCER

- CanArrest for quercetin and curcumin, augmented with extra quercetin and bromelain.
- green tea EGCG plus vitamin E
- melatonin
- indole-3-carbinol
- milk thistle extract
- grapeseed extract
- resveratrol
- Ginkgo biloba
- Selenomethionine
- Soy genestein
- Iscador or Helixor M type mistletoe
- Vitamin D3
- Ginseng

PANCREAS CANCER

- indole-3-carbinol
- R+ alpha lipoic acid
- low-dose Naltrexone
- co-enzyme Q-10
- green tea EGCG concentrate with vitamin E

- milk thistle extract
- Jingli Neixao
- CanArrest – particularly for quercetin and curcumin
- reishi mushroom extract
- Iscador or Helixor mistletoe
- soy genestein
- vitamin D3

PROSTATE CANCER

- milk thistle extract
- green tea EGCG plus vitamin E
- curcumin (with bromelain, bioperine or lecithin for absorption)
- resveratrol
- R+ alpha lipoic acid
- co-enzyme Q-10
- indole-3-carbinol from cabbage
- pomegranate and related sources of ellagic acid and proanthocyanidins such as grapes and berries.
- low intake of fat, particularly animal fat and hydrogenated fats.
- omega 3 marine oils
- modified citrus pectin
- control insulin levels with the Schwarzbein Principle diet, Mediterranean diet, low glycemic index diet.
- flaxseed
- goji berry extract
- soy genestein
- melatonin
- homeopathics such as *Conium* 6C or *Carcinosum* 30C.
- zinc citrate
- vitamin D3
- artemisinin

AVOID IN PROSTATE CANCER
- DHEA supplements as they boost growth factors and sex hormones.
- Sterols and sterolins as they can increase DHEA.
- Chondroitin supplements used for arthritis may increase the spread of prostate cancer.
- Ashwagandha, other than short-term during radiation therapy, as it may increase testosterone.
- Dairy foods and all animal fat.
- Selenium

SARCOMA

- curcumin with bromelain, or CanArrest
- green tea EGCG plus vitamin E
- grapeseed extract OPCs
- reishi mushroom extract
- milk thistle extract
- vitamin K2
- co-enzyme Q-10
- R+ alpha lipoic acid
- Iscador or Helixor P type mistletoe (or M type for osteomuscular sarcomas)
- artemisinin
- omega 3 marine oils; reduce omega 6 fats from grains, meat and vegetable oils.

SKIN CANCERS

- grapeseed extract OPCs – orally and topical NASOBIH *NutraCream*
- green tea EGCG plus vitamin E
- milk thistle extract
- CanArrest – for curcumin, quercetin and bromelain
- vitamin A as retinol palmitate
- co-enzyme Q-10.
- sterols and sterolins
- melatonin
- pomegranate
- Helixor or Iscador P type mistletoe

STOMACH CANCER

- Aloe vera gel
- CanArrest for curcumin and quercetin
- green tea EGCG concentrate with vitamin E
- grapeseed extract
- resveratrol
- R+ alpha lipoic acid
- reishi mushroom extract
- TCM: Liu Wei Di Huang Wan or Liu Wei Hua Jie Tang; Fare You cabbage extract
- indole-3-carbinol
- milk thistle extract
- vitamin C
- soy genestein

THYROID CANCER

- green tea EGCG concentrate with vitamin E
- milk thistle extract
- reishi mushroom extract
- resveratrol
- pomegranate
- quercetin with bromelain
- alkylglycerols from shark liver oil
- omega 3 marine oils
- vitamin A
- zinc citrate

UTERINE CANCER

- CanArrest – for curcumin and quercetin
- Green tea EGCG concentrate with vitamin E
- Indole-3-carbinol
- R+ alpha lipoic acid

VULVA – see Cervix…..

PART TWO – INTEGRATIVE ONCOLOGY

In this section you will see how naturopathic care dove-tails with medical oncology to give better results with less harm. Do not let any ignoramuses convince you these supports are unsafe or unsupported by scientific evidence. However, there are real concerns about interactions between medical drugs and procedures and natural medicines, and even foods. Therefore you need a naturopathic physician trained in integrative oncology to make sure everything you take is compatible and synergistic.

Chapter Three – Surviving Medical Oncology

The prevailing view in oncology, the regular medical approach to cancer, is that surgery, radiation, chemotherapy drugs, hormone blockers and some immune therapies are the only realistic treatments for cancer. They are often described as "evidence-based." Good scientific evidence is very expensive to generate, and so it turns out that most of what is considered "proven" to work to a high standard is drug medicine, which is owned by someone who will get a fat profit from the investment in major research. This is a serious bias.

Naturopathic oncology is not just "faith-based" though! We could be proud if we only held to the standard of "judgement-based" medical practice. That would be making decisions based on good judgement, training, and experience, informed by science but also rooted in common humanity, caring, heart, spirit, and other areas of consciousness. I am quite at ease proposing the use of entirely safe medicines which have a utilitarian value when used by reputable physicians – that do a great deal of good for a great number of people. "Clinically proven" we can say.

However, the really excellent news (and your oncologists and pharmacists may not even know to tell you), is that many of our successful therapies are also backed up by large scale placebo-controlled randomized trials done at universities and hospitals. Do not slavishly follow any out-dated injunction to avoid mixing dietary and supplement prescriptions with your medical oncology, because "We don't know if they are safe to combine or useful." This is ignorant rubbish. Oncologists and pharmacists are the least likely to use alternative medicines, to refer for alternative medicine, have relevant education or clinical experience, and are the least interested in reading the scientific literature or taking continuing education in alternative medicine, of all the licensed health professions. Yet their patient population is the greatest consumer of CAM or complementary and alternative medicine, or as we prefer to say, *integrative medicine*. Nearly 80% of cancer patients are using these healing arts and science, so it is ethically troublesome and clinically disappointing if the oncology system is unaware of the positive values that drive their use, and the actual risks involved. All too often they are simply not told by the patient, and did not ask. They are not always taken as authorities in this field, due to perceived, bias, bigotry and exaggeration of risks of CAM. There are very real concerns that need to be addressed regarding interactions between medical drugs and natural medicines.

Integration of naturopathic medicine, Chinese medicine and conventional medicine is common in China, the USA, Europe, and now in Canada. You deserve the best!

If you are getting surgery, chemotherapy or radiation you must review all your supplement and medications. I don't mind you checking your drug prescriptions with the pharmacists, but I do expect to have the last word on your naturopathic medicines.

We will need to focus on what will make these harsh therapies safer and more likely to actually help. Do as much as you can of the recommended supports, but do not embellish without the express permission of your naturopathic physician in oncology.

INTEGRATING SURGERY SUPPORT

Surgery is almost always the best chance for a cure of cancer. If the surgeon can catch it in an early stage and get it out with clean margins, it is possible the disease is removed from the patient.

Even if surgery cannot be curative, it is best to "de-bulk" tumour burden by surgery. This gives us a smaller tumour to fight, and that takes less drugs and natural medicines.

Surgeons will usually not remove a tumour if there are metastases to major organs. Removing the "mother" tumour sometimes results in the satellite tumours suddenly growing quite wildly. If the disease staging tests such as bone scans, MRI scans, CT scans or PET scans show the cancer has spread, usually surgery is off, and you can expect to be offered whole body (systemic) treatments like chemotherapy.

When a surgeon says "We got it all," that only means they removed all the visible cancer cell accumulations they looked for where scans detected them. There can be microscopic cancers already loose at the time of surgery. These can best be dealt with preventatively, before they can grow or mutate further.

There is always some risk of cancer reoccurrence. I do not think it is prudent to turn your back on cancer, and the conditions that gave rise to it. Therefore I advise seeking professional help in deciding on what therapies should follow surgery.

PRE-OP PREPARATION

Surgery or biopsy can spread cancer. This can involve seeding of cancer cells along a needle or catheter track, or shedding into vessels or cavities during tumour handling. It is not a common occurrence. Estimates of **port-site recurrence** vary from near zero for breast cancer to 17% for gallbladder cancer. I have seen cases of recurrence seeded in the surgery scars soon after surgery, including breast cancer cases. Reduce metastasis risk with **modified citrus pectin** MCP 1 teaspoon, or 4 capsules twice daily. Modified or fractionated citrus pectin, and larch arabinoglycans, work like putting flour on Scotch tape – mets can't stick to other cells, and if they cannot attach to the vasculature walls they cannot invade and grow. Have this at hand to <u>start the day before your surgery</u> or biopsy procedure, and continue for up to 6 months, then review. Green tea **EGCG** is also of service in reducing metastases from surgery.

<u>Avoid for a week</u> all herbs and supplements which interact with sedatives and

46

anaesthetics: St. John's Wort *Hypericum perforatum*; valerian root – *Valeriana officinalis*; kava kava, *Piper methysticum,* ginseng *Panax ginseng* and *Panax cinquefolium,* skullcap, passion flower, hops, melatonin, inositol, GABA and 5-hydroxy-typtophan 5-HTP.

Avoid ephedra herb as it increases sympathetic nerve tone. Avoid citrus, licorice root and lindera as they increase blood pressure. Avoid peony root, milletia and high-dose niacin as they dilate peripheral blood vessels.

Avoid natural medicines which can cause bleeding or clotting issues: EPA fish oils; garlic *Allium sativa*; gingko leaf *Gingko biloba*; ginseng root *Panax ginseng* or *Panax cinquefolium*; bromelain; vitamin K, salvia, rehmannia, ligusticum, ginger, atractylodes, carthamus, reishi, cordyceps, Coenzyme Q-10, resveratrol and green tea EGCG extract. Vitamin C and vitamin E are a risk if taken in high doses.

Surgery mix – 6C potency homeopathics *Hypericum, Staphysagria* and *Arnica* – this formula was given to me by Dr. Andre Saine, ND, a great homeopath. Being a classical homeopath, he dispensed them separately, but being an eclectic, I like to mix them in one bottle. He told me patients will come back and say their surgeon told them "I've never seen anyone heal so fast" and that is exactly what has happened in many cases. *Hypericum* treats nerve injury and pain, *Arnica* helps relieve trauma, edema, inflammation, and *Staphysagria* deals with the injury at an emotional and mental level. <u>Start this the day before your procedure.</u>

Wound healing support: **vitamin C** – 2,000 mg, **zinc citrate** – 60 mg; **vitamin A** – 3,000 IU daily; high protein – which might include a whey protein powder – 1 ounce (30 grams) twice daily. It is mandatory in cases with recent poor nutrition due to poor appetite, or mechanical issues such as oral or gastro-intestinal tumours. <u>Start these supplements 2 weeks pre-op</u> if you have been nutritionally compromised. This dose schedule may be reduced or even eliminated if you have been consistent with a very wholesome diet with fresh and raw fruits and vegetables, and have been taking food supplements.

Psychology – every cancer therapy can do harm, and it is necessary to describe the risks so patients can choose to give their informed consent, and go into it with eyes open. However, like food, one you have chosen this path, you must try to fully embrace it. Most problems that can arise can be moderated by expectations that it will go well. Like an Olympic athlete or an astronaut, rehearse getting the therapy many times. Visualize success and *feel* the benefits you are going to receive. If you can worry about side-effects and problems, you can visualize something better happening. Let it be like sunshine chasing away all your shadows.

POST-OP PROTOCOL

If you are concerned about cancer spreading during surgery or biopsy, take **modified citrus pectin** – 4 capsules or 1 teaspoon twice daily and **green tea EGCG** 700 mg. three times daily, with **Vitamin E** 400 IU daily, for two to six months, then discuss further use with your naturopathic physician.

Support wound healing with **zinc citrate** – 30 mg twice daily with food; **vitamin A** – 3,000 I.U. daily; and **vitamin C** – 1000 mg. 3 times daily, or get these nutrients by sufficient intake of fresh and raw fruits and vegetables. Discontinue when all incisions are well healed, in favour of a maintenance level of supplements or food concentrates.

Remember surgery is very immunosuppressive. This is the time for homeopathic, nutritional and herbal support for the immune system – *Engystol, Thymuline*, **vitamin A, vitamin C, zinc citrate**, cat's claw, Reishi mushroom.

Ferdinand Sauerbrach, a thoracic surgeon, has demonstrated improved surgical wound healing and increased resistance to infection with a **salt-restricted diet.** Again, continue this until all wounds are completely healed.

Reduce pain, edema and blood clot risk with **Bromelain** – 500 mg. 2 to 4 times daily, away from protein foods. For inflammation: **curcumin** 500 mg. 3 times daily or **Phytoprofen** 2 capsules up to 3 times daily; or **EPA omega 3 oils** 2 to 4 grams daily with food. Ramp up physical activity as soon as possible.

Centella asiatica or gotu kola herb will accelerate wound healing, and makes the healed tissue stronger. Take at least 500 mg of a quality extract yielding 50 to 100 mg of triterpenic acids, twice a day.

Prevent adhesions and excessive scarring with **catechins** 500 mg. 3 times daily and **vitamin E** – 400 to 800 I.U. daily with food. Once the incision has closed, use topical **Rosa mosqueta** (Rosehip) cream to reduce scars and keloids. **Aloe vera** leaf gel increases wound strength, flexibility on healing, decreases scars and reduces risk of metastasis. Vitamin E reduces and softens scars.

Deep wounds such as from punch biopsies can be filled with a sugar paste, which sterilizes while it promotes granulation tissue. Other vulneraries or wound healers include calendula – marigold flower, chickweed, and comfrey leaf

Probiotics are good bowel bacteria, essential to good health, and often diminished by stress and antibiotics. If you have a bout of diarrhea after surgery, take a capsule of enteric coated mixed bowel bacteria 2 to 3 times daily, away from food, for up to 2 months.

A positive attitude appears to make a real difference in outcome – less pain, less complications, faster healing, etc. Use the pharmacy in your head to create healing conditions.

RADIATION THERAPY FOR CANCER

Ionizing radiation is a standard treatment for cancer, despite significant risks and side-effects. About 1/3 of cases treated with radiation will not achieve good local control of tumours. The average is about 1 to 2% local reoccurrences per year. Radiotherapy is nonetheless often a reasonable option, though not to be entered into lightly. It can really burn tissue and leave permanent damage.

The beam energy is commonly measured in Grays (**GY**). Cancer treatments typically range from 3 to 10 Grays. If you have been given radiation therapy once, you may only receive it again if the total dose accumulated will be less than 70 to 80 Grays, as more is potentially fatal.

Human exposure to 4.5 GY all at once will kill 50% of persons. This is why a high therapeutic dose must be delivered in small fractions per day, spread over several days or weeks, not all at once.

Radiation dosing is all about the volume of tissue that must be treated. When the field of treatment is large, the amount of energy that needs to be delivered to get all the cancer cells goes up dramatically, and risk of injury and burns increases.

Cells, like our body as a whole, are about 70% water. Ionizing radiation usually forms hydroxyl radicals *OH and superoxide radicals from the water inside cells. These energized oxygen compounds break strands of DNA, the genetic code.

If both strands are broken, and go unrepaired, the cell may die. Cells injured by radiation will also die if abnormal connections between strands (dimers) are not repaired.

However, if one strand remains unrepaired, the cell survives, but in an altered form. Thus radiation can kill cancer cells, but can also cause normal cells to develop into cancer. These secondary cancers can take 20 years to develop into clinical disease.

You can get leukemia from the radiation of ten CT scans! If you are offered some other way to check up on your cancer, such as a magnetic resonance image MRI or a blood test for a tumour marker, you should take the opportunity to reduce your radiation exposure.

External beams such as X-ray devices, gamma ray "cobalt bomb," linear electron megavoltage accelerators (Linacs) and the "gamma knife" units bombard the body from the outside; so much of the energy gets absorbs into overlying tissues and doesn't reach the tumour. This is like sunlight going into water; it is absorbed near the surface and so can't get too deep. Newer types of radiation such as proton beam and pi meson beams overcome some of this problem, acting more like depth charges, delivering a big punch deep in the tissues while sparing more of the superficial structures.

Implants such as brachytherapy use high dose radioactive substances in pellets placed near a cancer to deliver a very high local dose. Many of these isotopes release high energy particles with large mass which cannot penetrate too far into healthy structures around the tumour.

Rapidly dividing cells are most susceptible to radiation damage: cancers, small lymphocyte immune cells, bone marrow where we make blood cells, the delicate linings of blood vessels and of the Gastro-intestinal tract, and hair follicles. That is why radiation kills cancer but also makes the hair fall out and the gut to be disturbed by sores, vomiting and diarrhea. If the bone marrow goes down, you can bleed to death from lack of platelets, die of infection due to lack of white immune cells, or go into organ failure due to lack of red blood cells to carry oxygen in and carbon dioxide out.

The classic symptoms of radiation toxicity: malaise, weight loss, nausea, vomiting, diarrhea, sweats, fever and headache.

Any tissue subject to the radiation doses used for cancer therapy can be permanently altered in its growth pattern. Initially there is a robust inflammatory response by the immune system. A slow but relentless fibrosis or scarring ensues, gradually reducing blood flow. After many years, irradiated tissue may be unable to heal from trauma or surgery. Radiation to the heart is associated with increased risk of coronary artery disease and congestive heart failure. Naturopathic therapies can assist with these conditions.

The 1/3 local failure rate in radiotherapy is mostly due to **the hypoxic cell problem** – 2.5 to 3 times higher doses are needed for the same biological effect in low oxygen parts of tumours than for fully oxygenated cells. My research area for several years at the British Columbia Cancer Research Foundation Medical Biophysics Unit was on this "hypoxic cell problem." We looked at new drugs and new radiation sources that would kill the cells living on the edge of survival in oxygen-deprived parts of a tumour.

I am pleased to tell you there are many natural agents which naturopathic doctors are trained to use which not only radio-sensitize, they increase the therapeutic benefit by also reducing the harm to non-cancerous cells!

I now know that pre-treatment with natural medicines like green tea EGCG temporarily increases tumour oxygenation, and thus improves responses to radiotherapy. It must be stopped during radiation therapy.

Nicotinamide increases local blood flow, and is a strong radio-sensitizer – it amplifies the effect of the radiation to kill more cancer cells. It is far better than the synthetic drug I was doing medical research on. It is suitable to use all through radiation therapy.

I am frequently asked about hyperbaric oxygen therapy and cancer. Using 100% oxygen under pressure certainly delivers a massive dose of oxygen. We know it cures "the Bends" in divers, but will it help to kill cancer? Well, the oxygen does increase chemical damage and cancer cell death from radiation. Oxygen in really high doses does increase immune activity against cancer cells. However, it increases blood vessel growth into the tumour too. The net effect is controversial. Some of my colleagues use HBO2T to increase the effectiveness of radiation therapy, and tell me it is safe.

Radiation works primarily by inducing oxidative stress. While moderate dose anti-oxidants during radiation therapy may be associated with increased survival time, increased tumour responses, and reduced toxicity, this issue remains controversial among radiation oncologists. Certainly **high dose anti-oxidants may reduce effectiveness of radiotherapy**. However, it is scientific humbug for oncologists to declare natural anti-oxidants unsafe while using high-potency synthetic anti-oxidants with radiotherapy such as Amifostine, Mesna and Dexrazoxane, and natural –origin Pentoxifylline. There may be a research gap between natural and synthetic products motivated by economics, but the scientific principle is established. Anti-oxidants have a role in radiation therapy, but require an experienced professional to make the correct prescription.

One anti-oxidant which is very well researched and shows positive effects combined with radiation therapy is melatonin. It certainly protects the GI mucosa, and regulates the bio-rhythms needed to coordinate healing.

After radiation therapies there can be a prolonged suppression of bilirubin, albumin and uric acid seen on the blood tests. This effect needs to be treated with a balanced program of anti-oxidant supplementation.

The blood-thinning drug Coumadin or Warfarin does not interact well with radiation therapy, so patients are encouraged to switch to low-molecular weight heparin anti-coagulation therapy. Other anti-coagulants actually improve the efficacy of radiotherapy.

Be proactive, as all doses of radiation cause injury, though the symptoms may only appear much later on.

Treating Radiation Exposure

Radiation can cause cancer. Radiation therapy is sometimes curative, but is most used as an adjunct to surgery or chemotherapy. It can be very toxic in the short term, and it can also trigger a relentless decline in circulation due to fibrosis or scarring of the lining of the blood vessels. Tissues can lose the ability to heal.

To reduce collateral damage to healthy tissue hit by the radiation, without losing the impact on the cancer cells:

Ashwagandha herb is a significant protector of healthy cells, yet increases tumour cell killing by radiation.

Shark liver oil alkylglycerols reduce secondary tissue damage by about 60%.

Homeopathic medicines are helpful to restore homeostasis. Consider *Radium bromatum, Radium iodatum, X-ray, Thuja occidentalis, Cadmium iodatum, Cadmium sulpuricum, Calcarea fluoricum, Fluoric acidum, Phosphoricum acidum, Cobaltum metallicum, Rhus venatum, Belladonna, Arsenicum bromatum* and *Causticum*.

Other radioprotectant agents to consider are quercetin, **vitamin A** as retinol palmitate, beta carotene, vitamin B2 – thiamine, vitamin B3 – niacin, vitamin B5 – pantothenic acid, selenium, glutathione, squalene, **curcumin**, green tea, melatonin, zinc aspartate, taurine, ginseng, reishi, cordyceps, bael fruit *Aegle marmelos*, marine omega 3 oils.

Dr. Christopher, master herbalist, recommended Oregon grape root *Berberis aquifolium* for radiation recovery. Berberine has now been shown to reduce radiation pneumonitis.

The traditional Vietnamese herb for detoxification *Vigna radiata* contains the flavonoid *vitexin* which has been shown to protect from radiation induction of weight loss, and damage to peripheral blood cells. Note that this herb treats the condition called "deficiency heat" seen by doctors of traditional Chinese medicine TCM in irradiated patients. I use **Da Bu Yin Wan** formula for this purpose. TCM formulas such as *Radio-Support* will address issues such as deficient qi, blood and yin, blood heat, and blood stasis.

To increase killing of the cancer cells by radiation and enhance chances of a cure consider ashwagandha herb, vitamin A, melatonin, holy basil, and maitake PSK extract.

Quercetin, apigenin, genestein and hypericin are PKC inhibitors which regulate p-glycoprotein, which acts as a pump to export drugs out of cells, as well as acting as radiosensitizers, increasing cell sensitivity to radiation.

COX-2 inhibitors selectively radiosensitize tumours. For example, curcumin is an Akt inhibitor - and the Akt / mTOR pathway mediates radio-resistance.

Niacinamide (nicotinamide) is a special form of vitamin B3 which increases blood flow to tumours to overcome hypoxic cancer cell resistance to radiation. The effect is very specific to tumour vasculature. I worked for years in research on this problem of hypoxia or low oxygen levels in tumours. Low oxygen areas are places cancer cells can hide out and survive radiation therapy. After millions of dollars spent on research, no drug is safer and more effective as a radiosensitizer than nicotinamide/niacinamide.

Red wine can reduce the risk of acute radiation toxicity, including high-grade skin toxicity, without affecting anti-tumour efficacy. It is suspected that resveratrol is the active ingredient. Enjoy one glass daily for good health!

Aged garlic extracts enhance DNA repair and reduce immune suppression by radiation.

Probiotics help protect the gut from radiation injury, and protect immune competence.

Super-oxide dismutase SOD repairs radiation injury to the bladder and GI tract. SOD can be elevated significantly by taking **goji berry**, also called wolfberry or *Lycium barbarum*.

Avoid during radiotherapy:

No sugar allowed! A strict low glycemic diet. can markedly increase effectiveness of radiotherapy. An American study showed an 8-fold difference in responses to radiation between patients with the highest intake of sugar and the lowest. This is huge! High sugar load increases insulin-like growth factor IGF-1, which suppresses apoptotic mode of death in cancer cells induced by ionizing radiation. One exception to this rule is the use of sips of honey during radiation to prevent mouth and throat ulceration (mucositis) in head and neck cancers.

Taking anti-oxidants during radiation therapy is a very controversial subject, although there is good evidence that moderate doses administered prior to radiotherapy may have a net positive effect. The most controversial are beta carotene, vitamin E and co-enzyme Q-10. Oncologists are comfortable with some antioxidants such as Pentoxifylline from xanthines, and synthetic anti-oxidant drugs such as Amifostine and Dexrazoxane, but are still biased against natural forms. I am absolutely sure melatonin is both safe and helpful with radiotherapy. Do remember that some anti-oxidants such as vitamin C become pro-oxidant therapies in high doses, such as by intravenous administration.

Radiation can induce a profound drop in anti-oxidant status, marked by signs of oxidative stress such as persistently low serum albumin, bilirubin and uric acid. I recommend only food-sources of anti-oxidants from fruits and vegetables during radiotherapy. Eat cabbage, broccoli, kale, cauliflower, chard, spinach, beans, lentils, miso, curry, seaweeds, tomatoes, yams, squash, raw carrots, grapes, pomegranates, and all berries.

Avoid use of supplemental manganese iron and copper, except as in a one-a-day multivitamin. Do not use rehmannia and cinnamon based herbal preparations during RTx without expert guidance.

Do not put any oil-based skin care products on the skin exposed to radiation during the entire course of your radiation therapy. Your skin could be fried to a crisp! Remember that lipid peroxidation from radiation hitting fats creates rampant cell killing. You cannot wash off enough to prevent damage, so don't use any.

Radiation Therapy Support Summary

Take only the following supports during the course of radiation therapy and for one month after the last dose of radiation. Any other medicines or supplements should only be considered during this time if prescribed by a physician.

One week before radiation therapy: pre-treat with anti-angiogenics including **green tea EGCG** and **Can-Arrest.** Stop the green tea extract when radiation starts. Continue Can-Arrest throughout the course of radiation treatment and for at least a month after the last dose.

Give also one week pre-treatment with **alkylglycerols**, and throughout the course of radiation, particularly if any marrow bones are exposed.

During radiation therapy:

Ashwagandha herb to make tumour cells more sensitive to radiation, but protects healthy cells! Rx – 2 capsules 3 times daily at meals.

Curcumin extract from turmeric to control inflammation and promote tumour oxygenation. Note that lecithin, bromelain or bioperine is required to ensure adequate absorption. **Can-Arrest** is an excellent product, because it has several anti-inflammatory and anti-angiogenic ingredients that synergize together. Rx – 2 capsules 3 times daily at meals. **Curcumin 7X** is also excellent, Rx 1 capsule 2 to 3 times daily.

Marine source omega 3 oils are also safe anti-inflammatories to use with radiation therapy.

Vital Victoria multivitamin with minerals Rx – 1 capsule daily at a meal. The vitamin A helps local regulatory cells maintain a more normal growth pattern.

No sugar! Scrupulously follow the low glycemic diet plan. This makes a huge difference.

Red wine – one glass daily will reduce skin damage during radiation, without reducing efficacy.

Mushroom polysaccharides such as JHS Naturals hot water extract of Reishi mushroom, called **Gano 161** Rx 1 -2 capsules 2 to 3 times daily.

Niacinamide 500 to 1,000 mg up to 3 times daily with meals. Niacinamide assists by increasing tumour blood flow.

Zinc citrate 30 mg at each meal reduces dermatitis and mucositis, boosts immune function, improves tissue repair and healing, while improving local control of the cancer. Mandatory for radiation to the head and neck.

Siberian ginseng Eleutherococcus *senticosus* is also a good radio-protectant recommended by Keith Block, at 500 mg daily. It controls lipid peroxidation and DNA damage.

Skin damage and burning can be treated with aloe vera leaf gel during therapy. Do not use any oils on your skin, even though you may think you can wash them off before the next radiation treatment. Oils lead to lipid peroxidation which can fry you to a crisp!

<u>After</u> the therapy is complete we can apply *Rosa mosqueta* oil with vitamin A and D3 to burnt areas, emu oil, or NASOBIH™ NutraCream with Protovin™. Homeopathic remedies which are particularly useful in healing radiation injuries include *X-ray 200C, Radium bromatum, Cadmium sulphuricum,* and *Causticum.*

TREATING COMMON RADIATION SIDE-EFFECTS WITH NATUROPATHIC MEDICINE

Despite our best efforts to prevent problems, people do get hurt by the radiation. Most issues will be well addressed by the oncology doctors and nurses. However, natural medicines can be less expensive and far more effective. Do not hesitate to ask for acute naturopathic care for any radiation side-effect.

ANEMIA – bone marrow damage takes 1 to 3 weeks to manifest after receiving a toxic dose of a chemo drug, but then may progress to complete failure to produce any of the blood cell types. If the marrow stops making red blood cells the patient becomes anaemic. Lack of red cells means not enough hemoglobin to carry oxygen out to the tissues and carbon dioxide back to the lungs to be breathed out as waste. Anemia makes a person tired and listless. Your doctor may order blood transfusions if your hemoglobin falls below 90. Use iron with caution as it is very oxidizing, making ROS which damage DNA. It is safer to check iron status by measuring serum ferritin before giving iron. Vitamin B-12 and folate given by intramuscular injection can kick up blood cell production. Support bone marrow nutrition with sesame oil 1 tsp., shark liver oil alkylglycerols 1 – 2 capsules three times daily, Marrow *Plus* from Health Concerns 3-4 capsules three times a day, *Shi Chuan Da Bu Wan* or Shiquan 8 pellets three times a day, *Panax ginseng* 500 to 1000 mg. twice daily. *AHCC* (active hexose correlated compound) is a proprietary Japanese low molecular weight compound from fermented shiitake and other medicinal mushrooms grown in rice bran, which has been found to prevent many chemo side-effects and increase the effectiveness of methotrexate, 5-fluorouracil and cyclophosphamide at doses of 3 grams daily.

Resistance to the blood-building drug Erythropoietin therapy is reduced by co-administration of L-carnitine and vitamin A. Erythropoietin can cause great harm in some patients, even killing them with blood clots.

ANOSMIA – Loss of smell leads to loss of taste, with degradation of quality of life, and appetite. Steroid hormones are used, and we may also use *Ginkgo biloba* extract, zinc citrate, and homeopathic *Zincum metallicum* or *Mercurius solubilis.*

APPETITE- loss of appetite or anorexia is helped by ginger, bitters, peppermint, thiamine, melatonin, Marinol and reishi mushroom extract, royal jelly. Make small meals, and control odours. Your acupuncturist may needle ST-36, SP-6, CV-12, BL-20 and 21 for appetite. For loss of taste add LI -4. The TCM herb formula Bu Zhong Yi Qi Wan is recommended by myself, and by the prominent integrative medical oncologist Keith Block. Other herbs include gentian, bitters, catnip, fennel, peppermint and ginseng. Exercise helps. Be aware that bromelain used in high doses as an anti-inflammatory can powerfully inhibit appetite. The amount in Can-Arrest or our curcumin and quercetin products will not bother.

ATTITUDE – Expectation plays a central role in the occurrence of side-effects. If the patient believes they can stay well, visualizes success, and positively affirms and embraces the therapy, they will likely do better than if they are fearful. However, it is not a trivial concern that chemo can cause great harm, even death. Anxiety is therefore normal, but high levels of depression, as measured by the Hospital Anxiety and Depression Scale (HADS) questionnaire, can predict pathological responses to chemotherapy. Such patients may display high emotional restraint and not appear severely depressed. This is a good reason to integrate mind-body medicine with orthodox protocols!

BURNS – Radiation can cause severe burning of the skin and underlying tissues in some individuals.

2 to 4 weeks: dryness, follicle epilation, erythema due to cytokine release, and melanin pigment changes.

3 to 6 weeks: dry desquamation, scaling and itching

4 to 5 weeks: moist desquamation: basal cells are lost, oozes fluid. Extreme burns cause dermal necrosis.

After 12 weeks: atrophy, fibrosis due to increased fibroblast activity, TFGß causes dermal thickening and edema.

After 6 months: telangiectasia.

Green tea extract or Ching Wan Hung Red Capital ointment may be used on burned skin, after radiation ends. Homeopathics *Apis mellifica, Cantharis, Radium bromatum, Causticum* and *Arsenicum bromatum* can assist healing radiotherapy burns.

After the last dose of radiation can we consider use of certain oils and emollients. Note: severe skin burns and inflammation from radiotherapy do not always respond well to emollients such as aloe vera, or to oils. Use only physician-approved products on skin damaged by radiation, and monitor responses closely. Rosa mosqueta (or rosehip oil /cream) prevents and treats burn scars. Use Ferlow Brothers aloe or Rosa creams – organic botanicals in a base of organic grapeseed oil, with vitamin E. Vitamin E oil may be sprayed on sloughing skin (moist desquamation). For skin discoloration use vitamins A and D3 topically and orally. Emu oil soothes mild burns and dermatitis.

CONSTIPATION – Number 42's are remarkable for relieving even the stubborn constipation from codeine and morphine painkillers. #42's are an old naturopathic remedy combining cape aloe root and wormwood. It may have originated with the esteemed O. G. Carroll, ND. We also consider Hoxsey herbal tincture, aloe vera juice, psyllium fibre, acupuncture "Prosperity treatment," enemas, and occasionally we refer for colonic irrigation by a certified colon therapist. We always advise good hydration, regular exercise and establishing a bowel habit.

I have no objection whatsoever to the use of stool softeners such as *Colace* or

Naturopathic Oncology

Grandma's Laxative

Pitted dates ½ cup 125 ml
Prune nectar ¾ cup 200 ml
Figs ½ cup 125 ml
Raisins ¾ cup 200 ml
Pitted prunes ½ cup 125 ml
Simmer dates in prune nectar until very soft. Spoon into a blender; add figs, raisins and prunes. Blend until smooth. Keep refrigerated. Use as a spread on toast or crackers, or eat by the spoonful. Yes. It is high-glycemic, but we have to balance competing interests in making clinical decisions. Another good formula: 2 cups bran, 2 cups applesauce, 1 cup unsweetened prune juice – take 2 to 3 tablespoons twice daily.

Docusate, glycerine or lactulose suppositories, or *Senokot*, which is just natural senna leaf extract.

We often suggest fruit such as prunes, papayas and rhubarb. We may recommend Grandma's fruit spread:

DEHYDRATION – treat aggressively with miso broth, mango juice and electrolyte drinks such as the WHO formula – 1/2 tsp salt, 3/4 tsp baking soda, up to 8 tsp sugar, and up to a cup of fruit juice to 1 litre water. Intravenous therapy is normal saline, 0.9% salt, with 5% glucose.

DERMATITIS – See also BURNS. Prevent injury with curcumin. My favourite remedy to correct the redness and blood vessel changes in the skin from radiation injury is the anti-oxidant NASOBIH NutraCream™, which contains the world's most potent grapeseed extract OPCs – Protovin™ – and also has alpha lipoic acid, vitamin A, MSM, CoQ-10, DMAE, EDTA, rosehip, essential oils, and many other brilliant natural components. Naturopathic oncologist colleagues suggest topical and oral remedies such as tea of calendula and rosemary, aloe vera inner leaf gel, lavender oil, emu oil, curcumin, honey, sea buckthorn, vitamin U, L-carnosine, green tea extracts.

DIARRHEA – BRAT diet (banana, rice, apple, toast). Replace probiotic gut bacteria. I use *Vitazan Ultimate Acidophilus* – a potent mixture of billions of acidophilus and other probiotics, which includes FOS food for the bugs, and is enteric coated. Replace electrolyte salts as well as water, with miso soup, broth, juices or an electrolyte drink– at least an 8 ounce glass per bowel movement. World Health Organization WHO approved electrolyte replacement formula is ½ tsp salt, ¾ tsp baking soda, a cup of fruit juice, sweetened to taste with the equivalent of up to 8 tsp sugar, in 1 litre water. Intravenous therapy is normal saline, 0.9% salt, with 5% glucose.

Bentonite clay can absorb toxins. L-glutamine gives energy to heal the lining of the gut. *Po Chai* pills are a tremendous Chinese herb for toxic diarrhea, but also consider

Xiang Sha Yang Wei Pian and *Ba Zheng Wan* formulas. Acupuncture points ST 25 and 37. Prosperity treatment is a special acupuncture technique using 4 needles around the belly button, and it can treat either diarrhea or constipation, with good results in about 5 minutes. Consider omega 3 oils.

FATIGUE – is linked to inflammation, NFkB, CRP, IL-1β and IL-6. Exercise – and start prior to therapy! Use L-carnitine 500 to 1000 mg three times daily for energy, or even better acetyl-L-carnitine. ALC crosses the blood brain barrier to help heal the brain from radiation injury. The Chinese ginseng root *Panax ginseng* is a wonderful tonic. I like to give 1 to 2 vials daily of the Chinese tonic herb formula Ling Chih Feng Wang Jiang with reishi mushroom, codonopsis, royal jelly and lychee fruit juice. If it is not available, give royal jelly, *Codonopsis*, reishi mushroom extract, or vitamin B5. Omega 3 marine oils reduce fatigue and depression by reducing interleukin IL-6. Naturopathic physicians may give intravenous drip or push of Myer's cocktail of vitamins and minerals to boost the immune system and revitalize. We may simplify this to a shot of vitamin B12 in the rump. Give by mouth chlorella algae or wheat grass juice for chlorophyll. Consider the herbs rhodiola, nettles, astragalus, Siberian ginseng *Eleutherococcus senticosus,* ashwagandha, shitake and cordyceps. Sometimes one must just conserve energy and ask for assistance on bad days. Prepare food ahead of time and bank some down time – then use it to rest, contemplate, and visualize positive results from the therapy. Reiki therapy will help!

FAT NECROSIS – Radiation can cause fatty tissues to suddenly die. Rx alkylglycerols from shark liver oil 600 to 1,200 mg daily.

HAIR LOSS – Some claim vitamin E will reduce hair loss, or at least stall it. AHCC compound also claims to protect the hair follicles. Acupuncturists may use ST 36, SP 6, LV 8, BL 20 and 23, and moxa to BL 17. Afterwards, we use Shou Wu Pian tablets of bearsfoot herb *Polygoni multiflori,* to re-grow hair more rapidly. You may have to learn to love your skull, or hats, headscarves and wigs.

LUNG INJURY – lung irradiation can result in inflammation (pneumonitis) leading to scarring (fibrosis) which becomes acute 1 to 6 months after treatment, causing cough with blood in the sputum, shortness of breath, chest pain, and even death. Give patients at risk high doses of vitamin E, vitamin C, N-acetyl cysteine, grapeseed extract OPCs and milk thistle extract.

MOUTH SORES – sores in the mouth and bleeding gums hurt, reduce eating and can get infected. Called mucositis, it can sometimes spread through the whole gastro-intestinal tract and cause GI bleeding. This can be the factor which limits using an effective dose of chemo, especially in leukemia cases. I have adapted a Chinese herbal product to this problem, with brilliant results. Fare You "vitamin U" 4 pills three times daily will generally prevent or rapidly heal mouth sores, or throughout the GI tract. It is a pharmaceutically pure form of the amino-acid methionine extracted from green cabbage. It is also terrific for stomach ulcers, colitis and diverticulitis, and completely safe. Vitamin E 800 IU is said to prevent mouth sores. Give L-glutamine at up to 10 grams per day or 2 gm/m², or one rounded teaspoonful dissolved in a warm drink three times daily. Consider liquid folic acid/folate, *Glycyrrhiza* as DGL licorice extract, chamomile tea or tincture, green tea with honeysuckle flower, marigold flower juice *Calendula officinalis succus,* chlorophyll, slippery elm bark *Ulmus fulva*, vitamin E gel, homeopathic *Traumeel*, and *RadiaCare* oral rinse. The BC Cancer Agency's "Magic Mouth Rinse" is distilled water, Nystatin anti-fungal, Benadryl elixir anti-histamine, and Solu-Cortef hydrocortisone sodium succinate. A simple oral rinse of ½ teaspoon each of baking soda and salt in a glass of warm water may be used several times a day. Adding N-acetyl-cysteine to the oral rinse improves effectiveness. Use a very soft toothbrush, or a finger or gauze pad, and consider baking soda rather than toothpaste. The mouth will be soothed by cold or frozen yoghurt and soft, bland food. Avoid over-the-counter mouthwashes such Listerine, Scope. Avoid crunchy, spicy and acid foods. Burning mouth neuropathy is treated with R+ alpha lipoic acid. Try ice-chips too. Some of my American peers swear by honey for mucositis. In radiation therapy for head and neck cancers 20 ml of honey is taken 15 minutes before radiation and this is repeated every 15 minutes for the next 6 hours. Dry mouth or xerostomia may be corrected with hyperbaric oxygen therapy, *SalivaSure* lozenges, or artificial saliva spray.

NAUSEA – ginger is very good, as 2 capsules of root powder, as ginger tea, even as ginger ale. SeaBand is an acupressure band with a button that presses on PC-6. Even more potent is acupuncture needling at the points ST-36, PC-6, HT-1, CV-12. Homeopathics *Arsenicum, Nux vomica, Tabacum, Ipecac* or *Cuprum metallicum* have often worked very well. Eat often in small amounts, especially starches such as dry crackers, and drink plenty of fluids. Medical marijuana cannabis tetrahydrocannabinols THC does work well for some, if they can tolerate the other effects. If nausea arises from a gut reaction to stress I prescribe Xiao Chai Hu Tang formula.

NERVE INJURY – Always use R+ alpha lipoic acid, time-release 150 to 300 mg three times daily for any nerve damage or neuropathy, from numbness, phantom sensations or pain. Burning mouth syndrome is a toxic neuropathy shown to respond very well to R+ alpha-lipoic acid. The Benfotiamine form of vitamin B1 is useful at doses of 160 mg twice daily. *Ginkgo biloba* leaf extract can help neuropathy and brain injury. Other adjuncts we may consider are L-glutamine -6 to 10 grams a day, vitamin B6 – 500 mg twice a day, vitamin B12, B-complex, calcium, melatonin, vitamin E, omega 3 oils, grapeseed extract and milk thistle extract. Homeopathics of interest are *Hypericum perfoliatum* and *Aconitum napellus*, as in *Traumeel* oral, topical or injectable. Some colleagues use Metagenics brand *Neurosol*, which contains borage GLA oil, B-complex vitamins and beta-carotene.

ORGAN DAMAGE – make sure you ask the radiation oncologist and technicians to set up as narrow a beam as possible, and mask or shield vital tissues and glands- remember the squeaky wheel gets the grease. You do not have to be embarrassed to remind your care givers to slow down and focus on your safety. You will be less hassle to them if you prevent problems before they occur. Use radioprotectants such as green tea, vitamin A, melatonin, glutathione and ashwagandha. Organs need supplemental Co-enzyme Q-10 to repair; it really makes a huge difference in healing. My American colleagues suggest melatonin 20 mg twice daily, boswellia 500 mg 4 times daily, selenium to 1,000 mcg daily, medium chin triglycerides 13- 26 grams, and *Oralmat* rye extract adaptogen. SOD from Goji berry repairs RTx injury. For brain injury from radiation add DHA from omega 3 marine oils.

PLATELETS – failure to make platelets or thrombocytopenia can make it impossible to form a clot, with a risk of severe haemorrhage. Your doctor may prescribe a transfusion of platelets if the count falls below 20. Yunnan Baiyao *Panax pseudo-ginseng* 1-2 capsules three to four times daily is a reliable and fast therapy which I have seen out-perform synthetic drugs. The pineal gland hormone melatonin helps regulate the production of platelets, with efficacy comparable to Neupogen, and it's a lot safer. Consider also shark liver oil alkylglycerols, and maitake mushroom extracts. High-dose vitamin C can help recovery. It is thought that eating fresh raw pineapple may help increase the platelet count.

Avoid aspirin (ASA) and Advil (ibuprofen), *Ginkgo biloba*, and other blood thinners. Keep vitamin E dose under 600 IU daily. Report to your physician any bleeding signs such as bruising, red spots on skin, bloody urine or black, tarry stools. Avoid ginger, which reduces platelet counts and is a direct anti-coagulant.

PROCTITIS – Give probiotic friendly bacteria culture. Inflammation of the rectum and anus from pelvic radiation can respond to hyperbaric oxygen therapy. So can urethritis or any other chronic inflammation from radiation. Use SOD, as from Goji berry.

VOMITING – treat dehydration aggressively – drink electrolyte (blood minerals) replacement, make a cup of miso soup, consider acupuncture. Replace salt and soda as well as water, or the water will not stay in the blood; the basic electrolyte replacement formula is ½ tsp salt, ¾ tsp baking soda, up to 8 tsp sugar and a cup of juice per litre water.

WEIGHT LOSS – 80% of cancer cases are malnourished, and 40% die of malnutrition. Weight loss is a cardinal sign of cancer, and must be monitored and managed aggressively. Loss of over 20% lean body mass is critically dangerous; increase carbohydrates & protein intake. Cancer can cause cachexia, a metabolic syndrome with profound weight loss. Use marine oils rich in the fatty acid eicosapentaenoic acid EPA – especially seal oil, 2 capsules twice daily with meals. You may use fish oils up to 1 tablespoonful daily. Consider melatonin, L-glutamine, bitter melon *Momordica charantia*.

WHITE BLOOD CELLS – Leukopenia or failure to produce enough white blood cells means a loss of vital immune cells, so the person's resistance to infection can plummet. The neutrophils are the first responders to infection, and so are the most critical to protect. The most aggressive product to raise the count is shark liver oil alkylglycerols; in doses to 1200 mg. Naturopathic doctors have long had great success rebuilding immune health with thymus and spleen glandular extracts. I really like to use Dolisos homeopathic Thymuline to balance the thymus-activated immune cells. My American colleagues use *Polyerg*a spleen peptides. I give chlorella algae, up to 20 grams daily. Botanicals to consider are poke root *Phytolacca decandra* or golden seal root

Hydrastis 30 drops of tincture twice daily. Consider the Chinese herbs Siberian ginseng, astragalus, ligustrum, codonopsis, milletia, white atractylodes, sage *Salvia miltiorrhizae*, lyceum, salix root, scutellaria and royal jelly. The classic TCM formula Shih Chuan Da Bu Wan stands out from the pack, but we also like *Marrow Plus* formula. Ayurveda suggests *Podophyllum hexandrum*. We may give dilute intravenous hydrochloric acid. Acupuncture points include TW-5. Supplement zinc, selenium, vitamins A, C, E, B6 and B12. An intramuscular injection of B12 will pump up the neutrophils, our first responders to infection. Avoid crowds, avoid people with infectious illness, and wash your hands often, especially after using the toilet and before eating. Exercise. Report to your physician any sign of infection such as fever over 38°C, chills, cough, sore throat, painful urination, or inflammation such as redness, swelling and pain anywhere.

LATE and CHRONIC EFFECTS OF RADIOTHERAPY

Radiation sets off a relentless loss of microcirculation in the field. Radiation permanently alters the extracellular matrix which surrounds and supports our cells and the memory immune cells and stem cells in the ECM which regulate all cell growth. The area irradiated will never be the same, and in fact may become a medical problem many years later. The process of altered growth and healing is relentless and insidious, but you can do a lot to correct it naturally. **To reduce the chronic fibrosis and other late effects in exposed tissues I prescribe** vitamin A, **vitamin D3, vitamin E, and vitamin C**, nicotinamide, milk thistle **extract, omega 3 marine oil** seal oil, bromelain and nattokinase. Really, some combination of these need to be taken for the rest of your life.

Remember to always express gratitude for the care and help you have been given by your radiation oncologist, while forgiving yourself for stresses it put your body to. Try to be filled with gratitude. It is healing.

CHEMOTHERAPY

Combining natural medicine with chemotherapy is the most controversial area for integrative physicians. There are so many complex drug combinations in the standard protocols and experimental trials. The bald fact is that they are hunting through a near infinity of combinations, with little success. For a rational look at which cancers can actually respond in a meaningful way to chemo please read *Questioning Chemotherapy* by Dr. Ralph Moss, Ph.D. Chemo patients are often already on complex multi-drug regimes, including meds for the side-effects of chemotherapy, so it is daunting to avoid drug interactions. Radiation and most chemo drugs activate the cancer cell death sequence and thus kill the cancer cells by generating oxidative stress and ROS damage. It was wisely suggested a few years ago that antioxidant supplements would prevent these chemo drugs and radiation from working against the cancer. This would clearly be a catastrophe for the patient. It turns out it is true that high-dose anti-oxidants reduce the effect of radiation on cancer cells, and should not be taken during radiation therapy

However, a recent review of 214 studies on this issue showed only 3 potentially unfavourable interactions of specific chemo drugs with specific antioxidants. In all the rest the antioxidants reduced harm from the drugs, increased effectiveness, or most often, gave both benefits. Studies continue to show that antioxidants are not usually a problem during chemotherapy, and are actually wise to take, under professional supervision. See the References section at the end of this book. Why has this science not being used as the basis for rational prescription of these adjuncts? Integrative care can move medical oncology forward and reduce costs.

Years ago the Canadian Cancer Society sponsored a conference at Vancouver General Hospital which brought in top scientists from China. These doctors presented over 50 large scale randomized and placebo controlled clinical studies from universities and hospitals demonstrating how Traditional Chinese Medicine formulae interact with chemotherapy drugs. The TCM herbs consistently increased responses to chemo, often doubled the remissions, and consistently reduced morbidity and mortality. I have been a cancer researcher and scientist and in my opinion these are solid studies, and are as rational a basis for therapy as the rationale for the orthodox therapies they support. Still, we do not see naturopathic physicians or TCM doctors in our public hospitals and cancer centers, nor do we even see oncologists being "permitted" by the College of Physicians and Surgeons to refer to Naturopathic Physicians for co-management.

In the post-chemo phase, patients need to be detoxified. Naturopathic doctors are expert at detoxification.

For a few generations now, whenever a really poisonous substance was found in nature or made in a drug laboratory, it was immediately sent to the cancer research establishments to be evaluated as a cancer drug. The orthodox or allopathic medical treatment of cancer has emphasized *cytotoxic* or cell-killing medications. Chemo drugs kill rapidly dividing cells, targeting their DNA. Most of the cytotoxic effect results from apoptosis triggered by sublethal DNA damage. This is good. However, they also tend to go beyond this level of damage into *necrosis,* the rapid death of cells, which is a messy, inefficient and risky process, producing inflammation which is itself a promoter of tumour growth.

"Chemo" side-effects limit dosage, limit efficacy, and even kill patients. Any step we can add which reduces these risks increases the potential for the chemo to achieve its intended result. I consider it a major success to help a patient live through chemo with a reasonable reserve of health. As Dr. Robert Atkins, M.D. has said in *Atkin's Health Revolution,* "The damage done to the body by an unsuccessful course of chemotherapy is often so great that the patient's immune system never recovers sufficiently to stand a fighting chance." Immune cells are damaged in the bone marrow and also via leaky gut syndrome and disordering of the gut-associated lymphoid tissue where 70 to 80% of our active immune cells reside. Naturopathic physicians often feel that if chemo is given and fails, the hope for a response to biological treatments is also likely lost. We just too often have nothing left to work with in these damaged bodies.

Cytotoxic or cell-killing chemo poisons actually promote the spread of cancer (metastasis) by injuring cells of the immune system and cells lining inside of blood vessels.

Naturopathic Oncology

Chemo drugs kill a constant percentage of cells in a tumour with every dose. When a drug kills 99.999% and the tumour burden is a mere billion cells, there will still be 10,000 surviving cells. It works out that only an infinite number of doses of the drug would kill the last cancer cell. Theoretically, chemo cannot ever cure a tumour, as even one cancer cell might re-grow a tumour. Fortunately, in some case the chemo so weakens the cancers cells, and the immune system turns on it attack mode and clears up the remaining cancer. This can only happen if the immune system survives the chemotherapy. Therefore, this is part of my job description – to maintain immune health during chemo.

A common myth is that chemo drugs are somehow selective for cancer cells. Common drugs such as taxanes, anthracyclines and 5-fluorouracil actually kill healthy cells better than they kill cancer cells. Doxorubicin is ten times deadlier to good cells than cancer cells.

Most chemo drugs are known to cause cancer! These carcinogens cross-link DNA in healthy as well as cancer cells. They can also bind a single DNA strand to a protein or metal, activating frame shift mutations responsible for turning on oncogenes such as *ras*. Some tie the telomeres on the ends of the chromosomes into four-strand knots, creating an immortal cell.

Chemo is more effective with leukemias and lymphomas than with solid tumours, possibly due to drug delivery issues. In the disseminated cancers chemo is so successful you would be daft to not try it. Other than these blood-borne cancers, and testicular cancer, which are only 3% of all cancers, chemotherapy is not as well proven to good scientific standards to have a positive influence on survival or quality of life as you may think. There is some support for its use in sarcomas, retinoblastoma, ovarian, breast and small cell lung cancer.

This is all well known to oncology doctors, 75% of whom say they would not participate in a chemotherapy trial if they had cancer, due to its "ineffectiveness and its unacceptable toxicity." Yet in North America 75% of cancer patients are prescribed chemo by these same doctors. In Canada, the same 75% majority of oncologists surveyed said they "would not undergo chemotherapy or recommend it to a loved one" for a majority of cancers! The more experience doctors and nurse have with chemo, the less they like using it on their own family. This sort of nonsense has cost the medical profession a lot of credibility with patients. Ultimately, we must have *integrity* – to be one and the same to all persons, all the time – to fulfill our professional duty to each patient. There are hard choices, to be made between the doctor and patient, in an atmosphere of trust. The question I ask myself with patients is would I take the treatment myself, or give it to my children or my dear wife.

Cells lacking a functioning p53 DNA repair gene cannot die from chemo. This applies to 50 % of cancers, especially late stage cancers. The tumours may go into remission, but they will be back.

- Chemo is commonly toxic to other rapidly growing normal cells
- epithelial or skin-like cells lining the mucous membranes of the mouth and entire gastro-intestinal tract, causing nausea, diarrhea, vomiting, GI and mouth

ulcerations.

- the lining of the blood vessels and muscle of the heart, causing congestive heart failure.
- hair follicles – thus hair often falls out to the point of baldness
- bone marrow, causing anemia through loss of replacement red blood cells, loss of platelets needed for clotting, and loss of white blood cells of the immune system with infections due to immune suppression
- nerve injury, kidney damage, lung pneumonitis, and tinnitus are also frequent problems. Many patients get "chemo brain" syndrome – confusion and mental deterioration.
- chronic late effects include persistent fatigue, persistent bone marrow suppression, infertility
- chemo drugs can cause cancer including leukemia and lymphoma. For example, high-dose chemo with epirubicin with cyclophosphamide can trigger secondary acute myeloid leukemia up to 10 to 20 years later.
- Multi-drug resistance develops in cancer cells treated with chemotherapy, and so tumours which develop after the primary therapy are very hard to treat.
- During chemotherapy do not take selenium in amounts over 200 mcg daily, or give any N-acetyl-cysteine, as these can promote chemo-resistance.

INTEGRATIVE SUPPORT FOR CHEMOTHERAPY

I will advise you on specific supports matched to your prescription. Do not take anything else without explicit permission. Take the prescribed supports during the entire course of chemo, and for 3 to 4 weeks after the last dose. If you encounter any difficulties during chemo, we have solutions, so do not hesitate to ask for further help. Some common supports are:

Mistletoe is scientifically proven to support chemo and radiation. It is prescribed by more than 2/3 doctors in Germany and Switzerland, in their hospitals and cancer clinics. Chemo cannot actually kill the last cancer cell and cure cancer. If the chemo removes the bulk of the cancer cells, and the immune and stem cells working to support and "repair" the tumours, it can create an advantage for the immune system. Unfortunately the immune system can also be damaged or even destroyed by chemo drugs and associated medicines. However, mistletoe injections can maintain immune competence and turn the immune response to "attack mode."

Asians use astragalus-based herbal formulas for the same purpose -to keep the immune system alive through chemo. *Shih Chuan Da Bu Wan* 12 pellets twice daily. Astragalus-based formulas are proven to the highest scientific standard to reduce harm from chemo in many larger-scale university and hospital based double-blind controlled studies. Unfortunately, most have been published in Asian languages only. Their claimed efficacy and utility have been confirmed through my many years of clinical practice. It can double the chance of a good response, while reducing side-effects by 1/3 to 1/2. One oncologist I know remarked that some of my patients actually had improving blood counts as chemo progressed, something absolutely unheard of before.

Naturopathic Oncology

My current favourite formula is ***Astragalus Combination*** from St. Francis Herb Farm. I prescribe 2 capsules 2 to 3 times daily to protect the bone marrow and blood cells. Other Traditional Chinese Medicine style formulas we may use are *Chemo Support* or *Marrow Plus*. In cases where blood counts fall despite astragalus therapy, we can institute other remedial therapies, which may have to include the medical oncologist reducing the dose of the chemo drugs to more tolerable levels.

The eminent integrative physician Dr. Keith Block, MD, is a medical oncologist with over 30 years experience, Medical Director of an integrative cancer hospital in Chicago, and editor-in-chief of the top journal in the field, *Integrative Cancer Therapies*. He suggests *Shih Chuan Da Bu Wan* during chemotherapy. I am glad to see such an influential person reading the same science and bringing it to the aid of cancer patients.

Dr. Block also will sometimes recommend supplemental melatonin, L-carnitine, rhodiola, L-theanine, R+ alpha lipoic acid and DHA omega 3 oil with various chemotherapy scenarios.

DHA omega 3 oil – is a chemo-sensitizer, improving chemo outcomes by regulating cytokines, immune cell signalling molecules. It is safe with all chemotherapy drugs. Use cautiously with blood thinning medications.

Ashwagandha – 1 to 2 capsules 2 to 3 times daily. This adaptogen or stress-modulator reduces adrenaline to increase the number of cancer cells throwing the off-switch (apoptosis). It is also an immune-modulator, protecting the immune system from collapse during steroid use and chemotherapy. Since Ashwagandha can raise DHEA, it is not good long-term in hormone-dependent cancers. In such cases consider the related adaptogens rhodiola *Rhodiola rosea* or Siberian ginseng *Eleutherococcus senticosus*.

Vitamin A –retinol palmitate – 10,000 I.U. daily supports all cytotoxic chemo drugs. This dosage neutralizes vitamin D effects at the X-R-X retinoid nuclear receptor. 3,000 IU is safe for long-term use.

Fasting on water only for 48 hours pre-chemo and 24 hours post-chemo improves tumour shrinkage and markedly reduces side-effects. This is very traditional hard-core naturopathic medicine, and should only be undertaken with close supervision by a naturopathic physician, and with due regard to the vitality and weight of the patient.

Hyperthermia can amplify chemo efficacy when used concurrently. This is not just a sauna or peat bath temperature, it is brutally hot. Beware bait-and-switch fraud! Really high temperatures require in-hospital management and after-care for proteolytic muscle and related tissue breakdown.

A complete program of integrative naturopathic supports must be specifically matched up to all the drugs prescribed by your medical oncologist and integrative medicine team, and your current medical condition!

Should you have side-effects or problems during chemo, which are not being taken care of by the usual drugs, please ask me or my colleagues for further help. We have some terrific tools to care for common toxicities. For example, to protect the lining of the mouth and entire gut *Fare You* "vitamin U" cabbage extract tablets up to 3 times daily.

Green cabbage and mung bean sprout juice protects the GI tract and improves appetite. For appetite, fatigue and immune function we use royal jelly with reishi mushroom extract *Ganoderma lucidum,* and other herbs – 1 vial 1 to 2 times daily. Many Gastro-intestinal upsets can be prevented or quickly relieved with the TCM formula "Eight Pearls Decoction" also called Ba Zhen Tang, and similar results are seen with Bu Zhong Yi Qi Wan. Ginger root is great for nausea – 2 capsules as needed. I may prescribe *Xiao Chai Hu Tang* to bring blood and yin to your center, for nausea and gut reaction to stress. Homeopathic Rx's also work well, for example *Arsenicum album, Tabacum, Colubrina,* or *Cuprum metallicum.*

Psychology is important. You can rehearse mentally, like an astronaut would, or an Olympic athlete. The more you believe this is the right choice, and that it will go well, the less likely you are to have problems during the therapy. Release any negative attitudes and expectations! Go for your choices with faith and with gusto.

Good foods to try during rough chemo days:

- Cream of rice (congee) or oatmeal porridge.
- Broth made from marrow bones, or stock made into a pureed soup.
- Poached or soft-boiled eggs.
- Milk or yoghurt from goats, rice, soy, almonds or oats. These can also be used as a base for smoothies blended with whey or rice protein powder and a greens product such as wheatgrass, barley green, chlorella, spirulina or blue-green algae, and fruit of your choice.
- Apple sauce, mashed banana, or dried fruit soaked and poached.
- Fresh fruit and freshly made fruit juices.
- Fresh vegetable juices of carrot, cabbage, kale, spinach, celery, beet roots and tops, parsley, chard, cilantro, watercress.
- Poached fish.

Antioxidants as supplied by food are in fact generally safe and beneficial with chemo drugs.

Oncologists were justifiably worried about the possibility that antioxidant supplementation during chemotherapy might prevent free radical formation by the oxidative chemo drugs. This would lower the number of cancer cells being damaged to the point were the cell death program (apoptosis) of the cancer cell would switch on. Antioxidants should interfere with chemo, because we are trying to oxidize the cancer to death. However, clinically it is clear that in general, antioxidants actually increase the ability of the chemo drugs to kill cancer cells.

As it turns out, uncontrolled reactive oxygen species formed in chemotherapy lead the formation of toxic aldehydes. These poisons arrest the cancer cell's movement through its cell cycle into the checkpoint where apoptosis can begin. Antioxidants reduce the formation of the aldehydes. The usual net result of giving antioxidants with chemo is more cancer cells move into a death cycle than with the chemo drug alone. This is called *the Conklin Hypothesis.* Antioxidants take you two steps forward and one step back – so the end result is still one step forward. Natural source products with a mixture of carotenoids, ascorbates, tocopherols, polyphenols and proanthocyanidins are ideal. Selenium is limited to 200 mcg. Beyond that, it may increase chemo-resistance. For mega-dose therapy consult an orthomolecular physician.

AVOID DURING CHEMOTHERAPY

Several foods and natural herbs in common use can interact poorly with chemotherapy drugs, by inducing liver enzymes which clear the drugs This can make the drug too weak and result in therapeutic failure, or make the drug too strong and increase toxicity. Definitely avoid St. John's Wort and grapefruit during any chemotherapy, and consider restricting use of garlic, rosemary, alcohol, tobacco, and yohimbe.

Be very cautious mixing chemo drugs with supplemental glutathione or products which increase it such as HMS 90 whey or N-acetyl cysteine. Curcumin, selenium and milk thistle may be used during chemo only on the direction of an experienced integrative physician. These products can do a lot of good, but may alter drug metabolism by the liver if directly mixed with the wrong drug. These can ruin the therapy, or make it more harmful, so get experienced and knowledgeable help.

NutraSweet or aspartame promotes drug resistance through phenylalanine derivatives. The amino acid Tyrosine does the same.

A high sugar /glycemic load diet can elevate insulin-like growth factor IGF-1, which is anti-apoptotic and blunts chemo efficacy. Safe sugar substitutes are discussed in the section on naturopathic diet for cancer.

INTEGRATIVE SUPPORT FOR SPECIFIC CHEMOTHERAPY DRUGS

A naturopathic physician in oncology or trained integrative physician can put together a concise plan to support a good response with less side-effect. The following information is one resource in selecting a natural health product protocol to safely interact with complex multi-drug chemotherapy, in a patient likely to be on several additional medications. If you experience side-effects despite these precautions, and the good care you will receive at the BC Cancer Agency and our hospitals, then please ask our clinic to assist. We have some very good options for care of mouth sores, nerve damage, nausea, pain, and many other conditions.

We are particularly concerned to avoid mixing natural supplements which use the same liver detoxification pathways as the synthetic drugs. However, sometimes there are over-riding effects which make us consider the use of natural agents, even if they do affect drug metabolism. For example, quercetin acts on a common drug detox pathway in the liver, but also activates a protective pump which bails toxins out of cells. For some chemo drugs, concurrent use of quercetin has a net positive effect, and more cancer cells get killed. This requires the counsel of a scientific professional who reads the totality of scientific and medical evidence available and makes a balanced decision.

ARABA-C – Araba-C is derived from sea sponges, and is likely to provoke mouth sores, so use Fare You tablets.

ANASTRAZOLE – Aromatase inhibitors are synergistic with natural aromatase inhibitors quercetin, grapeseed extract, and white button mushrooms *Agaricus bisporus*, as well as the hormone modulators indole-3-carbinol and melatonin. Manage risk of bone loss with MCHA calcium – microcrystalline hydroxyapatite ossein complex with added vitamin D3, vitamin C, and magnesium citrate. Increase exercise, and manage joint pains with omega 3 marine oils and topical emu oil.

AVASTIN (BEVACIZUMAB) – An anti-angiogenesis agent, so it will interfere with blood vessel construction in normal wound healing, and may also provoke bleeds of the gums, nose or female reproductive tract. It can cause hypertension, intestinal bleeding and bowel perforation. It also increases risk to kidneys of high-grade proteinuria and nephrotic syndrome..

BICLUTAMIDE (CASODEX) – Biclutamide can be enhanced with ginseng, gamma oryzanol, sage and motherwort.

BISULPHAN – Bisulphan is synergistic with quercetin against human leukemia.

BLEOMYCIN – Bleomycin increases free radicals, so it is less toxic and more effective in patients given supplemental vitamins A, C and E; selenium, taurine, squalene and green tea.

BORTEZOMIB (VELCADE) – Bortezomib is less effective if mixed with green tea or quercetin. It is positively synergistic with curcumin and modified citrus pectin.

CAMPTOTHECIN – Camptothecin is from the Chinese "Happy Tree." There is a risk of later developing a secondary leukemia, due to damage to the bone marrow stem cells which give rise to blood cells

Quercetin improves absorption of camptothecin by cancer cells. Bu Zhong YI Qi Wan or Ba Zhen Tang herbal formulas reduce gastro-intestinal side-effects. Never mix Camptothecin with curcumin.

CARMUSTINE (BCNU) – Beta-glucans from maitake mushroom increase effectiveness against prostate cancer. Synergistic with berberine as found in golden seal, barberry, coptis and other herbs.

CISPLATIN, CARBOPLATIN & OXALIPLATIN – Improve effectiveness with quercetin (30% more apoptosis), coenzyme Q-10, genestein, selenium, mistletoe, coriolus PSK, shitake lentinan, green tea EGCG, resveratrol, vitamins A, niacin or a B-complex, C, and E. Platinum drugs are an exception to the rule against curcumin, as it definitely enhances their efficacy.

Milk thistle and selenomethionine can blunt tumour resistance to cisplatin, increasing efficacy.

Platinum compounds can cause severe nerve damage, hearing loss, severe kidney toxicity, nausea, vomiting, and bone marrow suppression. Reduce toxicity with milk thistle (liver protectant), astragalus (kidney protectant), omega 3 DHA oil (prevents kidney damage and increases efficacy), L-glutamine (nerve & GI protectant), quercetin, melatonin, and vitamins C and E. Low vitamin E status correlates with severe peripheral nerve damage from cisplatin, so Rx 600 mg daily. Selenium at 200 mcg daily reduces bone marrow suppression, kidney toxicity, and development of drug resistance. Intravenous glutathione protects nerves from toxicity, but it is controversial whether or not this reduces effectiveness. The platinums reduce tissue stores of magnesium and vitamin D, so it is essential to replace these. Ba Zhen Tang – Eight Pearls Decoction – reduces gastro-intestinal GI side-effects, as does Bu Zhong Yi Qi Wan formula. Some of my colleagues use Jian-Pi Yi-Qi Li-Shui Decoction, all-trans retinoic acid ATRA, or Polyerga spleen extract.

Carboplatin is less toxic to the kidneys, but more damaging to the bone marrow and blood cell counts than cisplatin. It can provoke genetic mutation. Carboplatin produces electrolyte (blood minerals) imbalances, nausea and vomiting, abnormal liver function, nerve damage, and muscle pain. Consider extra glutamine and Polyerga with carboplatin, and cytokine modulators such as astragalus and ganoderma. Oxaliplatin is more effective when combined with thymoquinone from black seed *Nigella sativa.*

Do not mix platinum drugs with N-acetyl cysteine, glutathione, alpha lipoic acid, *Ginkgo biloba*, squalene, zinc or high dose vitamin B6, unless directed by a naturopathic physician skilled in oncology.

Italian MDs use intravenous glutathione IV-GSH with cisplatin and cyclophosphamide chemo in ovarian cancer cases.

CYCLOPHOSPHAMIDE (CYTOXAN) – CP or Cytoxan is a mustard agent related to mustard gas used in World War I, but now banned as a weapon – except against cancer. Cyclophosphamide may cause nausea, baldness, bleeding in the urinary bladder, bone marrow damage, reduced natural killer cell activity, and increased risk of metastatic spread of cancer.

Increase effectiveness with vitamin A, beta carotene, vitamin C, vitamin E, coenzyme Q-10, folic acid and B-complex vitamins, quercetin, omega 3 oils and aloe vera juice. TCM formula Yi Kang Lin is synergistic.

Reduce toxicity with ashwagandha, melatonin, green tea, Co-enzyme Q-10, omega 3 oils, AHCC, grapeseed extract, cordyceps, coriolus PSK, magnesium, selenium, N-acetyl cysteine, glutathione, Polyerga spleen extract and lots of water. Red ginseng ginsenoside Rg3 reduces haemolysin, protecting the red blood cells. The TCM formula Buzhong Yiai or Central Qi Pill reduces toxicity and improves effectiveness.

Curcumin must <u>not</u> be used. It reduces death of the cancer cells.

CYCLOSPORIN – Cyclosporine is a powerful immune suppressor, to prevent rejection of transplanted tissue, including bone marrow transplants. Grapefruit juice increases its toxicity. Do not use immune enhancing herbs or mushrooms, or plant sterols.

DOXORUBICIN – Originally called Adriamycin because it was extracted from a unique fungus found only in a ruined stone tower overlooking the Adriatic sea. Doxorubicin is an antibiotic which binds inside the spiral strands of DNA.

Doxorubicin is a pro-oxidant, and is particularly toxic to cells low in oxygen. It is highly toxic to the muscle of the heart. There is only so much you can tolerate in a lifetime, so it is not often repeated. It can provoke baldness, nausea, vomiting, and leaking of fluid out of the blood vessels. It suppresses bone marrow and therefore blood cell counts, especially white immune cells. It can cause acute myelocytic leukemia AML.

Improve effectiveness with vitamin A, vitamin C, grapeseed extract OPCs, vitamin E, DHA omega 3 oils, milk thistle, mistletoe, melatonin and soy genestein.

Green tea theanine 50 – 200 mg daily, and quercetin 500 – 100 mg 2 to 3 times daily, help the drug accumulate in cancer cells, while sparing the heart and other healthy tissues.

Reduce toxicity with garlic, selenium, melatonin, grapeseed proanthocyanidins, omega 3 oils, squalene, coriolus PSP, green tea EGCG polyphenols and catechin. Adriamycin depletes the tissues of vitamins A, beta carotene, B2, B6, C, E and zinc, and supplementing with these will improve safety and efficacy. Anti-oxidants in virgin olive oil also seem to help. Vitamin B6 particularly reduces hand-foot syndrome (PPED). Pre-treatment with vitamin E is reported to reduce hair loss, while improving efficacy. The most critical supports are vitamin E and Co-enzyme Q-10 to protect the heart muscle from damage, which can enlarge the heart and lead to congestive heart failure. The heart can be further supported by taurine, carnitine, hawthorn berry, lily of the valley, and rhodiola herb.

Do not mix with N-acetyl cysteine or glutathione antioxidants as they can increase drug resistance. Do not mix with feverfew herb parthenolides.

HER-2 positive breast cancer may respond to anthracycline chemo drugs including Doxorubicin, Epirubicin, Adriamycin, Daunorubicin, Idarubicin and Mitoxantrone.

However, HER-2 negative cases do not respond to anthracyclines, and they no longer represent the standard of care for these patients.

EPIRUBICIN – Epirubicin is less toxic to humans given melatonin supplementation. The omega 3 oil DHA at 1.8 grams chemosensitizes tumors to anthracyclines, improving time to progression and overall survival in FEC chemo for breast cancer. See Doxorubicin entry above.

ERBITUX (CETUXIMAB) – Erbitux is incompatible with high dose of vitamin C.

ETOPOSIDE – *Podophyllum* or mandrake root was the origin of this compound. Etoposide chemo is enhanced with quercetin, melatonin, vitamin A, and beta-carotene.

Avoid St. John's Wort which increases toxicity. Avoid glucosamine sulphate, glucosamine HCl and N-acetyl-glucosamine, which reduce its effectiveness.

5-FLUORO-URACIL / 5-FU – 5-Fluorouracil is an "anti-vitamin" agent which interferes with the metabolism of a nutrient needed to make DNA. 5-FU causes loss of appetite, nausea, mouth sores, diarrhea, baldness, kidney failure, loss of white blood cells of the immune system, rashes, skin darkening or increased tendency to burn in the sun.

Improve effectiveness with quercetin, melatonin, aloe vera, shitake lentinan and vitamins A, vitamin C, vitamin E.

Reduce toxicity with L-glutamine, glutathione, chamomile mouthwash, coenzyme

Q-10, and vitamin B6. Ginseng helps preserve immune function.

Caution: do not mix with high doses of carotenoids, including beta carotene, lutein, and lycopene.

GEMCITABINE – Gemcitabine is closely related to 5-FU. This is one of the most effective and relatively least toxic chemotherapy drugs, and we can easily help it do even more, with less harm. Many patients just breeze through chemo with this drug. However, a small percentage of persons will have a genetic variation which causes them to metabolize this pro-drug into a very noxious chemical, and they may find it intolerable.

Synergistic with GLA oils, B-complex vitamins, melatonin, squalene, shark liver oil alkylglycerols, astragalus (Shih Chuan Da Bu Wan is an astragalus-based TCM formula), green tea, gotu kola, black seed *Nigella sativa*, and *Ginkgo biloba* extract.

Green tea EGCG improves efficacy while reducing GI toxicity of Capecitabine.

Quercetin reduces tumour cell resistance. Do not mix with estradiol, soy or legume coumarins.

GOSERLIN (ZOLADEX) – Zoladex is a hormone suppressant, which can be improved with ginseng, cleavers herb and gamma oryzanol.

HERCEPTIN – Herceptin targets the growth factor amplified in patients expressing the HER-2/neu gene.

It also damages the heart quite severely. You must take hawthorn berry *Crataegus oxyacantha,* Lily-of-the-Valley *Convallaria majus*, vitamin E and co-enzyme Q-10 to prevent or correct heart damage. I often add the homeopathic remedy *Naja tripudians 6C*. I am proud to say this has rapidly restored heart function in patients who otherwise would never have qualified for this therapy, due to weakening of their heat from previous chemo with drugs like Doxorubicin, or due to other causes. This approach has definitely allowed many patients to recover, and continue on in therapy, after cardiac damage forced a halt to the Herceptin therapy. It has, of course, also consistently restored heart health following Herceptin therapy.

Improve efficacy against the cancer with quercetin, *Aloe vera*, *Polygonum* herb, and NFkB Reishi mushroom extracts *Ganoderma lucidum*. Emodin from *Aloe vera,* and quercetin, reduce HER-2/neu gene expression, the root of the problem. Evening primrose oil or black currant oil gamma-linolenic acid GLA inhibits mutant HER-2/neu protein, increasing Herceptin response 30 to 40-fold in these cases. Olive oil's oleic acid improves efficacy. Flax oil alpha linolenic acid (ALA) is a potent support for Herceptin, inhibiting epidermal growth factor receptor EGFR.

It is important to control insulin-like growth factor IGF-1, which strongly interacts with the HER-2/neu receptor, and Herceptin therapy. This means close adherence to the low-glycemic diet.

HYDROXYUREA – Hydroxyurea or hydroxycarbamide is a common chemotherapy, which induces apoptosis by inhibition of ribonucleotide reductase enzyme. It is used in chronic myelogenous leukemia CML, polycythemia vera, and meningiomas. It is relatively benign, and is often taken for long periods of time.

Prevent liver and kidney and bone marrow toxicity with Shih Chuan Da Bu Wan or Astragalus Combination, co-enzyme Q-10, and milk thistle extract.

IRINOTECAN – Irinotecan is a semi-synthetic compound – a natural compound altered by a chemist – from the Chinese "Happy Tree." Improve drug uptake about 30% with quercetin.

Improve effectiveness with melatonin, milk thistle extract, soy genestein and selenomethionine.

Do not mix with curcumin.

ITRACONAZOLE – This anti-fungal can damage the liver and the heart. Milk thistle can reduce this risk.

Do not eat grapefruit or drink grapefruit juice, it reduces efficacy.

LETROZOLE (FEMARA) – Letrozole or *Femara* is an aromatase inhibitor capable of reducing estrogen and estrone.

The most striking risk is thinning of the bones. Support bone health with MCHA calcium complex, vitamin D3 and exercise.

Support with natural AI's quercetin, grapeseed extract, indole-3-carbinol and white button mushrooms. Also supported by Bcl-2 inhibitors such as curcumin and green tea extract.

MEGACE – Megace therapy can be enhanced with licorice root, sage, red clover, vitamins B6 and B12, and gamma oryzanol.

MELPHALEN – Avoid combining melphalan with glutamine, leucine, tyrosine or methionine supplements, as these will reduce uptake into the bloodstream, and therefore decrease efficacy.

MERCAPTOPURINE – Avoid mixing with anti-gout drugs, quercetin, myricetin, kaempferol, cinnamon and propolis.

METHOTREXATE (MTX) – Methotrexate is an antimetabolite or anti-vitamin agent which blocks use of the B-vitamin folic acid, necessary for DNA and protein manufacture. It is sometimes given in a fatal dose followed by "leucovorin rescue" which is calcium folinic acid. 1 in 100 patients can die from this procedure.

MTX is toxic to the kidneys and liver. It causes nausea, vomiting, diarrhea, mouth sores, inflamed skin, blurred vision, dizziness, and loss of adequate white blood immune cells.

For safety counteract the intense production of reactive oxygen species with vitamin A, vitamin E and selenomethionine.

Improve effectiveness with milk thistle extract, licorice root and polygonum. L-glutamine increases uptake of MTX into tumours.

Do not combine with glutathione, tangeritin, or high doses of folic acid or vitamin C. Avoid mixing with echinacea, black cohosh root or salicylate-rich herbs such as bilberry, willow and wintergreen.

MITOMYCIN – Mitomycin is synergistic with Yi Kang Ling formula, melatonin and marine omega 3 seal oil.

PAZOPANIB (VOTRIENT) – Pazopanib is a blood vessel growth inhibitor. Watch for bleeding issues.

PREMETREXED – Premetrexed is less toxic if homocysteine levels are reduced, so give vitamin B-12 and folic acid.

RIBAVIRIN – Quercetin improves Ribavirin's efficacy.

RITUXIMAB – Beta glucans improve responses to rituximab, even creating responses in patients previously unresponsive. An excellent source is *Agaricus blazei* mushroom extract, or **reishi** mushroom extract.

SANDOSTATIN – Sandostatin or octreotide will irritate the gallbladder, so give bile salts, digestive enzymes and the TCM formula Li Dan. Induces hypoglycaemia, so prescribe a high protein, low fat diet with low glycemic carbs.

SORAFENIB (NEXAVAR) – Sorafenib inhibits several growth factors for cancer, but also impedes blood vessel growth. Be aware of the significant risk of bleeding. Do not mix with any blood-thinners. *Jingli neixao* can help the fatigue, diarrhea, nausea, anorexia, hypertension, and icterus. See hand-foot syndrome below.

SUNITINIB (SUTENT) – Sunitinib inhibits several growth factors for cancer, but also impedes blood vessel growth. Be aware of the significant risk of bleeding. Do not mix with any blood-thinners. *Jingli neixao* can help the fatigue, diarrhea, nausea, anorexia, hypertension, and icterus. See hand-foot syndrome below.

TAMOXIFEN – Tamoxifen blocks some types of estrogen receptors, and has other complex effects on hormones. It delivers about a 50% reduction in the risk of a reoccurrence of breast cancer.

Tamoxifen can cause some serious side-effects. Although I must admit most women tolerate it reasonably well, integrative naturopathic support is definitely needed for safety. Tamoxifen can increase risk of blood clots by 3%, particularly in the deep leg veins and lungs. This risk is most pronounced for obese or high body mass index persons. It increases risk of uterine cancer by about 1%. It also increases by about 1% the risk of retinal damage, rashes, leukorrhea, depression, liver damage and increased tumour pain. Be prepared for hot flashes and thinning hair. In the presence of bony metastases it can precipitate excess blood calcium.

Melatonin is highly synergistic, reduces risks and reinforces hormone blockade.

GLA oil (gamma linolenic acid) from borage or evening primrose oil at 2.8 grams daily improves effectiveness by reducing expression of estrogen receptors. Quercetin improves effectiveness by increasing bioavailability. Vitamin E and selenomethionine in moderate doses will improve effectiveness. Vitamin A is particularly useful, extending remission times and improving response rates.

The energy regulator Co-enzyme Q-10 makes Tamoxifen more effective by increasing expression of tumour suppressor gene manganese super-oxide dismutase MnSOD. Co-enzyme Q-10, vitamin B2 riboflavin and B3 as niacin or as niacinamide, reduce DNA methylation and induce DNA repair enzymes, boosting Tamoxifen efficacy. My *Vital Victoria* brand 1-a-day multivitamin is a good way to get the vitamin

A, selenomethionine, B-vitamins and vitamin E in the correct balance.

It is important to control insulin-like growth factor IGF-1, which strongly interacts with estrogen receptors, and Tamoxifen therapy. This means close adherence to the low-glycemic diet.

Indole-3-carbinol is complementary in estrogen receptor positive ER+ breast cancer cases as it suppresses estrogen receptor activity by a different signalling pathway, increasing the arrest of the cancer cell growth cycle.

The use of soy foods with Tamoxifen has been a controversy, but recent evidence indicates a high degree of synergy. High soy <u>food</u> intake is associated with an additional 60% reduction in risk of breast cancer occurrence in pre-menopausal women on Tamoxifen. High intake is over 40 mg of soy isoflavones daily. A better target is 60 to 80 mg. Do <u>not</u> use genestein supplements, only use food sources.

Do <u>not</u> combine Tamoxifen with high dose vitamin D (over 2,000 IU daily), flavonoids such as tangeritin or grapefruit, black cohosh root *Cimicifuga racemosa*, St. John's Wort *Hypericum perfoliatum*, or red clover blossoms *Trifolium repens*, including Hoxsey herbal tonic.

Tamoxifen activity may be reduced by certain medications, for example the anti-depressant selective serotonin reuptake inhibitors SSRIs. Effexor may be prescribed for the hot flashes. I think it wise to choose naturopathic options for mood such as 5-HTP.

Acupuncture reduces hot flashes well, and the effect persists after treatment.

Smoking should be stopped and alcohol minimized.

TARCEVA (ERLOTINIB) – Erlotinib or Gefitinib, commonly called Tarceva, will typically cause blistering and peeling skin disorders. Use topical sea buckthorn i.e. New Chapter brand with calendula and rosemary, and *Aveeno* colloidal oatmeal lotion, soap and bath soak.

It can also cause abnormal eyelash growth and dry eyes. In some cases it provokes ulceration and perforation of the cornea or of the digestive tract.

Cancer cell killing increases if combined with indole-3-carbinol and soy genestein.

Do not mix with quercetin or curcumin.

TAXANES – Taxol is from yew tree bark. Taxotere (Docetaxol) and Paclitaxel are synthetic taxanes. Taxanes can provoke anaphylactic shock reactions, so to avoid serious trouble you will be pre-treated with Benadryl and/or Decadron – an antihistamine and a steroid drug. Sensory nerve damage, muscle pain, joint pain, mouth sores, nausea, vomiting, loss of white blood immune cells, and heart toxicity can also occur.

B-complex vitamins improve effectiveness. Improve efficacy further with vitamin C – 4 to 6 grams daily, resveratrol, vitamin E, and Iscador mistletoe injections. Highly synergistic with essential fatty acids such as GLA from evening primrose oil, and with Ashwagandha herb *Withania somnifera*.

Strongly supported by vitamin D3, improving efficacy while reducing toxicity.

Soy genestein increases efficacy by reducing DNA binding with nuclear factor NFkB.

Taxanes cause joint and muscle pain by raising COX-2 enzymes which promote inflammation. Use natural COX-2 inhibitors such as omega 3 marine oils, boswellia and resveratrol.

L-glutamine at 2 to 3 grams up to three times daily reduces risks of nerve damage and muscle pain. This can be supported with acetyl-L-carnitine and vitamin B6 in the pyridoxal-5-phosphate form. Pyridoxine B6 also treats skin eruptions on the hands and feet, called palmar-plantar PPE.

Melatonin (21 mg) is neuroprotective against taxane neuropathy.

Curcumin <u>may</u> improve efficacy of Docetaxol.

Do <u>not</u> mix with quercetin, berberine, NAC or St. John's Wort as they may reduce efficacy.

TEMOZOLAMIDE/TEMODAL – Temodar or Temodal is a unique chemo drug for certain brain cancers. It induces autophagic cell death rather than the usual apoptosis pathway. The drug may lower platelet counts. Support with alkylglycerols, grapeseed extract, and if needed for platelets, Yunnan Baiyao.

THALIDOMIDE – Thalidomide a potent inhibitor of blood vessel in-growth to tumours and it may also be useful for wasting syndrome. May cause nerve injury, such as numbness and pain in the limbs, which is treatable with vitamin B6, benfotiamine and R+ alpha lipoic acid.

VINCA ALKALOIDS – Vincristine and Vinblastine from periwinkle flower can cause constipation, small bowel paralysis, baldness, mouth sores, inflamed skin and nerve toxicity such as foot drop, phantom sensations, and loss of tendon reflexes. This class of drugs increases inflammation.

Effectiveness is increased by vitamins A, C and E, as well as Cordyceps mushroom extracts.

Prevent or treat nerve toxicity with milk thistle extract, vitamins B6 and B12. Give COX-2 inhibitors to reduce side-effects such as joint and muscle pain, and to increase anti-tumour effects – for example omega 3 marine oils.

Give stool softeners or laxatives.

Quercetin overcomes resistance to Vincristine and Vinblastine therapy.

An Example of a Common Chemo Support Prescription:

With FEC – 5-Fluorouracil, epirubicin and cyclophosphamide for breast cancer
- Shih Chuan Da Bu Wan – 12 pellets twice daily (or Astragalus Combination 3 capsules twice daily).
- Co-enzyme Q-10 – 100 mg twice daily
- Melatonin 3 mg at bedtime – 8 pm to 12 midnight <u>only!</u>
- Ginkgo biloba extract – 100 mg twice daily
- Vital Victoria multivitamin with minerals – 1 daily
- Omega 3 marine oils 2,000 to 4,000 mg daily.

GRADING CHEMO TOXICITY

It is really unusual for anyone to die from chemotherapy now. You will be tested before each round of chemo to determine how your bone marrow is being affected, by counting and describing the red blood cell, white blood cells and platelets. You will also be tested to see how your vital organs, the liver and kidneys are tolerating the drugs. Your heart may sometimes be assessed, and as well, your gastro-intestinal upsets will be graded. The most common grading is on a scale to four:

0 = normal range
1 = mild toxicity, continue drug at 100% of the prescribed dose
2 = moderate toxicity, reduce dose to 75% of Rx
3 = severe toxicity, reduce dose to 50% of Rx, or wait for improvement
4 = critical toxicity, may be fatal if unchecked, suspend therapy

Usually therapy is only reduced, slowed or suspended if more than one organ or cell type is affected. However, the most important are low platelet counts, due to risk of haemorrhage, and low white blood cells, particularly neutrophils, the first-responder immune cells necessary to survive and infection.

It is important to monitor serum albumin, a protein required to keep fluids in the vessels. It is a sign of severe oxidative stress to see a drop in albumin, bilirubin and uric acid. Untreated, it gives a poor prognosis. Prescribe antioxidants and whey protein supplements.

Treating Common Chemo Toxicities with Naturopathic Medicine:

The simple chemo supports you were prescribed will not always prevent reactions and damage from toxic chemotherapy drugs. Fortunately there are many more naturopathic interventions which can stabilize fitness for therapy, relieve side-effects and heal organ failure. If you have any concerns during your medical therapies which are not being addressed by your medical doctors and nurses, or you do not get relief from the drugs you have been prescribed for side-effects, please ask you naturopathic physician for help. You may be pleasantly surprised to find there are many inexpensive, safe and very effective natural products for use in medical oncology.

After chemo most patients will benefit from detoxification for health restoration. Our goal is real vitality, not just the end of gross disease.

ANEMIA – bone marrow damage takes 1 to 3 weeks to manifest after receiving a toxic dose of a chemo drug, but then may progress to complete failure to produce any of the blood cell types. If the marrow stops making red blood cells the patient becomes anaemic. Lack of red cells means not enough hemoglobin to carry oxygen out to the tissues and carbon dioxide back to the lungs to be breathed out as waste. Anemia makes a person tired and listless. Your doctor may order blood transfusions if your hemoglobin falls below 90. Use iron with caution as it is very oxidizing, making ROS which damage DNA. It is safer to check iron status by measuring serum ferritin before giving iron. Vitamin B-12 and folate given by intramuscular injection can kick up blood cell production. Support bone marrow nutrition with sesame oil 1 tsp., shark liver oil alkylglycerols 1-2 capsules three times daily, *Panax ginseng* 500 to 1000 mg. twice daily. Key TCM herbs to look for are astragalus and tang kuei, as in formulas such as *Marrow Plus* from Health Concerns 3-4 capsules three times a day, *Milletia 9* from Seven Forests 6 tabs three times daily, *Shih Chuan Da Bu Wan* or Shiquan 8 pellets three times a day. *AHCC* (active hexose correlated compound) is a proprietary Japanese low molecular weight compound from fermented shiitake and other medicinal mushrooms grown in rice bran, which has been found to prevent many chemo side-effects and increase the effectiveness of methotrexate, 5-fluorouracil and cyclophosphamide at doses of 3 grams daily.

Resistance to the blood-building drug Erythropoietin therapy is reduced by co-administration of L-carnitine and vitamin A. Erythropoietin and its analogues can cause great harm in some patients, primarily thromboembolic events – in 17% of cases. They also fail to significantly reduce the need for blood transfusions.

Grandma's Laxative

Pitted dates ½ cup 125 ml
Prune nectar ¾ cup 200 ml
Figs ½ cup 125 ml
Raisins ¾ cup 200 ml
Pitted prunes ½ cup 125 ml

Simmer dates in prune nectar until very soft. Spoon into a blender; add figs, raisins and prunes. Blend until smooth. Keep refrigerated. Use as a spread on toast or crackers, or eat by the spoonful. Yes. It is high-glycemic, but we have to balance competing interests in making clinical decisions.

ANOSMIA – Loss of smell leads to loss of taste, with degradation of quality of life, and appetite. Steroid hormones are used, and we may also use *Ginkgo biloba* extract, zinc citrate, and homeopathic *Zincum metallicum* or *Mercurius solubilis.*

APPETITE- loss of appetite or anorexia is helped by ginger, bitters, peppermint, thiamine, melatonin, Marinol and reishi mushroom extract, royal jelly. Make small meals, and control odours. Your acupuncturist may needle ST-36, SP-6, CV-12, BL-20 and 21 for appetite. For loss of taste add LI -4. The TCM herb formula Bu Zhong Yi Qi Wan is recommended by myself, and by the prominent integrative medical oncologist Keith Block. Other herbs include gentian, bitters, catnip, fennel, peppermint and ginseng. Exercise helps. Be aware that bromelain used in high doses as an anti-inflammatory can powerfully inhibit appetite. The amount in Can-Arrest or our curcumin and quercetin products will not bother.

ATTITUDE – Expectation plays a central role in the occurrence of side-effects. If the patient believes they can stay well, visualizes success, and positively affirms and embraces the therapy, they will likely do better than if they are fearful. However, it is not a trivial concern that chemo can cause great harm, even death. Anxiety is therefore normal, but high levels of depression, as measured by the Hospital Anxiety and Depression Scale (HADS) questionnaire, can predict pathological responses to chemotherapy. Such patients may display high emotional restraint and not appear severely depressed. This is a good reason to integrate mind-body medicine with orthodox protocols!

CHEMO-BRAIN – Many patients complain of "brain-fog," a feeling of cognitive impairment, poor memory, poor concentration, and felling "too tired to think straight." In some cases there are severe mood changes, irritability and even frank psychosis. Chemo makes the cerebellum and cortex have to work harder on common tasks such as short term memory. Changes in the basal ganglia and frontal cortex are persistent for many years after chemo. Fortunately this responds brilliantly to acetyl-L-carnitine. Note that ordinary L-carnitine does not cross the blood-brain barrier nearly as well.

CONSTIPATION – Number 42's are remarkable for relieving even the stubborn constipation from codeine and morphine painkillers. #42's are an old naturopathic remedy – capsules of cape aloe root and wormwood.

We also consider Hoxsey herbal tincture, aloe vera juice, psyllium fibre, acupuncture Prosperity treatment, enemas, and occasionally we refer for colonic irrigation by a certified colon therapist. We always advise good hydration, and suggest fruit such as prunes, papayas and rhubarb. We may recommend Grandma's fruit spread:

Another good formula is 2 cups bran, 2 cups applesauce, 1 cup unsweetened prune juice – take 2 to 3 tablespoons twice daily.

I have no objection whatsoever to the use of stool softeners such as Colace or Docusate, glycerine or lactulose suppositories, or Senokot, which is just natural senna leaf sennosides.

DEHYDRATION – treat aggressively with miso broth, mango juice and electrolyte drinks such as the WHO formula – 1/2 tsp salt, 3/4 tsp baking soda, up to 8 tsp sugar, and up to a cup of fruit juice to 1 litre water. Intravenous therapy is normal saline, 0.9% salt, with 5% glucose.

DIARRHEA – BRAT diet (banana, rice, apple, toast). . Replace probiotic gut bacteria. I use *Vitazan Ultimate Acidophilus* as it is a potent mixture billions of acidophilus and other probiotics includes FOS food for the bugs, and is enteric coated. Replace electrolyte salts as well as water, with miso soup, broth, juices or an electrolyte drink– at least an 8 ounce glass per bowel movement. Bentonite clay can absorb toxins. L-glutamine gives energy to heal the lining of the gut. *Po Chai* pills are a tremendous Chinese herb for toxic diarrhea, but also consider *Xiang Sha Yang Wei Pian* and *Ba Zheng Wan* formulas. Acupuncture points ST 25 and 37. Prosperity treatment is a special acupuncture technique using 4 needles around the belly button, and it can treat either diarrhea or constipation, with good results in about 5 minutes. Consider omega 3 oils.

FATIGUE – exercise – and start prior to therapy! Use L-carnitine 500 to 1000 mg three times daily for energy, or even better acetyl-L-carnitine. ALC crosses the blood brain barrier to help "chemo-brain." The Chinese ginseng root *Panax ginseng* is a wonderful tonic. I like to give 1 to 2 vials daily of the Chinese tonic herb formula Ling Chih Feng Wang Jiang with reishi mushroom, codonopsis, royal jelly and lychee fruit juice. If not available, give royal jelly, *Codonopsis*, reishi mushroom extract, or vitamin B5. Omega 3 marine oils reduce fatigue and depression by reducing interleukin

IL-6. Naturopathic physicians may give intravenous "Myer's cocktail" of vitamins and minerals to boost the immune system and revitalize. We may simplify this to a shot of vitamin B12 in the rump. Give by mouth chlorella algae or wheat grass juice for chlorophyll. Consider the herbs rhodiola, nettles, astragalus, Siberian ginseng, ashwagandha, shitake and cordyceps. Sometimes one must just conserve energy and ask for assistance on chemo days. Prepare food ahead of time and bank some down time – then use it to rest, contemplate, and visualize positive results from the therapy. Reiki therapy will help!

HAIR LOSS – Alopecia is very common from chemotherapy. It cannot usually be prevented. Some claim vitamin E will reduce the loss, or at least stall it. AHCC compound also claims to protect the hair follicles. Acupuncturists may use ST 36, SP 6, LV 8, BL 20 and 23, and moxa to BL 17. You will likely have to learn to love your skull or hats, headscarves and wigs. Afterwards, we use Shou Wu Pian, which is bearsfoot herb, to re-grow hair more rapidly.

HAND-FOOT SYNDROME – palmar-plantar erythrodysesthesia PPED begins as a tingling, numbness or redness of the skin on pressure areas such as hands, feet, elbows or knees. It can progress to severe reddening and peeling of the skin at the extremities, which can impair function and lead to serious infections. Use topical emollients such as aloe vera lotion, or moisturizers such as Bag Balm. Take vitamin B6 as pyridoxal-5-phosphate, Rx 100 mg twice daily. Avoid rubbing the skin, pressure, hot showers and sun exposure. Apply cold ad lib. *Aller-C* and homeopathic *Apis mellifica* can help reduce the histamine release, and quercetin suppresses this at the source.

HEART DAMAGE – My preferred Rx: for heart injury by chemo drugs is Co-enzyme Q-10 300 mg daily, vitamin E 400 IU daily, *Convallaria majus*, *Crataegus oxyacantha* and *Naja tripudians* 6CH as a tincture 1 dropper-full 3 times daily. Naturopathic oncologists are also using grapeseed extract OPCs, *Ginkgo biloba*, omega 3 oils, L-carnitine, *Angelica*, *Lycium* and *Ginseng*.

KIDNEY DAMAGE – repair any organ damage with Co-enzyme Q-10, in doses of 100 to 300 mg daily. Renal tubule damage is helped by quercetin at about 1,500 mg daily. Support it with mixed anti-oxidants, astragalus herb, and omega 3 oils. The omega 3 docosahexaenoic acid DHA prevents cisplatin nephrotoxicity. Kidney failure is sometimes averted with Jin Gui Shen Qi Wan formula, also called Rehmannia Eight and Sexoton. We can also use astragalus, angelica, nettle seed, pellitory-of-the-wall and parsley-piert for kidney recovery.

LEUKOPENIA – failure to produce white blood cells means a loss of immune cells, so the person's resistance to infection can plummet. The most aggressive product to raise the count is shark liver oil alkylglycerols; in doses to 1200 mg. Naturopathic doctors have long had great success rebuilding immune health with thymus and spleen glandular extracts. I really like to use Dolisos homeopathic thymus – *Thymuline*. My American colleagues use *Polyerg*a spleen peptides. I give chlorella algae, up to 20 grams daily. Botanicals to consider are *Phytolacca* (poke root) or *Hydrastis* (golden seal root) – 30 drops of tincture twice daily. Consider the Chinese herbs Siberian ginseng, astragalus, ligustrum, codonopsis, milletia, white atractylodes, salvia miltiorrhizae, lyceum, salix root, scutellaria and royal jelly. Ayurveda suggests *Podophyllum hexandrum.* We may give dilute intravenous hydrochloric acid. Acupuncture points include TW-5. Supplement zinc, selenium, vitamins A, C, E, B6 and B12. An intramuscular injection of B12 will pump up the neutrophils, our fist responders to infection. Avoid crowds, avoid people with infectious illness, and wash your hands often, especially after using the toilet and before eating. Exercise. Report to your physician any sign of infection such as fever over 38°C, chills, cough, sore throat, painful urination, or inflammation such as redness, swelling and pain anywhere.

MOUTH SORES – sores in the mouth and bleeding gums hurt, reduce eating and can get infected. Called mucositis, it can sometimes spread through the whole gastro-intestinal tract and cause GI bleeding. This can be the factor which limits using an effective dose of chemo, especially in leukemia cases. I have adapted a Chinese herbal product to this problem, with brilliant results. *Fare You* "vitamin U" Rx: 4 pills three times daily – will generally prevent or rapidly heal mouth sores, or throughout the GI tract. It is a pharmaceutically pure form of the amino-acid methionine extracted from green cabbage. It is also terrific for stomach ulcers, colitis and diverticulitis, and completely safe. Vitamin E 800 IU is said to prevent mouth sores. Give L-glutamine at up to 15 grams twice per day or 2 gm/m², or one rounded teaspoonful dissolved in a warm drink three times daily. 5 grams in ½ ounce water makes a great mouth rinse – swish for 1 minute, then swallow. Use 4 times daily. For children give 1 gm / m² body surface area. Consider liquid folic acid/folate, *Glycyrrhiza* as DGL licorice extract, chamomile tea or tincture, green tea with honeysuckle flower, marigold flower juice *Calendula officinalis succus,* chlorophyll, slippery elm bark *Ulmus fulva,* vitamin E gel, homeopathic *Traumeel,* and *RadiaCare* oral rinse. The BC Cancer Agency's "Magic Mouth Rinse" is distilled water, Nystatin anti-fungal, Benadryl elixir anti-histamine, and Solu-Cortef hydrocortisone sodium succinate. A simple oral rinse of ½ teaspoon each of baking soda and salt in a glass of warm water may be used several times a day. Use a very soft toothbrush, or a finger or gauze pad, and consider baking soda rather than toothpaste. The mouth will be soothed by cold or frozen yoghurt and soft, bland food. Avoid over-the-counter mouthwashes such Listerine, Scope. Avoid crunchy, spicy and acid foods. Burning mouth neuropathy is treated with R+ alpha lipoic acid, and Liu Wei Di Huang Wan formula. Try ice-chips too. Some of my American peers swear by honey for prevention of mucositis. This violates my low-glycemic rule in radiotherapy, but I can support it in radiation therapy for head and neck cancers: 20 ml of honey is taken in small sips starting 15 minutes before radiation, and this is repeated every 15 minutes for the next 6 hours.

NAIL DAMAGE – Fingernails and toenails can be discoloured and deformed by chemotherapy drugs, with risk of pain, infection and loss of mobility. Good hygiene is important and regular pedicure and manicure by a professional is sometimes needed. Disinfectants, antibiotics and corticosteroids are sometimes used, and cushioning, petroleum jelly emollition and sticking to roomy and comfortable shoes may be needed. I use oil of oregano topically for infection, while for repair I use chickweed cream and methylsulfonylmethane MSM.

NAUSEA – <u>ginger is very good</u>, as 2 capsules of root powder, as ginger tea, even as ginger ale. SeaBand is an acupressure band with a button that presses on PC-6. Even more potent is acupuncture needling at the points ST-36, PC-6, HT-1, CV-12. Homeopathics *Arsenicum, Nux vomica, Tabacum, Ipecac* or *Cuprum metallicum* have often worked very well. Eat often in small amounts, especially starches such as dry crackers, and drink plenty of fluids. Medical marijuana cannabis tetrahydrocannabinols THC does work well for some, if they can tolerate the other effects. If nausea arises from a gut reaction to stress I prescribe Xiao Chai Hu Tang formula.

NERVE INJURY – Always use R+ alpha lipoic acid, time-release 150 mg three times daily for any nerve damage or neuropathy, from numbness, phantom sensations or pain. Burning mouth syndrome is a toxic neuropathy shown to respond very well to R+ alpha-lipoic acid. The Benfotiamine form of vitamin B1 is useful at doses of 160 mg twice daily. Other adjuncts we may consider are L-carnitine or acetyl-L-carnitine – 2 to 3 grams daily, L-glutamine -6 to 10 grams a day, vitamin B6 – 500 mg twice a day, vitamin B12, B-complex, calcium, melatonin, vitamin E and milk thistle extract. Homeopathics of interest are *Hypericum perfoliatum* and *Aconitum napellus,* as found in *Traumeel.* Contrast hydrotherapy and cold-sock treatments are often helpful. Nattokinase fibrinolytic therapy may help chemo neuropathy.

PLATELETS – failure to make platelets or thrombocytopenia can make it impossible to form a clot, with a risk of severe haemorrhage. Your doctor may prescribe a transfusion of platelets if the count falls below 20. Yunnan Baiyao *Panax pseudo-ginseng* 1-2 capsules three to four times daily is a reliable and fast therapy which I have seen out-perform synthetic drugs. The pineal gland hormone melatonin helps regulate the production of platelets, with efficacy comparable to Neupogen, and it's a lot safer. Consider also shark liver oil alkylglycerols, and maitake mushroom extracts. High-dose vitamin C can help recovery. It is thought that eating fresh raw pineapple may help increase the platelet count. Sesame oil nourishes the marrow. Some use Standard Process *Cataplex T.*

Avoid aspirin (ASA) and Advil (ibuprofen), *Ginkgo biloba*, and other blood thinners. Ginger root reduces platelet counts, and is a direct blood thinner. Keep vitamin E doses less than 600 IU daily. 400 IU daily is generally quite safe. Report to your physician any bleeding signs such as bruising, red spots on skin, bloody urine or black, tarry stools.

VOMITING – treat dehydration aggressively – drink electrolyte (blood minerals) replacement, make a cup of miso soup, consider acupuncture. Replace salt and soda as well as water, or the water will not stay in the blood; the WHO basic electrolyte replacement formula is ½ tsp salt, ¾ tsp baking soda, up to 8 tsp sugar and a cup of juice per litre water.

WEIGHT LOSS – 80% of cancer cases are malnourished, and 40% die of malnutrition. Weight loss is a cardinal sign of cancer, and must be monitored and managed aggressively. Loss of over 20% lean body mass is critically dangerous; increase carbohydrates & protein intake. Cancer can cause cachexia, a metabolic syndrome with profound weight loss. Use marine oils rich in the fatty acid eicosapentaenoic acid EPA – especially seal oil, 2 capsules twice daily with meals. You may use fish oils, up to 1 Tablespoon daily. Consider melatonin, L-glutamine, bitter melon *Momordica charantia*. Intravenous vitamin C can help stabilize weight.

WHITE BLOOD CELLS – see LEUKOPENIA

DETOXIFYING FROM CHEMO DRUGS

I will examine you 3 to 4 weeks after the last dose of chemotherapy, and will typically want to detoxify you and restore immune health. I usually start with this simple program I learned from Dr. Craig Wagstaff, ND:

THREE TO SIX DAY ELIMINATION DIET
NO MEAT, NO DAIRY, NO EGGS, NO FISH, NO GRAINS
Breakfast

Apple or Grape juice – 8 ounces. You can make more if you desire, but be sure that you take 8 oz at least.
Fresh fruit – ½ pound. You may eat more, but try to eat at least ½ pound. You can eat any fruit(s) but please **no bananas.**
Herbal Tea. One cup if desired
Between breakfast and lunch you should drink all the **pure, unsweetened** fruit and vegetable juice you can hold. Also eat fresh raw vegetables and fruit. The more food you put down, the more thorough the cleansing. If you cannot get fresh juices, use the unsweetened **pure** canned/frozen variety. Make up a lot of Vegetable Broth (See recipe below). This is better than any of the canned vegetable juices. Drink lots of this broth, it is full of minerals!

RECIPE FOR BROTH

- 7 Carrots
- 1 small bunch Celery (cut finely)
- Place these ingredients in 2 quarts (8cups) of hot water and boil for 15minutes.
- Add:
- One-third bunch of parsley
- Large handful of fresh spinach (cut finely)
- Boil for 10 minutes more and drain off the juice or broth.
- Flavour with onion, okra, green peppers or garlic.

The purpose of this broth is to **FLUSH**. Drink lots of it during the days of this diet, it is full of minerals from the vegetables. If you cannot make your own broth, Organic Vegetable Broth is available in tetra packs in most grocery stores.

Lunch

<u>Vegetable Broth.</u> –up to two cups during the meal.
<u>Salad.</u> Make a chopped salad of fresh raw vegetables. Use a dressing of olive oil and sea salt. Use four or more vegetables from the list below:
- Artichokes Cucumbers Lettuce Rutabagas
- Asparagus Celery Lotus Spinach
- Beans Dandelion Greens Okra Squash
- Beets Endive Onions Swiss chard
- Brussels Sprouts Fresh Green Peas Parsley Tomato
- Cabbage Green Peppers Pumpkin Turnip
- Carrots Kale Radishes
- Cauliflower Kohlrabi

Other vegetables can be added, except no **potato or avocado**
<u>Dessert</u> Fresh fruit, if desired
<u>Herb Tea</u> After the meal, if desired
Between lunch and supper drink all the fruit and vegetable juice you desire. Eat all the fresh fruit and vegetables you want. Fill up, its medicine for you. The purge comes from the vitamins and minerals in the food so <u>be sure to eat plenty.</u>

Supper

<u>Vegetable Broth.</u> Drink two cups during the meal, more if you desire. This recipe makes about a one-day supply. You can make more if desired and place in the refrigerator, but it can be used hot or cold.

<u>Cooked Vegetables.</u> Select two or three of the different kinds of veggies listed above and cook them with oil or steam them. Eat a generous helping – vegetables are rich in salicylates, which inhibit NFkB and therefore reduce inflammation.
<u>Dessert.</u> A salad of fresh fruits
<u>Tea.</u> After meal if desired. If you feel hungry after dinner, eat fresh fruit and drink **pure** fruit or vegetable juice – all you want!

LIVER DETOX

Vitazan Milk Thistle Combination is the ideal liver cleanser formula– 2 caps, 3 times daily with food. This is available in our clinic. Note the curcumin in this formula to slow Phase1 and speed up Phase 2, reducing build-up of toxic intermediates, reducing symptoms of a "healing crisis." Ellagic acid as found in berries and pomegranate also accomplishes this important task,

Indole-3-Carbinol: 200 mg 3 times daily really helps clear chemicals such as formaldehyde and solvents, and is particularly valuable for the very chemically sensitive patient.

Dream Protein: whey powder is sugar and fat free. Quality whey supplies "conjugators" which neutralize toxic intermediates from Phase I stage. One scoop, one or two times daily. May be added to the juice/soups. Once a sulphur compound or amino-acid is conjugated or bound to a toxin, the body will not recycle it back and it will pass out in the urine or bowel movement. If dairy is not tolerated we can use soy or rice protein concentrates.

Fibre: if you are constipated or suspect you have parasites add 1-2 Tablespoons daily of **psyllium** husks and fresh-ground flaxseeds.

What to expect from this cleanse:

The first day you may feel a slight discomfort by having changed your regular mode of eating, but do not allow this to disturb you for it is natural. On about the <u>third or fourth day</u> the bowels and kidneys will begin to move freely. Much toxic material will be passed. There will be symptoms of headache, perhaps nausea, gas, a few aches and pains but <u>do not</u> be alarmed, this is Natures way of cleaning you out. These symptoms are quite natural and to be expected. About the fifth day you will feel a surge of energy, you'll be surprised at yourself! Your complexion will become clear and your eyes will brighten and you'll feel wonderfully clean inside. The little cells that were so full of toxins are not clean and they begin crying out for another food. Continue on until the end of the sixth (or last) day; then seek advice about balancing your diet. If you start this diet – **STICK TO IT**. Don't try it one day then quit, if you follow the instructions you will reap a wonderful reward of <u>HEALTH</u> again.

"The Seven Day Rice Diet" is a good transition back to a regular diet.

Seven Day Brown Rice Diet

General instructions:

This diet will give you all the nutrition you will need while your body cleanses and heals itself. You don't have to go hungry, and you don't have to count calories, weigh food or pay much attention to the selection of food. You eat whenever you are hungry, and as often as you like. While on this diet, you may experience some weight loss.

- Eat until you feel full but not engorged. It is better to eat several small meals per day rather than 3 large ones.
- Do not drink with your meals, as this dilutes the enzymes in the stomach needed to properly digest the food eaten. Wait about 10 to 15 minutes before or after eating to drink.
- Try to keep the consumption of fruits, vegetables and rice separate. Food combining is based on the discovery that certain combinations of foods may be digested with greater ease and efficiency than others. Therefore, eat only fruits at one time, vegetables at another and rice at different time as well. This also

- goes for fruit and vegetable juices.
- If you find brown rice alone to be too bland you may flavour with Ginger, Garlic, or Bragg's Aminos – a delicious **unfermented** salt-free soy sauce, available at grocery stores.

What's allowed on the diet?

- Brown rice, preferably organic. Basmati, red and wild rice may be added for variety.
- Fresh vegetables, any kind you like, lightly steamed if you wish. Onions are especially good for cleansing and are very sweet and tasty when steamed.
- Fresh fruits, any kind, except oranges and orange juice. With fruits and vegetables, it is best to consume only organic produce whenever available. However, this is not always possible, buy in season and locally grown fruits and vegetables, wash them thoroughly before eating. When buying dried fruit, purchase only un-sulphured dried fruit.
- Fresh garlic, onion and ginger.
- Cayenne or chili pepper and/or a non-salt herbal seasoning (e.g. "Vegit"), turmeric (curry)
- Vegetable and fruit juice – the best is fresh pressed from a juicer and consumed within 20 minutes, otherwise buy quality juices with no additives, sugar, chemicals, and little or no salt.
- Green tea.
- Other foods allowed are: lentils, rice cakes, sesame seeds, ocean-going fish, free-range chicken, chickpea humus, soy tofu and tempeh.
- Absolutely <u>no shellfish</u> (shrimp, oysters, scallops, clams, lobster etc) or catfish.

Cooking instructions for brown rice:

Rinse rice well, five or six times in warm water. Proportions of water to rice for cooking are 2-2 ½ cups of water to 1 cup of rice. Bring water to a boil, add rice, stir, cover and reduce heat to simmer for 45minutes, or until the water has been fully absorbed. Do not lift the lid until cooking is finished, after which the rice will be doubled in volume and fluffy-looking.

Alternate Method: Add rice + cold water in a rice cooker. Most models have a light that goes off when rice is perfectly cooked.

Other elements we may consider for drug detox include:

- Laxatives. Once the bowels are clean and balanced the liver can be more aggressively cleansed.
- Enemas or colonic irrigation for severe cases.
- Probiotic gut bacteria

- Liver herbs such as dandelion root, burdock, milk thistle, globe artichoke, black radish and chelidonium.
- Anti-oxidants, including alpha lipoic acid and N-acetyl-cysteine.
- Infrared sauna – up to 40 minutes 1 to 2 times daily for 4 weeks. Twice a week is healthful.
- Dry skin brushing.
- Acupuncture detox: LV-3, ST-36, KI-3 and 7, LU-7, LI-4, GB-20, PC-6, HT-7, GV-20 and 23, BL-13 (LU), 18 (LV) and 23 (KI); ear points: Shen men, Sympathetic, Kidney, Liver, Lungs.
- Purified water – the best is Nikken optimized "pi-mag" water, which features microcluster water structure, making it a more powerful solvent than ordinary water.
- Start your day with fresh lemon juice in water.
- Lots of steamed vegetables.
- Daily aerobic exercise, such as yoga, pilates, weight training, or pole walking.
- An orderly personal schedule with adequate sleep.
- Relaxation, spiritual practice, self-expression.

Another excellent naturopathic detox protocol is described in Dr. Peter Bennett's book the *7-Day Detox Miracle*, 2001, Prima Publishing.

Herbal kidney cleanses are often needed. Skin brushing and deep breathing contribute to waste removal. The more **emunctories** or organs of elimination we can enlist, the quicker and easier it goes.

Before detoxifying for heavy metals, you need to have any mercury-silver amalgam dental fillings taken out.

This process is potentially quite harmful, if not done by a dentist with specialized equipment and training. You can really stir up a hornet's nest in your immune system if too much mercury is released into the patient. Heavy metals are often removed by intravenous chelation therapy with agents such as EDTA, DMPS and DMSA. These are sometimes given orally, and may be supported by supplements such as chlorella algae, garlic, cilantro and N-acetyl-cysteine.

It is possible to detoxify emotionally as well as physically. You may suddenly feel old traumas, anger, have disturbed dreams or see old scars get inflamed. Report any discomfort to your naturopathic physician.

PART THREE

Chapter Four – A Deeper Look Into The Biology Of Cancer And The Science Of Oncology

In this part we explore the scientific language and medial concepts of oncology – the arts and science of cancer care. For those with an interest in science and medicine, this will be fascinating. You will learn some of the fundamental facts about the nature of cancer. It is full of medical terms used by doctors and research scientists.

You will find my descriptions very brief. Once you know the terminology and the concept, you can readily find more details in the many fine textbooks in oncology. There is also a wealth of knowledge readily accessible online from a huge variety of medical databases. See: Web Resources. My goal is to give a clinician's overview of the field.

Most patients are content to be told what to do by their naturopathic and orthodox medical physicians. You may skip this if you find technical jargon and science make your head hurt. However, I find many patients want to know what causes cancer, what is the nature of the enemy, and how do we think we can control it. Understanding of these concepts will guide us to rational therapies now, and future directions for cancer care.

You cannot become an oncologist with a few weeks of study of the internet. Do not embarrass yourself by trying. You are the CEO of your body, and have the right to give or withhold informed consent – you should be able to get all the information you feel you need to make good decisions on treatments you will accept. *This does not mean we have to educate a patient to the level of a doctor.*

I hope this chapter will give educated lay people the fundamentals to make good decisions, including insight into selecting a team of qualified professionals.

Overview of Cancer Occurrence and Causes

Cancer is not a benign or self-limiting disease. It is unstable, dangerous, and unforgiving of poor choices.

Cancers are the second leading cause of death. Only cardiovascular disease – heart attack and stroke – kills more people in North America – but cancer is very close to overtaking CVD as the #1 killer.

Epidemiology is the study of disease trends in large populations. It gives a way to sort out the multiple factors which act to create or prevent diseases. As an example, you can look at the occurrence of heart disease in those who smoke cigarettes and compare it to the rate for non-smokers, and you can see it is much worse in smokers. You can then tell a smoker how much risk they are taking by smoking. Since real individuals often do some things which are good and several things which are bad – at least bad for <u>their</u> biology – it is only by this method that the relative role of each action can be discerned.

Epidemiology research into cancer has led many experts and textbooks to state that "Remarkable differences can be found in the incidence and death rates of specific forms of cancer around the world." The biggest differences arise from cultural factors, especially diet.

In the USA in the year 2001 – over 1,300,000 new people were diagnosed with cancer; treatment costs were over $100 billion US dollars. Divide by 10 to get the Canadian figures.

Cancer will affect more than 1 in 3 persons alive today in Canada. To be precise, about 1 in 2.7 females and 1 in 2.3 males will have a serious cancer. About 1 in 5 Canadians will die of cancer. Overall survival at 5 years for all cancers at all stages is about 63%, but by excluding common treatable skin cancers, the numbers flip to 64% of those diagnosed from cancer still dying of cancer.

Since I was born in 1952, the incidence of cancer in the USA rose approximately 50%. When I graduated from university the chance of a Canadian woman getting breast cancer in her lifetime was 1 in 11. Now it is about 1 in 7.

10 % of deaths of children under age 15 are due to cancers, notably acute leukemias and brain tumours. Many of these are preventable, if we would only clean up our environment and bodies of chemical poisons.

While early detection and small advances in treatment mean the death rate is slightly lower now, the number of people getting cancer and dying of cancer has risen steadily. Canadian death rates from cancer in the last 20 years have climbed 48%, twice the rate of growth of the population (if not "corrected for age and gender"). We have an increasing elderly demographic in Canada. Aging increases cancer risk. It is a major killer of the elderly.

There are at least 300 distinct neoplastic diseases we call cancer. Aside from the balky off-switch issue in common, the various cancers differ widely in their primary growth factors and overall biology. Cancer is not a simple disease, it has many forms, many causes, and therefore there is no simple cure. What works for one cancer at one stage in one person will not always do the same for another person, another cancer type, or the same cancer in the same person at a later stage.

Despite the best of medical care, people are right to fear it. People greatly fear both the disease and treatments Mortal fear is to be expected if something can kill you.

Cancer has very high morbidity, meaning it causes great sickness and harm, again despite the best of modern medical care. Some are so lacking in grace as to say that a lot of the suffering of cancer patients is caused by applying the best of modern medical care. This is called iatrogenic harm. However harsh modern oncology is, and it can be savage, remember these good doctors know how awful the disease can be if untreated, and are trying their best to help with what they know. In fact nearly 100% of those diagnosed with cancer will suffer some harm from the treatment. They may be disfigured or maimed by the surgery, suffer various complications, be burned by the radiation and scar up, or be made very ill by the chemotherapy drugs. Orthodox treatment can kill patients, and it can trigger cancer cell formation, resulting years later in another cancer even if the first type was cured by the treatment.

Is it any wonder sensible, educated and cautious people are using all possible adjuncts to reduce the harm from cancer therapy, to restore their full health, and to prevent a reoccurrence?

Most **benign tumours** do not become cancerous. However, if they get large in the wrong place they can be as damaging as cancer.

The role of genetics in cancer is surprisingly minor, considering the central role of DNA abnormalities in cancer. Studies with twins show inherited factors increase risk for stomach, colorectal, lung, breast and prostate cancers by 26 to 42%. Certain races have increased risk of certain cancers, although it is really a saw-off as they often have lower risk from other conditions.

Asian women have low risk of breast cancer, but when they move to the USA and adopt the American diet and lifestyle their risk increases by 60%. Overall, immigrants to our Western civilization lifestyle see increased cancer risk of 80% after 10 years exposure. The same diet and lifestyle habits of the Western world also give rise to heart disease, stroke, arthritis, diabetes, auto-immune diseases, and Alzheimer's dementia.

However, a whopping 70 to 90% of cases are attributable to environmental and cultural factors rather than genetic predisposition, and are therefore theoretically preventable. For example risk arises from exposure to xenobiotics – chemicals which accidently mimic our hormones, from man-made (exogenous) hormones, tobacco, alcohol, amines, polyamines, polycyclic aromatic hydrocarbons formed by burning sugars, excess sun exposure, heavy metals, pesticides, and excess sugar intake.

When I worked in cancer research at the B.C. Cancer Research Foundation, Medical Biophysics Unit, there was a new laboratory set up to measure the potential to cause genetic mutation (mutagenicity) and cancer causing potential (carcinogenicity) of environmental toxins. There had been an unusual cluster of cancers in a seaside town, and it turned out they were eating mussels off of creosote-treated pilings at the wharfs. In all the years they tested compounds for mutagenicity and carcinogenicity the substance that was the most dangerous was caramel candies, such as the little caramel cubes we always get as Halloween treats. It turns out scorching or burning sugars generates some serious toxins.

You should not assume Health Canada, or anyone else is actually protecting you from carcinogens. Their puny efforts are proving ineffectual at lowering our toxic burden. Our DNA is unravelling in a chemical soup approved for our consumption by agencies such as Health Canada, based on research submitted largely by the chemical, food and drug industries. If you were not aware of it before, now understand that your health and safety has been sold out to commercial interests in the food, chemical and pharmaceutical industries.

I advocate use of the PRECATIONARY PRINCIPLE – if it is carcinogenic, remove it from our diet and environment. Guy Dauncy explores this admirably in his book *101 Ways to Prevent Cancer*

Our air is being fouled and poisoned with tars, soot, asbestos and organic oils which cause lung cancer. Vinyl chloride and phthalates from plastics are damaging our livers.

Polycarbonate plastics release estrogenic bisphenol –A. The FDA in America says 2 parts per million of bisphenol-A are safe, but one thousand times less than that – 2 parts per billion – is measurably estrogenic in humans. Recently we have seen a movement away from using plastic bottles for drinking water, and this trend now has to spread to all food and beverage containers. Use food-grade stainless steel, glass, ceramic or wooden vessels.

We eat toxic dioxins – formed from burning organic compounds – in everything. The whole planet, including the oceans is fouled with them. We all have residues of pesticides on our tissues, even if we live on an organic farm and eat only organic food. Herbicides and pesticides can end up acting like hormones and growth factors in our bodies. These xenobiotics or xenohormones are major disruptors of normal growth and development.

Food may be contaminated by highly carcinogenic fungal aflatoxins and nitrosamines, polycyclic aromatic hydrocarbons, and the ubiquitous benzopyrenes.

Cancer has many causes and it therefore must have many possible paths to a cure.

Cancer is a disorder of the control of growth of cells. Cancer cells grow faster than normal cells from the same tissue or organ.

Cells have the genetic code on their chromosomes, in the form of DNA. Each cell has about 2 meters of DNA, coiled incredibly tightly in a double spiral with links like steps on a ladder formed by 4 alkaline chemicals called bases. Using 4 letters (bases) arranged into 3 letter words (codons) the DNA library has all the information needed to create all the different cell shapes, sizes and products to form tissues, organs and the whole individual human being. Normal cells read only parts of the whole library, and become specialized or differentiated for a particular job in a particular place.

Cells should grow until they touch another cell, and then stop – this is called contact inhibition. Cellular adhesion molecules (CAM) touching another cell results in a signal being sent from the cell's outer membrane surface to the DNA in the nucleus of the cell. It tells the DNA to stop growth of the cell, as it has reached its neighbour's property line. Reducing ICAM-1 expression in solid tumours improves resistance to leukocyte invasion.

Cells should have a limited lifespan, duplicating themselves a few dozen times. Repeated copying of the genetic information produces errors and missing bits in the DNA, so it begins to look like a bad photocopy. The aging normal cell removes a bit of the end of the chromosomes called a telomere every time it is copied. When that telomere is gone, the cell cannot be copied, just like a videocassette with the little plastic tab removed cannot be recorded anymore. When the cell is old and has some errors that cannot be repaired, it will then quietly dissolve away in a natural process called apoptosis, to be replaced by a new cell.

Cancer cells develop their abnormal characteristics from changes in the DNA called **mutations**. Most mutations do not work out to be good for a cell's survival, but

sometimes the cell gets lucky with a **non-lethal mutation** and develops the core skills that make cancer cells malignant or hostile to life:
- Excess rate of growth and cell doubling
- Invasion into normal tissues
- Spread to distant sites – metastasis

Immortality – cancer cells also become "immortal" in the sense that they have no set lifespan. They can double and double and never throw the apoptosis off-switch to die. This means they make far more copies of their DNA than they were designed to, so the DNA becomes riddled with errors and abnormalities, making them unstable and bizarre acting. Tumours are unpredictable because various cell lines are genetically unstable and constantly evolving new genetic variations.

Mutations can arise from DNA instability triggered by oxidative damage. The average cell must repair over 10,000 oxidative hits per cell per day.

Free radicals of oxygen (ROS) release lightning bolts of energy which break up the DNA. Healthy levels of antioxidants like vitamin A, C, E, selenium, and glutathione reduce the free radical ROS levels, and DNA repair enzymes in the cell nucleus cope with the damage if it is not too severe.

ROS also produce disulphide bonds between sulphur atoms as on cysteine moieties in DNA bases. This makes a chemical cross-link between DNA strands to form a dimer, rendering both strands unreadable. Repair of some DNA dimers is possible, but if too many accumulate, the cell will die. Antioxidants protect the DNA from these sulphur bonds gluing the pages of the genetic book shut. Antioxidants which help the DNA include vitamin C, vitamin E, carotenes, selenium, glutathione, alpha lipoic acid and grapeseed extract.

ROS deplete the stem cell pool, allowing the accumulation of senescent cells. These old cells are at higher risk of cancerous transformation, due to shortened telomeres, accumulated mutations and errors, and genomic instability.

Carcinogenesis can be just a deletion or a translocation away.

Cancer cells can counter-attack our immune cell ROS by producing immune suppressive factors such as cytokines IL-10, TGFß and prostaglandin PGE-2.

Genomic instability is associated with carcinogenesis, and cells can have these internal defects while still appearing histologically abnormal under a microscope. Instability includes allelic imbalance, unbalanced loci, and shortened telomeres, particularly affecting glycolytic genes. One implication of this is the "field of cancerization effect" where these genetic problems occur up to a centimetre out from tumours, providing a potential source of new cancer cells in areas that look normal, and may be described by the pathologist as clean surgical margins.

Micro-RNA contributes to carcinogenesis by reducing tumour suppressor gene expression while increasing expression of proto-oncogenes.

Redox (reduction or oxidation) reactions occur when cells are exposed to excessive levels of trace minerals such as iron and copper. Redox agents produce dangerous free radicals and reactive oxygen species ROS which can activate or deactivate proteins – including genetic control proteins such as transcription factor STAT-3, nuclear factor kappa-B NFkB and activator protein one AP-1.

Normally the **tumour suppressor gene phosphatase and tensin homologue PTEN** opposes activation of the P13K / Akt / mTOR pathway, the gatekeeper for tumour growth. PTEN has an up-regulating feedback loop with tumour suppressor gene p53, and prolongs the half-life of p53 protein, protecting it from degradation. PTEN down-regulates VEGF expression, IGF-1 signalling and modulates G2/M cell cycle arrest. PTEN function can fall off due to deletion, mutation or epigenetic silencing. It is very sensitive to small chromosomal rearrangements, and is often inactivated when BRAC-1 mutations reduce DNA repair.

The **P13K/Akt** signalling pathway is a central regulator of critical cellular functions such as cell adhesion, angiogenesis, migration and drug resistance. It regulates crucial proteins and genes including p53, NFkB, cyclin D, *Bad* and mTOR. Heat shock protein ninety HSP90 can bind to Akt and chaperone it past degradation pathways and allow the cancer cell to evade apoptosis.

mTOR kinases phosphorylated by Akt are activated to the state where they can increase protein synthesis and translation, if they sense glucose and amino acid nutrient availability. mTOR will increase building of VEGF receptors. mTOR is inhibited by curcumin.

Nuclear factor kappa-light-chain-enhancer of activated B-cells or NFkB is a DNA transcription or copying factor which controls the expression of proteins involved in cell adhesion, migration, invasion, cell death (apoptosis), oncogenes, angiogenic factors and growth factors. It is constitutively up-regulated in most advanced cancers. It can promote cancer cell survival by preventing apoptosis. It increases risk of metastasis by increasing matrix proteases such as MMP-9. It increases adhesion factors such as galectin 3. It increases angiogenesis via increased vascular endothelial growth factor VEGF. It increases fibroblast growth factor two FGF-2. NFkB stimulates myeloid-derived immune cells in tumours to make excessive pro-inflammatory substances such as IL-1, IL-6 and IL-8. IL-1 increase release of PGE-2, increases leukocyte activity and number, stimulates endothelial cells and fibroblasts critical to angiogenesis. IL-6 is associated with fatigue from cancer. IL-8 attracts leukocytes and stimulates angiogenesis. NFkB generates tumour necrosis factor alpha TNFa. It regulates pro-inflammatory substances such as COX-2.One strategy for blocking NFkB is to inhibit EGFR – epidermal growth factor receptors. Vitamin E turns off NFkB and other pro-inflammatory genes.

p53 is known as the Guardian of the DNA because it arrests the cell cycle at the G1-S checkpoint, assesses for DNA damage, attempts to repair damage and mutations, and initiates cell suicide if it is unable to make repairs.

Apoptosis follows the release of cytochrome C after the oligomerization of the mitochondrial protein *bak*.

p53 inactivates mitogenic oncogenes, promotes genomic stability and resistance to chemical carcinogens. It suppresses tumour growth by inhibiting angiogenesis via release of anti-angiogenic collagen fragments by activating alpha (II) collagen prolyl-4-hydroxylase. Dangerous and intractable cancers – melanoma, prostate, lung, bladder, cervix, breast and colorectal cancers – have early occurrence of p53 mutations which reduce apoptotic removal of abnormal cells, increasing cell proliferation and longevity. Other cancers also can develop this problem, and so become more difficult to cure.

Fortunately, sometimes the p53 can be encouraged to resume more normal levels of control over cell growth. Natural agents supporting p53 activity can reverse the abnormal control of cell growth which is the very core of the cancer problem – these include quercetin, folic acid, selenium and zinc.

Normalizing p53 is a prime target for the general prevention of cancers. Aging in general is now linked to lowered anti-oxidant response damaging the tumour suppressing p53-ARF pathway.

Reduced apoptosis in cancer cells increases malignancy – how dangerous a cancer is – by increasing cell survival and longevity. Old cancer cells accumulate DNA damage, DNA instability, and mutations. They get tougher to treat and are faster growing!

Anti-apoptotic signalling results from activity of the *bcl-2* -B-cell leukemia-lymphoma two, *bcl-xL*, *rhoA* and *ras* genes.

Ras integrates regulatory signals. Mutant k-ras translates EGFR activity into Map kinase pathway growth signalling. Ras is particularly vulnerable to mutation by chemical carcinogens such as dyes, heavy metals and polycyclic aromatic hydrocarbons. The *ras* protein attaches to the inner cell membrane via farnesyl lipid (an intermediate in cholesterol synthesis), then is phosphorylated by tyrosine kinase, causing a kinase cascade leading to increased cell growth. Mutant *ras* leads to continuous growth signalling. Mutant *ras* increases angiogenesis and lymphangiogenesis by VEGF, PDGF and FGF. *Ras* can be inhibited by bromelain, D-limonene, vitamins A, E, D3, quercetin, green tea EGCG, and Rasfonin from the fungus *Trichurus terrophius*.

Apoptosis is increased by *bax* and *bad* genes.

Bad gene, and therefore apoptosis, is strongly inhibited by epinephrine (adrenaline). This is how chronic mental and emotional stress inhibits clearance of cancer cells. This is exaggerated in those with emotional repression marked by a hyper-rational attitude which refuses to process and express stressors. If we can't let it out and let it go, it eats away at us.

Inflammation reactions by the immune cells produce ROS, which increase mutation rates, DNA transcription (copying), and cell growth factors. These increase proliferation of more cancer cells.

In 2005 Italian scientists noted that one of the most common mutations associated with the transformation of a cell to cancer, called the MET oncogene, leads to a disturbance in the clotting factors, and increased fibrin production. Fibrin is the protein net which sticky platelets cling to make a clot. Fibrin is also a major trigger of inflammation, which makes cancer grow wildly. The other key role of fibrin in cancer progression is that cancer cells move out of tumours by eating the fibrin strands. As they pull it in, they drag themselves beyond the tumour boundary, into the extra-cellular matrix ECM, and beyond.

Activator protein one AP-1 is a constitutively active and inducible transcription factor which regulates cytokines. It relies on the **MAPK** pathway – mitogen activated protein kinases. Activator protein AP-1 is activated by hypoxia, a low oxygen level, which is seen in fast growing tumours which outstrip their blood supply.

AP-1 activation is associated with progression from pre-neoplasia to malignancy, including the acquisition of invasiveness and accelerated proliferation.

Steroid receptor co-activator SRC-3 is also known as A1B1 oncogene. When amplified or over-expressed it initiates tumorigenesis, it is a potent growth promoter, and up-regulates matrix metalloproteinases MMP-3 and MMP-13, which promote cell migration, invasiveness and metastasis. It is often active in squamous esophageal carcinomas, and cancers of the stomach, prostate and breast. It is particularly activated in HER-2+ breast cancer, as HER-2 signalling phosphorylates A1B1. SRC-3 can create resistance to Tamoxifen therapy.

STAT 1, 3 and 5 are signal transducers and activators of transcription – they speed copying of the DNA in cancer cells. STAT-1 is strongly inhibited by green tea EGCG, while STAT-3 is strongly inhibited by indole-3-carbinol_and curcumin. STAT-5a/b modulates prolactin hormone.

Beta-catenin modulates genes for VEGF, PPARΔ, MMP-7, MTI-MMP, Survivin and transcription factors. The β-catenin protein stimulates cell-to-cell adhesion and proliferation. It is stabilized by Wnt proteins made by cancer stem cells, which use it for their self-renewal. It is reduced by the omega 3 fat DHA, and by regulating casein kinase.

Genetic expression becomes abnormal in many ways in a cancer cell. The cell may produce less than normal of growth inhibitors or may increase and facilitate DNA copying (transcription) factors. Overproduction of growth factors can also occur, such as **transforming growth factor alpha TGFa** which binds to epidermal growth factor receptors, and can transform the cell growth pattern and "immortalize" a cell when over expressed.

Transforming growth factor beta TGFß transforms fibroblasts to myofibroblasts. It is an acute phase anti-inflammatory cytokine which inhibits the immune system. It is released from a protein complex called stable latency associated peptide, by pH under 3, proteases, and radiation injury.

TGF is a potent immunosuppressor, making it harder for immune cells to find and kill cancer cells. TGFß stops differentiation of T-cells into active cytotoxic or helper cells. TGFß blocks production of the interleukin IL-2 needed to proliferate T-cells. It is supported in blocking immune function by interleukins IL-4, IL-5 and IL-10. TGFß inhibits secretion of tumour necrosis factors TNFa and TNFß, inactivating cytotoxic NK cells and lymphokine-activated killer cells. When activated by stromal cell thrombospondin-1 TGFß suppresses T-cell effectors activated against tumour antigens, creating local immune tolerance.

TGF is both a sensor and a signaller of oxidative stress. TGF also induces angiogenesis, making blood and lymphatic vessels grow into the tumour to feed it oxygen and nutrients, and carry away wastes.

TGF de-regulates pericellular proteolysis – it allows cells to make enzymes which dissolve the protein barriers around it – which can allow the cancer cell to creep away and spread to new sites. Cancers which produce more of this compound are extremely dangerous.

TGFß is generally pro-apoptotic, via several mechanisms, including the Smad pathway, p53, up-regulation of Bax, down-regulation of Bcl-2 and Bcl-Xl, and enhancement of Fas-induced apoptosis.

Transforming growth factor alpha TGFß is a primary ligand of epidermal growth factor receptor, an erb/HER receptor tyrosine kinase.

TGFß is over-expressed in cancers of the breast, stomach, pancreas, colon, rectum, prostate, ovary, non-small cell lung cancer, melanoma and glioma.

TGFß has been found to be active in single cancer cells metastasizing throughout the body, but must switch off for the cell to grow in its new location. TGFß signalling is increased by surgery, radiation and chemotherapy, raising concerns these therapies may contribute to cancer spreading.

TGFß is not active in clumps of cancer cells moving around, which tend to lodge in lymphatics and not travel as far as single metastatic cells.

Tumour necrosis factor TNF and Fas gene protein ligands bind to plasma receptors to activate apoptosis initiator caspase enzymes, which then trigger "execution" caspases, which activate endonucleases and catabolic enzymes. This dissolves the damaged DNA and kills the cell.

TNFa is an acute pro-inflammatory cytokine which stimulates the immune system. TNFa is made by macrophages, proliferating T-lymphocytes, B-cells and NK cells. It is supported in immune stimulation by interferon INFγ and interleukins IL-2, IL-6 and IL-12.

TNFa up-regulates protease MMP-9 expression and therefore angiogenesis.

TNF is linked to headaches including migraine.

DNA methylation controls which parts of the genetic code are active. One DNA base can accept a methyl group –CH3 a carbon with a few hydrogens attached. When methylated, that part of the DNA cannot be opened, read and used. Reduced cytosine base methylation in cancer cells increases the rate of DNA transcription and therefore expression of most genes, including the bad ones.

The "methylation paradox" is that when regulatory regions of tumour suppressor genes are hypermethylated, this triggers hypomethylation of most of the cancer cell genome.

This phenomenon increases as tumours progress and become more invasive. Hypomethylation causes chromosomal instability including translocations and deletions of genes and loss of genomic imprinting._Fortunately dietary methyl group donors and antioxidants can increase methylation, reducing malignant gene over-expression. These include vitamins B12, B2, B6, folic acid, and betaine, all found in whole foods and vegetables. Folate is critical for the synthesis of s-adenosylmethionine SAMe which is the final methyl donor to DNA. Methylation deficits produce excessive gene transcription. We can monitor serum homocysteine and urinary methylmalonic acid (MMA) as markers of this problem. Demethylation will unmask viral gene and oncogene sequences embedded in our DNA, which may be a critical step in the development of cancer. Also "unsilenced" by demethylation are many growth promoter genes. These make existing cancers grow even faster.

Conversely, methylation can shut off any of about 1,000 tumour suppressor genes.

Acetylation -CH3CO- of histone proteins is another epigenetic regulator of DNA

94

function. Inhibiting histone deacetylation reverses epigenetic aberrations responsible for chemotherapy resistance and other problems.

Tyrosine kinases are major regulators of cell growth and survival. The TK super-family of cell surface receptors transduce external signals into internal signals. These transmembrane glycoproteins bind a ligand on the outer surface, which then activates phosphorylation of the intrinsic tyrosine kinase on the inner membrane surface. The tyrosine residue becomes a docking site for messenger molecules, which create a cascade of signals to the nucleus, altering gene expression, cell proliferation, and apoptosis. This in turn alters cell migration, invasion, and angiogenesis. The signalling pathway involves the *ras, raf* and mitogen activated protein kinase MAPK systems, i.e. P13K – Akt-m-TOR – p7056k- Ras-Erk-1/2. A prominent TK is the *erb* family of receptors, including epidermal growth factor receptor EGFR and HER-2/neu. TGFa and EGF bind exclusively to *erb* receptors. More than 90% of solid tumours express at least one member of the *erb* family. For example about 1/3 of breast cancers over-express HER-2/neu (erb2) which correlates with a poorer prognosis due to increased invasiveness and reduced response to chemo or hormone therapies. EGFR/HER1 are treated with tyrosine kinase inhibitors Tarceva (erlotinib) and Iressa (gefitinib) as well as the monoclonal antibodies Erbitux (cetuximab) and Vectibix (panitumumab).

Topoisomerase enzymes I and II tend to be elevated in cancer cells. These enzymes open up DNA strands to be read, including oncogenes and proto-oncogenes. They break and later rejoin DNA strands, resolving strains in the helix during replication.

Virus activation of oncogenes can turn on changes in the DNA which lead a good cell to become permanently transformed into the cancer lifestyle. Many oncogenes appear to be identical to retrovirus sequences thought to have been spliced into our human ancestor's DNA by viral infection many thousands of years ago. Other retroviruses may have entered the human race more recently, in vaccines extracted from animal cells infected with viruses. These new viruses are not yet oncogenic, but may evolve in that direction, as have their predecessors.

The human DNA genome library locked in the nucleus of every human cell is now cluttered with millions of viral sequences: 1.3% is complete viral genomes – including oncogenes – which can trigger cancer directly.

Ten percent of our genome consists of hundreds of thousands of copies of the viral promoter Alu, each only 280 base-pair sequences long. If these get turned on, all kinds of viruses lurking in the body, perhaps even lurking inside the cell's nucleus can become active. An immune system overwhelmed by viruses cannot fight cancer.

Fifteen percent of our genes code for the viral enzyme reverse transcriptase. This turns on viruses made of RNA.

We have lots of RNA viral sequences in our human DNA. The Salk polio vaccine saved many lives, but exposed us to the SV40 DNA virus from polio virus grown on rhesus monkey kidney cells.

Viruses can cause some cancers:
- squamous cancers such as cervical carcinoma – human papilloma virus HPV. HPV oncoproteins target p53 protein for degradation, deregulating cell cycling, impairing tumour-specific T-cell response, and increasing immune suppressor

cell activity.

- Burkitt's lymphoma, Hodgkin's Disease and nasopharyngeal carcinoma – EBV – Epstein-Barr virus
- Inflammatory breast cancer – mouse mammary tumour virus MMTV-like virus.
- Kaposi's sarcoma – herpes virus.
- Hepatocellular carcinoma / hepatoma – Hepatitis B or C virus
- T-cell leukemia and lymphoma – T-cell lymphotropic virus-1
- lymphoma, brain, bone and mesothelioma – SV-40 simian virus.
- Merkel cell neuroendocrine skin carcinoma – Merkel cell polyomavirus.

Survival or anti-apoptotic signals arising from hormones, growth factors and cytokines may be altered by mutations affecting their cell surface receptors.

Growth factor receptors on the cell membranes may mutate and deliver continuous mitogenic (growth) signals, like a gas pedal that jams, putting growth on full throttle. Mitosis is another word for the doubling of the DNA and its separation and division into 2 new cells. Transmembrane receptors for growth factors, such as epidermal growth factor receptor EGFR, have an extracellular binding region (on the outside of the cell) and an intercellular kinase (on the inside of the cell wall). Ligand binding (contact with its target molecule) results in homo- or hetero- dimer formation with activation of the associated tyrosine kinase inside the cell. This triggers several intracellular pathways, such as **mitogen-activated protein kinase MAPK** and AKT / P13K, which result in increased growth, resistance to apoptosis and increased angiogenesis. All of this means more cancer cell growth.

Cell division is normally regulated by cell **growth factors** such as epidermal growth factor EGF, platelet-derived growth factor PDGF, transforming growth factor beta one TGFβ-1 and insulin-like growth factor one IGF-1. It should be obvious that we do not want cancer cells to have any more growth factors, given that it is a disease of excessive cell growth.

Normal signal transduction from the cell surface receptors to the nucleus occurs by way of **phosphorylated tyrosine kinases PTK**. A receptor activated by its growth factor will make the PTK add fats on the inside of the cell. Lipid isoprenyloid tails on PTKs activate ras proteins which become trapped in their excitatory guanidine tri-phosphate-bound GTP forms.

This activates **cyclin-dependent kinases**. Cyclins tell the cell to enter its cell cycle, its reproduction process. Cell cycle entry and progression results in cancer cell division – the cell copies itself and splits in two – and tumour growth. This step is normally regulated by Rb, Wt-1 and p53 tumour suppressor genes.

Abnormal cell-to-cell communication at **cell adhesion molecules** CAM and gap junctions causes loss of contact inhibition, so the cells keep growing even after they bump up against another cell and should stop. This makes cells pile up into hard tumours – and still they grow! An independent cell is malignant, unable to act in the interest of the common good of the body network. An example is the role of the Von Hippel-Lindau VHL tumour suppressor gene. VHL normally promotes transcription of

E-cadherin cell adhesion molecule. Loss of VHL results in loss of **E-cadherin**, with subsequent development of aggressively growing and spreading cancer. The surface of a cancer cell sends its nucleus "do not die" signals more than "do die" messages, so it never dies.

Cells get replaced al the time, and lots of human tissues replace very rapidly. Most cells eventually die off voluntarily, when damaged or when old enough to have accumulated a high risk for serious errors. When I grew human cells for research, we could only keep them going a few dozen generations of doubling, then they would expire. In a living person the cells also shut down after just a few dozen copies. No one can make a normal human cell live longer. This is called **the Flickman limit**, and is usually about 50 cell doublings. However, we also grew Hela cells, which are human cervical squamous fibroblast cancer cells from a woman named Helen Lane. She died of this disease in Baltimore, Maryland in 1951. Her cancer cells appear to be immortal. They grow incessantly, and never shut themselves off. All over the world, research labs have these and similar cancer cells which can be kept going indefinitely, as long as they are fed and properly cultured.

Humans have a built in off-switch for bad cells. Every cell can turn itself off permanently and get recycled and replaced. This gentle process is **apoptosis** or programmed cell death. Normal cells check their DNA before they copy into two potentially flawed cells. Apoptosis should result in cells being quietly and safely removed and recycled if they are over 50 doublings old – the Flickman limit. Chromosomes have a structure called a **telomere** on their end, which shortens with every copying. When the telomere runs out, the cell can no longer copy the DNA. It locks down and goes into senescence, followed by recycling of the cell by its neighbours. It sacrifices itself for the greater good. Sometimes the neighbour cells grow into the space, or a stem cell replaces it with a fresh new cell. DNA can be prematurely damaged by ultraviolet light, ionizing radiation and oxidative stresses. DNA can accumulate dangerous errors, deletions and translocations, well before the Flickman limit. Apoptosis will typically switch on if there are more than 50,000 to 60,000 nicks and strains on the DNA – the limit a cell can usually repair. Old or damaged cells turn inside out and get themselves recycled and replaced.

Cancer cells can be made to undergo apoptosis if treated with natural agents!
SWITCH OFF THE BAD CELLS
This is the primary objective in treating all cancers!

Autophagy is an alternative way for cells to die. It means to eat oneself. The cells sequester cytosol or cytoplasmic organelles within double membranes, called autophagosomes. These autophagic vacuoles fuse with endosomes and then with lysosomes, and digestion ensues. This is presumed to be a mechanism to cope with damaged organelles and recycle them. Autophagy can be induced in cancer cells by catastrophic inhibition of growth signals such as mTOR and other kinases.

Loss of differentiation means the cell forgets what it is supposed to be doing – and usually ends up concentrating on growth for its own sake. The more undifferentiated a cell is, the more likely it will lose its sense of place and purpose, and lose the controls put on it by the specialized cells around it. It also means it can be less specific about the conditions under which it can live, so it will be better able to spread and grow in the wrong places. If a cell is completely de-differentiated it is called anaplastic. If it is only partly dedifferentiated it is dysplastic. Natural agents which support cell differentiation can help a cancer cell remember how to behave appropriately, and reduce its survival in other tissues. Vitamin C is known to be a regulator of embryonic stem cell differentiation, and vitamin D regulates differentiation throughout life.

How does any cell know what part of the huge library of DNA information it is expected to use? Cells have the whole library, but open up a small part by unmasking part of the DNA. Imagine a cell entering a library, opening up a book, studying it, using the information, and becoming trained to have a certain career. Just as an electrician studies electricity while a lawyer studies law, each cell uses only part of the available library. An eye cell acts like an eye cell and a stomach cell acts like a stomach cell because each makes different special enzymes from specific parts of the DNA. These enzymes make chemical reactions happen to give that cell what it needs for its specialized or "differentiated" way of life. So how does it know what part to open up and read? By where it is in space relative to other cells, within electrical, magnetic and especially chemical gradients. The signals from its surrounding network vary by how far from the top, front or middle it is. Normal cells know where they are, and behave accordingly. In fact, if they are moved too far away they may fail to grow. Cancer cells becoming undifferentiated specialize in one thing only – growing fast and spreading to new places. They can open up all sorts of new parts of the DNA code, to adapt to new surroundings. They can also open up parts of the code, using topoisomerase enzymes, to make chemicals which are toxic, or which allow other bad behaviour.

BRAC-1 and BRAC-2 are general DNA repair genes, preventing tangles in the strands of genetic material. Carriers of mutations have distinctly increased risk for cancers of the breast, pancreas, prostate, bone, pharynx and GI tract. If your family has clusters of these cancers you can be tested. If you carry the mutation, selenium can help reduce its expression.

PARP or poly-ADP-ribose polymerase is another DNA repair gene, which needs vitamin B3 to operate.

Angiogenesis is the growth of new blood vessels to growing tissue. It happens in healing cuts and wounds and it happens for growing cancerous tumours. Arteries run into little capillaries which supply vital blood and nutrients to nearby cells. Angiogenesis is required for growth of a tumour past a very small size – 1 to 2 millimetres in diameter. This size tumour is undetectable, still safely localized at the in situ stage. New endothelial cells in the vascular buds secrete growth stimulating polypeptides such as IGF, Gm-CSF, PDGF and IL-1. Once a cancerous tumour has mastery over angiogenesis, it can grow large enough to kill the patient.

Placental growth factor (PGF) binds to vascular-endothelial growth factor receptor one VEGFR-1, also called FLT-1, to promote angiogenesis and tumour progression independently of VEGF.

Cells stressed by heat, cold, hypoxia or low glucose produce **heat shock proteins HSPs** which prepare the cell for additional stress. Cancer cells make HSPs to try to stay alive despite imbalanced oncoprotein signalling that would otherwise be lethal. HSPs are in a class called chaperone proteins, which regulate client proteins such as kinases, kinase receptors (cell proliferation), MMP-2 (invasion), steroid receptors, telomerase, Akt (apoptosis) and HIF-1α (angiogenesis).

HSP-90 can resist apoptosis from radiation or chemotherapy by regulating the strongly apoptotic 17AAG protein folding client. Blocking HSPs will increase cancer cell death. Natural HSP inhibitors include quercetin and alpha lipoic acid.

HSPs form a complex with mutant forms of p53 protein, produced by mutations on the p53 gene, and this complex disrupts normal mechanisms which would arrest the cancer cell growth cycle.

Heat shock factor one HSF-1 allows cells with malignant mutations to adapt and survive. HSF-1 modulates two oncogenic signalling pathways – extracellular signal-regulated kinase ERK downstream of Ras, and activation of protein kinase-A PKA downstream from G-coupled receptor activation. HSF-1 also blocks translation of proteins by inhibiting the mammalian target of rapamycin mTOR pathway. HSF-1 promotes glycolysis.

Release of heat shock proteins into the circulation stimulates an immune response. This is one of the few things a cancer cell can do which will attract the attention of an immune cell. All too often the cancer cell looks normal to the immune cells, and goes unchecked until it is so deranged it cannot be stopped. Necrotic cells release HSP-peptide complex, which stimulates cytotoxic T-cells and non-specific NK cells. Apoptotic cells expressing HSPs are taken up by dendritic cells, which then present antigens to T-cells, leading to a tumour-specific immune response. Hyperthermia (heating) treatments may work in part by increasing immune system awareness of the cancer cells.

HSP-90 inhibitors such as cisplatin can also induce cell cycle arrest, via mechanisms independent of p53

Fibrin: My Chinese medicine training taught me that cancer is associated with "blood stasis." The Chinese knew this over a thousand years ago, and it is easily diagnosed by TCM pulse and tongue assessment. About 150 years ago Western physicians began to notice cancer patients had a very high risk of forming blood clots – depending on the cancer, 7 to 30 times normal risk.

In 2005 Italian scientists noted that one of the most common mutations – on the MET oncogene – is associated with the transformation of a cell to cancer leads to a disturbance in the clotting factors, and increased fibrin production. Fibrin is the protein net which sticky platelets cling to make a clot. Fibrin is also a major trigger of inflammation, which makes cancer grow wildly.

The other key role of fibrin in cancer progression is that cancer cells move out of tumours by eating the fibrin strands. As they pull it in, they drag themselves beyond the tumour boundary, into the ECM, and beyond.

Genes = Life

We have 97% the same genes as a chimpanzee. We have 90% of the same genes as a corn plant. In fact only 3% of our genetic material in every one of our cells is actually needed to code for uniquely human proteins! It is astonishing how much every living thing on the planet has in common at a genetic and biochemical level. This is the crux of why we believe remedies from the natural world are generally safer, because they have to be compatible with the same basic life processes.

Non-mutagenic factors in carcinogenesis include wounding, misregulation of proteases such as MMP-2 and stromelysin, and increased expression of platelet-derived growth factor PDGF.

SUMMARY OF CARCINOGENESIS

Tumour progression is characterized by progressive evolution of clones of cells with faulty DNA repair mechanisms, declining sensitivity to growth inhibition signals, reduced immune surveillance, evasion of apoptosis, sustained tumour-mediated angiogenesis, and an evolving ability to invade and metastasize.

As DNA monitoring and repair breaks down, and oncogenes are unmasked, the mutation rate of cells outstrips the genetic and immune controls. A cell must accumulate several peculiar biochemical skills before it can be a cancer. Many cells die trying, making fatal mutations or missing key steps. Those that do succeed in becoming cancerous continue to mutate and develop more and more ways to grow faster than their normal neighbours.

A million cells is the size of the head of a pin – undetectable, and so is called occult cancer, meaning "hidden." By a billion cells, it is the size of a small marble and possibly detectable by touch or scans. This is called clinical cancer and it is as few as 30 doublings old. This mass weighs about 1 gram. After just 10 more doublings it can grow to 1 kilogram, which can often be fatal.

PHASES OF TUMOUR GROWTH

There are 3 distinct phases in the growth of a tumour.

1. Induction – Genetic, viral, and environmental factors trigger malignant patterns of cell growth. Ultraviolet light and radiation causes DNA base fusion. ROS add oxygen compounds to the bases. Persistent oxidative stress and synergy with promoters such as hormones, phenols, and phorbol esters contribute to mutation and dedifferentiation. Chemical alkylating agents add methyl groups to the bases. Irreversible DNA damage or mutation occurs, especially to tumour suppressor genes Rb, CDK4, cyclin d and p16. Oncogenes turn on, DNA repair and apoptosis genes are turned off, and a cancer is born.

2. Progression – After loss of 2 or more suppressor genes and activation of several oncogenes there follows a period of growth of the transformed malignant cell clones. The environment must continue to support mutation and development of angiogenesis, invasion of adjacent tissues, immune evasion and other malignant characteristics. The descendants or clones of the original cancer cell change into a variety of mutants, so in fact there are several types of cancer within every large tumour.

3. Proliferation – 30 doublings produce 1 gram or about a billion cells, the threshold

of detection, and in 10 more doublings produce 1 kilogram of tumour, which may be incompatible with life. Heterogeneous (mixed cell type) tumours are capable of rapid growth, invasion and metastasis. These are the hallmarks of cancer.

CANCER BY CELL TYPE

Carcinomas originate in epithelial tissue, and include squamous cell, transitional cell, basal cell and adenocarcinoma. These are the most common types of cancers, and the ones the immune system is most likely to miss detecting and responding to until quite late in the course of the disease. Dermal use of immune stimulants is always indicated.

Sarcomas arise in mesenchymal tissues such as muscles, skeleton, blood vessels, lymph vessels and reticular tissue; e.g. osteosarcoma, myosarcoma, fibrosarcoma. Homotoxicology drainage remedies for the mesenchyme are always indicated.

Lymphomas and leukemias begin in lymphatic reticular tissue, a subset of mesenchyme stem cells from the bone marrow, giving rise to Hodgkin's disease, lymphatic & myeloid leukemias. In Chinese medicine we look at the kidney and spleen to regulate blood building.

Neuromas develop in nerve tissue, and include glioblastoma multiforme, astrocytoma, neuroblastoma, meningioma, and pheochromocytoma. Dietary fats, fat-soluble toxins and antioxidants are often key issues.

Other malignancies – hydatidiform mole, teratoma. As for all tumours, in Traditional Chinese Medicine a lump results from stagnant blood, which stopped moving due to deficiency of chi flow, arising from constrained liver chi.

Whatever the spot on the DNA or the cell surface or where in the body, cancer arises from living beyond the safe limits of cell chemistry. This incredible self-repairing organism can take a lot of abuse. It forgives a lot of exposures and it tolerates a lot of malnutrition.

Once cancer arises, the environment around the cell can be detoxified, the cells can be nourished, and the immune cells activated to create healing conditions.

It can take up to 20 years from the time the DNA damage reaches the point where the cell is permanently transformed into a lifestyle of uncontrolled growth to the point where it starts to harm organs and the whole person. Note that tumours grow kinetics are logarithmic, meaning they grow faster and faster as they get bigger.

Cancerous or malignant tumours are dangerous, toxic and parasitic. Cancer cells are out of touch with their neighbours and community, like dangerous renegades. The immune system is usually trying to repair the cancer, but cannot overcome the genetic damage, and immune cells in tumours protect it from immune attack.

SURVIVAL RATES

The most generally useful measure is 5 year survival disease-free. This allows comparison of the effects of different treatments. Often a patient who lives 5 years without a sign of the original cancer is truly cured. However, such survival statistics do include people who will die of their cancer due to delayed re-occurrences, who have enjoyed a long remission or pause in the disease.

Individual survival is NOT predictable with much accuracy! No one can really say with certainty how long a patient will survive. All we can predict is the average survival time, based on present standards of care. There is naturally always hope of increased life and quality of life with natural medicine support to enhance regular medical care.

There is always hope of a miracle by Divine intervention, luck, or whatever you can find to believe in. Do not ever give up! A wise man once said "Fear is faith in evil." Believe in good and the grace of peace will come to you.

Quality of life may be severely and irrevocably diminished by medical oncology. Natural and drug adjuncts are supportive therapies which reduce harm and increase the potential for successful treatment outcomes.

Allopathic medicine has reasonable success treating leukemias and lymphomas, and skin cancers. Localized in situ cancers are typically 50 to 80% curable. Spread into regional lymph nodes is a sign of aggressive disease with a poorer prognosis, often less than 50% survival. Distant metastases are rarely curable but effective palliation can give 5 to 20% 5 year survival. For the most common and majority of cancers there has been no significant change in survival rates in modern times. Cancer remains a traumatic disease with a generally unfavourable outcome.

GRADING

Grading is done by a pathologist looking at cancer cells stained to make them visible under a microscope. The severity of the cancerous changes is given based on the degree of differentiation of tumour cells, and on the number of mitoses with highly condensed chromatin figures – the number of cells caught in the act of making an extra copy of their DNA. More differentiation means more normal specialization for a particular job. More mitoses mean it is growing fast.

Grades I to IV are usually assigned, a higher number meaning increasing anaplasia – loss of recognizable differentiation. Anaplastic cells are wild and dangerous.

Histology (cell architecture) does not necessarily determine the clinical behaviour of the tumour. In other words, you cannot see through a microscope exactly how the cancer will behave in the body, so grading is only part of the information needed to decide on therapies.

The practice of medicine is informed by data, but clinical judgement is based on the subjective elements of perception, experience and belief.

STAGING

Staging is based on the key characteristics of cancer:
- proliferation – uncontrolled growth
- invasion – pushing into neighbours
- metastasis – spread to other organs

Size of the primary lesion (T)

Extent of spread into regional lymph nodes (N)

Blood-borne metastases to distant locations (M)

This is clinically critical information in selecting therapies and making a prognosis – an estimate of the outcome of the disease.

APOPTOSIS

Apoptosis is an off-switch for bad cells, built into every human cell. This is the ideal way to remove problem cells or cells no longer needed in the body. It is a "Magic Bullet" which gently takes out unwanted cells with no harm to any other cell. They are simply recycled. It is the future of curing cancer in a humane way.

"Programmed cell death" or cell suicide is rapid, orderly, and removes individual cells. Nearby cells are not harmed. This is a normal part of the growth and maintenance of healthy tissues. Before a cell will split into two new cells it must arrive at a checkpoint in the cell cycle, and run a test to see if the DNA is in suitable condition to be copied. A program is run which is much like "Scandisk" utility on a computer, which checks your hard-drive for errors. The cells use the p53 gene to run a check, and if it finds over 50,000 to 60,000 nicks, breaks, errors, deletions or mutations, it knows this much damage cannot be repaired. It will throw the off-switch to kill the cell, instead of ending up with two bad cells. The cell turns inside-out, gets recycled, and is replaced by a fresh new cell derived from a local stem cell.

Energy-dependent, apoptosis requires the basic energy molecule adenosine tri-phosphate (ATP), usually made by burning sugars. This combustion of sugars for energy occurs in the mitochondria.

There are about 1,000 **mitochondria** in every cancer cell, inherited from your mother's egg. There is no DNA in mitochondria from your father. The mitochondria have their own DNA copying and repair systems. They seem to be able to throw the apoptosis death switch in cancer cells. Apoptosis pathways converge on the mitochondria after activation of the interleukin-2 converting enzymes ICE and the expression of cytoplasmic proteases trans-glutaminases and endonucleases.

p53 tumour suppressor protein directly promotes apoptosis by interacting with the mitochondrial protein *bak* to cause its oligomerization and thus the release of cytochrome C. A cascade of death signals follows. Apoptotic control by mitochondria is lost when they shut down due to hypoxia. Inhibiting the enzyme pyruvate dehydrogenase kinase restores the function of the mitochondria, and can have a very dramatic tumour-killing effect.

Cells undergoing apoptosis show cell shrinkage, chromatin condensation making the DNA visible in the nucleus, surface blebbing (bubbles), and fragmentation into apoptotic bodies -membrane-bound bits of the stuff from inside the cells – the cytoplasm (liquid) and organelles (structures).

Phagocytosis, or the eating and digestion of whole cells or apoptotic bodies (cell fragments), is carried out by parenchymal cells in tissues or macrophage immune cells. Digestion in their enzyme-filled organelles called lysosomes is rapid.

No inflammation or immunological reactions are created. There is no release of iron or other metallic ions that can cause oxidative stress.

Apoptosis is triggered by a preponderance of "do die" signals over "do not die" signals sent to the DNA. This is a dynamic balance, like yin and yang, both are always present – it is the overall balance that determines the net outcome.

Apoptosis is increased by *bax* and *bad* genes. As mentioned before, stress markedly inhibits the *bad* protein.

Anti-apoptotic signalling results from activity of the *bcl-2* (B-cell-leukemia-lymphoma 2), *bcl-xL*, *rhoA* and *ras* genes. Curcumin sharply shifts *bcl-2* proteins to promoting apoptosis. Garlic and hibiscus proto-catechuic acid reduce bcl-2 expression, inducing apoptosis.

Other apoptosis promoters from Nature: quercetin, EGCG, melatonin, indole-3-carbinol, ellagic acid, betulinic acid, caffeine, genestein, berberine, vitamin E succinate, selenium, glutathione, and mistletoe (viscum) lectins. These are antioxidants and bioflavonoids from apples, onions, garlic, turmeric, soybeans, coffee, green tea and other food grade plants as well as herbs or botanical medicines such as mistletoe. Perillyl alcohol is found in essential oils of lavender and palmarosa. Limonene is found in essential oils of lemon, lemongrass, orange and celery.

There is a blood test for serum cytochrome C which measures the global level of apoptosis in the body. The technique relies on an enzyme-linked immuno-absorbent assay. Above normal range suggests a high tumour mass with a low apoptotic rate, and double the risk of dying within 3 years.

ANGIOGENESIS

Cancers by definition are growing faster than the normal cells of their type. They can have 30 to 40 times normal basal metabolic rate. Therefore they must have even greater than normal amounts of oxygen and nutrients, requiring a blood supply greater than normal for that tissue.

Normal cells are never more than a millimetre away from a blood vessel, as oxygen can only passively diffuse through that much tissue. Therefore, past 2 mm diameter, zones of low oxygen or hypoxia will develop in tumours. If the cancer cells in tumours of about 3 mm diameter cannot recruit local support cells – stroma, immune and stem cells – to generate a higher than normal rate of blood and lymph vessel in-growth, they will fail to maintain a pathological growth rate, and probably cease to be a disease..

Hypoxic cells release chemicals which trigger new blood vessels to sprout and extend into tissues that are low in oxygen. Capillary basement membranes dissolve, a bud grows, and elongates along collagen scaffolding into the hypoxic zone.

This is called angiogenesis, and it is driven by **angiogenic factors** such as hypoxia-inducible factor one HIF-1, lipoxygenases LOX, insulin, insulin-like growth factors one and two IGF-1 & 2, tumour necrosis factor alpha TNFa, granulocyte macrophage colony-stimulating factor GM-CSF, focal adhesion kinase FAK, basic fibroblast growth factor bFGF, platelet derived endothelial growth factor PDGF, interleukin eight IL-8, interleukin one beta IL-1β, heptocyte growth factor, lactic acid, histamine, fibrin, prostaglandins, epidermal growth factor EGF, heat shock protein HSP-90, lipoxygenase 12-LOX, c-Src, AT-1, cyclooxygenase COX-2 and vascular-endothelial growth factor **VEGF**.

Obviously, complex and redundant mechanisms drive the induction of blood vessel growth. This duplication and layering of controls makes it a complex business to alter angiogenesis, and even more difficult to sustain the effectiveness of anti-angiogenic therapies.

Ischemia (hypoxia caused by reduced blood flow) and inflammation activate an endogenous cholinergic angiogenic pathway. This pathway is independent of VEGF and bFGF, and is stimulated by nicotine. Tobacco products cause blood vessels to constrict for hours after exposure, and this adds insult to injury.

Formation of new blood supply to hypoxic cells is a normal part of wound healing. Cancer is "the wound that will not heal."

Tumour stromal or structural support cells become activated by cancer cells to secrete VEGF, protein dissolving MMPs and osteonectin, all of which remodel the extracellular matrix and make fibroblasts lay in the protein scaffolding into which new blood vessels can develop. Matrix metalloproteinases MMPs are zinc-dependent endopeptidases which mediate the accumulation and release of vascular-endothelial growth factor VEGF in the extracellular matrix ECM. New lymph vessels form to carry away wastes, at the same time as new blood vessels bring in nutrients.

HIF-1 occurring in the hypoxic regions of the tumour plays an important role in VEGF expression, angiogenesis, and tumour growth. IL-1β and TNFa activate NFkB to induce HIF-1 to trigger the release of VEGF. Furthermore, hypoxia induces the expression of Rac. Rac and Id-1 inhibit differentiation and DNA synthesis, increasing the stabilization of HIF-1α, resulting in the up-regulation of VEGF. HIF-1α is a new target for the anti-angiogenic therapy of hepatic (liver) cell carcinoma HCC. Curcumin (a natural compound isolated from the commonly used spice turmeric), green tea extract and its major component (-)-epigallocatechin-3-gallate, and resveratrol (a natural product commonly found in grapes and various other fruits), 3-(5'-hydroxymethyl-2'-furyl)-1-benzyl indazole (YC-1), TX-402 (a quinoxaline N-oxide), vitexin (a natural flavonoid compound identified as apigenin-8-C-b-D-glucopyranoside), CK2α siRNA, and rapamycin significantly inhibit hypoxia-induced angiogenesis via down-regulating the expression of HIF-1 and VEGF.

The expression of tumour suppressor von Hippel-Lindau VHL gene and p53 DNA Guardian gene are down-regulated by hypoxia.

The primary angiogenic triggering compound is vascular endothelial growth factor VEGF, a highly conserved heparin-binding glycoprotein which induces endothelial cell mitogenesis and migration, increases vascular permeability and vasodilatation, induces proteinases which remodel the extracellular matrix, inhibits antigen-presenting dendritic immune cells, and inhibits endothelial cell apoptosis. VEGF expression is regulated by hypoxia, and mediated by 3 distinct cell surface receptors as well as 2 co-receptors. The tyrosine kinase domain Flk-1 and Flt-1 play a critical role in tumour angiogenesis, and have been the targets of research with humanized recombinant monoclonal antibodies.

Tumours may make excessive vascular endothelial growth factor, enslave local immune cells and stem cells to make abnormal levels of VEGF, or release platelet-derived endothelial cell growth factor alpha PDGFa to recruit stromal fibroblasts to make VEGF. However, they do not generate matching levels of angiopoietin APN, a relative of MMP. APN recruits pericytes to remodel crude blood and lymph vessels into mature forms. Therefore in tumours the vessel loops formed tend to be chaotic, thin-walled, and leaky, increasing risk of spread of cancer cells into the general circulation. The fluid build-up (edema) leaking into the tumour increases the osmotic fluid pressure in the tumour, which can squeeze off blood flow, and trigger a new round of hypoxia and angiogenesis.

By the time a cancer is of a detectable size, it is often getting most of its energy from fermenting sugars throughout the cancer cell, rather than the usual burning with oxygen in about 1,000 little structures called mitochondria. These little combustion chambers shut down when oxygen levels in the tumour drop. Fermentation or anaerobic glycolysis is about 18 times less efficient than the aerobic burning in the mitochondria. Fermentation also produces lactic acid as a waste product, turning the tumour quite acidic. Unfortunately lactic acid is a growth factor, so soon the tumour is growing again. Dr. Otto Warburg won a Nobel Prize for discovering this anaerobic behaviour, which is absent in adult tissues, and only faintly active in embryonic tissue and benign tumours. This is called the Warburg effect. The cancer cells will continue to make energy from sugars without oxygen, even if oxygen levels are restored in their part of the tumour by renewed angiogenesis. The mitochondria membranes remain hyper-polarized, suppressing activity in ion channels. Mitochondrial suppression leads to suppression of apoptosis – the cancer cell cannot throw the off-switch for bad cells, and becomes immortal.

Anti-angiogenic therapy initially will paradoxically increase blood flow in a tumour! Suppression of VEGF leads to an increased ratio of vessel re-modeling protein APN relative to VEGF. Unopposed VEGF makes somewhat rudimentary, leaky and inefficient blood vessels. With relatively more APN, the vessels are more organized and efficient, and with less leakage there is less back-pressure against in-flow of blood. This is a good thing to do just before radiation therapy, to overcome the hypoxic cell problem.

Surgery is never done on a tumour if there is evidence of smaller metastatic lesions. Removing the original or "mother" tumour can cause the remaining tumours to grow very quickly. As long as the mother is left in place, it puts out signals which slow angiogenesis in the others, keeping them smaller.

The abnormal stomach bacteria *Helicobacter pylori* induce angiogenesis via VEGF and IL-8. This increases risk of stomach cancer as well as upper GI ulcers and cardiovascular disease. *H. pylori* also induce EGF via AP-1.

Copper is an essential mineral, an obligatory co-factor, for many angiogenesis promoters. It is proven to reduce circulating levels of vasculoendothelial growth factor VEGF, fibroblast growth factor two FGF-2, and interleukins 6 and 8 (IL-6, IL-Angiogenesis promoters angiotropin, angiogenin, and cysteine-rich proteins are copper dependent. Copper can be removed by chelating with tetrathiomolybdate TM. Treatment for three months will usually reduce copper to about 20% of baseline levels, which will often arrest tumour growth. The TM is given with food to bind the copper in the food, and also given between meals to bind-up blood copper. As copper is involved in heme synthesis and red blood cell proliferation, a side effect can be anemia and mild leukopenia, reversible on easing up the therapy. A low copper diet and zinc supplements can keep levels steady. Monitor ceruloplasmin in the blood, a protein made in the liver, incorporating 6 to 7 atoms of copper, which transports iron from the liver to the bone marrow. Use purified water if your home has copper pipes. Zinc supplementation can lower copper absorption. Green tea chelates copper, inhibits endothelial cell growth, and very significantly inhibits VEGF. Anti-copper therapies like TM only inhibit small tumours; larger ones tend to escape its effect via alternative angiogenic pathways.

Placental growth factor (PGF) binds to vascular-endothelial growth factor receptor one VEGFR-1, also called FLT-1, to promote angiogenesis and tumour progression independently of VEGF. Antibodies against PGF may be a good strategy, as they do not cause pruning of capillaries in healthy tissue, not do they induce angiogenic rescue genes such as Fgf-1, Fgf-2, Sdf-1, MMP-9 and Cxcl-1.

The tumour endothelial marker TEM CD-276 is specifically over-expressed in the blood vessels of human tumours, but not in normal tissue and wound-healing angiogenesis. My naturopathic colleagues in the USA have developed a drug C-Statin from the common bindweed *Convolvulus arvensis*.

Anti-angiogenesis agents induce tumour stasis, not tumour regression – they stop the cancer from growing bigger but may not get rid of the cancer.

Powerful anti-angiogenic drugs such as Avastin – bevacizumab, an antibody that neutralizes VEGF, can cause big problems with blood vessels in normal tissues. For example, the highly vascular choroid plexus membrane on the brain ventricles can be damaged, impairing production of cerebrospinal fluid. The result can be headaches, blurry vision, and even fatal seizures and brain swelling. Other adverse effects may include high blood pressure, loss of protein from the kidneys, and blood clots.

Natural anti-angiogenic compounds include catechin, EGCG from green tea, catechins, curcumin, vitamins A, C, D & E, mushroom shikonin, soy genestein isoflavone, milk thistle silibinin, alpha lipoic acid, quercetin, indole-3-carbinol, beta carotene, salicylates, taurine, melatonin, ellagic acid, grapeseed oligomeric proanthocyanidins, resveratrol, N-acetyl cysteine, MSM, flaxseed, IP6, omega 3 oils and shark liver oil. Use COX-2 inhibitors and inhibitors of NFkB to down-regulate inflammation.

INVASION

Cancer does little harm growing into a simple lump. It could be just removed by a surgeon and tossed away if that were all it could do. Because cancer cells stop communicating normally with their neighbours, they can push past them and spread into surrounding structures, and beyond. This is where the tumour becomes a serious problem.

Cancer cells lose contact inhibition, primarily through changes to cell adhesion molecules and gap junction proteins. Membrane APN enzyme regulates invasion.

Invasion is also regulated by urokinase type plasminogen activator uPA. Green tea

EGCG controls this factor.

AP-1 activation is associated with the acquisition of invasiveness, including the induction of Fos to express cytokine-induced metalloproteinases.

Cancer cells may over-produce proteolytic enzymes, which dissolve the extracellular matrix ECM which binds cells together. Matrix metalloproteinases MMPs are collagenases and gelatinases which digest connective tissue and allow invasion. Collagens, glycoproteins and proteoglycans in the ECM are enzymatically digested.

Breakdown products of the ECM are growth-promoting, angiogenic, and chemotactic. These increase tumour growth and movement in a vicious cycle. MMP's stabilize tumour vasculature via regulation of platelet-derived-growth factor PDGF.

- MMP-1: an interstitial collagenase
- MMP-3: stromelysin, breaks basement membranes
- MMP-9: active in angiogenesis
- MT-1 MMP: membrane type 1 matrix metalloproteinase

Inhibitors of MMP's include curcumin, Scutellaria baicalein, green tea EGCG, resveratrol, digestive enzymes, Zeel, Hormeel S. Collagenase inhibitors include Curcumin, green tea EGCG, quercetin, grapeseed oligomeric proanthocyanidins, gotu kola, genestein, emodin, luteolin, PSK, EPA, vitamin A and vitamin C.

Growing tumours can then progressively infiltrate through the basement membrane that normally forms a boundary for a tissue. This is like a prisoner digging an escape tunnel out of where it supposed to stay – now it can get loose and do harm.

Single tumour cells or clusters are shed from tumours as normal cell-to-cell adherens are down-regulated, by mechanical and hydrostatic pressure, central necrosis, and by proteolytic enzymes. Adherens are like a glue or clamp that keeps cells stuck to each other.

Invasion is associated with hypercoagulability, usually the result of the met oncogene encoding a growth factor receptor which up-regulates plasminogen activator's inhibitor type 1 and COX-2. This makes a lot of fibrin. Motility can involve creeping along ECM protein fibres such as fibrin, as they are pulled into the cancer cell for digestion. Its food becomes a path of escape. Receptors on the tumour cells learn to adhere to laminin and fibronectin proteins in the extracellular matrix ECM rather than just to other cells. The matrix fills in the space between cells, and learning to ride the matrix gives cancer cells a highway out of town.

IL-6 is associated with hypercoagulation.

Cell motility and invasiveness increases in hypoxia. Low oxygen stimulates lipoxygenases LOX, leading to ECM collagen fibre deposition, activation of focal adhesion kinase FAK, and finally altered B1 integrin.

Abnormal gut bacteria such as some *E.Coli, Salmonella typhimurium and Listeria monocytogenes* can turn beta-casein-derived peptides into pro-invasive factors which allow tumour cells to move through collagen in the connective tissue. This is one reason some doctors advise cancer patients to avoid eating milk and cheese.

Penetration into blood vessels, lymphatic channels and body cavities allows the opportunity to spread.

Invasion is a thoroughly malignant process. Cancer cells becoming invasive is a sharp turn for the worse. Tumours showing invasiveness are dangerous. Actual invasion of vessels and tissues is destructive. Invasion needs to be actively suppressed. This requires modulation of the entire immune and stem cell network supporting the malignant phenotype.

METASTASIS

Metastases or mets are the most dangerous aspect of a malignant tumour. Successful colonization of a distant part of the body with cancer usually means much poorer chance of recovery.

Once certain organs are metastasized with cancer, life expectancy may be reduced to months. There is an urgent necessity to find a treatment that works.

A metastasis is a discontinuous secondary tumour made of one of the cell types found in the original tumour. For example, a metastasis of breast cancer to the brain means the "brain met" is still made of breast cancer cells, not brain cells.

Generally a "met" will be clones or descendants of cancer cells which are particularly mutated to be aggressive, rapidly growing, treatment-resistant, and anaplastic.

Medical procedures can increase risk of tumour cell spread. A large-needle core biopsy of breast tumours increases risk of having a positive sentinel node on biopsy by an odds ratio of 1.48, while a fine needle aspiration increases the odds ratio by 1.53, compared to surgical excision of the entire undisturbed lump of tumour. Surgery causes significant seeding of other areas in 1 to 2 % of cases. Using anti-angiogenics such as green tea EGCG can reduce survival of the cancer cells let loose by surgery.

Primary sites of metastases and screening methods:

- bone – radioisotope bone scans
- liver – elevated LDH enzyme in serum
- lung – CT scan or cytology from bronchoscopy
- brain – CT or MRI scan

Metastasis is very actively promoted by TGFß. Transforming growth factor turns fibroblasts into motile myofibroblasts.

Hypoxia induces LOX, which increases collagen fibre formation in the extracellular matrix. This activates focal adhesion kinase FAK, altering B1-integrin, increasing cell motility which can lead to metastasis.

Cancer cells secrete inflammatory factors such as versican, which stimulate immune cells to promote metastasis. This is mostly carried out by macrophages, via toll-like receptor TLR-2 and its co-receptors TLR-6 and CD-14.

Disseminated metastases must evade immune surveillance. Immune cells may be killing millions of these wandering cells daily. It is likely that all tumours shed millions of cells daily, but it is actually quite rare for such wanderers to survive.

STAT-3 transcription activator influences the spread of cancer into bones, providing a homing signal into a suitable secondary site. Indole-3-carbinol and curcumin inhibit STAT-3. Other factors active in spread of cancer to the bones include TGFß, RANKL and Src tyrosine kinases.

TGFß has been found to be active in single cancer cells metastasizing throughout the body, but must switch off for the cell to grow in its new location. TGFß signalling is increased by surgery, radiation and chemotherapy, raising concerns these therapies may contribute to cancer spreading. TGFß is not active in clumps of cancer cells moving around, which tend to lodge in lymphatics and not travel as far as single metastatic cells.

A metastatic cell must then adhere to endothelial cells lining the blood vessels in the target organ. Insulin-like growth factors I and II are chemoattractants for metastases. The cell will stop and attach where it "smells" this chemical. These are high when the diet is rich in sugars and simple carbohydrates.

The metastatic cells attach to the blood vessel wall via adhesion integrin molecules. Fibronectin from fibroblasts derived from mesenchymal stem cells, and P-selectin and E-selectin from activated endothelial cells promote metastatic cell adhesion and extravasation. Endothelial cells are activated to make matrix metalloproteinase MMP-9, allowing the metastatic cells to leave the blood vessel through the basement membrane of the endothelium lining, and thus to enter the new tissue. Once in the niche, metastatic cells probably use cell-to-cell adhesion molecules such as CD-44 to attach, giving them the ability to begin cell doubling. Only an attached cell can pull two sets of chromosomes apart via a micro-tubule spindle, to form two new cells.

Metastases only grow significantly if they can stimulate angiogenesis or new blood vessel growth into their new home. It is suspected that immune cells such as macrophages, platelets, fibroblasts and local as well as bone-marrow derived progenitor stem cells are essential recruits to complete this process. Endothelial progenitor cells mediate the angiogenic switch that enables progression to a macrometastasis. Progenitors make VLA-4 which reacts with fibronectin, a fibroblast protein up-regulated by tumour growth factors.

Metastasized cells probably require bone-marrow-derived progenitor/stem cells to express VEGF1, and may not succeed without these support cells. VEGFR-1 myeloid cells are recruited by inflammatory and angiogenic cytokines such as VEGF-A, placental growth factor PlGF, and soluble KIT ligand. Stem cells migrate to tumours as they become larger and local immune and stem cells fail to arrest inflammation around the tumour. This is likely when they reach about 1 centimetre in diameter, when hypoxia is often developing, and around the time they become detectable by current common diagnostic tests.

Micrometastases in the bone marrow are very common after definitive treatment of even minimal and localized breast cancers. These can persist for many years, and increase risk of early reoccurrence.

CD8+ effector memory immune cells infiltrate tumours and restrict perineural and vascular invasion, and thus squelch metastasis.

Membrane-bound APN enzyme regulates invasion and metastasis. It is blocked by curcumin.

Natural anti-metastatics include fractionated or modified citrus pectin (MCP), larch arabinogalactan, aloe vera juice, eicosapentaenoic fatty acid (EPA), conjugated linoleic acid (CLA), bromelain and heparin. Rx a very low fat diet, as a high fat diet makes cancer cell membranes aggressive, and dramatically raises risk of mets

IMMUNE EVASION

Healthy adults may produce 500 to 1000 new cancer cells daily. Dr. Kobayashi screened asymptomatic adults and estimates only 1 in 1000 is completely cancer free. 70.6% had precancerous cells, about 25% had pre-clinical cancers, and about 5% had undiagnosed clinical cancer – tumours over 1 gram.

NK cells and apoptosis remove most cancers as they arise. Natural killer NK cells are large lymphocytes specialized to kill viral infected, solid tumour or leukemic cells. Up to 15% of total lymphocytes are NK's. Exercise increases NK cell counts.

Remedies which increase NK activity, as measured from bioactivity assays from the patient's blood, have no reliable significant clinical effect on cancer outcomes. Beware of claims that a product will cure cancer based only on its impact on NK cell number or activity. Natural Killer cells can only kill cancer when other immune cells such as macrophages support them or at least refrain from blocking them. Tumour cells tend to attract immune and stem cells to make angiogenic and growth factors, while suppressing immune targeting of tumour cells. Macrophages are large lymphocytes which move into tumours, support its growth, and even release enzymes to help the cancer cells invade and spread.

We shed cells profusely from every tissue, such as about 50 million skin cells sloughed off per minute! Tumours may shed up to 3 to 4 million cancer cells per gram of tumour per day, yet successful metastasis is relatively rare.

However, when one does escape to a new part of the body, it can produce diagnosable malignant disease in about 5 to 20 years. It is usually metastatic cancer deposits which cause the worst effects of cancer, and tend to responsible for most cancer deaths.

Cancer cells evade NK cells by expressing high levels of MHC-1 protein on their surface.

Fortunately, immune cells do usually recognize cancer cells as being out of place when loose in the bloodstream. Most cancer cells shed into the lymph and blood vessels will be targeted and killed.

The immune system can easily be overwhelmed by cell clusters and clumps. These may arise from a traumatic blow to a tumour, cutting into the cancer for biopsy, in surgery, etc. It is relatively rare, but cancer occasionally explodes into rapid growth and spread when disturbed. To reduce or eliminate this risk I prescribe modified citrus pectin and green tea EGCG concentrate around the time of biopsy and surgery, and for 2 to 6 months after.

Immune cells, stem cells and specialized mesenchymal cells literally build a zone in which cancers can hijack normal homeostatic growth restraints. Key immune compounds in this process are ROS, histamine, metalloproteinases, and cytokines.

Cytokines include interferons, lymphokines, chemokines and haematopoietic growth factors. AP-1 is an important modulator of cytokines. Cytokines which modulate inflammation and angiogenesis include MCP-1, MIP-1b and IL-8. Cytokines associated with HER-2 / neu + status include MIP-1b and IL-8. Cytokines associated with high-grade breast cancer include MCP-1, MIP-1b, IL-1b, IL-8, IL-10 and IL-12.

IL-6 is associated with increased risk of blood clots, stimulates VEGF, triggers low hemoglobin (anemia) and is a major growth factor for haematological malignancies. IL-6 is strongly inhibited by beta carotene.

Interstitial immunoglobulin deposition can activate the complement cascade, creating inflammatory growth factors.

The tumour microenvironment is marked by chronic inflammation, which may lead to impaired T-lymphocytes and accumulation of activated myeloid suppressor cells and regulatory T-cells, shutting off the immune response to the tumour. The normal ratio of suppressor to helper T-cells is about 4:1Impaired T-lymphocytes are always higher in the circulation and tissues of persons with malignant tumours. A key pro-inflammatory cytokine is TNFa; it is dependent on activation of NFkB to create an anti-apoptotic condition.

When tumours get quite large and hypoxic, the inflammation is so intense it will attract bone-marrow derived stem cells. These stem cells can become enslaved to make new full-blown tumour cells *de novo*, and are associated with increased risk of metastasis.

Cancer cells develop the ability to block the processing of their antigens, proteins which tell the immune cells they are not behaving normally. Tumour cells evade recognition by modulation of surface proteins, antigenic degradation, absorption or shedding, shedding of TNF receptors, and induced immunosuppression. Two major factors in immune-suppression are transforming growth factor beta TGFß and prostaglandin PGE-2.

Thymus activated immune T-cells can destroy tumour cells only with adequate tumour antigen presentation by macrophages and dendritic cells. Dendritic cells carry antigens to lymphoid tissue to present to adaptive immune cells. Naturopathic physicians always use thymus for cancer care: glandulars, extracts, peptides or homeopathics. I like to prescribe the homeopathic *Thymuline* to modulate the T-cells.

Matrix metalloproteinase inhibitors such as green tea polyphenols improve antibody-binding to target cells, and reduce cleavage of antigens, supporting immunotherapy. MMPs are also regulated by reduction of AP-1, TNFa and IL-1β, such as by curcumin therapy.

Viral-associated cancers such as cervical squamous cell carcinoma, inflammatory breast cancer, Kaposi's sarcoma, Burkitt's lymphoma and T-cell leukemias and lymphomas are also associated with immune suppression such as in Acquired Immunodeficiency Syndrome, Human Immuno-deficiency Virus, and AIDS Related Complex AIDS/HIV/ARC.

Mistletoe lectin injection therapy helps suppress Epstein-Barr virus EBV and activate immune response against tumour viruses.

Melanoma, lymphoma and renal (kidney) cell carcinoma express tumour-associated antigens, and have been known to respond to immune modulating therapies such as monoclonal antibodies and vaccines. Other cancer types are less likely to respond to immune therapies.

Current active immunotherapy techniques are still crude and expensive, but progress is being made identifying antigenic targets (molecular profiling of cancer cells), overcoming negative regulatory mechanisms, and making antibodies with attached toxins, radionuclides, and light-activated poisons. About 400 monoclonal antibodies are in clinical trials.

Note that the fatigue, depressive mood and cognitive function characteristic of advanced cancer is largely due to the release of the immune cell cytokine IL-6. Other cytokines contribute to loss of appetite, and that "sick" feeling. TNF is associated with anorexia.

Fatigue and weakness is also associated with blunting of small intestine villi and resultant malabsorption, secondary to gut inflammation and dysbiosis – disturbance of the gut bacteria flora and fauna. This in turn causes a host of immune dysregulation issues as leaky gut syndrome disrupts the gut-associated lymphoid tissue GALT. An estimated 60 to 80% of the active immune cells in the human body live in this lymphatic network around the gastro-intestinal tract.

In summary, the immune system can eliminate cancer cells, if in surveillance-attack mode, but sometimes gets recruited to enter repair mode, and supports tumour growth and spread. Advanced cancers can completely evade immune control and run rampant. Immune modulation or re-balancing is the goal of naturopathic oncology. We want to immuno-edit and get tumour dormancy, and once stable, we push on for tumour destruction and cure.

INFLAMMATION & CANCER SURVIVAL

Inflammation results in the release of cytokines, as described above. Cytokines are chemical signals which trigger normal cells to grow to repair and replace tissues as they age or those damaged by infection or trauma. Cytokines can also trigger cancer cells to grow. The immune system seems to regard cancer cells as injured cells, needing support and nurturing. They set up an inflammatory response, around "the wound that will not heal."

High levels of inflammation correspond to the Chinese medicine concept of "fire poison" or "heat toxin." When this is present, the patient is in great danger, and uncontrolled, death often follows soon. This is becoming recognized in Western medicine. The measurement of blood markers for systemic inflammation such as serum

C-reactive protein (CRP) is now being used to assess survival prognosis. Note that high levels correspond to increase risk of death from cancer, heart disease and many other risks. The hazard rating from all causes increases about three fold with every ten fold increase in CRP.

In post-menopausal women elevated white blood cell counts, with no known infection, is potentially a warning of the onset of cancer. Leukocytes invade the tumour, but more often than they overcome the tumour cells, they are enslaved and encoded by the tumour to make growth factors such as VEGF angiogenesis factor and interleukins.

Cancer cells also recruit local (peripheral) stem cells to make VEGF and other growth factors. Tumour cells co-opt immune signalling molecules such as selectins, chemokines and their receptors to foster proliferation, survival, invasion, migration and metastasis. When inflammation in and around a tumour reaches a critical point, bone-marrow derived stem cells are then called in to manage the cell growth pattern and inflammation. Rather than healing the wound, these BMD stem cells perpetuate the tumour growth, and may contribute even more strongly to treatment resistance, re-occurrences and metastasis.

Cancer cells loose in the circulation can return to the site of origin after presumed curative therapy, attracted by interleukins IL-6 and IL-8 involved in the inflammation/ repair response. They can then re-seed and cause a reoccurrence.

History of chronic use of non-steroidal anti-inflammatory drugs NSAIDS is associated with up to 50% reduced risk of breast and colon cancers. These drugs block cytokines such as prostaglandins. Prostaglandins are eicosanoids made from dietary polyunsaturated fatty acids by the action of cyclooxygenase enzymes COX -1 & 2.

COX-2 makes series-2 prostaglandins PGE-2 and PGE-2a, which are hormone-like compounds acting locally to produce pain, inflammation and swelling. COX-2 and its product PGE-2 contribute to tumour viability and progression by increasing cell proliferation, inhibiting apoptosis, increasing angiogenesis, increasing invasiveness, increasing metastasis, and by immunosuppression.

CUGBP-2 protein helps normal cells regulate COX-2 production, but it is abnormally low in cancer cells.

COX-2 is stimulated by tumour promoters, growth factors, angiogenesis factors such as VEGF, and cytokines. Inducers include oncogenes Ras and Src, ultraviolet radiation, hypoxia, IL-1, EGF, TGFß, TNFa and benzo(a)pyrene.

COX-2 mRNA and protein overexpression is found in epithelial tumours, colorectal cancer tissue, gastric, pancreatic and many other carcinoma biopsy samples, and in brain gliomas. Increased expression is significantly correlated with unfavourable clinico-pathological characteristics such as worse tumour size, stage, de-differentiation, lymph node involvement, vascularisation (angiogenesis) and metastases.

Low COX-2 expression and receptor levels strongly correlate with extended survival in cervical carcinoma – 75% 5 year survival for patients with low values versus 35% 5 year survival for those with high levels.

The hormones progesterone and estradiol estrogen up-regulate COX activity. Healthy bodies produce these hormones, but they are also taken as drugs and in our food from use in farm animals. Many agricultural pesticides, herbicides and chemical fertilizers mimic estrogens when they enter the human body. These chemicals which act like hormones, even though they are not intended to, are called "xenobiotics." "Xeno" means foreign, man-made substances used for convenience, which turn on us and poison us.

COX-2 is linked to aromatase gene expression. PGE-2 activates aromatase to increase biosynthesis of estrogen in fat cells. This can produce a vicious cycle of estrogen dysregulation in breast cancer. Blocking the HER-2/neu signalling reduces COX-2 expression.

COX-2 up-regulates metallo-proteinases such as MMP-2 which increase tumour cell migration and invasion. Inflammation makes cancer spread.

Zinc has been found to regulate COX-2 expression in cancer better than the drugs Celecoxib or Indomethacin.

Tumour derived PGE-2 promotes the production of the potent immunosuppressive cytokine IL-10 by lymphocytes and macrophages, while simultaneously inhibiting IL-2 production, a cytokine which dampens inflammation. PGE-2 also inhibits natural killer cells and lymphokine-activated killer cells.

Lipoxygenase (LOX) enzymes create inflammation, pain, vasoconstriction and thrombosis promoting compounds from arachidonic acid (AA). These include hydroxyeicosatetraenoic acids 5-HETE, 12-HETE and 15-HETE. A third pathway produces 12-HETE and 16-HETE directly using cytochrome p-450.

5 and 12-HETE and LOX product LTB4 are longer acting than COX products, strongly stimulate cancer cell growth and progression, and inhibit apoptosis. 12-HETE is associated with reduced cell adhesion, invasion and metastasis, and correlates with advanced stage and poor differentiation.

Hyperinsulinemia increases PGE-2 synthesis from dihomo-gamma-linolenic acid (DGLA). Another good reason to limit sugar and refined foods in the diet!

C-Reactive protein CRP is a marker in the blood for inflammation occurring somewhere in the body. High levels before cancer surgery indicate a worse prognosis, shorter disease-free intervals, advanced tumour stage, higher tumour grade and poorer overall survival. Abnormal CRP is always a danger sign. Inflammation indicates the tumour is getting growth factors from the immune system, and support for invasion and spread. It does not mean the immune system is attacking the tumour cells, but rather is in "repair" mode, which enables the tumour to survive and prosper.

Fibrinogen levels in the blood can also be tested to quantify the level of inflammation.

Dietary measures to limit inflammatory eicosanoids

- Restrict arachidonic acid rich foods – meat, dairy, poultry – a vegan diet does help, if correctly constructed.
- Reduce refined carbohydrates – processed starches, simple sugars and alcohol
- Eliminate hydrogenated fats and trans fatty acids – margarine, shortening and lard.
- Reduce intake of omega 6 plant oils – especially corn oil and corn-silage fed animal foods.
- Increase omega 3 oils from nuts, seeds, fish and sea mammals, and grass-fed land animals.
- Ingest adequate zinc, magnesium, vitamins A, B3 and B6, C and E.
- Botanical LOX inhibitors include green-lipped muscle extract, boswellia and scutellaria.
- Quercetin, curcumin and EPA marine oils inhibit both LOX and COX. Food sources include onions, apples, curry and fish.
- Other COX-2 inhibitors are green tea EGCG, licorice, grapeseed

proanthocyanidin and garlic.

Acid/alkaline balance and cancer:

Tissue/fluid Acceptable pH Ideal pH

Blood 7.35 - 7.45 7.41
Urine 4.5 – 8.46.4 – 6.8
Saliva 6.0 – 7.5 6.60 – 6.75
Colon5.0 – 8.4
Stomach 1.0 – 3.5

Signs and symptoms of excess acidity:
- Gallbladder pain, neck and shoulder pain
- headache
- acidic stomach
- coated tongue
- swollen tonsils
- cold, moist hands
- clammy skin
- skin rashes
- increased nasal mucus
- irregular, scanty or heavy menstruation
- osteoporosis

To alkalize:
- avoid excess protein intake, particularly red meat
- increase intake of fruits and vegetables
- reduce carbohydrates to a low-glycemic load
- reduce stress
- Capra goat milk whey minerals
- Alkaline salts – carbonates and bicarbonates of sodium, potassium, calcium and magnesium.

I believe I made it abundantly clear in the naturopathic diet section what I think of alkalizing as a cancer therapy. In short, tumour acidity is far more complicated than simply lactic acid formation from the Warburg effect. Anaerobic glycolysis proceeds in cancer cells even in the presence of normal oxygen tension. Tumours are surrounded by efficient pH buffers, and growth of human tumours is independent of intra-tumoral pH. Alkalizing a tumour is not realistic, nor useful. Alkalizing human tumours may actually increase their growth!
While there is evidence one can alkalize and thereby suppress tumours in mice,

this is not substantiated in humans. All that can be expected is extracellular changes in pH on a small scale. Alkalizing the extracellular milieu has been shown to increase cancer cell proliferation in many cancers. Alkalizing promotes an increase in insulin, glycolysis, growth factors, mitogens and tumour promoters. Conversely, acidification can be demonstrated to elicit tumour regressions via cytotoxic reductions in heat shock proteins and lactate transport.

However, alkalizing the human body may have anti-aging, restorative and healing potential. Alkaline-ash foods are to be emphasized over acid-ash foods, but for reasons not linked to pH. A diet rich in fruits and vegetables, low in meat, and low sugars and high-glycemic starches is sufficiently alkalizing to support recovery from cancer.

TUMOUR MARKERS

Cancer cells are so abnormal in so many ways, it is likely they will make and leak abnormal chemicals which we may detect in the blood. For generations now, researchers have noticed the striking similarity between cells growing as a cancer and the early cells growing in the trophoblast – the early embryo stage where our lives begin. Many cancers make chemicals that should not be seen in a person who is not pregnant or not a foetus.

Tumours often produce characteristic metabolites, antigens & hormones which are measurable in the blood by radio-immunoassays. Rarely is a single tumour marker test sensitive or accurate enough to be diagnostic, or even an effective screening method for early warning of the onset or return of a cancer. However, some attempts have been made to use panels of several of these tests for early detection, such as the Kobayashi panel of ten markers. This idea deserves further study.

Tumour markers are being used, with some caution, to guide diagnosis, prognosis, the initial therapeutic strategy and changes in therapeutics. They tend to fall if treatment response is good, and rise if the cancer is reoccurring. While they imply a certain level of "tumour burden," the amount produced by a cancer can vary, so a doubling of the level of tumour marker doesn't necessarily mean twice as many cancer cells are present. We like to see these numbers low or zero, but people can survive well with high numbers too. Your physician may choose to not tell you these numbers, as they can cause needless concern. What you need to hear most is that the physician is monitoring you and providing definitive, rational and comprehensive care.

Carcinoembryonic antigen CEA – non-specific, this chemical indicates undifferentiated cells are present, similar to those found in an embryo, where the cells are not yet committed to being a certain tissue. CEA can be raised in benign conditions and is not sensitive in early malignancy. Elevated in 20 to 70% of cancer patients, depending on tumour site and stage. For example levels should fall to zero after complete resection of colon cancer, or at least into the normal range within 4 weeks, rising levels tend to suggest re-growth, and high levels are associated with a poorer prognosis. It rises sharply when there are liver mets. Normal is under 4.0 but it may be up to 6 in smokers.

Prostate specific antigen PSA – PSA is a glycoprotein enzyme made by the prostate gland, and its expression is conserved in nearly every case of prostate cancer, no matter how undifferentiated. Thus it is a moderately useful prostate cancer screening tool, with the rate of doubling being the most significant indicator of tumour aggressiveness. Normal is under 4.0, ideal is under 2.5. Requires expert interpretation and clinical context.

Ca class of tumour markers are carbohydrates (starches) produced by cancer cells:

- **Ca 19-9** – elevated in some cancers of the breast, pancreas, liver, biliary tract, stomach and colon. Normal is under 37. May be increased in inflammatory diseases of the Gastro-intestinal tract including pancreatitis, and may be falsely negative in patients with Lewis negative blood group.
- **Ca 15-3** – Elevated in some breast cancers. Normal is under 31.
- **Ca 125** – rising levels can indicate relapse and level of tumour burden in breast cancer. The CA stands for carbohydrate antigen, as this is a glycoprotein mucin produced by epithelial cells in the breast, ovary, and peritoneum. Normal is under 35. It can be elevated in peritonitis, injury to the peritoneal membrane by laparoscopy, and in infections such as mononucleosis.

Human chorionic gonadotropin beta subunit β-**HCG** – is useful in germ cell tumours such as testicular cancer to monitor effect of treatment and reveal relapses. Home pregnancy tests detect this hormone.

Alpha-fetoprotein **AFP** – should not occur except in foetal blood, indicates hepatoma (up in 72% of cases), pancreatic (23%), gastric (18%) or germ cell tumours (75% of nonseminomatous testicular tumours). Post-therapy return to normal levels usually correlates with effective therapy. Normal is under 8.6 ng/ml.

Lactate dehydrogenase **LDH** – fast growing tumours in high S-phase outstrip their blood supply and become anaerobic, producing toxic lactic acid. LDH monitors cell death in oxygen starved tumours, and is also a marker for tumour lysis (break-up). It is elevated in liver disease and blood haemolysis.

TUMOUR MARKER BY ORGAN OR CELL TYPE

Bladder – TCC: Survivin; urinary telomerase assay TRAP; urinary nuclear matrix protein twenty-two NMP-22.

Bone – alkaline phosphatase

Breast – CEA, CA 15-3, CA 125, CA 549, CA M26, CA M29, CA 27.29, MCA, PSA, isoferritin, tissue polypeptide antigen TPA, mammary tumour-associated glycoprotein, and kappa casein. CK-19 cytokeratin is associated with a poorer prognosis.

Carcinoma – CK-7 CK stands for cytokeratin, a protein on the outside of cells originating in the lung, mesothelium, salivary gland, breast or peritoneum.

Colon – CEA, Ca 19-9, TPA, CK-20+, CK-7-, CDx-2+. Gastro-intestinal – kappa casein, Ca 19-9.

Epithelium – AE1 / AE3.Gastro-intestinal epithelium – CK-20

Leukemia – β2-microglobulin, isoferritin

Liver – AFP, CEA, Ca 19-9. Liver mets – alkaline phosphatase, 5'-nucleotidase, glycolytic enzymes

Lung – CEA, TPA, TTF-1; small cell – NSE, CK-BB. Bronchial epithelium – CK-7+ and TTF-1+; Ki-67 bimarker of proliferation in the parabasal layer.

Lymphoid – CD-45

Lymphoma – β2-microglobulin, monoclonal immunoglobulins; Epstein-Barr viral antibodies in Burkitt's lymphoma. CDK9/Cyclin T1 protein complex detects an aggressive form of Hodgkin's disease.

Mesothelium – calretinin

Myeloma – Bence-Jones protein immunoglobulins, monoclonal immunoglobulins

Nasopharyngeal – Epstein-Barr viral antibodies

Neuroblastoma – VMA, NSE, catecholamines; CNS – β2 microglobulin

Ovary – CEA, HCG, AFP, LPA, Ca-125, apo-lipoprotein A1, truncated transthyretin, galactosyl transferase, serum glycoprotein YKL-40, and a cleavage fragment of inter-alpha-trypsin inhibitory heavy chain H4.

Pancreas – CEA, TPA, Ca 19-9, Ca 50, pancreatic onco-foetal antigen

Prostate – prostate specific antigen PSA, standard, ultrasensitive or free PSA, and prostatic acid phosphatase PAP

Squamous cell carcinoma antigen – Normal is under 1.5

Stomach – Ca 19-9, foetal sulfoglycoprotein antigen

Testes – LDH, placental-like AP; germ cell: AFP, beta-chorionic gonadotropin β-HCG

Thyroid – calcitonin, thyroglobulin

Vascular – CD-31 and CD-34 antigens.

A DEEPER LOOK AT RADIATION THERAPY FOR CANCER

The naturopathic support program for patients undergoing radiation therapy is given in Chapter Two. In short, all medications and supplements need to be reviewed, some supports need to be taken during and for about 3 weeks after the last dose of radiation, and any side-effects or problems that arise can be addressed with naturopathic care.

Ionizing radiation is a standard treatment for cancer, despite significant risks, side-effects, and about 1/3 of cases failing to achieve good local control of tumours. The average is about 1 to 2% local reoccurrences per year. You may be shocked how little high-level scientific evidence there is for survival benefits from many applications of radiotherapy. Its clinical usefulness is simply sufficient to assume that radiation can be a reasonable option, though not to be entered into lightly. Here is a primer on radiotherapy:

Radiation used for cancer therapy delivers a large amount of energy in a small, localized volume along the beam line (linear energy transfer or LET). Photons or nuclear particles are used.

This energy is commonly measured in Grays (GY) – 1 joule of energy absorbed into 1 kilogram of matter.

Cancer treatments range from 3 to 10 Grays. If you have been given radiation therapy once, you may only receive it again if the total dose accumulated will be less than 7,000 to 8,000 CentiGrays or 70 to 80 Grays, as more is usually fatal. The human LD50 for acute radiation exposure is 4.5 Gy – half of those exposed to this level will die. Therefore any high dose must be delivered in small fractions per day, over several days or weeks, not all at once.

A second "boost" dose may be added to the usual once a day dose, late in the regime, to overcome the accelerated repopulation of tumour cells induced by radiation injury. Like all living things, these cancer cells struggle hard to survive.

Radiation dosing is all about the volume of tissue that must be treated. When the field of treatment is large, the risks are large.

Electromagnetic photonic energies such as X-ray, gamma ray, or ultraviolet light produce indirect ionized particles of high energy and excited atoms with electrons in higher orbits, which are more chemically reactive. This creates havoc in our life chemistries. Oxygen is crucial to transduce the radiant energy into chemical form.

High speed sub-atomic particles – electrons, protons, neutrons, pi mesons. If they have over 10 electron volts of energy –they can produce direct ionization by ejecting electrons from atoms, which then break covalent chemical bonds, produce free radicals of oxygen (ROS), and secondary particle cascades. The large particles have a short range that is dependent on their initial kinetic energy or velocity.

Ionizing radiation disturbs several phases of the cell cycle. Cyclins and their respective CDKs are disrupted, leading to genomic instability. The CDK inhibitor p21 is a primary mediator of p53-dependent G1 cell cycle arrest from DNA damage from radiation. Mitotic (doubling) delay at G2 in the cell cycle is proportional to the radiation dose, prolonging the generation time, producing non-dividing cells, chromosome aberrations, giant cells and cell death.

Cells are about 70% water. Ionizing radiation usually forms hydroxyl radicals [*OH] and superoxide radicals from the water inside cells, which break strands of DNA, the genetic code. If both strands are broken, and go unrepaired, the cell may die. However, if one strand remains unrepaired, the cell survives, but in an altered form.

DNA strand breaks induce transcription factors NFkB and p53. The NFkB will up-regulate Bcl-2 genes, cell adhesion molecules, pro-apoptotic Bax, TNFa, IL-6, IL-1b, AP-1 and MMPs. It regulates over 200 genes involved in the inflammation response.

p53, the guardian of the DNA, co-ordinates cell cycle arrest, manages apoptosis and modulates the DNA repairs process, primarily through induction of the antioxidant enzyme glutathione peroxidase. p53 activates other anti-ROS proteins, suppresses oxidation from nitric oxide synthase, and induces DNA repair enzymes.

We do not want the cancer cells to be able to repair the radiation damage, but we do want healthy cells to survive. Unfortunately the radiation disrupts important regulatory cells, creates a chronic disturbed pattern of growth, and can give rise to significant fibrosis and necrosis in all cells within the field of the radiation.

External beams such as X-ray devices, gamma ray "cobalt bomb," linear electron megavoltage accelerators (Linacs) and the "gamma knife" units bombard the body from the outside; so much of the energy gets absorbs into overlying tissues and doesn't reach the tumour. This is like sunlight going into water, – most of the energy is absorbed near the surface and so the deeper one goes, the less energy has penetrated.

Implants such as rapid cesium pellet brachytherapy use high dose radioactive substances placed near a cancer to deliver a very high local dose. Many of these isotopes release high energy particles with large mass which cannot penetrate too far into healthy structures around the tumour.

Rapidly dividing cells are most susceptible: cancers, small lymphocytes, bone marrow, vascular endothelium, Gastro-intestinal endothelium & hair follicles. That is why radiation kills cancer but also makes the hair fall out and the gut to be disturbed by sores, vomiting and diarrhea.

Radiation activates sphingomyelinase or ceramide synthetase which hydrolyzes the cell membrane lipid sphingomyelin, increasing ceramides, resulting in apoptosis – the cell dies.

Radiation kills more cells at low doses than one would predict from the direct impacts, as if cells not hit by the radiation receive panic signals from the injured cells, and turn on their own death cycle. Even if only 1% of cancer cells are directly hit by radiation, up to 30% of cells will show reactive sister chromatid exchanges. Conversely, high-dose radiotherapy kills less cells than one might expect. This paradox is thought to be due to "**bystander effects**." This phenomenon is an indirect action on cells distant to the radiation field, thought to be mediated by alteration in epigenetic regulation. The bystander effect becomes saturated at doses under 1 Gray, but is most prominent in high-dose radiation exposures. The abscopal or out-of-field effects injure DNA and macromolecules, causing neighbouring cells to mutate, transform and die. Bystander damage involves CX43 gap junctions responsible for cell-to-cell communication. Also involved is a factor released by the thymidine phosphorylase-5'-deoxy-5-fluoridine suicide gene system. Lipid peroxides and inosine nucleotides may be released, as well as cytokines such as TNFa, IL-6, IL-8. This will impact tumour cells, and normal endothelial cells, fibroblasts and lymphocytes. As a result, side-effects can occur well outside the area actually hit by the therapeutic radiation.

Radiation is oncogenic, causing normal cells to become cancerous. This is the consequence of un-repaired single-strand DNA breaks. There is up to a 20 year induction phase. Even 0.5 Gy exposures can trigger cancer. Decades after treatment there is a 6 –fold increased risk of a new solid tumour from radiotherapy for Hodgkin's disease, 4 to 5 times increased risk of esophageal cancer after radiotherapy of breast cancer, and increased occurrence of secondary leukemia, lymphoma, breast, thyroid, lung and GI cancers.

Even the dose of one CT scan to the abdomen, pelvis or chest, 10 mSv units, gives a 1 in 1,000 chance of developing cancer. Ten CT scans give a significant risk of developing leukemia or lymphoma. It is estimated that 38 CTs will increase risk of cancer by about 12%. During radiologic diagnostic imaging we can freely use anti-oxidant protectants such as grapeseed extract OPCs, melatonin, vitamin C, bioflavonoids, resveratrol, green tea extract, vitamin E, N-acetyl-cysteine, glutathione, vitamin A, pomegranate, milk thistle extract, and curcumin.

Sclerosis, or scarring and contraction of vascular endothelium (the lining of blood vessels), is slowly progressive, leading to endarteritis (inflamed lining), fibrosis &

thrombus (clot) formation. Transforming growth factor beta one TGFβ-1 is involved in the injury response and subsequent persistent stromal changes in the collagen and hyaluronic acid of the extra-cellular matrix. TGFß can be modulated with vitamin A, R+ alpha lipoic acid, berberine, sulforaphane, rehmannia and rhubarb root. Inhibition of TGFß by berberine is potent enough to increase the efficacy of radiation therapy. Radiation induced-fibrosis, xerostomia and other injuries can be repaired with anti-oxidants and blood vessel dilators.

Radiation to the heart is associated with increased risk of coronary artery disease. This scarring goes on relentlessly for years after the therapy. Given enough time, it will always degrade the ability of the tissue to heal. Omega 3 oils may help slow this effect by thinning the blood, increasing capillary perfusion.

Radiation to the chest area, including breasts and mediastinal lymph nodes, can induce a restrictive cardiomyopathy leading in time to heart failure. Radiation to the neck and mediastinum doubles risk of stroke and triples risk of transient ischemic attacks. I respond with omega 3 marine oils.

One-third local failure rate is mostly due to **the hypoxic cell problem** – 2.5 to 3 times higher doses are needed for the same biological effect in low oxygen parts of tumours than are used for fully oxygenated cells. My research area for several years at the British Columbia Cancer Research Foundation Medical Biophysics Unit was on this "hypoxic cell problem." We looked at new drugs and new radiation sources that would kill the cells living on the edge of survival in oxygen-deprived parts of a tumour.

The biradical nature of oxygen makes it the most important electron acceptor in biological systems. Without oxygen the radiation damage is repaired in $1/100,000^{th}$ of a second. The potent radiolytic products of water, the hydroxyl radical OH* and bare protons H+ react with molecular oxygen and other reactive oxygen species ROS to form stable enough radicals to generate lipid peroxidation. Polyunsaturated fats combined with oxygen-stabilized hydroxyl radicals are the most potent bio-killers from radiation therapies.

Hypoxia-inducible factor HIF-1 activates p53, promoting ATP metabolism and increasing resistance to radiation therapy. Using inhibitors of HIF-1 <u>after</u> RT may improve efficacy.

Pre-treatment with anti-angiogenics normalizes VEGF-APN ratios, thins the basement membranes, increasing tumour oxygenation, and thus improves responses to radiotherapy. Nicotinamide increases capillary perfusion, and is a strong radiosensitizer – it amplifies the effect of the radiation to kill more cancer cells. Heat shock protein 90 HSP90, Cox-2, P-glycoprotein PKC and Akt/mTOR signalling pathway inhibitors are radio-sensitizers.

It is interesting to note that children are given Carbogen gas to breathe before radiation therapy to make their tumours more sensitive to the therapy. This is 80% oxygen (O2) mixed with 20% carbon dioxide (CO2). Normal air is 21% oxygen and the rest is mostly nitrogen (N2).

I am frequently asked about hyperbaric oxygen therapy and cancer. Using 100% oxygen under pressure certainly delivers a massive dose of oxygen. We know it cures "the Bends" in divers, but will it help to kill cancer? Well, the oxygen does increase chemical damage and cancer cell death from radiation. Oxygen in really high doses will increase immune activity against cancer cells. However, it increases blood vessel growth into the tumour too. The net effect is neither good nor bad. I simply do not recommend it as a curative cancer treatment. If hyperbaric therapy is needed for another life-threatening condition in a patient who has, or may have cancer, I would not hesitate to use it.

Some of my colleagues use HBO2T to increase the effectiveness of radiation therapy, and tell me it is safe.

A novel idea in contemporary radiation care is photodynamic therapy with ionized oxygen. Light of a specific wavelength is used to activate the ion-charged oxygen at the tumour only.

Radiation works primarily by inducing oxidative stress. While moderate dose anti-oxidants during radiation therapy may be associated with increased survival time, increased tumour responses, and reduced toxicity, this issue remains controversial among radiation oncologists. High dose anti-oxidants can theoretically reduce effectiveness of radiotherapy. However, it is scientific humbug for oncologists to declare natural anti-oxidants unsafe while using high-potency synthetic anti-oxidants with radiotherapy such as Amifostine, Mesna and Dexrazoxane, and natural –origin pentoxifylline. There may be a research gap between natural and synthetic products motivated by economics, but the scientific principle is established. Anti-oxidants have a role in radiation therapy. Melatonin is the best researched, with clear benefits. I recommend it. Many of my colleagues give intravenous vitamin C during radiation therapy. Do not self-prescribe – these adjunct therapies need expert planning and supervision.

Lithium mineral protects neurons from radiation injury by reducing the number of double-strand DNA breaks.

Curcumin is very valuable, reducing the inflammatory response and increasing the cancer cell kill, while protecting normal cells from damage. This increases the "therapeutic differential." The primary action is reduction of the cytokine TGFß, which in turn reduces fibrosis due to TGFβ-1 and the release of circulating tumour cells and therefore metastases.

Some of my colleagues are also supporting radiation therapy with astragalus, L-glutamine, green tea EGCG, soy isoflavones, omega 3 DHA, sea buckthorn, Siberian ginseng *Eleutherococcus senticosus*, and *Gingko biloba*. Demulcent herbs such as marshmallow root and licorice root DGL are often used to protect the throat. Berberine has now been shown to reduce radiation pneumonitis via inhibition of sICAM-1 and TGF-β1

After RT there can be a prolonged suppression of bilirubin, albumin and uric acid, which can be treated with a balanced program of anti-oxidant supplementation.

The blood-thinning drug Coumadin or Warfarin does not interact well with radiation therapy, so patients are encouraged to switch to low-molecular weight heparin anti-coagulation therapy.

In all forms of cancer therapy it is important to support the clearance from the body of damaged cells and their debris. This means giving antioxidants, liver support, and help for the circulating and the reticulo-endothelial immune system, which digest bad cells. Toxic therapies like radiation kill patients directly and indirectly, and often render them so debilitated they cannot then respond to complementary and alternative natural therapies. Integrating both orthodox and natural adjuncts (supports) helps keep the options open by protecting a reserve of vitality.

An interesting phenomenon is the beneficial and immune stimulatory effect of small doses of radiation. This is called radiation hormesis, and is like a homeopathic response. This is the Arndt-Schulz Law, that below a certain threshold, toxic substances can be bio-protective. In fact a very small dose of radiation before, or even hours after an exposure to a toxic dose of radiation will reduce DNA damage. It seems we have an adaptive response to miniscule radiation doses, with induction of DNA repair, apoptosis, anti-oxidant protection, and enhanced immune function.

Be proactive, as all doses of radiation cause injury, though the symptoms may only appear much later on. Natural protectants and healers of radiation injury include green tea, vitamin A, curcumin, vitamin E, N-acetyl-cysteine, glutathione, resveratrol, grapeseed proanthocyanidins, milk thistle silymarin, vitamin C, melatonin, carotenoids, lycopene, selenomethionine, pomegranate, apigenin and Triphala.

A DEEPER LOOK AT CHEMOTHERAPY

The naturopathic support program for patients undergoing chemotherapy is given in Chapter Two. Here we will explore some of the deeper issues raised by giving cell-killing drugs to humans composed entirely of cells.

For a few generations now, whenever a really poisonous substance was found in nature or made in a drug laboratory, it was immediately sent to the cancer research establishments to be evaluated as a cancer drug. The orthodox or allopathic medical treatment of cancer has emphasized *cytotoxic* or cell-killing medications. Chemo drugs kill rapidly dividing cells, targeting their DNA. Most of the cytotoxic effect results from apoptosis triggered by sublethal DNA damage.

"Chemo" side-effects limit dosage, limit efficacy, and even kill patients. Any step we can add which reduces these risks increases the potential for the chemo to achieve its intended result. I consider it a major success to help a patient live through chemo with a reasonable reserve of health. As Dr. Robert Atkins, M.D. has said in *Atkin's Health Revolution*, "The damage done to the body by an unsuccessful course of chemotherapy is often so great that the patient's immune system never recovers sufficiently to stand a fighting chance." Immune cells are damaged in the bone marrow and also via leaky gut syndrome and disordering of the gut-associated lymphoid tissue where 70 to 80% of our active immune cells reside. Naturopathic physicians often feel that if chemo is given and fails, the hope for a response to biological treatments is also likely lost. We just too often have nothing left to work with in these damaged bodies.

Cytotoxic or cell-killing chemo poisons actually promote metastasis by injuring immune cells and vascular cells. Always support and follow chemo with anti-metastatic therapies. Examples include fractionated or modified citrus pectin, green tea EGCG, Co-enzyme Q-10, aloe vera juice, EPA omega 3 marine oils, melatonin, quercetin, and mistletoe.

Chemo drugs obey first-order kinetics – a constant percentage of cells are killed by a given exposure, i.e. if a drug kills 99.999% and the tumour burden is a billion cells, there will be 10,000 surviving cells, causing an apparent clinical remission but guaranteeing a reoccurrence in time. It is nearly impossible for chemo to kill every last cancer cell.

A common myth is that chemo drugs are somehow selective for cancer cells. Common drugs such as taxanes, anthracyclines and 5-fluorouracil actually kill healthy cells better than they kill cancer cells. Doxorubicin is ten times deadlier to good cells than cancer cells.

Most chemo drugs are known to cause cancer! These carcinogens cross-link DNA in healthy as well as cancer cells. They can also bind a single DNA strand to a protein or metal, activating frame shift mutations responsible for turning on oncogenes such as *ras*. Some tie the telomeres on the ends of the chromosomes into four-strand knots, creating an immortal cell.

Chemo is more effective with leukemias and lymphomas than with solid tumours, possibly due to drug delivery issues. In the disseminated cancers chemo is so successful you would be daft to not try it.

Other than these blood-borne cancers, and testicular cancer, which are only 3% of all cancers, chemotherapy is not as well proven to good scientific standards to have a positive influence on survival or quality of life as you may think. There is some support for its use in sarcomas, retinoblastoma, ovarian, breast and small cell lung cancer. This is all well known to oncology doctors, 75% of whom say they would not participate in a chemotherapy trial if they had cancer, due to its "ineffectiveness and its unacceptable toxicity." Yet in North America 75% of cancer patients are prescribed chemo by these same doctors. In Canada, the same 75% majority of oncologists surveyed said they "would not undergo chemotherapy or recommend it to a loved one" for a majority of cancers! The more experience doctors and nurse have with chemo, the less they like using it on their own family. This sort of nonsense has cost the medical profession a lot of credibility with patients. Ultimately, we must have *integrity* – to be one and the same to all persons, all the time – to fulfill our professional duty to each patient. There are hard choices, to be made between the doctor and patient, in an atmosphere of trust. The question I ask myself with patients is would I take the treatment myself, or give it to my children or my dear wife. I wonder if most oncologists could answer this question truthfully with their patients.

In some states such as California and New York, it is illegal for a physician to treat cancer by any method other than chemotherapy drugs, surgery and radiation! I always think it unfortunate when the courts get involved in our health care! I don't even fully understand why Health Canada exists – Canada has a constitution which makes health a Provincial jurisdiction.......

Fractionated chemo – using small doses more often over a longer time – tends to give better outcomes, as do multi-drug protocols. I was in cancer research when this radical concept of multi-drug chemo was first explored. It has made chemo more effective, but not nearly as effective as we would like to see. There is plenty of room for lots more improvements. I think integrated naturopathic supports are the biggest advance in chemotherapy we are likely to see in the near future.

Other techniques to improve the risk to benefit ratio include intra-arterial infusions, chemo resistance screening tests, monoclonal antibody chemo targeting, and chromotherapy light-activation.

An American naturopathic doctor I know had the same osteosarcoma that cost Terry Fox his leg, but who had a better therapy than Terry. He had the chemo delivered in extremely high doses only into his leg, while the circulation to his leg was isolated from the rest of the body and run through a heart-lung bypass to keep it oxygenated. He is alive and walking on both his legs decades later.

Chemo is commonly toxic to other rapidly growing normal cells – bone marrow , epithelium, GI mucous membranes, hair follicles – thus causing anemia through loss of replacement red blood cells, loss of platelets needed for clotting, loss of white blood cells of the immune system, baldness, nausea, diarrhea, vomiting, GI and mouth ulcerations, and so on. Heart damage, nerve damage, kidney damage, infections due to immune suppression, tinnitus, and pneumonitis, are also frequent problems. Many patients get "chemo brain" syndrome – confusion and mental deterioration. Chronic late effects include persistent fatigue, persistent bone marrow suppression, infertility, and increased risk of other cancers such as leukemia and lymphoma. For example, high-dose epirubicin with cyclophosphamide chemo can trigger secondary acute myeloid leukemia, which can arise after 10 to 20 years latency.

MULTI-DRUG RESISTANCE

Cancer cells can become resistant to many chemo drugs. Any cancers the reoccur after chemotherapy are possibly drug resistant, primarily through activation of P-glycoprotein PgP, an ion pumping system which uses an ATP-binding cassette protein to expel cellular toxins. PgP is an ATP-dependent efflux pump, and is also called ABCB-1 and MDR-1. Cancer cells activate the porter system to pump out chemo drugs as quick as they come in. Quercetin modulates the P-glycoprotein porter system, keeping more drug in the cancer cells. Cells lacking a functioning p53 gene cannot undergo apoptosis after chemo. This applies to 50 % of cancers, especially late stage cancers. The MDRI gene is also modulated by NFkB, STAT 3, PGE2 and COX-2 inhibitors.

Natural agents which can reverse resistance are quercetin, green tea EGCG and theanine, ginseng, curcumin, *Salvia, Euphorbia*, melatonin, vitamin C and vitamin K3.

Electrical therapy with 50 Hz AC current at 7.5 amps pulsed can down-regulate multi-drug resistance in tumour.

INTEGRATIVE SUPPORT FOR CHEMOTHERAPY

Prescribe supports for the entire course of chemo, starting from the first day and continuing for 3 to 4 weeks after the last dose. Some common supports are described in Chapter Two.

Oncologists were justifiably worried about the possibility that antioxidant supplementation during chemotherapy might prevent free radical formation by the oxidative chemo drugs. This would lower the number of cancer cells being damaged enough that apoptosis or programmed cell death of the cancer would switch on. Antioxidants should interfere with chemo, because we are trying to oxidize the cancer to death. However, clinically it is clear that antioxidants actually increase the ability of the chemo drugs to kill cancer cells. As it turns out, uncontrolled reactive oxygen species formed in chemotherapy lead the formation of toxic aldehydes which arrest the cancer cell's movement through its cell cycle into the stage where apoptosis can begin. The usual net result of giving antioxidants with chemo is more cancer cells move into a death cycle than with unsupported chemo. Natural source products with a mixture of carotenoids, ascorbates, tocopherols, polyphenols and proanthocyanidins are ideal. Selenium is fine up to 200 mcg, beyond that it may increase chemo-resistance. For megadose therapy consult an orthomolecular physician.

Avoid: Several foods and natural herbs in common use can interact poorly with chemotherapy drugs, by inducing liver enzymes which clear the drugs. This can increase toxicity or result in therapeutic failure. There is no confirmed data, but some things to consider avoiding during chemo: St. John's Wort, grapefruit, garlic, rosemary, alcohol, tobacco, and yohimbe.

Be very cautious mixing chemo drugs with supplemental glutathione or products which increase it such as HMS 90 whey or N-acetyl cysteine. Curcumin, selenium and milk thistle may be used during chemo only on the direction of an experienced integrative physician. These products can do a lot of good, but may alter drug metabolism and by the liver if directly mixed.

Hyperthermia can amplify chemo efficacy if used concurrently.

INTEGRATIVE SUPPORT FOR SPECIFIC CHEMOTHERAPY DRUGS

A naturopathic physician in oncology or trained integrative physician can put together a concise plan to support a good response with less side-effect. The following information is one resource in selecting a natural health product protocol to safely interact with complex multi-drug chemotherapy, in a patient likely to be on several additional medications. If you experience side-effects despite these precautions, and the good care you will receive at the BC Cancer Agency and our hospitals, then please ask our clinic to assist. We have some very good options for care of mouth sores, nerve damage, nausea, pain, and many other conditions.

We are particularly concerned to avoid mixing natural supplements which use the same liver detoxification pathways as the synthetic drugs. These are usually cytochrome P-450s such as CYP3A4, CYP1A2, CYP2D6, CYP2Ea, or glucuronosyltransferases UGT1A1.

We also are concerned about interactions with transport proteins such as P-glycoprotein PgP, a pump which bails toxins out of cells to protect them. Many cancer cells are able to up-regulate this pump during severe chemical stress, such as cytotoxic chemotherapy.

For example, quercetin, grapeseed extract and kava kava induce CYP3A4 expression in human hepatocytes (liver cells), which metabolizes chemo drugs such as cyclophosphamide, irinotecan, etoposide, vincristine and paclitaxel. This potentially reduces their effectiveness, by increasing the speed at which they are cleared from the bloodstream. However, quercetin makes drugs like Tamoxifen more bio-available and will also help keep chemo drugs inside the cancer cells, increasing efficacy. This is due to quercetin's modulation of p-glycoprotein – more drug is trapped inside the cancer cell, making the chemo more effective. It is a case of two steps forward, one step back – you are still one step ahead. The therapy is more effective while less toxic – perhaps we are two steps ahead after all. Therefore one must look at the overall action and determine if the net effect is positive or negative. This requires the counsel of a scientific professional who reads the totality of evidence available and makes a balanced decision.

A few natural products which do not ever seem to combine well with anything – chemo, most other drugs, most botanicals and nutraceuticals – are grapefruit and St. John's Wort *Hypericum perfoliatum*.

ARABA-C – Araba-C is derived from sea sponges, and is likely to provoke mouth sores, so use Fare You tablets.

ANASTRAZOLE – Aromatase inhibitors markedly increase risk of bone loss. Manage risk of bone loss with MCHA calcium – microcrystalline hydroxyapatite ossein complex with added vitamin D3, vitamin C, and magnesium citrate. Increase exercise, and manage joint pains with omega 3 marine oils and topical emu oil. Aromatase inhibitors are synergistic with natural aromatase inhibitors quercetin, grapeseed extract, and white button mushrooms *Agaricus bisporus*, as well as the hormone modulators indole-3-carbinol and melatonin.

AVASTIN (BEVACIZUMAB) – A potent angiogenesis inhibitor, it can interfere with normal wound healing, and increase risk of bleeds of the gums, nose or female reproductive tract. It may cause intestinal bleeding and bowel perforation. It also increases risk of hypertension, high-grade proteinuria and nephrotic syndrome.

BISULPHAN – Bisulphan is very toxic to highly oxygenated cells due to production of superoxide free radicals. It is synergistic with quercetin against human leukemia.

BLEOMYCIN – Bleomycin is very toxic to highly oxygenated cells due to production of superoxide free radicals, but is less toxic and more effective in patients given supplemental vitamins A, C and E; selenium, taurine, squalene and green tea.

BORTEZOMIB (VELCADE) – Bortezomib – a proteasome inhibitor, is less effective if mixed with green tea or quercetin.

It is positively synergistic with curcumin.

CAMPTOTHECIN – Camptothecin is a topoisomerase enzyme inhibiting alkaloid from the Chinese "Happy Tree" *Camptotheca accuminata*, Topoisomerase helps cancer cells double by relaxing the DNA spiral, opening it up for copying.

All topoisomerase poisons increase risk of later developing a secondary leukemia, because they promote chimeric fusion of non-homologous DNA strands in hematopoietic progenitor stem cells, the bone marrow stem cells which give rise to blood cells

Quercetin improves absorption of camptothecin by cancer cells.

Bu Zhong YI Qi Wan or Ba Zhen Tang herbal formulas reduce gastro-intestinal side-effects.

Never mix Camptothecin with curcumin.

CARMUSTINE (BCNU) – Carmustine is a nitroso-urea compound 1, 3-bis (2-chloro-ethyl)-1-nitrosourea) – thus the alternate name BCNU. Beta-glucans from maitake mushroom increase efficacy against prostate cancer by inhibiting a glutathione dependent detoxifying enzyme glyoalase I (Gly-1).

Synergistic with berberine as found in golden seal, barberry, coptis and other herbs.

CASODEX (BICLUTAMIDE) – Biclutamide can be enhanced with ginseng, gamma oryzanol, sage and motherwort.

CISPLATIN, CARBOPLATIN, OXALIPLATIN – Platinum complexes cross-link DNA, and deamidate the Bcl-xL gene, which inactivates a switch that could trigger apoptosis.

Platinum compounds can cause severe neurotoxicity, severe nephrotoxicity (kidney damage), nausea, vomiting, ototoxicity (hearing loss) and myelosuppression. Monitor electrolytes for low sodium, calcium, potassium and magnesium.

Reduce toxicity with milk thistle (liver protectant), and astragalus (kidney protectant), omega 3 DHA oil (prevents kidney damage and increases efficacy), quercetin, melatonin, and vitamins C and E. Low vitamin E status correlates with severe peripheral nerve damage from cisplatin, so Rx 600 mg daily. Selenium at 200 mcg daily reduces bone marrow suppression, kidney toxicity, and development of drug resistance. Intravenous glutathione protects nerves from toxicity, but it is controversial whether or not this reduces effectiveness. The platinums reduce tissue stores of magnesium and vitamin D, so it is essential to replace these. Ba Zhen Tang – Eight Pearls Decoction – reduces gastro-intestinal GI side-effects, as does Bu Zhong Yi Qi Wan formula. Some of my colleagues use Jian Pi Yi Qi Li Shui Decoction, all-trans retinoic acid ATRA, or Polyerga spleen extract.

Cisplatin is a heat shock protein HSP-90 inhibitor, inducing cell cycle arrest independent of p53. It can be a significant radio-sensitizer, given about 6 hours pre-radiation.

Carboplatin is less renal toxic but more myelosuppressive than cisplatin; produces electrolyte imbalances, nausea and vomiting, abnormal liver function, neuropathy, myalgia (muscle pain) and is mutagenic. Consider extra glutamine and Polyerga with carboplatin, and cytokine modulators such as astragalus and ganoderma.

Improve effectiveness with quercetin (30% more apoptosis), coenzyme Q-10, gingko biloba, genestein, selenium, mistletoe, coriolus PSK, shitake lentinan, green tea EGCG, resveratrol, vitamins A, niacin or a B-complex, C, and E.

Platinum drugs are an exception to the rule against curcumin, as it definitely enhances their efficacy. Milk thistle and selenomethionine can blunt tumour resistance to cisplatin, increasing efficacy.

Do not mix platinum drugs with N-acetyl cysteine, glutathione, alpha lipoic acid, *Ginkgo biloba*, squalene, zinc or high dose vitamin B6, unless directed by a naturopathic physician skilled in oncology.

Italian MDs use intravenous glutathione IV-GSH with cisplatin and cyclophosphamide chemo in ovarian cancer cases.

CYCLOPHOSPHAMIDE (CYTOXAN) – Cytoxan is a mustard agent related to mustard gas used in World War One, but now banned as a weapon – except against cancer. Cyclophosphamide (CP) cross-links DNA, potentially causing nausea, baldness, bleeding in the urinary bladder, bone marrow damage, reduced natural killer cell activity, and increased risk of metastasis.

Increase effectiveness with vitamin A, beta carotene, vitamin C, vitamin E, co-enzyme Q-10, folic acid and B-complex vitamins, omega 3 oils and aloe vera juice. TCM formula Yi Kang Lin is synergistic.

Reduce toxicity with ashwagandha, melatonin, green tea, Co-enzyme Q-10, omega 3 oils, AHCC, grapeseed extract, cordyceps, coriolus PSK, magnesium, selenium, N-acetyl cysteine, glutathione, Polyerga spleen extract and lots of water. Red ginseng ginsenoside Rg3 reduces haemolysin, protecting the red blood cells. The TCM formula Buzhong Yiai or Central Qi Pill reduces toxicity and improves effectiveness.

Curcumin and quercetin must **not** be used. By reducing reactive oxygen species ROS and JNK inhibition, they reduce death of the cancer cells by apoptosis.

CYCLOSPORIN – Cyclosporine is a powerful immune suppressor, to prevent rejection of transplanted tissue, including bone marrow transplants. Grapefruit juice increases its toxicity. Do not use immune enhancing herbs or mushrooms, or plant sterols.

DOXORUBICIN (ADRIAMYCIN) – Originally called Adriamycin because it was extracted from a unique fungus found only in a ruined stone tower overlooking the Adriatic Sea. Doxorubicin is an anthracine antibiotic which intercalates DNA (binds inside the spiral strands), inhibiting DNA and RNA synthesis and can cause chromosome breaks.

Doxorubicin is a pro-oxidant, and is particularly toxic to cells low in oxygen. It is highly toxic to the muscle of the heart over total doses of 500 mg/m2. Cardiomyocyte apoptosis is induced by endocannabinoid ananamide, preventable by CB-1 receptor inhibitors. Grapeseed extract OPCs can completely eliminate myocardial oxidative stress.

It causes myelosuppression – grossly inhibits bone marrow cells and therefore blood cell counts, especially white immune cells, i.e. leucopenia. It can provoke post-treatment acute myelocytic leukemia (AML), alopecia, nausea, vomiting, and extravasation (leaking of fluid out of the blood vessels).

Improve effectiveness with vitamin A, vitamin C, grapeseed extract OPCs, vitamin E, DHA, milk thistle, mistletoe and melatonin. Soy genestein reduces DNA binding with nuclear factor NFkB.

Green tea theanine 50 – 200 mg daily, and quercetin 500 – 100 mg 2 to 3 times daily, help the drug accumulate in cancer cells, via the p-glycoprotein drug porter system, while sparing the heart and other healthy tissues.

Reduce toxicity with garlic, selenium, melatonin, grapeseed proanthocyanidins, omega 3 oils, squalene, coriolus PSP, green tea EGCG polyphenols and catechin. Adriamycin depletes the tissues of vitamins A, beta carotene, B2, B6, C, E and zinc, and supplementing with these will improve safety and efficacy. Anti-oxidants in virgin olive oil also seem to help. Vitamin B6 particularly reduces hand-foot syndrome (PPED). Pre-treatment with vitamin E reduces hair loss while improving efficacy.

The most critical supports are vitamin E and Co-enzyme Q-10 to protect the heart muscle from damage, which can enlarge the heart and lead to congestive heart failure. The heart can be further supported by taurine, carnitine, *Crataegus oxyacantha*, *Convallaria majus* and *Rhodiola rosea*.

Black cohosh herb *Cimicifuga racemosa* improves *in vitro* cancer cell cytotoxicity by 100-fold. I have not seen it tried on humans.

Do not mix with N-acetyl cysteine or glutathione antioxidants as they can increase drug resistance. Do not mix with feverfew herb parthenolides or glucosamine.

HER-2 positive breast cancer may respond to anthracycline chemo drugs including Doxorubicin, Epirubicin, Adriamycin, Daunorubicin, Idarubicin and Mitoxantrone.

However, HER-2 negative cases do not respond to anthracyclines, and they no longer represent the standard of care for these patients.

EPIRUBICIN – Epirubicin is less toxic to humans given melatonin supplementation. See Doxorubicin entry above. The omega 3 oil DHA at 1.8 grams chemosensitizes tumors to anthracyclines, improving time to progression and overall survival in FEC chemo for breast cancer.

ERBITUX (CETUXIMAB) – Erbitux inhibits the epidermal factor receptor EGFR. It is a monoclonal antibody from a human/mouse chimera. It is used primarily for head and neck and metastatic colorectal cancers. It is not useful in advanced colorectal cancer if the patient has a κ-ras mutation at codon 12 or 13. It is incompatible with high dose of vitamin C.

ETOPOSIDE – *Podophyllum* alkaloid toxins from mandrake root were the origin of this compound. The alkaloids are now made synthetically by a pharmaceutical company, so now they are OK as a medicine.

Etoposide chemo is enhanced with quercetin, melatonin, vitamin A, and beta-carotene.

Avoid St. John's Wort which increases toxicity. Avoid glucosamine sulphate, glucosamine HCl and N-acetyl-glucosamine, which reduce effectiveness of topoisomerase II inhibitors.

5-FLUORO-URACIL / 5-FU – 5-Fluorouracil is a pyramididine anti-metabolite which inhibits DNA synthesis. This is an "anti-vitamin" agent.

5-FU can cause anorexia, nausea, stomatitis, diarrhea, alopecia, renal failure, leukopenia, rashes, pigmentation changes – darkening and sunburning easily.

Improve effectiveness with quercetin, melatonin, aloe vera, shitake lentinan and vitamins A, vitamin C, vitamin E.

Reduce toxicity with L-glutamine, glutathione, chamomile mouthwash, coenzyme Q-10, and vitamin B6. Ginseng helps preserve immune function.

Caution: do not mix with high doses of carotenoids, including beta carotene, lutein, and lycopene.

GEMCITABINE – Gemcitabine is closely related to 5-FU. Gemcitabine inhibits manufacture of DNA. It also down-regulates CYP 2C9. This is one of the most effective and relatively least toxic chemotherapy drugs, and we can easily help it do even more, with less harm. Many patients just breeze through chemo with this drug. However, a small percentage of persons will have a genetic variation which causes them to metabolize this pro-drug into a very noxious chemical, and they may find it intolerable. A deficiency of cytidine deaminase (CDA) is a good predictor of early severe toxicities. This can include myelosuppression, and a rare fatal haemolytic-uremic syndrome.

Quercetin reduces tumour cell resistance.

Synergistic with GLA oils such as evening primrose oil, B-complex vitamins, melatonin, squalene, shark liver oil alkylglycerols, astragalus (*Shih Chuan Da Bu Wan* is an astragalus-based TCM formula), green tea EGCG, soy genestein, resveratrol, curcumin, DIM, sulfaphorane, gotu kola, *Ginkgo biloba* extract and thymoquinone from black cumin seed *Nigella sativa*.

Do not mix with estradiol, soy or legume coumarins.

GOSERLIN (ZOLADEX) – Goserlin is a LHRH hormone agonist, and can be improved with ginseng, cleavers herb and gamma oryzanol.

HERCEPTIN – Targets the receptor for the growth factor associated with the HER-2/neu gene, but also damages the heart.

You must take hawthorn berry *Crataegus oxyacantha*, Lily-of-the-Valley *Convallaria majus*, vitamin E and Co-enzyme Q-10 to prevent or correct heart damage. I often add the homeopathic remedy *Naja tripudians 6C*.

I am proud to say this has rapidly restored heart function in patients who otherwise would never have qualified for this therapy, due to weakening of their heat from previous chemo with drugs like Doxorubicin, or due to other causes. This approach has definitely allowed many patients to recover, and continue on in therapy, after cardiac damage forced a halt to the Herceptin therapy. It has, of course, also consistently restored heart health following Herceptin therapy. My naturopathic oncologist colleagues in the United States may suggest these additional heart supports: L-carnitine, *Ginkgo biloba* extract, grapeseed extract, angelica, lyceum, ginseng.

Improve efficacy against the cancer with quercetin, *Aloe vera*, *Polygonum* herb, and NFkB Reishi mushroom extracts *Ganoderma lucidum*. Emodin from *Aloe vera*, and quercetin, reduce HER-2/neu gene expression, the root of the problem. Evening primrose oil or black currant oil gamma-linolenic acid GLA inhibits mutant HER-2/neu protein, increasing Herceptin response 30 to 40-fold. Olive oil (oleic acid) improves efficacy. Flax oil alpha linolenic acid is a potent support for Herceptin, inhibiting epidermal growth factor receptor EGFR.

It is important to control insulin-like growth factor IGF-1, which strongly interacts with the HER-2/neu receptor, and Herceptin therapy. This means close adherence to the low-glycemic diet.

HYDROXYUREA – Hydroxyurea or hydroxycarbamide is an inhibitor of ribonucleotide reductase, used in chronic myelogenous leukemia, polycythemia vera, and meningiomas.

Support liver and kidney and bone marrow from toxicity with Shih Chuan Da Bu Wan, an Astragalus-based TCM herb formula, Co-enzyme Q-10, and milk thistle extract.

IRINOTECAN – Irinotecan is a semi-synthetic compound – a natural compound altered by a chemist. The natural compound originates from the Chinese "Happy Tree" *Camptotheca accuminata*. Topotecan and related drugs block topoisomerase I enzyme, which relaxes and opens the DNA spiral during cell division. If the cancer cell cannot open up the DNA, it cannot double into two cells.

Improve drug uptake about 30% with quercetin. Improve effectiveness with melatonin, milk thistle extract, soy genestein and selenomethionine.

Do <u>not</u> mix with curcumin.

ITRACONAZOLE – This very liver-toxic anti-fungal, mainly used in stem cell transplant cases. It can also damage the heart.

Milk thistle can reduce these risks. Do not eat grapefruit or drink grapefruit juice, it reduces efficacy.

LETROZOLE – Letrozole or *Femara* is an aromatase inhibitor capable of reducing estrogen and estrone twice as much as Anastazole. When Letrozole fails, about 15% of cases can be rescued by the related drug Exemastane or *Aromasin*. Support with natural AI's quercetin, grapeseed extract, indole-3-carbinol and white button mushrooms, and Bcl-2 inhibitors curcumin and green tea extract. Support bone health with MCHA calcium complex, vitamin D3 and exercise.

MEGACE – Megestrol acetate or progestogen is an estrogen receptor disruptor. Megace therapy can be enhanced with licorice root, sage, red clover, vitamins B6 and B12, and gamma oryzanol.

MELPHALEN – Avoid combining melphalan with glutamine, leucine, tyrosine or methionine supplements, as these will reduce uptake into the bloodstream, and therefore decrease efficacy. Melphalan can produce a very prolonged haematological toxicity, particularly in elderly patients. Be proactive with astragalus formulas and alkylglycerols.

MERCAPTOPURINE – Avoid mixing with xanthine oxidase inhibitors, which block purine metabolism. This includes some anti-gout drugs, quercetin, myricetin, kaempferol, cinnamon and propolis.

METHOTREXATE (MTX) – Methotrexate is an antimetabolite or anti-vitamin agent which inhibits dihydrofolate reductase, blocking reduction of the B-vitamin folic acid, necessary for DNA nucleic acid and protein synthesis.

It is sometimes given in a fatal dose followed by "leucovorin rescue" which is calcium folinic acid. 1 in 100 patients can die from this treatment.

MTX is nephrotoxic and hepatotoxic (damages the kidneys and the liver). It causes nausea, vomiting, diarrhea, mucositis (mouth sores), dermatitis (inflamed skin), blurred vision, dizziness, and leukopenia (drop in immune cells).

Improve effectiveness with milk thistle extract, licorice root and polygonum. L-glutamine increases uptake of MTX into tumours.

For safety counteract the intense production of reactive oxygen species with vitamin A, vitamin E and selenomethionine.

Do not combine with glutathione, tangeritin, or high doses of folic acid or vitamin C. Avoid mixing with echinacea, black cohosh root or salicylate-rich herbs such as bilberry, willow and wintergreen.

MITOMYCIN – Mitomycin is synergistic with Yi Kang Ling formula, melatonin and marine omega 3 seal oil.

Do not mix with beta carotene, as it reduces efficacy.

PAZOPANIB (VOTRIENT) – Pazopanib is a dual inhibitor of EGFR and PDGFR, and an inhibitor of angiogenesis. Watch for bleeding issues.

PREMETREXED – Premetrexed is less toxic if homocysteine levels are reduced, so give vitamin B-12 and folic acid.

RIBAVIRIN – Quercetin improves Ribavirin's efficacy.

RITUXIMAB – Beta glucans improve responses to rituximab, even creating responses in patients previously unresponsive. An excellent source is ***Agaricus blazei*** mushroom extract, or **reishi** mushroom extract.

SANDOSTATIN – Sandostatin or octreotide inhibits several kinase growth factors, but will irritate the gallbladder, so give bile salts, digestive enzymes and the TCM formula Li Dan. Induces hypoglycaemia, so prescribe a high protein, low fat diet with low glycemic carbs.

SORAFENIB (NEXAVAR) – Sorafenib inhibits several tyrosine protein kinases, including platelet-derived growth factor PDGF, vascular endothelial growth factor receptor VEGFR kinases 2 and 3, the stem cell factor receptor cKit, and Raf kinase – which links to the MAP Kinase via the Raf/Mek/Erk growth signalling pathway. Be aware of the significant risk of bleeding. Do not mix with any blood-thinners.

SUNITINIB (SUTENT) – Sunitinib is a tyrosine kinase receptor inhibitor, capable of hitting multiple targets. It blocks signalling at all the platelet-derived growth factor receptors PDGFR and the vascular endothelial growth factor receptors VEGFR. By cutting off the blood supply and proliferation, it can shrink tumours. Be aware of the significant risk of bleeding. Do not mix with any blood-thinners.

TAMOXIFEN – Tamoxifen is a non-steroidal anti-estrogen which binds to cytoplasmic beta estrogen receptors ERß, and has other complex effects on hormones. It delivers about 15% reduction in the risk of a reoccurrence of breast cancer.

Tamoxifen can cause some serious side-effects, so although I must admit most women do very well on Tamoxifen, integrative naturopathic support is definitely needed for safety. It can cause a 3% increased risk of blood clots, such as a deep vein thrombosis or pulmonary embolism. This risk is most pronounced for obese (high body mass index) persons. It increases risk of uterine cancer by about 1%. It also increases by about 1% the risk of retinal damage, rashes, leukorrhea, depression, liver damage and increased tumour pain. Be prepared for hot flashes and thinning hair. In the presence of bony metastases it can precipitate hypocalcaemia (excess blood calcium).

Tamoxifen activity may be reduced by certain medications (e.g., selective serotonin reuptake inhibitors [SSRIs]), which are potent inhibitors of the cytochrome P-450 CYP2D6 enzyme, which is necessary for activation of the drug. Effexor may be prescribed for the hot flashes. The use of soy foods with Tamoxifen has been a controversy, but recent evidence indicates a high degree of synergy. High soy food intake is associated with an additional 60% reduction in risk of breast cancer occurrence in women on Tamoxifen.

Melatonin is highly synergistic, reduces risks and reinforces hormone blockade.

GLA oil (gamma linolenic acid) from borage or evening primrose oil at 2.8 grams daily improves effectiveness by reducing expression of estrogen receptors. Quercetin improves effectiveness by increasing bioavailability. Vitamin E and selenomethionine in moderate doses will improve effectiveness. Vitamin A is particularly useful, extending remission times and improving response rates.

The energy regulator Co-enzyme Q-10 makes Tamoxifen more effective by increasing expression of tumour suppressor gene manganese super-oxide dismutase MnSOD. Co-enzyme Q-10, vitamin B2 riboflavin and B3 as niacin or as niacinamide, reduce DNA methylation and induce DNA repair enzymes, boosting Tamoxifen efficacy.

It is important to control insulin-like growth factor IGF-1, which strongly interacts with estrogen receptors, and Tamoxifen therapy. This means close adherence to the low-glycemic diet.

Indole-3-carbinol is complementary in estrogen receptor positive ER+ breast cancer cases as it suppresses estrogen receptor activity by a different signalling pathway, increasing the arrest of the cancer cell growth cycle.

The use of soy foods with Tamoxifen has been a controversy, but recent evidence indicates a high degree of synergy. High soy food intake is associated with an additional 60% reduction in risk of breast cancer occurrence in women on Tamoxifen. High intake is over 40 mg of soy isoflavones daily. Do not use genestein supplements, only use food sources.

Do not combine Tamoxifen with high dose vitamin D (over 1,000 IU daily), flavonoids such as tangeritin or grapefruit, black cohosh root Cimicifuga racemosa, St. John's Wort Hypericum perfoliatum, or red clover blossoms Trifolium repens, including Hoxsey herbal tonic.

Tamoxifen activity may be reduced by certain medications, for example the anti-depressant selective serotonin reuptake inhibitors SSRIs. Effexor may be prescribed for the hot flashes. I think it wise to choose naturopathic options for mood such as 5-HTP. Acupuncture reduces hot flashes well, and the effect persists after treatment. Always include the acupoint LV-2 for hot flashes. Smoking should be stopped and alcohol minimized.

TARCEVA – Erlotinib or Gefitinib is an EGFR inhibitor. Tarceva is cleared from the body by CYP 3A4.

Tarceva will typically cause blistering and exfoliative skin disorders. For the skin use topical sea buckthorn, for example New Chapter brand with calendula and rosemary, and *Aveeno* colloidal oatmeal lotion, soap and bath soak.

It can also cause abnormal eyelash growth and dry eyes. In some cases it provokes ulceration and perforation of the cornea or along the GI tract.

Apoptosis increases if combined with indole-3-carbinol and genestein. Support with berry and pomegranate flavonoids.

Do not mix with quercetin or curcumin.

TAXANES – Taxol is a mitotic inhibitor from yew tree bark. It depolymerizes microtubules such as mitotic spindles into tubulin. Taxotere (Docetaxol) and Paclitaxel are synthetic taxanes.

Taxanes can provoke anaphylactic shock reactions, so to avoid serious trouble you will be pre-treated with Benadryl and/or Decadron – an antihistamine and a steroid drug, to try to avoid serious trouble. Sensory nerve damage, muscle pain, joint pain, mouth sores, nausea, vomiting, loss of white blood immune cells, and heart toxicity can also occur.

B-complex vitamins improve effectiveness. Improve efficacy further with vitamin C – 4 to 6 grams daily, resveratrol, vitamin E, and Iscador mistletoe injections. Highly synergistic with essential fatty acids such as GLA from evening primrose oil, and with Ashwagandha herb *Withania somnifera*. Curcumin <u>may</u> improve efficacy of Docetaxol.

Strongly supported by vitamin D3, improving efficacy while reducing toxicity. Soy genestein increases efficacy by reducing DNA binding with nuclear factor NFkB.

Taxanes cause joint and muscle pain by raising COX-2 enzymes which promote inflammation. Use natural COX-2 inhibitors such as omega 3 marine oils, boswellia and resveratrol.

L-glutamine at 2 to 3 grams up to three times daily reduces risks of nerve damage and muscle pain. This can be supported with acetyl-L-carnitine and vitamin B6 in the pyridoxal-5-phosphate form. Melatonin (21 mg) is neuroprotective against taxane neuropathy.

Do <u>not</u> mix with quercetin, berberine, NAC or St. John's Wort as they may reduce efficacy.

TEMOZOLOMIDE – Temodar or Temodal is a unique chemo drug for certain brain cancers. It induces autophagic cell death rather than the usual apoptosis pathway. It can cause thrombocytopenia. Support with alkylglycerols, grapeseed extract, and if needed for platelets, Yunnan Baiyao.

THALIDOMIDE – Thalidomide a potent inhibitor of angiogenesis – blood vessel in-growth to tumours. It may also be useful for wasting syndrome. May cause nerve injury, such as numbness and pain in the limbs, which is treatable with vitamin B6, benfotiamine and R+ alpha lipoic acid.

VINCA ALKALOIDS – Vincristine and Vinblastine, from periwinkle flower, bind tubulin, and destroy mitotic spindles. The cancer cell cannot pull apart its chromosomes into two new cells.

Microtubule inhibitors up-regulate COX-2 enzymes, increasing inflammation.

They can cause constipation, small bowel paralysis, baldness, mouth sores, inflamed skin and nerve toxicity such as foot drop, phantom sensations, and loss of tendon reflexes.

Prevent or treat nerve toxicity with milk thistle extract, vitamins B6 and B12. Give COX-2 inhibitors to reduce side-effects such as joint and muscle pain, and to increase anti-tumour effects – for example omega 3 marine oils.

Give stool softeners or laxatives.

Effectiveness is increased by vitamins A, C and E, as well as Cordyceps mushroom extracts. Quercetin overcomes resistance to Vincristine and Vinblastine therapy.

COMMON CHEMO COMBINATIONS

ABV- doxorubicin, bleomycin and vinblastine

ABVD – doxorubicin, bleomycin, vinblastine and dacarbazine

ACTT – Adriamycin, cyclophosphamide, taxol and herceptin

BACOP – bleomycin, doxorubicin, cyclophosphamide, vincristine and prednisone

BEACOPP – bleomycin, etoposide, doxorubicin, cyclophosphamide, vincristine, procarbazine and prednisone.

BEP – bleomycin, etoposide and cisplatin.

BRAJACCT – Adriamycin, cyclophosphamide, taxol, herceptin, tamoxifen and adjuvant radiotherapy.

BRAJCAFPO – uses CAF on days 1 and 8. – cyclophosphamide, adriamycin and fluorouracil.

BRAJCAF-G – Cyclophosphamide, adriamycin (doxorubicin), 5-fluorouracil and filgrastim G-CSF

BRAVDOC – Docetaxol

BRAVTRAP and BRAVTRNAV – Trastuzumab / Herceptin for HER-2 + breast cancer

CAMP – cyclophosphamide, doxorubicin, methotrexate and procarbazine.

CHOP-B – cyclophosphamide, doxorubicin, vincristine, prednisone and bleomycin.

CHOP + R – cyclophosphamide, doxorubicin, vincristine, prednisone, and rituximab.

CMFVP – cyclophosphamide, methotrexate, 5-fluoruracil, vincristine and prednisone.

CNAJATMZ –Temozolomide chemo as an adjunct during radiation.

COP-BLAM – cyclophosphamide, vincristine, prednisone, bleomycin, doxorubicin and procarbazine.

CVP – cyclophosphamide, vincristine and prednisone

FAC – 5-FU, adriamycin, cyclophosphamide Also called CAF.

FAM – 5-fluoruracil, doxorubicin and mitomycin.

FEC – 5-FU, epirubicin, cyclophosphamide. Also called CEF.

FOLFOX- 5-FU, oxaliplatin, leucovorin.

FOLFIRI – 5-FU by infusion, irinotecan and leucovorin.

GIFOLFIRI – Irinotecan, 5-fluorouracil and leucovorin folinic acid.

GIFUR3 – 5-fluorouracil, leucovorin and radiation for high-risk rectal cancer.

Naturopathic Oncology

GOCXRADC – Cisplatin and radiation concurrently for cervical cancer.
GUBEP – bleomycin, etoposide, cisplatin.
HNCMT2 – chemo and radiation for squamous cell cancers of the head and neck.
ICE – ifosfamide, cyclophosphamide and etoposide.
IFL of Salz: 5-FU, irinotecan and leucovorin.
LUSCCAV – adriamycin, vincristine, cyclophosphamide.
LYCHLOR – Chlorambucil for low-grade lymphoma.
LYALEM – Alemtuzumab / Campath for lymphomas and leukemias
LYRITUX – Rituximab / Rituxan for lymphomas.
MACC – methotrexate, doxorubicin, cyclophosphamide and lomustine.
MOPP – mechlorethamine, vincristine, prednisone and procarbazine.
MVPP – mechlorethamine, vinblastine, procarbazine and prednisone.
MYMYP – Melphalan and prednisone for multiple myeloma.
ProMACE-CytaBOM – cyclophosphamide, doxorubicin, etoposide, prednisone, cytarabine, bleomycin, vincristine, methotrexate and leukovorin.
UGIAJFFOX – 5-FU, leukovorin, oxaliplatin, plus a 5-FU bolus.
ULUGEF – Gefitinib / Iressa as a 3rd line therapy for NSCLC.
UGOOVVIN – Vinroelbine as a palliative
VAC – vincristine, dactinomycin and cyclophosphamide.

GRADING CHEMO TOXICITY

It is really unusual for anyone to die from chemotherapy now. You will be tested before each round of chemo to determine how your bone marrow is being affected, by counting and describing the red blood cell, white blood cells and platelets. You will also be tested to see how your vital organs, the liver and kidneys are tolerating the drugs. Your heart may sometimes be assed, as well as your gastro-intestinal upsets will be graded. The most common grading is on a scale to four:

0 = normal range
1 = mild toxicity, continue drug at 100% of the prescribed dose
2 = moderate toxicity, reduce dose to 75% of Rx
3 = severe toxicity, reduce dose to 50% of Rx, or wait for improvement
4 = critical toxicity, may be fatal if unchecked, suspend therapy

Usually therapy is only reduced, slowed or suspended if more than one organ or cell type is affected. However, the most important are low platelet counts, due to risk of haemorrhage, and low white blood cells, particularly neutrophils, the first-responder immune cells necessary to survive and infection.

It is important to monitor serum albumin, a protein required to keep fluids in the vessels. It is a sign of severe oxidative stress to see a drop in albumin, bilirubin and uric acid. Untreated, it gives a poor prognosis. Prescribe antioxidants and whey protein supplements

Chemo toxicities can often be reversed with traditional Chinese TCM herb formulas, available in pills and capsules. Naturopathic and integrative supports can make all the difference when faced with a dose reduction and therefore a reduced chance of effectiveness of a chemotherapy program.

PART FOUR – A DEEPER LOOK AT NATUROPATHIC ONCOLOGY

Chapter Five – Diet & Food Supplements In Cancer

"The scientific and medical literature and theorists fail to vividly portray issues which are patently obvious to clinicians, especially those who work with nutrition."--Dr. Mark Gignac, N.D., Cancer Treatment Centers of America

Many nutrients are associated with lowered risk of certain cancers, and are therefore preventative. Most are antioxidants and flavonoids; some are minerals, vitamins, proteins and oils. They abound in the traditional foods of our ancestors that can be hunted, milked, fished, picked or gathered.

Lowered risk from all cancers, and longer survival with cancers, is associated with low caloric intake. Over-eating is a major risk that is all too commonly taken in our modern society with its energy rich agricultural foods. Over-fuelling causes insulin resistance, hyperinsulinism, hormonal shifts, blood fat imbalances, and metabolic aging. Periodic fasting extends the human lifespan.

Good nutrition naturally supports healing as well. Dietary interventions with cancer patients appear to remove obstacles to cure.

When used in concentrated form, nutrients become nutraceutical drugs. I believe food and plant concentrates as dietary supplements are essential to overcome cancer. Once well, a whole foods diet may be sufficient to maintain a remission.

There are about 200 documented cases of spontaneous remissions from advanced cancer each year in the U.S.A. These often correlate with dietary factors, including a switch to vegetarian diet and use of supplements.

The Grape Cure, Gerson Diet Therapy, the Macrobiotic diet, Dr. Kelley's Nutritional Metabolic Therapy, Dr. Brusch's Diet, the Hallelujah Acres – God's Way Diet and Moerman Diet all have their supporters, and may be useful adjuncts to more definitive therapies.

The clinical bottom line is that diet alone may not cure cancer, but bad nutritional management will contribute to reduced repair and healing, weight-loss, cachexia, fatigue and complications. Malnutrition and inanition (not eating) are the direct cause of death in 22% of all cancer patients.

The absolute taboos in the diet of cancer patients are high-sugar foods and red meat raised by contemporary agri-business methods. We forbid tobacco products. I strongly urge reduction of chemical intake in all forms, by washing food better, choosing organic food, raising your own food, and by cleaning up chemicals in the home and workplace. Beyond this point we need to get personal, and tailor the diet to the individual constitution, tastes, culture, condition and disease.

The modern agricultural-based diet is significantly different from the diet of our hunter-gatherer ancestors. Our ancestors had very low rates of cancer. The protective elements they had which we now tend to lack in our diets are largely due the reduction in consumption of coarse vegetation, especially the herbaceous or aerial parts of plants. These lost protectants include calcium, potassium, fibre, omega 3 fatty acids, polyunsaturated fats, trace minerals, antioxidants, flavonoids, isoflavones and polyphenols.

For example, covalent DNA binding is associated with malignant transformation of genes, but is inhibited by phenethyl isothiocyanate in broccoli and cabbage, ellagic acid in fruits, nuts, berries, seeds and vegetables, and by polyphenolic acid flavonoids in fruits and vegetables. Tumour promoters are inhibited by retinol and carotenoids in orange, yellow and green fruits and vegetables, vitamin E in nuts and wheat germ, organosulphur compounds in garlic and onions, curcumin in turmeric (curry) and by the vanillyl alkaloid capsaicin in chili peppers.

Estrogen, progesterone and thyroid hormones are biotransformed into benign forms by indole-3-carbinol in cabbage, Brussels sprouts, broccoli, cauliflower and spinach, and by selenium in garlic and seafood.

Absorption of carcinogens is reduced by fibre in fruits, vegetables, grains and nuts, and by riboflavin and chlorophyll in fruits and vegetables.

The modern diet is an experiment in nutrition which is not going well for us. The hybridized plants that are now staples in our diet have been genetically manipulated to be big and sweet and juicy, release more sugar faster because they have simpler starches and less fibre.

Foods may be heavily contaminated with chemical carcinogens and xenobiotics. Our estrogen and insulin growth factors are going wild!

Grain silage and "by-product" filth fed to animals are also higher in compounds associated with higher cancer risk, such as xenobiotics, saturated fat, herbicides and pesticides.

Until wholesome nutrition is at the core of cancer therapy and prevention, the disease will remain largely unbeatable.

SUGAR, BLOOD GLUCOSE, INSULIN & CANCER RISK

High dietary sugar intake is associated with many cancers, including breast, colorectal, biliary and melanoma. The worst sugar is sucrose from sugar cane. Sucrose, fructose and many other food sugars are mostly converted into glucose, the major sugar found in the blood-stream and the primary energy fuel for most cells in the body.

Insulin is a protein made in the pancreas and put into the blood to move fats, sugars and proteins into cells. It must attach to the receptors on the cell membrane in order to pump nutrients into the cell. Its attachment is assisted by glucose tolerance factor (GTF), which is composed of chromium, zinc, and some B-vitamins. Insulin increases fat storage and therefore promotes excess body fat. Insulin also activates the liver enzyme HMGCoA reductase to overproduce cholesterol from carbohydrates. Exercise and stress reduction can lower insulin levels.

Insulin resistance is a complex metabolic problem where the insulin cannot get nutrients into the cells. Insulin resistance is linked to increased incidence of cancer of the colon, breast, pancreas, esophagus, uterine endometrium, and prostate. A marker for insulin resistance is the apple-shape body type with prominent abdominal obesity. Insulin resistance can also lead to "Syndrome X" with high blood pressure, cholesterol disorders, cardiovascular disease – atherosclerotic plaque, stroke and heart attacks, and other major health risks such as osteoporosis, osteoarthritis, and premature aging.

Cancer patients increase glucose production in the liver by 25 to 40%, similar to non-insulin dependent adult onset diabetics (NIDDM), also known as type 2 diabetes. Unlike diabetics, cancer patients will continue to increase sugar production even while undergoing starvation, accelerating loss of body mass. Cancer cells metabolize glucose sugar at a rate 4 to 5 times that of normal cells.

Adenosine-mono-phosphate AMP is the energy storage molecule to which phosphate groups are added when cells collect energy from "burning" sugars or fats. The phosphates are then taken away, releasing energy to drive all activity and chemical reactions in the body, and the AMP goes back to be recharged. AMP-activated protein kinase AMPK is a critical cellular energy sensor and regulator. AMPK is inhibited by the accumulation of carbohydrates in cells, most notably in obesity, diabetes mellitus, and pre-malignancy. This confers a replicative advantage, inhibiting apoptosis. In malignancy, substrate limitation is mitigated by AMPK activation, and combined with defective tumour suppressors; the cancer cell undergoes a glycolytic switch.

When there is not enough oxygen to burn sugars in the usual way, cancer cells switch to fermentation. Loss of p53, activation of Akt and hypoxia-inducible factor one HIF-1 (induced by hypoxia or starvation) contributes to glycolysis.

Fermentation is not very efficient, making about 20 times less energy from the sugar than if it were burned in the usual way by oxidation, and leaving more harmful residues in the process. Lactic acid from fermentation is highly toxic and a tumour growth promoter.

Anaerobic glycolysis allows energy production without oxygen, but also provides the tumour cells with precursors for the synthesis of proteins, amino acids, nucleotides, phospholipids and triglycerides. The net effect is that glycolysis actually improves tumour cell survival.

Tumour dimeric pyruvate kinase M2PK is a marker for anaerobic glycolysis, which can be detected in EDTA plasma or in feces in cancer. It is also increased in inflammatory bowel disease IBD.

Malignant tumours have 1.9 to 3.0 times the insulin and related compounds seen in normal tissue. Most cancer cells have an abnormally high number of insulin receptors, compared to normal cells of the same type nearby.

Insulin is a general growth promoter. Hyperinsulinism and insulin resistance are highly pro-inflammatory, increasing IL-6, C-reactive protein, and NF kappa-B. Hyperinsulinism is seen in about 45% of early cancers, but rises to about 75% of advanced cancer cases.

C-peptide is a marker for pancreatic insulin secretion, accurately reflects the mean level of circulating insulin, and associates with cancer risk.

Post-prandial hyperinsulinemia – high blood insulin after eating – produces a significant surge in the doubling rate of hepatocellular carcinoma cells, which last for several hours after a meal that spikes up the blood sugar. Insulin excess in the bloodstream is not consistently correlated to the glycemic index of the foods due to great individual variability in digestive function and absorption faculty.

Chronic hyperinsulinism and insulin resistance increases delta-9-desaturase activity, which alters the ratio of stearic to oleic fatty acids, which may contribute to post-menopausal breast cancer.

Tumour cells can even secrete factors which block glucose uptake in healthy cells, provoking higher insulin secretion from the pancreas, stimulating further tumour growth and proliferation!

Diabetes increases risk of many cancers, such as pancreas, liver, colon, breast and uterine endometrium. Diabetes makes it harder to control many cancers, with increased rates of reoccurrence and higher mortality. However, diabetes lowers risk for prostate cancer, as low insulin leads to low testosterone levels.

Persons with Diabetes type 2 will have lower risk of cancer if they are on prescription Metformin, compared to those on sulfonylurea or insulin therapy.

All efforts to control blood sugar through diet and exercise will support reducing cancer risk. Naturopathic interventions for high blood sugar and insulin dysregulation include B-complex vitamins, chromium, zinc, vanadium, vitamins C and E, flaxseed, omega 3 oils, and alpha lipoic acid.

Insulin-like growth factor is produced in the liver. It has a very similar structure to insulin. IGF-1 is 70 amino acids long, and IGF-2 is 67.

Insulin-like growth factor one (IGF-1) or somatomedin C is a mitogenic peptide which promotes cell proliferation, anabolism, clonal expansion and inhibits apoptosis. IGF-1 is involved in the decision by the cell to progress from G-0 to G-1 phase of the cell cycle. Elevated levels are associated with a several fold increase in risk of ovarian, prostate, colorectal and lung cancer.

IGF reduces apoptosis, and so high levels interfere with both radiation and chemotherapy, including cytotoxic drugs and EGFR inhibitors. The influence on response rates is quite profound, so it is critical to follow a low-glycemic diet during these medical therapies.

Insulin inhibits IGF binding proteins (IGFBP 1 & 2) and this increases IGF bioavailability. Insulin and IGF may be directly mitogenic, interact with ras protein mutations, stimulate farnesyl transferase, modulate apoptosis, and stimulate angiogenesis by increasing production of vascular endothelial growth factor.

Usually only the IGF gene inherited from the father is active, but in persons with the maternal IGF gene also activated, risk for colorectal cancer is higher. Hypomethylation of DNA in cancer cells leads to a loss of imprinting of the IGF-1 gene.

Estrogen increases IGF-1 receptors on breast cells, increasing their rate of cell division. In turn, insulin and IGF-1 increase ovarian output of estrogen, and increase free estrogen by inhibiting liver production of sex-hormone binding globulin proteins. Free IGF-1 may stimulate estrogen receptors. It's a vicious cycle.

IGF-1 & 2 are stimulated by human growth hormone (HGH) produced in our pituitary gland. Therefore I forbid taking human growth hormone supplements, HGH releasers, or colostrums products. IGF-1 is excessive in milk from cows given recombinant bovine growth hormone (rBGH) to increase milk production.

IGF signalling is suppressed by vitamin D – another good reason to take extra vitamin D3, and to get some reasonable exposure to sunshine.

IGF-1 is strongly inhibited by green tea EGCG. Grapeseed oligomeric proanthocyanidins up-regulate IGF binding protein three IGFBP-3, which reduces IGF activity. Lycopene reduces blood levels of IGF-1.

Barnard, et al showed that the Pritiken regime – a very low fat whole food diet with exercise – markedly reduces liver production of IGF-1 and boosts IGFBP-1.

A relatively new treatment uses injections of high doses of insulin to induce a profound hypoglycaemic state in the cancer cells, concurrent with chemotherapy or intravenous alternative therapies. This is risky, but does potentiate the other therapies.

In naturopathic medical school I was told "sugar paralyzes the immune cells on contact." I have visualized it like putting salt on a slug – just nasty. As it turns out, sugar has an immediate and toxic effect on immune cells, including those responsible for surveillance on cancer cells. The effect is called glucose-ascorbate antagonism. High sugar intake reduces activity in the hexose monophophate shunt or pentose phosphate pathway, which reduces available NADPH. This lowers glutathione reduction, reducing recycling of vitamin C (ascorbate), allowing oxidative stress to build to levels which injure immune cells. They cannot produce a respiratory burst of superoxide and hydrogen peroxide against cancer cells and infectious organisms.

Above all, sugar and insulin and insulin-like growth factors are normalized by a wholesome diet and by creating a favourable ratio of lean body mass (sugar burning) to body fat (sugar storage).

The oral anti-diabetic drugs Rosiglitazone maleate – Avandia- or Pioglitazone reduce invasiveness and tumour growth by blocking peroxisome proliferators-activated receptors gamma PPARγ. Unfortunately, they also markedly increase risk of stroke and heart attack.

An interesting unproven remedy is Salicinum. This natural glycome sugar can only be split by the enzyme beta-glucosidase, which is only active in cells which are fermenting sugars by anaerobic glycolysis. The resulting fragment binds irreversibly to NAD+, stopping energy production from fermentation. In theory this should slow down cancer cells.

WEIGHT LOSS & METABOLIC CACHEXIA

Cachexia is the wasting away of the body triggered by metabolic changes of cancer. It is far more than just loss of appetite (anorexia) and digestive power. It is a critical shift into a chemical imbalance where the body consumes itself to feed the tumour with nitrogen and other elements. It is a cause of great distress, weakness, and robs the person of dignity. It is often manageable, which can prevent premature death and suffering.

Involuntary loss of 5% of lean body mass in the past 3 months or a 10% weight change in the past 6 months is a high risk negative prognostic indicator. A 20% loss is a critical condition.

Cachexia is a response to overwhelming oxidative stress. Tumour products such as lipid-mobilizing factor LMF directly stimulate lipolysis (fat burning) in a cAMP dependent system. NFkB activates a specific inflammatory syndrome in skeletal muscle fibres, which in turn initiates catabolism of skeletal muscle. Proteolysis-inducing factor PIF involves activation of NFkB and the acute phase protein STAT-3 transcription activator. Cachexia is also triggered by host immune factors such as the cytokines IL-1, IL-1B, IL-6, INF-gamma, TNF-alpha.

Tumour necrosis factor alpha TNFa produced by macrophages, lymphocytes and NK cells, is also called cachectin because it causes anorexia and weight loss, via the hypothalamic satiety center in the brain and by inhibition of gastric emptying. It increases glucose uptake, insulin resistance, protein catabolism in skeletal muscle, depletes fat stores, and is associated with fatigue and alterations of the sense of taste. TNF also induces reactive oxygen species, which are involved in tissue wasting.

TNF can be inhibited in a clinically significant way by appropriate doses of curcumin, green tea epigallocatechins EGCG, eicosapentaenoic fatty acid omega 3 oil EPA, melatonin, vitamin E or vitamin E succinate VES, coconut oil and flour, and the botanicals *Uncaria tomentosa* – cat's claw and *Silybum marianum* – milk thistle. Royal jelly with ginseng is a pleasant and effective nutritive general tonic for the qi and blood, strengthens and invigorates the fatigued cachexic patient. Best results are seen when combined with ganoderma (reishi) mushroom. These can restore appetite, nutrient and medication absorption, and body weight. If they are very Yang deficient add more Chinese ginseng *Panax ginseng*, or Siberian ginseng *Eleutherococcus senticosus*. Homeopathic *Arsenicum iodatum* is helpful in cachexia. *Phytolacca* helps emaciation and rapid exhaustion. The esteemed Dr. Dan Rubin ND has recommended *Oralmat* activated rye grass extract, 3 drops sublingually thrice daily, for appetite and weight gain. Another American colleague once recommended extra virgin coconut oil and coconut flour.

Cachexia in cancer patients is consistently responsive to eicosapentaenoic acid EPA supplements such as fish oil or seal oil. This omega 3 oil will improve quality of life, appetite and weight gain. EPA is the most effective supplement to manage weight loss, Rx at least 2 grams EPA daily. I prescribe harp seal oil, 2 capsules twice daily. There are some distilled fish oils from sardines and anchovies, which are of acceptable quality.

Dr. David Baker, MD has developed an effective cure for cachexia in AIDS patients, including the anti-oxidants R+alpha lipoic acid, grapeseed extract OPCs, vitamin C , pumpkin seed and Brazil nuts. Dr. Baker was a family doctor in Victoria, who now works primarily with AIDS patients, locally and in Africa.

Progesterone has a proven track record of benefiting appetite, and subjective well-being. It is presumed to down-regulate the synthesis and release of cytokines. It increases body weight, but unfortunately it is only water retention, not a change in lean body mass. It may stimulate PR+ breast cancers to grow. Progesterone receptors alongside estrogen receptors is known to give a better prognosis, but not if you feed the progesterone receptors! Progesterone therapy can lead to blood clots such as deep vein thrombosis, as well as menstrual spotting, and sexual dysfunctions.

Thalidomide has shown some potential benefits on appetite, nausea and well-being. Other drugs being studied are Ibuprofen at 50 mg twice daily to reduce C-reactive protein; pentifylline I.V. to reduce TNFa; and COX-2 inhibitors celecoxib or rofecoxib to modulate prostaglandins involved in cachexia as well as in the development of cancer. There are many natural COX-2 inhibitors.

Corticosteroids are used to inhibit prostaglandins and to suppress TNF production. The results on appetite, food intake and quality of life are short-lived, and there are significant risks of adverse effects. Steroids are best reserved for end-stage palliation.

The drug hydrazine sulphate was developed by Dr. Joseph Gold to stop the cachexic process. It was the first non-toxic chemotherapy developed, only causing some nausea and limb weakness in some cases. It is very inexpensive. It inhibits gluconeogenesis, slows or stops tumour growth, and produces significant improvement in subjective symptoms in at least half of terminal cases – in other words patients just feel better, have less pain, more energy, and increased appetite. Despite strong science from America and Russia, the cancer institutions such as the National Cancer Institute and the American Cancer Society have systematically blocked research efforts and have marginalized this drug. Being on hydrazine sulphate does require a lot of dietary restrictions, as it interacts with many other mono-amine oxidase inhibitors in common foods and drugs. I think **omega 3 EPA** is a much better choice.

PROTEIN and CANCER

Protein intake is a huge modifier of outcomes. Tumours become nitrogen sinks by catabolizing skeletal muscle, recruiting amino acids for gluconeogenesis via the lactic acid Cori cycle. If we do not feed protein consistently, protein will be drawn from the patent's flesh. Your doctor will probably test regularly for total blood protein, and the liver output of albumin and globulin proteins.

Your doctor may want to assess protein digestion by measuring stomach acid hydrogen chloride HCl, gastric and pancreatic digestive enzymes, and protein absorption. Falling albumin levels may indicate oxidative stress in the liver,

Some integrative oncology doctors advise against dairy foods. One reason cited is that the casein protein triggers invasiveness in tumours. Casein is milk curd – what turns solid when you curdle milk. It is the basis of all cheese. An enzyme that ramps up to digest it is casein kinase, which unfortunately can increase *beta-catenin*. This induces *survivin*, suppressing apoptosis while triggering hyper-proliferation of cancer cells.

Fish are generally fine if caught in the wild and eaten while still fresh. Highly recommended are salmon, pollock, sardines, sablefish, hake, herring and Pacific cod. Some farmed seafoods are acceptable, such as mussels, clams, oysters, trout, tilapia – just do some <u>due diligence</u> before you pick a brand.

L-glutamine is a principle fuel of cancer cells, generating 30 ATP energy molecules per glutamine. It is a critical stimulant of protein and nucleic acid (DNA and RNA) synthesis. L-glutamine protects the body from ammonia build-up, absorbing this toxic by-product of proteins, acting as a "nitrogen shuttle" to divert ammonia into amino acids, amino sugars, urea, and nucleotides. Theoretically it promotes production of glutathione also, but in fact it can cause glutathione depletion in leukemia bone marrow transplant cases.

It protects the gut lining from radiation and chemotherapy, suppresses prostaglandin PGE2 synthesis, stimulates NK natural killer cells. It reduces gut absorption and permeability changes and diarrhea caused by 5-fluorouracil. It protects from taxane neuropathy.

L-glutamine is used medically in healing from surgery, injury, sepsis (widespread infection), and starvation. It is not commonly found in intravenous feeding (total parenteral nutrition – TPN) solutions as it rapidly hydrolyzes so supplement with up to 30 grams daily by mouth or add to a parenteral bag for cachexia. Even 2 grams can make some difference.

It is critical to immune competence against infection, fuelling neutrophils, monocytes lymphocytes, improving the Th1/Th2 ratio.

L-glutamine is very useful to reduce cravings for alcohol.

L-carnitine drives mitochondrial energy production. Steve Levine, PhD is researching it as a "bio-energetic" regulator of mitochondrial dysfunction in cancer cells. It can help fight fatigue, and help fuel tissue repair. Acetyl-L-carnitine is a fat-soluble form of the amino acid, which allows it to readily cross the blood-brain-barrier. Therefore it is mush more useful than plain carnitine for healing nerve injury and for brain health, such as correcting "chemo-brain" – toxic cognitive impairment. It re-myelinates and reduces nerve cell apoptosis.

Rx 1 to 2 grams, 2 to 3 times daily.

Serum albumin under 3.5 is high risk, and survival falls 33% for every point decrease. Serum albumin falls with metastases, liver disease, expanded serum volume, and renal dysfunctions, so it does not just reflect loss of lean body mass. It is either poor protein intake from the diet or oxidative stress, or both. Serum half-life of albumin is 3 weeks, so it changes slowly on the labs. Albumin protein holds fluid in the vessels by colloid pressure, turning blood plasma into a thin gel. When albumin is very low in the blood, fluid balance throughout the body can be compromised.

Alpha-lactalbumin in human breast milk induces apoptosis in malignant trophoblastic cells in the infant digestive tract. Medical whey protein supplements retain this in an active form.

Whey protein lactalbumin in cow's milk is an excellent source of supplemental protein for cancer patients. Take 1 ounce or 30 grams of powder in liquid drink twice a day. Whey strips glutathione out of cancer cells, but raises it in normal cells! Dr. Keith Block, MD is a medical oncologist of over 30 years experience, and a leader in integrative oncology. He is not pro-dairy, but supports the use of whey supplements in nutritionally challenged patients. Some sensitive patients using whey may experience elevated markers of inflammation, such as ESR and CRP. These cases will do better on rice protein supplements.

SeaGest is a peptide concentrate from fresh lean white fish of the North Pacific, at 12 to 20 capsules daily for wound healing, to arrest cachexia, and for general vitality. The fish is bio-converted to peptides and amino acids by bacterial fermentation. Assimilation is nearly 100%. Related products include Foundation, formerly known as SeaCure.

Haelen is a nitrogen-enriched fermented soy protein drink developed in Chinese hospitals to supercharge their cancer patients with protein. It tastes yucky and is really expensive.

I have seen some very good responses quite consistently from amino acid balancing therapy. Blood levels are tested, and supplements specifically matched to the individual to correct any deficiencies. This is conducted through a clinic in Ottawa. See www. aminomics.com

MINERALS

I am a great admirer of the late medical geographer Dr. Harold Foster, PhD. He studied the mineralization of soils around the world, and correlated dietary intake of minerals with hundreds of medical conditions. His website www.hdfoster.com was one of my favourites. He felt the keys to controlling cancer are
- avoid mercury, and detoxify if exposed
- take adequate amounts and forms of selenium – i.e. selenomethionine 200 – 400 mcg.
- take adequate amounts and forms of calcium
- avoid chronic exposure to ferrocyanide from road salt, including water from polluted aquifers.

BORON – Boron is ubiquitous in food, including apples, pears, grapes, bananas, peanuts, beans, salad greens, broccoli, coffee, wine. Boron is protective of bone health, in part by increasing 17-beat estradiol levels in healthy post-menopausal women, and in men. Adequate dietary boron lowers risk of prostate, breast, cervical and lung cancer. It influences apoptosis, receptor binding mimicry, serine proteases, NAD hydrogenases, cell division and mRNA splicing.

CALCIUM – Dr. Harold Foster, PhD the renowned medical geographer has found high calcium in soils and water corresponds to populations with lower cancer rates. The benefits of hard water were amplified if selenium was also abundant.

Calcium at 1,200 mg daily of common forms such as calcium citrate or calcium carbonate reduces cancer cell proliferation, assists re-differentiation, and binds unconjugated bile acids. It is shown to reduce risk of colon cancer, and this effect lasts long after periodic dosing. In women, it reduces risk from all cancers.

The *Calcium Paradox* is that a toxic build-up of calcium inside cells or cellular hyper-calcinosis, results from low dietary intake of calcium, and/or deficiency of vitamin D3 -which assists calcium's absorption, metabolism and retention. Free calcium inside a cell moves protein kinases to the plasma membrane for phosphorylation, switching on growth and proliferation. High calcium inside the cells alters inflammatory eicosanoids via activation of NFkB, increasing lipid peroxides and thus oxidative stress in the mitochondria. The mitochondria fail, apoptosis is inhibited, and cell replication speeds up.

Low dietary calcium increases expression of the inflammatory molecule COX-2.

Microcrystalline hydroxyapatite ossein complex or **MCHA calcium** will harden the bones, reducing risk of metastases to the bones. If bone mets have occurred, this calcium will reduce or arrest the spread of cancer within bone, and generally reduces bone pain rapidly and significantly. It has bone growth factors which lay strong new bone in where it is needed, as well as preserving old bone. It increases bone density, bone mass and bone strength.

MCHA formulas are best with added magnesium citrate, vitamin C, vitamin D3, magnesium citrate, and boron. We give 2 caps twice daily. The therapeutic dose of 4 capsules yields 600 mg. of elemental calcium. There is no need to go higher than 4 capsules daily as the product does not work by its calcium alone, but by building the protein and proteoglycan scaffolding to which the minerals are attached in the bone matrix. This is like the steel re-bar in concrete or wire mesh in a glass window. It makes the brittle minerals into a strong and flexible structure.

CESIUM – Cesium resembles and substitutes for potassium in biological systems. It is taken up strongly by cancer cells, where it can raise intracellular pH to the point of cell death and necrosis. Doses less than 3 grams per day increase tumour growth – recall that alkalizing a tumour can accelerate its growth. Doses over 6 grams are purported to treat cancer. Doses should never exceed 9 grams daily. Reactions include hypertension, diarrhea, increased salivation, nausea, locomotor impairment, and injury to the heart and kidneys. I have met a few people who appear to have benefited from cesium, but due to toxicity concerns, I am not willing to recommend it at this time.

COPPER – Copper increases blood vessel growth into tumours (angiogenesis), so excess is to be avoided strictly. Copper also suppresses mitochondrial oxidative phosphorylation, inhibiting apoptosis. Beware copper water supply pipes, kettles, pans, and other sources of exposure. Use a good water treatment system if you have copper pipes. Copper can be chelated out of the body by supplementation with R+ alpha lipoic acid, N-acetyl-cysteine, MSM, curcumin and taurine. However, copper as a trace mineral in the diet is required for the proper function of a protein called ceruloplasmin, an iron transporter. Ceruloplasmin down in the 10 to 20 mg/dl range can impair the ability of bone marrow to make red blood cells, leading to anemia. This type of anemia looks like iron deficiency, but will not respond to iron supplements.

IODINE – Iodine as found in potassium iodide, is a tonic to the thyroid gland. Low thyroid is associated with poor immune function and healing. Hypothyroid is also linked to constipation, which is very detrimental to a cancer patient. I have seen patients pulled back from the brink of death by getting their bowels moving, and the relief of pain that accompanies this is also remarkable. The thyroid interacts in complex ways with sex hormone balance. For example, we will use iodine supplements to reliably get rid of fibrocystic breast lumps. Iodine helps adjust mitochondrial membrane function, supporting apoptosis.

Dr. Max Gerson felt that iodine counteracts the neoplastic effects of the sex hormones such as estrogen Iodine is used to make thyroid hormone, which sets the body thermostat, and how fast all the metabolic systems will run. Adequate thyroid function is critical to detoxifying the body of toxins produced by cancer cells, by the often toxic therapies for cancer, and especially to clear off the wastes and cell fragments as cancer cells die from a good therapy. Even natural therapies can result in a huge burden on the reticulo-endothelial system and liver detox systems, so it is critical to support the body in throwing off the diseased tissue. Potassium iodide was found in the Hoxsey formula at 3% W/V. Gerson used Lugol's iodine solution or desiccated thyroid extracts. The recommended therapeutic dose of elemental iodine is 2 to 4 mg. daily. One drop of Lugol's yields 2.083 mg, so the usual dose is 1 to 2 drops daily. See the comments on iodism given below in the discussion of potassium (iodide.)

IRON – Iron is the mineral that makes us able to deliver oxygen around in the blood, and to carry off carbon dioxide waste. The iron is the core of the hemoglobin protein, the red in the red blood cells.

Chronic illnesses such as cancer tend to induce a chronic, low grade anemia. If your red blood cells RBCs are reduced in number, and smaller than normal in size MCV, you may have iron-deficiency anemia. However, it is important that your doctor check your blood ferritin level to check on your iron transport activity. Iron supplements are only prescribed if the ferritin is low, and only for a specific period of time. I like to Rx 30 mg of iron citrate at every meal for one month, then retest. Iron is pro-oxidant, tends to stimulate tumours, and can aggravate bacterial infections.

Iron in plant foods, such as beans, is in an electronic state that makes it hard to absorb in our digestive tract. The heme form of iron in animal foods, particularly red meat, is absorbed much more readily. Unfortunately, red meat intake is linked to increased cancer risk.

I do allow patients to have some clean animal protein in their diet, if they wish. Their meat must always be grass pasture fed, and will be rich in healthy fats such as the anti-inflammatory omega 3 oils and CLA. Ordinary commercial and restaurant grade meat, finished in feedlots with corn silage and artificial diets, is higher in saturated fat and omega 6 oils. It is believed that the heme iron in meat induces intense lipid peroxidation in the presence of these pro-inflammatory agri-business animal fats, causing cancers of the breast, colon and other organs.

Cancer cells use more iron than normal cells, and so therapies that reduce iron actually can be very useful – such as artemisinin from wormwood. Perhaps the anemia in cancer cases is a natural defence mechanism. Certainly we do not want to give iron to cancer patients unless it is really necessary, as demonstrated by microcytic anemia and low ferritin.

To reduce an iron overload drink black tea at meals, without milk. Tea tannins bind dietary iron and prevent its absorption. Turmeric in curry and chili peppers bind iron and keep it from cancer cells. Lactoferrin and artemisinin rob the cancer cells of iron.

LITHIUM – Lithium can substitute for sodium in many cellular reactions. It inhibits glycogen synthase kinase GSK-3. It will increase circulating neutrophil granulocytes and platelets. It is known to help manage melanoma, prostate and uterine cancers, and the bony lesions of multiple myeloma. High dose inhibit promyelocytic and hairy cell leukemias, but beware – low doses increase leukemic cell proliferation. It is not recommended for lung cancer or parathyroid adenomas.

MAGNESIUM – Magnesium correlates with protection from prostate cancer, perhaps because it inhibits the secretion of insulin. It is also used in the mitochondria, important regulators of apoptosis. It is very important for heart health. Always take magnesium citrate when taking calcium supplements, for bone and heart health.

POTASSIUM – Potassium salts are perhaps the most critical minerals in controlling normal cell function, and it is absolutely certain that his ancestors ate a lot more potassium than does modern man. The agricultural diet has inflicted a huge reversal of the ratio of sodium to potassium seen in hunter-gatherer diets. Potassium is found in all vegetables, and it is a good idea to drink the water in which vegetables are cooked. Excellent food sources are potatoes and bananas. For those of you into energetics of medicines, this one has a very high "bovis" frequency, meaning it regulates homeostasis and supports vital life functions. The sodium to potassium balance – $Na+/K+$ – influences cellular protein configurations, and shape equals function and performance in proteins. Sodium distorts and slows many metabolic enzymes, while potassium straightens them out and revs up their functionality.

Today we call this proteasomal regulation, and it is an important issue in controlling the growth of cancer cells.

From Dr. F.W. Forbes Ross in early twentieth century London, to the Americans Professor Andrew C. Ivy, Dr. Max Gerson, and Harry Hoxsey in our time, the use of potassium iodide, potassium citrate, and potassium phosphate has been associated with cancer cures.

Potassium iodide is routinely used at 5 grains weekly, or about 50 mg daily. Certainly it is generally safe in these dosages, as it has long been used at twice this dose as an expectorant for coughs. Sometimes a patient will experience Iodism – pimples on the face, forehead or shoulders, watering eyes, and a runny nose. Rarely, allergic reactions can occur, with vomiting, cramps, fever, palpitation, and emaciation. Potassium iodide will pass in breast milk and will cause nursing babies to lose weight.

SELENIUM – Selenium is an anti-oxidant strongly associated with cancer prevention. At intakes of at least 200 mcg daily, selenium normalizes expression of BRAC gene mutations, restoring DNA repair and preventing cancer. It is required by the Guardian of the DNA – the p53 gene protein.

Some consider it to be a useful <u>pro-oxidant</u> therapy at 400 to 800 mcg. It may be given intra-muscular at 1,000 mcg every second day for 3 weeks. Dr. Foster likes yeast selenium – inorganic selenium fed to yeast and then reclaimed in an organic form. Some suggest methyl-seleno-cysteine. Organic forms of selenium may inhibit angiogenesis. I prefer to prescribe selenomethionine. Selenomethionine is synergistic with the 5-LOX inhibitor *Boswellia*.

It has been suggested recently that selenium is actually quite counter-productive in cases of prostate cancer, so we no longer use it as a therapy. I only recommend it to patients with BRAC mutations.

SODIUM – Salt delays wound healing after surgery. It induces swelling due to water retention by the kidneys. It can trigger fatigue. Putting extra salt on food is an addiction. Wean off it gradually, and in time you neither want it not need it. Sodium in salt antagonizes potassium, and in the modern diet we eat a lot less potassium and a lot more sodium than our ancestors did – and this is a major factor in many chronic and degenerative diseases.

ZEOLITE – Volcanic lava running into sea water is a natural source of zeolite. It can be liquefied with acid and heat. Zeolites detoxify the liver, remove heavy metals and xenobiotics, alter cell membrane charge, absorb antigens, block viruses, and is said to inhibit cancer cells. The anti-cancer action is primarily attributed to activation of gene p21, a universal inhibitor of cyclin-dependent kinases. It may induce apoptosis. I have seen it give clinical relief of cancer pain. I am not sure if it does any more than that. Natural Cellular Defence is a brand taken orally at doses of 10 to 15 drops 3 to 4 times a day. This requires 4 bottles a month, but maintenance doses of 3 drops 3 times daily require 1 bottle per month. It is harmless, but contraindicated if you are taking prescription lithium or a platinum chemo drug.

ZINC – Zinc is anti-angiogenic by competitively reducing copper absorption. Zinc enhances apoptosis and DNA repair mechanisms. Zinc deficiency has been linked to squamous cell cancers. Zinc replenishment prevents and reverses oral and esophageal cancers, likely by regulating COX-2 inflammatory growth factor and human papillomavirus. It prevents and treats radiation dermatitis and mucositis in head and neck cancers. Zinc activates thymus gland maturation of T-cells immune function. Zinc is vital to collagen formation for normal tissue repair.

DIETARY FIBRE

Adequate fibre intake is associated with lower risk of colorectal cancer. Pre-agricultural "hunter-gatherer" diets were very much higher in fibre than modern diets.

Fibre contains lignans and phytoestrogens which are anti-estrogenic. Lignans, phytoestrogens and isoflavonoids in food fibre stimulate production of sex hormone binding globulins (SHBG) which bind free estrogen. Gut fibre will diminish re-uptake of sex hormones, binds hormones and xenohormones and carries them out in the feces. Lignans can also disrupt cancer cell mitochondrial membranes.

Phytoestrogens can be anti-estrogenic, and actually reduce growth of estrogen-sensitive cancers. Many plant estrogens bind very poorly to human estrogen receptors – they have a low affinity, due to their shape and charge variations. They can plug up a receptor; fail to stimulate a growth signal, while keeping out any high affinity estradiols.

Take a daily fibre supplement such as psyllium husks and ground flaxseed. Start with a teaspoon of each a day, and gradually increase to a heaping tablespoonful each a day. It can cause increased gas at first, and later the bowel movements can become slimy, so work to find the right dose for your best bowel function.

Flaxseed is the richest known source of lignans which bowel bacteria can convert into entrolactones. These are strongly anti-estrogenic phytoestrogens. Even one teaspoonful of flaxseed daily raises the 2-OH estrone blood levels, and improves the ratio of good to bad estrogens. This is why the recommended dose of 2 tablespoons daily of fresh-ground flaxseed has been able to slow breast cancer growth, reduce invasiveness and impede the spread into lymph nodes. Flaxseed lignans induce production of sex-hormone binding globulin SHBG proteins, and reduce the number of receptors on cancer cells for insulin-like growth factor one IGF-1. They are also anti-angiogenic, anti-inflammatory, anti-oxidant, detoxifying, and anti-parasitic.

Psyllium husks are an excellent fibre supplement, being of a type preferred by gut bacteria to make butyrates and other beneficial short chain fats. These fats are essential for repair and normal function of the lining of the gut, and are not part of the human diet. They only can be made by probiotic bacteria from whole food fibre.

Psyllium husks will interact with some prescription drugs. It reduces absorption of lithium and carbamazepine, and alters the cardiotropic effect of digitalis, beta blockers and calcium channel blockers. Never administer these drugs at the same time as fibre supplements. Fibre supplements require professional supervision if there is a risk of bowel obstruction or other GI diseases.

PGX™ fibre from Natural Factors brand is an excellent way to mange blood sugar, reduce insulin resistance, and manage weight. Increase slowly due to potential to cause increased bowel gas. Take up to 3 to 5 before meals.

IP-6 or phytic acid up-regulates p21 and p53 genes while down-regulating mutant p53. Blocks tumour initiation and progression. At 5 to 8 grams daily it may inhibit breast and colon tumour growth. Phytic acid strongly chelates dietary minerals and medications, so take fibre away from all medicines. It tends to aggravate iron deficiency anemia in cancer patients, which can manifest as fatigue, sleepiness or feeling faint. One of my reputable and learned naturopathic colleagues co-wrote a book about IP6 titled "Too Good to Be True?" Unfortunately, I have to say my clinical experience with it has not been notable. I find there are more fruitful therapies which are easier and cheaper. NOT RECOMMENDED.

Modified Citrus Pectin Halts the Spread of Cancer!

The most dangerous thing a cancer cell can do is spread to distant parts of the body and grow into a new tumour. Often it is the spread into the vital organs such as the liver, lungs or brain which causes the most suffering and is often fatal. This ability to metastasize and live in a new environment depends on the cancer cell attaching itself to the new site. If it cannot attach, it cannot double and grow. Imagine if something as ordinary and cheap as the pulp left over from making orange juice could be turned into a fool-proof cancer medicine.

Ordinary fruit pectin can be modified by high heat and acid treatment to form small water-soluble carbohydrates which bind to proteins on cancer cells and stop them from attaching. The modified or fractionated pectin binds to galectin-3 proteins on the cancer cell surface, the major non-integrin cellular laminin-binding protein. This acts like putting flour on Scotch tape. The cancer cell coated in this small carbohydrate cannot stick anywhere to the vascular endothelium. If it cannot arrest by binding selectins on blood and lymph vessels, it cannot move out into new tissues.

Studies in mice and rats, against breast, prostate, colorectal, lung, melanoma, sarcoma and other cancers show consistent results in reducing the spread of cancer, the rate of tumour growth and blood vessel formation in new tumours. Because all cancers have these sugar-binding proteins for adhesion, it is expected to be useful in all solid tumour cancers. Phase I trials in humans have been very successful, and phase II trials are underway.

MCP is essential protection for patients undergoing tumour biopsy, surgery or therapy that may cause the tumour to shed cells. There is a 1 to 2% risk of spread of cancer by biopsy or surgical procedures.

MCP is appropriate also for tumours such as melanoma skin cancer which tend to spread very early in the course of the disease.

Recent studies indicate MCP taken long-term can slow the growth of some tumours. MCP antagonizes heparin-dependent fibroblast growth factor 1 (FGF-1) and its receptor FGFR-1. MCP blocks nm23 gene expression. There is evidence it can increase the cytoxic response of NK cells. There is emerging evidence that it removes toxic heavy metals from the human body. I have observed generally better survival in patients who take it long-term, compared to similar cases who do not take it.

MCP may inhibit substances associated with capillary leakage, which would be helpful in treating ascites.

Quality is critical. Most of the pectins need to be very small – a low molecular weight of only about 10 to 12 thousand Daltons. Vital Victoria MCP is made to this specification by a compounding pharmacist. Products with larger fragments are useless.

The dose is 6 to 30 grams daily, divided in 2 doses. The effect is dose-dependent, so most doctors recommend at least two teaspoons or about 8 grams of the powder daily. The bulk powder may be dissolved in some water using a blender, or electric whisk, as it is quite sticky. This may be further diluted in juice. Most prefer to take it in vegetarian gelatin capsules, Rx 4 caps twice daily. Four of the common size "00" size capsules equals one teaspoonful. MCP is a food grade substance, and completely non-toxic. Bowel movements may at first be a little looser than normal.

DIETARY FATS

Low fat diet <u>before</u> diagnosis is associated with 70% lower risk of mortality in breast cancer cases; changing to low fat diet after diagnosis has no measurable survival benefit. While it may be too little too late, a reasonably low fat diet with a balance of fats is healthful and may reduce risk of heart disease, stroke, diabetes, and most other diseases.

Tumours increase fatty acid oxidation and lipolysis to provide the gluconeogenesis substrates glycerol and free fatty acids. This allows them to make energy without sugars.

GOOD FATS – Omega 9, GLA, and Omega 3 EPA, DHA, DPA

Extra virgin grade or cold-pressed olive oil has the omega 9 monounsaturated oleic fatty acid, squalene and phenolic antioxidants known to protect against cancer of the prostate, breast, colon or skin. Polyphenolic compounds such as the secoiridoid oleuropein or the lignan 1-[+]-acetoxypinoresinol) dramatically reduce HER-2 expression and specifically induce apoptotic cell death in cultured HER-2 positive breast cancer cells, with marginal effects against HER-2 negative cells. Oleic acid inhibits conversion of arachidonic acid AA to the highly inflammatory and carcinogenic prostaglandin PGE-2. In prostate cancer this conversion is ten times that in benign prostatic hypertrophy BPH or enlarged prostate gland.

Linoleic acid is also a dietary replacement for saturated animal fats, to reduce risk of prostate cancer. Cold pressed vegetable oils with this fatty acid include sesame, grapeseed, olive and coconut

Conjugated linoleic acid CLA from meat and milk of grass-fed animals inhibits tumour initiation and reduces metastases at 1% of dietary calories. CLA is cytotoxic and cytostatic, modulates cellular responses to tumour necrosis factor alpha, enhances cell-to-cell communication, reduces hyperinsulinemia, benefits cachexia, and increases IL-2 production. Loading dose is 100,000 to 3,000,000 units. There is a small risk of dry skin, headaches and changes in liver enzymes.

Monosaturates and gamma linolenic acid (GLA) from nuts and seeds. GLA is associated with induction of cAMP, which re-differentiates cancer cells, and restores contact inhibition. GLA reduces angiogenesis by inhibiting vascular endothelial cell motility. GLA decreases the tumour promoter prostaglandin PGE-2. GLA reduces estrogen receptor expression, synergizing with Tamoxifen. Evening primrose, black currant or borage oil are all good sources.

Omega 3 fats are found in soy, canola, walnut, almonds, flaxseed (ALA), fish, and fish liver oils – especially eicosapentaenoic acid EPA and dihexanoic acid DHA.

EPA reduces PGE2 production by competing for arachidonic acid AA with LOX, COX-1 and COX-2. EPA alters many other cytokines and prostaglandins such as 4-series and 5-series leukotrienes, thromboxane A-3,

PGI-3. The resultant anti-inflammatory, vasodilating and blood-thinning effects reduces cachexia, inhibits metastasis, promotes apoptosis, modifies cell-cell signalling, and improves immune helper-suppressor cell ratio. EPA appears to down-regulate VEGF ligands and receptors, inhibiting tumour angiogenesis.

DHA alters proteasomal regulation of beta-catenin, which modulates genes for VEGF, PPARΔ, MMP-7. MTI-MMP and Survivin. DHA changes the cardiolipin lipid composition, hence changing the mitochondria membrane voltage and the cytosol membrane flexibility, adding more receptivity to other agents like cytotoxic drugs or natural agents like butyrate and R+ alpha lipoic acid. DHA inhibits TNFa, lipid peroxidation as measured by malondialdehyde MDA, and reduces inflammation as measured by CRP. It can prevent kidney damage by cisplatin chemotherapy. It increases chemo efficacy generally, by regulating cytokines such as IL-1 and IL-6.

Grass fed beef has a 2:1 ratio of omega 6 fats to omega 3 fats. This shifts to 10:1 $\Omega6:\Omega3$ if the cattle are fed grain such as corn silage.

Omega 3 oils increase survival time in generalized malignancy. $\Omega3$s modulate T-cell balance, markedly increasing the helper: suppressor ratio. Support with a little vitamin E, to retard oxidation/rancidity.

SHARK LIVER OIL

Shark liver oil contains alkylglycerols which are powerful stimulants to humoral and cellular immunity, including a marked effect on NK cell activity, protein tyrosine kinases and angiogenesis. It helps recovery from bone marrow suppression after chemotherapy or radiation. Animal studies show a great synergy with probiotics. Use 6 of 200 mg capsules for up to 30 days maximum. Excess use may over-stimulate platelet production.

BUTYRATES

Butyrates are four carbon fatty acids first found in butter. Butyrates are formed naturally in the gut by friendly bacteria (probiotics) digesting fibre, such as the fibre in psyllium seed husks. Butyrates stabilize the DNA and genetic code by regulating histone proteins; inhibits histone deacetylases, especially H4. Butyrates inhibit Bcl-2, increasing apoptosis. Butyrates increase p21 cyclin-dependent kinase inhibitor by 30 to 50 times, even in the presence of mutated p53. Butyrates increase nuclease access to chromatin, relaxing the strands, increasing the rate of transcription, most notably the MAPK cascade, ERK1/2 phosphorylation and induction of AP-1-like transcription factors for GSTP1 gene expression leading to increased cell glutathione-S-transferase. Butyrates may induce re-differentiation in colorectal and other cancers, reduce gut inflammation and improve absorption of magnesium. Salts of butyric acid can be made with sodium, potassium or other minerals e.g. TriButyrate sodium 4-phenylbutyrate. The taste and odour is similar to rancid butter, which naturally some find objectionable. Butyrates were found to increase colorectal cancer in some animal studies, but most showed great promise. Human clinical studies show minimal benefits from butyrate supplements. I prefer to prescribe psyllium husks and probiotics and let them make the butyrates where they are needed.

BAD FATS

Arachidonic acid AA, trans-fatty acids, excess linolenic acid LA, saturates, and omega 6 fatty acids -corn, soybean and safflower oils. Omega 6 fats are too high in the modern Western diet, such as from corn oil in margarine and shortening and in meat fed on corn silage. These promote inflammation.

Trans-fatty acids TFA in hydrogenated oils and polyunsaturated fatty acids PUFAs are pro-oxidants and promote mutation. The presence of too many TFAs occurs commonly in oil that has been over-heated, especially in frying foods or grilling. PUFAs go rancid fast, and do not stand up well to cooking either.

Cattle fed grain such as corn silage have fat with a 10:1 ratio of omega 6 fats to omega 3 fats, compared to a 2:1 ratio in purely grass fed beef. The saturated and mono-saturated fats induced in animals fed silage and artificial diets are very prone to peroxidation, which renders them rancid and toxic. The heme iron in red meat catalyzes this oxidation of these very fats, and is probably why modern agri-business red meat is linked to higher risk of cancer occurrence, and accelerated rate of growth and progression of tumours. Meat from grass fed wild game or pasture-only fed animals is less prone to provoke lipid peroxidation and inflammation, due to a shift to omega 3 fats and CLA. Bison and lamb are generally only grass-fed. Regards other meats, you must be selective, and apply due diligence. If you cannot find appropriate wholesome meat, I ask you to choose clean poultry, fish or vegetarian alternatives. If you are offered no other choice in a social situation, please eat only a small portion if it is ordinary commercial grade red meat.

VITAMIN D3

The active form of vitamin D is D3, also called 1, 25 dihydroxy –cholecalciferol or 1-25(OH)D. Taking vitamin D2 may actually lower blood levels of active D3. Vitamin D is partly activated in the kidney and becomes fully active as a vitamin and hormone on exposure to ultraviolet rays of sunshine on the skin.

Blood levels have been found to be low in the vast majority of people, even those living in sunny places like Hawaii and Arizona. Strict sun avoidance and use of sunscreens to avoid skin cancer has contributed to the low UV exposure, and the resultant epidemic of joint problems, chondromalacia, sub-clinical rickets, and rising occurrence of cancer. Exposing some skin to sunlight can provide over 10,000 IU per day, in the Canadian summer – based on whole body exposure to a dose that provokes slight redness of the skin in healthy Caucasians. However, from October through March the ultraviolet light intensity is not strong enough to make <u>any</u> vitamin D3! A study on women in Toronto found 3 in 4 were markedly deficient. Put another way, only 25% of Canadians have optimal D3 in their blood. Adequate vitamin D levels are also correlated with reduced risk of "death from all causes," including cardiovascular and immune diseases.

- Activates CYP-mediated xenobiotic detoxification in the gut
- helps bone metabolism, calcium absorption
- prevents intra-cellular hypercalcinosis – a trigger of carcinogenesis.
- acts directly on DNA to promote normal cell differentiation
- improves cell adhesion and gap junction communication.
- inhibits angiogenesis
- suppresses IGF-1 signalling
- up-regulates cyclin-dependent kinase inhibitors p27 and p21 (tumour suppressor).
- promotes apoptosis
- may inhibit metastasis by reducing tumour secretion of collagenase enzymes.
- topically, it can reverse early pre-cancerous lesions. Combines well with grapeseed OPCs, vitamins A, retinoids, curcumin, green tea extract, vitamin C and aloe acemannan for skin healing.
- cancer cells dislike vitamin D so much that mature tumours actively neutralize this vitamin and block its activation. This anti-vitamin activity in tumours can

be modulated by calcium, folate and genestein from soy. Genestein potently increases D3 and reduces it breakdown.

Vitamin D3 reduces the risk of cancer by up to 60% when at adequate levels in the blood, i.e. 75 to 90 nmol/L or 30 to 40 ng/mL. Year-round minimum levels of 100 to 150 nmol/L or 40 to 60 ng/ml. are optimal for prevention. It particularly reduces risk of breast, colorectal and pancreatic cancer, but is not particularly preventative of prostate cancer.

Vitamin D3 therapy reduces joint and muscle pain from aromatase inhibitor drugs.

Supplement routinely for prevention at 1,000 to 1,200 IU daily, as recommended by the Canadian Cancer Society, and in my opinion, take 2,000 I.U. in the winter. In fact, I and all the medical and naturopathic doctors I know take 2,000 IU daily all year round. Evidence shows that 3,000 IU daily is safe for long-term use. To raise levels rapidly, imbibe sublingually. 40 IU intake will raise serum 25OHD by about 1 nM or 0.4 ng/ml. The new "tolerable upper intake level" for almost all persons is 10,000 IU daily, for periods of medically supervised therapy. I advise staying at or below 3,000 IU daily for long-term use. Some American doctors are giving a single loading dose of 500,000 IU, followed by monthly doses of 50,000 IU. Surprisingly, it appears to be quite safe.

Contraindications to vitamin D supplementation include tuberculosis or other granulomatous diseases, metastatic bone disease, sarcoidosis, or William's syndrome.

Toxicity is not likely at serum levels under 75 ng/mL. Mega-dose vitamin D3 therapy, i.e. 5,000 IU twice daily, can provoke **hypercalcaemia** when plasma levels exceed 240 ng/ml or over 600 nM free 1-25(OH)D. Some cases may get in trouble at a serum concentration of 125 ng/ml. Monitor closely, within the first two weeks of therapy, and ensure a good fluid intake. Serum calcium phosphate product must not exceed 70 mg/dL to minimize metastatic tissue and blood vessel calcification and avoid hypercalcaemia.

A prescription drug form of 1, 25 vitamin D is *Calcitriol*, given weekly by injection of 0.5 mcg or more. It is the most biologically active form of vitamin D known. Weekly dosing avoids the hypercalcaemia seen with daily use.

Calcitriol is a potent inhibitor of prostaglandin production. In prostate cancer responses are amplified if combined with a non-steroidal anti-inflammatory drug NSAID such as Naproxen or Ibuprofen.

The persons at highest risk of developing hypercalcaemia have cancer of the lung, breast, or multiple myeloma.

At moderate risk are cases of lymphoma, leukemia, renal, gastro-intestinal, head and neck cancers.

The signs and symptoms of hypercalcaemia:
- Anorexia
- Thirst
- Nausea / vomiting
- Constipation
- Abdominal pain

- Frequent urination
- Muscle weakness
- Fatigue
- Confusion, disorientation, difficulty thinking
- If severe enough: heart arrhythmia, heart attack, kidney stones, coma.

VITAMIN A

Vitamin A as retinol palmitate and other retinoic acids are regulators of epithelial cell growth, and important immune modulators. Vitamin A penetrates into the very nucleus of the cell to receptor sites which regulate normal growth and differentiation. This is where the genetic mutations lurk inside a cancer cell. Retinol –

- promotes cell differentiation
- inhibits angiogenesis
- promotes apoptosis
- highly protective against viral infection – retinoic acid reduces viral DNA inside cells
- increases NK cell activity
- decreases serum insulin-like growth factor 1 – IGF-1
- inhibits 5-alpha reductase, reducing testosterone levels
- up-regulates transforming growth factor beta – TGFß.
- improves tumour response to radiation and chemotherapy
- protects the gut from chemotherapy
- reduces lipid peroxidation, a critical factor in radiation injury.
- prolongs survival in advanced cancers, particularly colorectal cancer.

Vitamin A is safe in doses up to 50,000 I.U. daily, for short periods, but must be under medical supervision, including monitoring serum triglycerides and bone mineral density. Ingesting over 3,000 IU of retinol daily long-term, will interact poorly with vitamin D3, causing bone loss, and neutralize vitamin D's anti-cancer effects.

Beta carotene is pro-vitamin A, meaning it can be metabolized into true vitamin A. Generally about 10% of beta carotene we take in ends up being converted into vitamin A.

COD LIVER OIL

Cod liver oil is <u>not</u> recommended for cancer patients. It has been used for over 200 years "to support the immune system." It is rich in vitamin A, vitamin D, squalene, EPA and DHA, all of which are theoretically antineoplastic. However, vitamin A – as retinol – and vitamin D compete for the XRX-retinoid receptor.

Consequently, retinol vitamin A in high doses (over 3,000 IU daily) over some months will block all the health effects of vitamin D, including its effects on bone, heart, cancer, and so on. This explains some of the high rates of osteoporosis in Scandinavian countries, where cod liver oil use is part of the culture.

REVICI'S LIPIDS

Emanuel Revici, MD was an innovative and revolutionary thinker who developed non-toxic therapies for cancer and other diseases. Revici began researching the role of fats in cellular metabolism in the mid-1920's, and continued this work in Manhattan at the Institute of Applied Biology from 1947 to his death in 1998 at the age 101 years. He made house calls at the age of 100!

He tested urine pH to individualize "biologically guided chemotherapy" based on the normal daytime acidification from catabolic processes and the nightly alkalinity from anabolic processes. He described the catabolic phase as increasing entropy by electrostatic charges and fatty acid predominance. He described the anabolic phase as quantum forces which oppose degeneration and increase order. Anabolism provides "negentropy" or negative entropy, opposition to the tendency of all things to become unorganized and dispersed. Anabolism is directed by sterols such as estrogen, progesterone and adrenal hormones. Recall that body builders use anabolic steroids to bulk up. The opposite of anabolism is catabolism, the actions in the body which break down materials or cells. He used "guided lipid" therapy to balance any extreme of either phase, consisting of fatty acids, sterols, animal tissue extracts and minerals incorporated into lipids. His opus was the 1961 text *Research in Pathophysiology as Basis for Guided Chemotherapy with Special Application to Cancer*.

This work is being carried on by Dr. Lynn August, MD who continues research on creating food grade fats as medicines. Fundamental to her work is the thesis that the fats at the cell membrane are the final defence of the immune system, and that cellular fats regulate the cell's behaviour and health. Dr. August runs a consultation service called Health Equations which interprets standard medical blood tests to yield "biological indices" of the relative dominance of catabolism (breaking down), anabolism (building up), and other aspects of metabolism. Even if all the lab values for a patient are in the "normal" range, some indices may be outside a range that is consistent with stability and balance. As a general rule of thumb a lab value that is within one third of the range from the middle of the normal values to the limits of normal is within the ability of the homeostatic control mechanisms to keep things stable. However, in the outer two thirds of the normal range there is increasing instability. When several biochemical pathways become unstable, risk of disease can become significant. Thus the analysis can show degenerative tendencies so preventative corrective action can be taken before gross illness occurs. The emphasis is on correcting the diet with whole foods, and if necessary, nutritional supplements.

Revici's belief in the health value to the immune system of natural cholesterol in foods such as meat, eggs and butter is echoed in the work of Diana Schwarzbein, MD in her excellent dietary book The Schwarzbein Principle. Many chronic diseases such as diabetes, autoimmune diseases, cardiovascular disease, arthritis and cancer were not common in cultures which ate a lot of these now politically incorrect foods. Recall the "French Paradox" which is a low rate of heart disease in French people eating a lot of cheese, butter and meat cholesterol. As in all things, it is the balance and quality of the foods in the diet which is the real issue.

I certainly believe in the "Palaeolithic Diet" principles, that we should eat the way our ancestors did: whole foods that could be taken from Nature by picking, gathering, digging, hunting, fishing, milking. This Stone Age style of eating is proven to result in less cancer, heart disease, stroke, and auto-immune diseases than the modern agricultural foods diet.

We need fear what the farmer does to the animal, not meat itself. Wild game is a health food. Grass fed domesticated red-meat animals are nearly as good.

A chicken allowed to live the life allotted to a chicken by its Creator is a wonderful food, on which our races have thrived, until a farmer with a degree in chemistry was put in charge of feeding them.

It is time to admit that veterinary and nutritional science has led us down the garden path and is spoiling our animal foods as certainly as chemicalization is despoiling the environment at large. Until they can show modern agri-business is decreasing and reversing the horrendous rates of cancer we are facing, most people will reasonably remain suspicious of the latest creations.

CALCIUM-D-GLUCARATE

A salt of glucaric acid, calcium-D-glucarate CDG naturally occurs in citrus fruits such as oranges and in vegetables such as the Cruciferae cabbage family and potatoes. It also is naturally produced by friendly gut bacteria in the colon or large intestine, where it inhibits beta-glucuronidase activity. CDG increases net elimination of fat soluble carcinogens, toxins, steroid hormones.

Glucarate increases glucoronidation in Phase II liver detoxification pathways, lowering lipids, regulating estrogen metabolism, decreasing estradiol levels, preventing hormone dependent cancers such as breast, prostate and colon. Human dose range is 1.5 to 3 grams daily, e.g. 3 capsules 1 to 2 times daily of Tyler brand, a professional product line.

The B-VITAMIN COMPLEX

B-vitamins are widely used throughout the body as enzyme co-factors, particularly in energy metabolism. The need for B-vitamins increases during stress, illness, cancer, chemotherapy and radiation therapy.

B1 or thiamine is important in energy production, and helps regulate the mitochondria, the energy combustion chamber in cells. Mitochondria also act as a second line of control to turn off bad cells. The fat soluble form benfotiamine has been found to enter the mitochondria better, and also enters the fatty nerve cells better. This is why it is the best choice in treating nerve damage, and numbness after chemotherapy.

B2 or riboflavin is also a regulator of energy production.

B3 or niacin helps the function of the DNA repair gene polyADP ribase polymerase PARP. B3 as niacinamide is a terrific radio-sensitizer.

Vitamin B12 is very helpful in the repair of nerve injury. I will often give a shot of it intramuscularly at the nerve root, or just in the buttocks. It is also a boost to red blood cell building in anemia. It is a useful tonic for fatigue in elderly patients, who usually don't absorb it well by mouth.

Folic acid is needed by p53 to regulate apoptosis. Folate, as found in green leafy vegetables, reduces risk ovary, breast and colorectal cancers.

ANTI-OXIDANTS

Always use antioxidants in mixtures! Single anti-oxidants are like drugs – they can unbalance homeostasis – the tendency of our bodies to remain stable – and actually cause harm. Take them the way they are found in Nature, working together as a team to detoxify, fight infection, and to rejuvenate. They work together in a beautiful synergy.

Oxygen began to be available in the environment when bacteria developed blue-green pigments for photosynthesis. Later these tricks passed to algae as the little miracle of chlorophyll, which takes light and stores it into chemical energy. Now all plants use the technology, store the sun as food for all other living creatures, and release oxygen. Oxygen makes up 21% of the air we breathe.

About 2% of all the electrons moved through the electron transport system in the process of normal energy metabolism, and end up as free radicals of oxygen. Also called reactive oxygen species (ROS), they are highly toxic to all cells. The most common ROS is superoxide radical which becomes hydrogen peroxide, and in the presence of iron or copper ions, becomes the highly toxic hydroxyl radical.

Oxygen reacts with almost every other element. It "oxidizes" by moving electrons, making high energy compounds. Oxygen chemistry makes possible the higher life forms which are very active. However, it not only reacts, it burns. To keep it in check, plants make a lot of antioxidants, which squelch its harsher characteristics. When we have a good balance between the forces of oxidation, and its opposite, reduction, we enjoy a harmonious state of good health. Abundant plant foods in our diet give this balance.

Do we even need expensive research to tell us foods that prevent cancer and support health and healing processes are good for cancer care? There is a convincing body of evidence that antioxidants actually help patients feel better, and in fact help them to survive. See the book *Foods That Fight Cancer* by Doctors Gingras and Beliveau from McGill University. They have also made a cancer-fighting cookbook.

Antioxidants can induce selective apoptosis of cancer cells, leaving normal cells unharmed, induce differentiation in cancer cells, making them behave more normally, and reduce cancer cell proliferation – so tumours grow more slowly. I do not for one minute believe that all the anti-cancer properties of anti-oxidants are solely due to their anti-oxidant properties. The ability to cause an oxygenation or a reduction reaction (redox) is but one property of many biological molecules. Being an anti-oxidant neither qualifies nor disqualifies a food or supplement as a cancer remedy. The critical issue is balancing redox potential in healthy cells, tissues and organs to optimize the health and survival of the patient, while stressing the cancer cells. Selecting the right anti-oxidant at the right point in your care requires a deep knowledge of biochemistry.

Dr. Tim Birdsall, ND of Cancer Treatment Centers of America says that cancer cells accumulate anti-oxidants due to poor "gating control," which makes them more acidic and increases their rate of apoptosis.

Oncologists have been arguing that antioxidants are risky with chemotherapy since reactive oxygen species formed in chemotherapy are downstream mediators which may be needed to trigger apoptosis. In other words the doctors think taking vitamins and anti-oxidants might stop their drugs from working to kill cancer. However, there is no science to prove this hypothesis. This does not stop scientists from promulgating the fear of mixing safe vitamins with dangerous drugs. They err on the side of leaving patients under-nourished and subject to the full brunt of the drugs anti-nutrient effects. Why? The political and economic system sees nothing much to gain from researching something which anyone can make and sell. If no big drug company wants to invest big money, no real work gets done. Scientists sell their services for research grants. No grants, no answers to simple questions, therefore no inclusion in evidence-based medical practice. However, it is not actually the case that most of orthodox medicine is proven to a high standard to be safe or effective, nor is it true that naturopathic medicine is not supported by a wealth of good scientific evidence. We do need and welcome more research, however.

Reducing oxidative stress during chemotherapy shifts cell killing from necrosis towards apoptosis. Caspase activation and apoptosis follow cytochrome C release from mitochondria, which is an early event in cancer cells undergoing chemotherapy, therefore cancer cells may be committed to apoptosis well before ROS (reactive oxygen species or free radicals of oxygen) are generated. ROS also inhibit caspases, enzymes which disassemble the cell once pro-apoptotic signals are given. Anti-oxidants would de-inhibit the caspases, so would tend to drive apoptotic cancer cell killing.

The Conklin Hypothesis explains why anti-oxidants actually do not have a negative impact on the safety or efficacy of chemo drugs. In fact, studies run about 100 to 1 in favour of anti-oxidants providing real improvements in the performance and tolerability of various chemo regimens in common use. Conklin notes that cytotoxic chemotherapy typically induces massive oxidative stress – this is how it forces cancer cells into apoptosis. However, rampant lipid peroxidation ensues, creating poisonous aldehydes. Aldehydes prevent cancer cells from moving throughout the cell cycle to the checkpoint where apoptosis can begin. If we inhibit oxidation and aldehyde levels, we get more cancer cells able to enter apoptosis. There is slightly reduced oxidative pressure to throw the apoptosis off-switch, but more cells are entering the zone where the death switch can be thrown in the cancer cell. The net effect is two steps forward, and one step back – you are still one step ahead!

Evidence is clear that chemotherapy leaves patients vulnerable to severe deficits of anti-oxidants.

Intrinsic anti-oxidants such as albumin, bilirubin and uric acid will often be depleted by chemo. Watch the lab tests for these indicators, for they are clinically very significant. Actively restore anti-oxidant balance in these patients!

The chemo drugs which create the maximum oxidative stress are anthracyclines, followed by platinums, alkylating agents, epipodophyllotoxins, camptothecins, cytoarabinoside. Less oxidative are purine and pyrimidine analogues, anti-metabolites, taxanes and vinca alkaloids.

Anti-oxidants may actually help promote apoptosis, may protect normal cells from the drugs, and may help coordinate the entire sequence. Apoptosis after radiation and chemotherapy agents depend on death ligand receptors. Antioxidants can help many chemotherapy agents, X-ray and hyperthermia treatments ligate or tie into these receptors – in other words, helps them kill cancer cells.

Naturopathic physicians use antioxidants discreetly with drugs, as there are a few poor interactions. However, good research evidence supports our clinical observations of favourable interactions. I hope in time enough science is done to validate this approach to the satisfaction of all.

Dr. Prasad has recommended during chemo a basic protocol of 4 to 8 grams of vitamin C, 800 IU vitamin E as VES, 30 to 60 mg natural beta carotene, exercise, stress reduction, and a low fat, high fibre diet.

High fat diets often have a lot poly-unsaturated fatty acids (PUFAs) which are already rancid from reacting with air or can oxidize within the body. PUFA oxidation forms strongly electrophilic aldehydes which bind to cysteine-rich extracellular domains of death ligand receptors. Antioxidants prevent PUFA oxidation, so the death receptors can stay open for business – and kill cancer cells.

The foods that have the highest natural anti-oxidant levels are, in order: red beans, red kidney beans, pinto beans, blueberries, cranberries, artichokes, blackberries, prunes, raspberries, strawberries, red delicious apples, Granny Smith apples, pecans, cherries, black plums, russet potatoes, black beans, plums, and Gala apples. Carrot juice will reduce oxidative stress measurably in humans, whereas beta-carotene pills won't.

Hippocrates said it well: "Food shall be your medicine!"

VITAMIN C

Vitamin C is an essential dietary factor, accelerating hydroxylation reactions in bio-synthetic pathways.

It is important for immune health, connective tissue, and a myriad of vital functions.

Vitamin C status is commonly very low in persons with advanced cancer, and this deficiency is associated with shorter survival time, higher inflammatory marker C-reactive protein CRP in the blood, and low serum albumin.

Vitamin C or ascorbic acid selectively increases peroxide poisoning of cancer cells, without harming non-cancerous cells. Tumours produce less than normal of the catalase enzyme which removes naturally occurring peroxides, allowing a deadly build up of hydrogen peroxide H_2O_2.

Vitamin C regulates embryonic stem cell differentiation. Vitamin C also inhibits p53-induced replicative senescence through suppression of ROS production and p38 MAPK activity.

Vitamin C is also sometimes anti-apoptotic, inhibiting caspase-9 activity and suppressing induction of apoptosis by TNFa and angiotensin II. Working with vitamin

E, it up-regulates anti-apoptotic Bcl-2 protein and down-regulates pro-apoptotic Bax in normal tissue. Fortunately, the opposite happens in cancer cells.

Vitamin C improves mitogen responses and increases production of IL-2.

Vitamin C is very effective in reducing chemical toxicity to DNA and to the liver. Vitamin C and glutathione recycle each other.

If vitamin C is able to return to its unoxidized form after ultraviolet light exposure, sunburn cannot occur. This is best achieved with oral and topical grapeseed extract. I use the NASOBIH™ protocol with oral NutraCaps and topical NutraCream. See www.nasobih.com

In moderate doses it alters hyaluronidase activity, slowing the spread of cancer.

Doses of 500 to 1,000 mg are as effective as 5,000 mg doses to increase natural killer NK cell activity, reduce apoptosis and increase mitogenesis of immune cells, restoring functionality to the immune system. Ascorbic acid is essential for the synthesis of immunoglobulins.

Large oral doses can cause gas and crampy intestinal pains. Itchy skin is sometimes seen. In these cases consider the non-acidic "buffered" form of vitamin C, which is the mineral salts of ascorbic acid, such as calcium, potassium, sodium and magnesium ascorbates.

Serious harm can occur using high-dose vitamin C in patients with glucose-6-phosphate dehydrogenase (G6PD) deficiency, an in-born error of metabolism. It is mandatory to screen patients for this condition before prescribing intravenous vitamin C therapy.

High-dose vitamin C therapy can deplete copper levels. This inhibits angiogenesis.

Taper off high oral dose regimes slowly to avoid rebound scurvy. Allow two weeks to bring off 12 grams a day, reducing by about 1 gram daily.

Vitamin C can also act as a pro-oxidant at higher doses, and so is the most problematic anti-oxidant to mix with many of the chemotherapy drugs.

Vitamin C therapy is incompatible with the EGFR inhibitor drugs such as Erbitux / Cetuximab.

High-dose vitamin C can stimulate progression of leukemias. Use with great caution.

Intravenous Vitamin C – Used palliatively, in large IV doses, it will extend life in terminal patients. Linus Pauling promoted use of really high doses of vitamin C for many health problems, and suggested that 50 grams a day would impact human cancer. Only 10 to 20 grams can be taken orally before provoking diarrhea. At 12 grams by mouth the blood level peaks and taking more is pointless. Therefore he proposed putting 50 grams or more into the veins by a slow drip. In these doses it is pro-oxidant, forming hydrogen peroxide via mobilization of nuclear copper. This induces apoptosis selectively in cancer cells. Healthy cells can neutralize the peroxide with catalase enzyme.

In the early studies circa 1973 in Vale of Leaven Hospital in Scotland, Dr. Ewan Cameron and his associates found intravenous vitamin C did arrest some very advanced, terminal stage cancers. It must be noted 1 in 10 of these cases treated with IVC died abruptly from tumour lysis or internal bleeding. It is suspected that the blood came from the sudden lysis or dissolving of tumours – in other words, perhaps the therapy worked too well. The risk of tumour lysis is highest in patients with very rapidly growing and large cancers, or a very high tumour burden. The only treatment for tumour lysis syndrome is the prescription drug Allopurinol, and aggressive alkalization with intravenous bicarbonate.

Because of this reported danger of provoking sudden death, it was my policy for several years to only recommend this therapy in terminal cases, where the benefits may outweigh the risks. However, I am now reassured by my peers that this risk is extraordinarily rare, so rare that not a single death has occurred in the last decade.

The risk of tumour lysis and haemorrhage can be readily managed by starting with a trial dose of 15 grams, followed by blood testing for LDH, creatinine, serum C saturation and markers of oxidative stress. If this test dose is well tolerated, the dose can then be safely ramped up to 25, then 50 and even into the 60-75 gram range.

All patients need to be screened for the inherited metabolic problem glucose-6-phosphatase deficiency G6PD.

People with G6PD will become very ill from high dose vitamin C. Most cases will have discovered this issue in early childhood and will advise their doctors, but we still order blood tests to be sure.

The target serum level is about 400 mg/dl blood, the point of maximum cite-toxic effect. Exceeding this level does not increase efficacy. A normal serum level is 1-2 mg/dl.

IV vitamin C can stabilize a majority of cancer cases, arresting growth and spread of tumours. It can occasionally cure advanced cancer. It does this by producing hydrogen peroxide in cancer cells, making oxidative stress which forces the cancer cells into apoptosis – they die off and are recycled. This is also how chemo drugs and radiation kill cancer. IV vitamin C can also vastly improve quality of life by increasing appetite, raising platelet counts, easing fatigue, and reducing pain. Side-effects are therefore extraordinarily rare, but can include haemolytic anemia, bleeding, reduced competence of white blood cells, kidney stones.

Catechins in green tea rapidly transfer electrons or hydrogen from ROS damage sites on DNA, preventing the development of strand breaks. Tea catechins are very active against hydrogen peroxide, so <u>don't use green tea extracts during IV vitamin C therapy.</u>

Medical history:

- Glucose-6-phosphatase deficiency haemolysis– test through MDS labs (Children's Hospital)
- Kidney disease, renal insufficiency, including edema – recent serum creatinine and eGFR labs
- Potassium deficiency – recent Chemscreen of blood
- Congestive heart failure and fluid overload disorders such as ascites
- Iron overload – recent serum ferritin
- Kidney oxalate stones – recent urinalysis

IV Solutions:

- Use sodium ascorbate 500 mg/ml.
- Withdraw an equal volume of IV solution from the IV bag before adding the vitamin C
- Keep osmolality below 1,200 milliOsmals
- Ringer's lactate if 15 to 30 grams ascorbic acid
  - 250 to 1,000 ml bag for 15 grams
  - 500 to 1,000 ml bag for 30 grams
- Sterile water is used for doses 30 grams and higher
- 500 to 750 ml bag for 30 grams
- 500 to 1,000 ml bag for 60 grams
- 750 to 1,000 ml bag for 75 grams
- 1,000 ml bag for 100 grams
- Add- Magnesium:1,000 mg
  - B6:100 mg
  - B-complex:1 ml
  - B12:1 ml or 1,000 mcg

Administration:

- Start with 15 grams twice in the first week
- Week two use 30 grams
- Week three, raise to a maximum of 65 grams. Most do well at 30 to 60 grams.
- Check for ankle edema pre-treatment, during and after removal of the IV line
- Weigh the patient at each visit
- Check serum potassium, creatinine, etc. at about 3 weeks of therapy
- Infusions are given twice a week for 3 to 6 months, then may be reduced to once weekly
- for another 6 months, then once every 2 weeks for a year, then once monthly to maintain
- Suggested flow rate is 0.5 grams per minute, and must never exceed 1 gram per minute
- Target serum level of ascorbic acid is about 400 mg/ dl. Saturation falls off rapidly after infusion
- Shaking during infusion indicates low serum calcium – slowly push 10 ml calcium gluconate at less than 1 ml per minute.

Infusion Duration by Dose:

The time you will need to be at the clinic, and the cost per treatment, depend on the dose. High doses take quite a long time to administer, so patients need to be prepared – bladder empty, recently fed, and with some music of book or TV to pass the time. It takes a few minutes to hook up the IV, a few minutes to take it out, and you must remain in the clinic for at least 15 minutes after the IV, to ensure you are safe to be active and vertical again.

Assuming an infusion rate of 0.5 grams per minute:

15 grams takes 30 minutes to run, total time in care will be about 1 hour.
25 grams takes 50 minutes to run, total time in care will be about 1 hour and 20 minutes.
50 grams takes 100 minutes to run, total time in care will be about 2 hours and 10 minutes.
60 grams takes 120 minutes to run, total time in care will be about 2 hours and 30 minutes.
75 grams takes 150 minutes to run, total time in care will be about 3 hours.
100 grams takes 200 minutes to run, total time in care will be about 3 hours and 50 minutes.

Supportive therapy:

- Oral vitamin K2 menaquinone – 45 to 90 mg daily, plus seal oil 2 capsules twice daily.
- Oral vitamin C to bowel tolerance, maximum 12 grams or 1 level tablespoon daily
- Selenomethionine 200 mcg 1 to 2 times daily

Do not take high-dose green tea EGCG therapy or N-acetyl-cysteine NAC during IV Vitamin C therapy, as they counter-act the hydrogen peroxide effect. NAC is anti-apoptotic under some conditions.

VITAMIN K and CANCER

In general, vitamin K is pro-oxidative, and will stress cancer cells by generating free radicals of oxygen ROS.
Vitamin K = phylloquinone – also called K1
- made by plants and animals
- a cofactor in normal blood coagulation, involved in post-translational modification of factor II (prothrombin), VII, IX, X and proteins C, S and Z.
- when reduced to its hydroquinone form it's a cofactor in carboxylation of plasma protein glutamic acid residues via gamma-glutamyl-carboxylase.
- A cofactor in bone metabolism
- Inhibits cancer cell growth, transformation, differentiation, immortalization and resistance to apoptosis.

Oral K1 in doses of 40-45 mg daily produces mild responses in some cancers. Several vitamin K-dependent proteins are ligands for receptor tyrosine kinases. RTKs regulate cell signalling in cellular survival, transformation and replication; for example epidermal growth factor receptors, ras, ERK and MAPK pathways

K2 is the **menaquinone** form,
- aka MK-n where n describes the number of isoprene side chains at the 3rd carbon.
- made by bacteria and animals.
- benefits heart, bone and liver. Slows the loss of bone, increases bone density, strength and fracture resistance. Reduces the risk of liver cancer in hepatitis C cases.
- co-factor for K-dependent proteins responsible for cell-cell-adhesion, signal transduction and cell-cycle arrest.
- activates p21.
- inhibits liver cancer cell growth and invasion via activation of protein kinase A.
- active against myelodysplasia and leukemia, in oral doses of 45-90 mg daily, e.g. MK-4 15 mg tid.

K3 or **menadione** is a synthetic provitamin.
- a radiosensitizer at IV doses of 150-200 mg per day. It also synergizes with chemo and overcomes drug resistance. Maximum dose is 250 mg/m2. A common dose is 25 mg time-release K3 twice daily.
- pro-oxidant, and synergistic with intravenous vitamin C in a ratio of 100:1. For example 25 grams ascorbic acid with 250 mg menadione, diluted in an IV bag of D5W given as a slow infusion. This combination restores DNase activity essential for apoptosis. It depletes intracellular glutathione and other sulphydryl rich proteins by direct arylation of thiols. Because K3 is fat-soluble, most doctors prefer giving it by intramuscular injection or oral dosing, rather than in an IV.
- K3 induces cell cycle arrest via cyclin dependent kinases, such as myc and fos. The proto-oncogene c-myc codes for a nuclear protein transcription factor, while c-fos codes for a nuclear protein which is a component of AP-1 transcription complex regulating growth and tumour transformation promoters.
- Combining vitamin C with K3 causes cancer cells to die by autochizis. K3 + C are only to be used in patients who have had a laboratory test of their blood to determine that they do not have a deficiency of the enzyme glucose-6-phosphate dehydrogenase G6PDH. K3 is a potent inhibitor of G6PDH.

Do not give N-acetyl-cysteine during a pro-oxidative agents such as vitamin K oral or IV therapy.

Adapted from "The Anticancer Effects of Vitamin K" by Davis Lamson, MS, ND and Steven Plaza, ND, LAc, **Alt. Med. Rev**. 2003; Vol. 8 No. 3: 303-318.

GLUTATHIONE

GSH is the most powerful antioxidant substance, critical to good immune function, particularly against viral infection. However, it does not perform medically when taken by mouth. We make it from pre-cursors such as the amino acids glutamine, methionine and cysteine.

Glutathione is a detoxifier of alcohol, drugs, tobacco, pesticides, herbicides, xenobiotics, petroleum hydrocarbons, smog, pollution, heavy metals, many carcinogens and tumour promoters.

Glutathione is protected and regenerated by anthocyans as found in grapeseed extract, and interacts in an antioxidant network with selenium, vitamin C, vitamin E and alpha lipoic acid. It is the hub of the network, like a crown gear in a transmission. The dangerous energy latent in a free radical of oxygen is not neutralized completely until glutathione has dealt with it. All other anti-oxidant-free radical combinations are in themselves still free radicals, and still capable of dropping a lightning bolt on critical bio-molecules. Induces normal p53 activity by redox modulation, which induces apoptosis in tumours. Is a protectant in radiation and chemotherapy.

Milk whey protein has the glutathione precursor cysteine. Alpha-lactalbumin in fresh human milk induces apoptosis in malignant trophoblastic cells. Studies show whey protein reduces risk of getting cancer.

I do not recommend HMS90 whey powder from Immuno-Cal Labs, as it is not cost-effective for cancer, as might be claimed by some of its multi-level marketing "associates." No matter how many packets a day they take there has never been a clear response, nor do they worsen discontinuing it. I will say that it is useful for neurological conditions. I prefer to prescribe *Dream Protein* brand whey powder, which is sugar-free, and is rich in un-denatured alpha-lactalbumin and associated immune factors.

N-acetyl cysteine is the most commonly used supplement to raise GSH levels in humans, and despite propaganda by HMS-90 advocates, is perfectly safe in reasonable doses. All types of doctors have prescribed it for decades to thin mucus in bronchitis and pneumonia. It turns thick mucus to water. NAC may interfere with some pro-apoptotic therapies in the care of lung cancer. At this time, I do not use it in lung cancer cases.

Glutathione is reliably increased in human liver and other tissues by supplements of milk thistle herb, polygonum, grapeseed extract, pine bark pycnogenol, resveratrol, bilberry, turmeric and melatonin.

Glutathione levels drop when supplementing long-term with high doses of vitamin K3, vitamin C, L-glutamine vitamin D megadoses and *Salvia miltiorrhizae.* Glutathione depletion will inhibit or kill melanomas and cancers of the prostate, pancreas and colon.

Glutathione can be given in doses of up to 1,600 mg daily

Some naturopathic physicians provide intravenous administration of orthomolecular doses of pure glutathione in a normal saline drip, concurrent with chemotherapy. IV GSH can provoke pulmonary edema, and so must be stopped at the first sign of persistent coughing or shortness of breath.

See comment below regarding opposing views on the safety of IV GSH with chemotherapy. Some believe it can increase drug resistance, and increase risk of metastasis.

Glutathione is significantly lowered by smoking a single cigarette. Glutathione is particularly low in cancers of the lung and liver. People under toxic burden should always be striving to protect their glutathione reserves.

It is very controversial right now, but some of my most respected peers fear that glutathione will interfere with most of our active cancer therapies, which are dependent on a pro-oxidant effect. For this reason I recommend it during detoxification and recovery, but not during an active anti-tumour phase of treatment.

N-ACETYL-CYSTEINE

NAC is a supplement which can be converted in the body into the ultimate antioxidant cancer fighter glutathione GSH.

Contrary to what is said by persons trying to market cysteine-rich whey supplements, which may increase glutathione levels in humans, NAC is not toxic or dangerous in the oral dose range of 2 to 3 grams usually prescribed by physicians. At a therapeutic dose exceeding 4 grams a day, it is possible to see runny nose, mouth sores and skin rashes, gastro-intestinal upset, nausea. The primary side-effect of excess use is diarrhea. Rare instances have been seen of encephalopathy, thought to be due to mobilization of heavy metals, increased hippocampal excitotoxin release triggering dementia, bronchospasm and hypotension i.e. anaphylactic shock.

A significant lung protectant, it markedly thins excess mucus. It has long been prescribed by physicians treating emphysema, asthma, bronchitis, tuberculosis.

NAC elevates p53 activity in transformed cells but not in normal cells. NAC may increase apoptosis in cancer cells, but there are reports of it acting as an anti-apoptotic agent. This has put a chill on using it for lung cancer, among others.

I am not convinced that NAC, or glutathione itself, as single agents, have a significant role in controlling most cancers. Experience suggests that if combined with appropriate anti-oxidants such as grapeseed extract, selenomethionine, R+ alpha lipoic acid, and vitamin E, its redox potential would be better balanced. Networks of anti-oxidants do perform better and more safely.

I currently prescribe it primarily for severe lung congestion, and as part of short-term detoxification protocols, including heavy metal detoxification.

Supports liver detoxification in Phase 2 conjugation reactions.

Suppresses NFkB activity, as does glutathione GSH and vitamin C

Inhibits viral transcription and boosts cellular immunity

Directly inhibits TNFa.

Chelates out toxic heavy metals and copper.

It is likely to interfere with most cancer therapies in the same way we described for glutathione, so is to be avoided until the detoxification and recovery phase of care.

Do not mix with therapeutic doses of vitamin C, vitamin K3, vitamin D3, melatonin, green tea EGCG, quercetin, resveratrol, feverfew, sage and curcumin.

Never mix with the platinum chemo drugs such as Cisplatin and Carboplatin.

Naturopathic Oncology

Top researchers and physicians in the field of integrative oncology such as Prasad, Block and Conklin advise against using NAC during chemotherapy, and also against taking the other endogenous (made in the body) anti-oxidants glutathione and alpha lipoic acid during chemo. They feel safer with the exogenous anti-oxidants, as found in food, such as vitamins C, E and natural carotenes.

GRAPESEED EXTRACT

Oligomeric-proanthocyanidins (OPC) including resveratrol in grape skins and seeds are powerful antioxidants, perhaps 50 times that of vitamin C and 20 times that of vitamin E. They are highly chemoprotective, and have significant effects on the vascular endothelium. OPC from pine bark was brought to Canada by Dr. Allen Tyler, ND, MD by way of the French scientist Professor Jacques Masquelier, who investigated its use by Quebec First Nations people.

Modern Chinese research has shown this antioxidant to be a balanced cancer treatment.

- Potent anti-oxidant, OPCs activate and restore/ recycle R+ alpha lipoic acid, glutathione, vitamin E and vitamin C.
- Reduces ROS activation of AP-1 protein
- OPC are significantly cytotoxic to human breast, lung and gastric adenocarcinomas, while at the same time enhancing the growth and viability of normal cells.
- OPC can regulate cell cycle/apoptosis genes p53, bcl-2, and c-myc. OPC increase expression of Bcl-2 gene and reduce expression of p53 and c-myc genes. This is how they reduce healthy cell apoptosis caused by chemotherapy drugs, reducing their toxicity.
- Inhibits DNA synthesis
- Anti-angiogenic, reduces VEGF induction by TNFa.
- Inhibits EGF
- Inhibits MAPK pathway
- Activates JNK protein, a regulator of apoptosis
- Induces cyclin kinase
- Inhibitor of p21 and Cip1.
- Up-regulates insulin-like growth factor one binding protein three IGF-BP-3 by several-fold.
- Aromatase inhibitor and suppressor of aromatase expression. Procyanidin B dimmers suppress estrogen biosynthesis, reducing circulating estrogen by about 80%, on par with some aromatase inhibitor drugs.
- Anti-inflammatory, inhibits NFkB, COX-1 and COX-2.
- Anti-viral. Increases lymphocyte immune cell proliferation.
- Increases natural killer cell NK activity
- GSE causes endothelium-dependent NO-mediated relaxations of arteries. This effect involves the intracellular formation of ROS in endothelial cells leading to the Src kinase/phosphoinositide 3-kinase/Akt-dependent phosphorylation of

eNOS. This may explain its effect on hot flashes, and asthma.
- Restores the integrity of the blood-brain barrier.
- Grapeseed extract is incompatible with N-acetyl-cysteine.

The daily therapeutic dose should be at least 400 mg daily. Usually this would be two of 100 mg capsules twice daily. Dr. Baker suggests using up to 4 capsules 4 times daily (1600 mg) for the first week, for a potent anti-inflammatory effect. This is synergistic with omega 3 marine oils. The dose is brought down to 3 caps 4 times daily the second week, 2 caps 4 times daily the next week, then 2 caps 3 times daily thereafter. Dr. Baker and I prefer the NASOBIH™ NutraCaps with 100 mg Protovin™ grapeseed extract, 20 mg resveratrol, 100 mg citrus bioflavonoids, and 100 mg vitamin C.

Similar compounds are found in the TCM herb Polygonum cuspidatum, Lycium fruit, better known as Goji or wolfberry, hawthorn berries, cocoa and almonds.

One of my primary motivations to write the first edition of *Naturally There's Hope* was to convey the importance of a combination of grapeseed extract, curcumin and green tea EGCG for the control of growth and spread of many cancers. There is a wonderful synergy between these non-toxic agents. Used in adequate doses of appropriate quality, responses can be quite gratifying.

I do not believe the absurdly primitive concept that some herbalists put forward that OPCs enhance metastasis simply because they are a "circulation enhancer." Even the concept of circulation enhancement is a nebulous one.

These bioflavonoids astringe the vascular endothelium, reducing leaks and building vessel wall integrity.

RESVERATROL

Resveratrol is a lipophilic anti-fungal called 3, 4,'5-trihydroxy-trans-stilbene phytoalexin.

Commonly derived from grape skins, therefore it is present in red wine at about 9 to 28 micromoles per glass. Grape juice is high in resveratrol and quercetin. Small amounts are also found in rice, peanuts, mulberries, giant knotweed and *Polygonum* herb.

- antioxidant which modulates manganese-super-oxide dismutase MnSOD.
- Chemo-preventative, increases glutathione retention
- Anti-angiogenic, inhibits VEGF activity.
- Inhibits DNA synthesis in S-phase of the cell cycle
- Inhibits MMP-2 matrix metallo-proteinase, blocking invasion and spread.
- increases lymphocytic anti-cancer cytokines.
- inhibitor of nuclear transcription factor NFkB, COX-2, JNK, Bcl-2, IGFR-1.
- antioxidant which modulates MnSOD
- pro-apoptotic via activation of caspase 3, and by a reduction in the Bcl-2/Bax ratio in favour of apoptosis.
- regulator of cyclin-dependent kinase CDK, induces its inhibitor p21WAF1/CIP, inhibits cyclin D1 and cyclin E

173

- blocks formation of estrogen-DNA adducts responsible for initiating breast cancer.
- Stimulates transcription of endogenous estrogen receptor.
- Inhibits BRCA-1 mutant cancer cells via reduced Survivin expression
- Suppresses CYP 1B1

Aggarwal has done quite a bit of research on resveratrol. Not all studies suggest *in vivo* efficacy. It is a phytoestrogen, and safety in post-menopausal ER+ breast cancer remains to be determined.

Dan Rubin suggests the pterostilbene methylated forms are the most effective, and so has used *Xymogen* brand, Rx: 2 caps, and adds 750 mg of the trans-form in the *Biotivia* brand. At higher doses we need to monitor for a possible reduction in platelets, and kidney stress including cast nephropathy.

BILBERRY

Vaccinium myrtillus or bilberry is a relative of the blueberry, cranberry and huckleberry. All are rich in anthocyanosides which are known to strengthen collagen. The anthocyanidin delphinidin in bilberry is a very powerful redox recycler of glutathione.

Delphinidins strongly inhibit EFR kinases, VEGF-2, ERK1/2, and chemotactic motility.

Anthocyanidins combined with glutathione in the product Recancostat has been found to suppress advanced chemo-resistant colon carcinoma, with increased survival and weight gain.

Daily dose should be over 100 mg of an extract standardized to 25 to 37% anthocyanosides.

POMEGRANATE

Pomegranate juice contains quercetin, ellagic acid, anthocyanidins, EGCG catechin, sterols, gallic acid, caffeic acid, vitamin C and iron. It has a unique ellagitannin punicalagin, the largest molecular weight polyphenol known.

Anthocyanidins and tannins in pomegranate fruit and juice inhibit tumorigenesis, inhibit angiogenesis, modulate UV-mediated phosphorylation of mitogen-activated protein kinases MAPK, and strongly inhibit activation of nuclear factor kappa B NFkB. Pomegranate down-regulates pro-inflammatory eicosanoids.

Ellagitannins in pomegranate are often hydrolyzed and absorbed as ellagic acid.

The ellagic acid content is also responsible for much of pomegranate's inhibition of prostate cancer, in doses as low as 8 ounces daily of the juice. Gut flora metabolize ellagitannins into bioactive urolithins which inhibits prostate cancer by suppressing testosterone synthesis and androgen receptor gene expression.

Pomegranate flavonoids inhibit aromatase, preventing synthesis of estrogen from adrostenedione and testosterone. They also strongly inhibit 17-estradiol growth signalling in breast cancer cells.

ELLAGIC ACID

Ellagic acid is found in many plant foods, including algae, but is highest in fruits and berries such as pomegranates, raspberries, blueberries, strawberries and grapes.

This is a potent anti-oxidant phenolic, with great value as an inhibitor of DNA mutations, including the "Guardian of the DNA, the p53 gene. This is the crux of cancer prevention.

It can act as a pro-oxidant in cancer cells, generating free radicals of oxygen ROS. This can restore the off switch in the cancer cell –the apoptosis suicide and recycling program.

It is also somewhat liver protective, anti-viral and anti-bacterial.

A significant portion of the protective effects of a diet rich in fruits and vegetables is attributable to this compound. Ellagic acid helps us to eliminate carcinogens such as fungal toxins, polycyclic aromatic hydrocarbons and nitrosamines.

Human studies show a potent action in prostate cancer – a single eight ounce glass of unsweetened pomegranate juice daily can arrest and even reverse early prostate cancer. From cell and rodent studies one can predict with certainty the same benefit will be seen when other cancers are treated with this nutraceutical.

BLACK RASPBERRIES

Raspberry anthocyanidins can prevent oral and esophageal pre-cancerous lesions from progressing to squamous cell cancer by activating tumour suppressor genes and restoring differentiation.

SALVESTEROLS

Salvesterols are a group of resveratrol-related plant anti-fungals which Dr. Gerry Potter has proposed are pro-drugs, bio-activated in cancer cells into a toxin called piceattanol. This is possible because only cancer cells have an active enzyme CYP1B1. Salvesterols may be found in organic plants stressed by fungi and molds. Sources include artichokes, rosehips, agrimony herb, hawthorn berries, plantain, burdock, chamomile grapes, strawberries and cranberries. They are claimed to inhibit tubulin synthesis, inhibit tyrosine kinase, etc. They are said to be incompatible with flaxseed, kiwi fruit, almonds, tobacco smoke, grapefruit, lima beans, and other foods.

Despite great promise, and impeccable basic science leading up to the human trials, I fail to see any responses with this product. NOT RECOMMENDED

Natural plant pesticides are very biologically active in cancers. We have better results and research to support prescribing resveratrol, curcumin, epicgallo-catechin gallate EGCG, allicin and sulforaphane.

QUERCETIN

Quercetin is a natural polyphenolic bioflavonoid found in many foods and herbs, such as white oak bark, apples and onions. The average diet provides about 25 mg daily. It is the primary dietary bioflavonoid. Quercetin is 3,3,'4,'5,7-pentahydroxyflavone, a sugarless (aglycone) form of rutin, and it can easily oxidize to a quinoid form which is a redox agent. Quercetin modulates the redox state and oxidative metabolism. Inhibits high aerobic glycolysis of tumour cells and thus inhibits ATP synthesis

Quercetin is significantly higher in plants grown in organic compost versus chemical fertilizer. The plants use it to extract nitrogen from the soil.

Bioflavonoids like quercetin inhibit thyroid peroxidase, which adds the iodine to thyroid hormone, and will aggravate hypothyroidism in patients with inadequate iodine consumption. For this reason we may combine it with potassium iodide supplementation.

An aromatase inhibitor, it reduces estrogen hormone formation in adipose tissue (fat cells). The aromatase gene CYP19 expression is promoted by prostaglandins sensitive to COX -2 inhibitors.

Binds type II estrogen receptors in breast, colon, ovary, melanoma, leukemia and meningeal cancer cells, inhibiting growth. ER-2 receptors have only a weak affinity for estrogen, and probably inhibit growth when stimulated by flavonoids. ER-2 expression is independent of ER-1 status, and the effective growth inhibition in breast cancer is equal to Tamoxifen.

Quercetin activates aryl hydrocarbon receptor AhR –dependent breast cancer resistance protein BCRP. It can be supported in this action by resveratrol, indole-3-carbinol and curcumin. It inhibits proteasomal degradation of AhR by green tea EGCG.

Down-regulates expression of mutant p53 protein, arresting human breast cancer cells in G2-M phase of the cell cycle and human leukemia cells T-cells and human stomach cancer cells in G1-S phase. DNA replication is thus markedly reduced.

Inhibits heat shock proteins, which disrupts formation of complexes of mutant p53 and HSPs which would allow tumour cells to bypass normal cell cycle checkpoints. No HSPs means no mutant p53 activity. If HSPs are left unchecked there is a risk of shorter disease-free survival and increased chemotherapy drug resistance in breast cancer.

Enhances NK cell activity and is immune stimulating. Inhibits replication of RNA and DNA viruses. Inhibits DNA polymerases B and I.

Induces apoptosis; blocks tumour export of lactate, resulting in a lethal drop in tumour pH, triggering pH-dependent apoptosis endonucleases. Normalizes mitochondrial control of apoptosis.

Cytotoxic effect is dose-dependent. When giving quercetin, always include an absorption adjunct such as bromelain or bioperine, or the quercetin may not be absorbed sufficiently to be medically useful. While quercetin is mutagenic to bacteria, it is not carcinogenic in humans.

Inhibits cyclooxygenase COX-2 transcription and lipoxygenase especially the LOX-5 / 5-HETE eicosanoid pathway. Reduces pro-inflammatory NFkB nuclear transcription protein.

Arrests p21-ras proto-oncogene, expression, a mutation found in 50% of colorectal cancers. The p21-ras mutation impairs cellular GTP-ase, allowing continual activation of the signal for DNA replication in colon cancer and many other tumour types.

Blocks peroxide inhibition of cell-cell signalling. Inhibits invasion and metastasis.

Suppresses signal transduction pathways such as protein kinase C and casein kinase II, preventing these signals from the cell surface to the nucleus from over-riding normal growth controls.

Interferes with the porter system ion pump, also called P-glycoprotein, which can pump drugs right out of cancer cells. This is like bailing water out of a sinking boat. Giving quercetin with many chemo drugs helps hold enough chemo inside the cancer cells to overcome multi-drug resistance MDR to effect a cure. It also restricts drug resistance by inhibition of heat shock protein HSP-70.

Increases effectiveness of radiation and chemotherapy, especially doxorubicin, ribavirin and tamoxifen.

Quercetin blocks epidermal growth factor receptor EGFR and reduces activity in the HER-2 signal pathway.

My learned colleagues at the Cancer Treatment Centers of America (**CTCMA**) prescribe a quercetin combination BCQ – bromelain, curcumin and quercetin – from Vital Nutrients at doses of 2 capsules three times daily. I use a Canadian version called Can-Arrest, or quercetin plus bromelain as compounded by my pharmacist. Dr. Leanna Standish, ND, PhD prescribes 1,000 mg twice daily. That is typically 2 capsules twice daily.

*AppleBoos*t is an interesting new product rich in free phenols and polyphenols, including quercetin and quercetin conjugates. It is a concentrate from apple peels, with a very high anti-oxidant ORAC score. Apple extracts appear to have particular benefit in squamous cell cancers. *An apple a day keeps the doctor away.*

Quercetin induced apoptosis via inhibition of Akt/PKB phosphorylation, an upstream kinase of pro-survival protein kinase cascade. Inhibition of Akt phosphorylation was coupled with a significant decrease of anti-apoptotic Bcl-2 and Bcl-XL. Quercetin caused a down-regulation of Cu-Zn Superoxide Dismutase which perhaps led to an increase of reactive oxidative stress (ROS). The decrease of Bcl-2 and Bcl-XL along with this oxidative stress caused release of mitochondrial cytochrome c into the cytosol and subsequent induction of pro-caspase-9 processing.

Quercetin inhibits the proliferative effect on breast cancer cells of environmental xeno-estrogens such as bis-phenol A and diethylstilbestrol DES.

Quercetin is highly synergistic with ellagic acid. The combination markedly increases activation of p53, p21 (cip1/waf1), MAP kinases, JNK1, 2 and p38. This results in apoptosis in cancer cells.

Quercetin inhibits lymphocyte tyrosine kinases.

Reactions are extremely rare, but just to illustrate the odd things one must expect in clinical practice, one patient experienced a dull headache, band-like around the head, became very spacey, losing words and thoughts, had a general sick and nauseated feeling, with shaky, wobbly legs making it hard to stand. This repeated several times until quercetin was stopped.

Extreme doses are toxic to the kidneys.

CAROTENOIDS

Beta carotene (provitamin A), lycopene, lutein, and other carotenoids in the diet are strongly associated with reduced risk of various cancers. There may be a therapeutic role in breast, prostate and cervical cancers.

Lycopene reduces IGF-1 stimulation of cancer cell growth in hormone dependent tumours, and is best derived from cooked tomatoes. L.O.M. is an exciting new high dose supplement of lycopene and lycopene-like carotenoids phycoene and phytofluene, from a specially bred tomato. The dose is 1 tablet twice daily. Take care to keep this product out of the light.

Lutein is found in spinach, broccoli, oranges, carrots, lettuce, tomatoes, celery and green vegetables.

Synthetic beta-carotene or as a high-dose supplement without other natural carotenoids is not recommended in cancer care. These can become a catalytic pro-oxidant in high-oxygen tissues – thus an increase risk for lung cancers when given to smokers. However, retinoids reduce risk of developing cancer when given after quitting smoking. Vitamin E supports lung repair as well. Grapeseed extract is stable in the lungs, and gives an opposite, positive effect in reducing risk of lung cancer in active smokers. Of course we must urge smokers to quit, since it is the single most preventable cause of cancers.

MELATONIN

Melatonin is the natural indoleamine hormone produced in the pineal gland in the brain. The daily variation in light received by the eye tells the pineal gland to make bursts of melatonin. In more technical detail: the enzyme N-acetyltransferase emitted in a circadian cycle from the suprachiasmatic nucleus after photic stimulation through the retinohypothalamic tract converts serotonin into melatonin. This internal body clock, designed to work under natural light, makes a daily hormone tide which creates a biological rhythm.

Outdoors on a bright sunny day we are exposed to a light intensity of about 100,000 Lux. Outdoors on a dull rainy day this falls to about 10,000 Lux. However, a well-lit classroom only provides about 400 Lux of ambient light. Obviously living under artificial light is not stimulating our pineal system the way natural light does.

Pinealectomy (removal of the gland) enhances tumour growth and metastasis in experimental animals. Pineal extracts, even if melatonin-free, inhibit human cancer cells.

Working rotating night shifts or going to bed after 2 am increases risk of breast cancer, presumably due to suppression of melatonin production. Normally melatonin levels peak between 2 and 3 am. Melatonin suppresses the synthesis and secretion of sex hormones by promoting the release of gonadotropin-releasing hormone.

Melatonin production is suppressed by morning light, and that promotes alertness. The ideal light to switch off melatonin is blue light at 480 nanometres wavelength. We only see down to about 555 nm, but the closest light to 480 we see is the bright blue color of the sky on a sunny day. Beta-blocker drugs for blood pressure and fast heartbeat depress melatonin secretion.

Long-term safety as a supplement is well established – for example melatonin has long been used in Europe in oral contraceptives. For insomnia and jet-lag we use 1 to 3 mg at bedtime. It can treat gastro-esophageal reflux disorder GERD. For cancer we use 10 to 20 mg at "bedtime" only!

IMPORTANT NOTE: <u>Never</u> take melatonin at any other time than at bedtime – what we call "the hour of sleep" – in the late evening. This is 8 pm to 12 midnight only! This is an example of chronobiology, the timing of administration of medicines to match natural biological cycles. If you forget to take it during the prescribed time of day, do not take any. Wait until the next evening. The dose is reduced if the patient has nightmares or feels groggy in the morning. Rare persons experience agitation or depression when over-dosed. After about 3 years of use the dose should drop to a maximum of 5 to 6 mg at bedtime.

Avoid melatonin for patients with disseminated cancers such as leukemia, lymphoma and multiple myeloma. It may be used short-term during chemo or radiation, but only as prescribed by a physician experienced in integrative oncology.

Melatonin inhibits corticotrophin-releasing factor, reducing cortisol levels and that of other adrenal corticoids. For this reason its use may be contra-indicated in patients on Prednisone or Dexamethasone or other steroid medication, or for persons with asthma, auto-immune diseases, infertility or adreno-cortical insufficiency.

There is a small theoretical risk of interaction if combined with SSRI antidepressant drugs such as Paxil – it could provoke serotonin syndrome, with a sudden rise in blood pressure.

Melatonin is a balancer and stabilizer in all stages of solid tumours: Melatonin is very helpful in most cancers, not just hormone dependent types.

- improves survival time as a sole agent in terminal cancer.
- doubles survival time and response rate to conventional therapy in all hormone sensitive cancers.
- antioxidant in low doses, protecting DNA, RNA and cellular membranes from oxidation.
- pro-oxidant in cancer cells at higher doses
- inhibits cancer initiation, anti-carcinogen.
- modulates hormones – estrogen, testosterone, prolactin and may make tumours more hormone dependent, which is more amenable to treatment
- blocks mitogenic effects of hormones and growth factors.
- Melatonin directly and indirectly inhibits epidermal growth factor receptor EGFR.
- increases effectiveness of radiotherapy, reduces myelodysplasia
- increases gap junction intercellular communication
- controls fatty acid uptake, transport and metabolism, by suppression of cAMP at plasma membranes.
- improves glucose tolerance.
- increases p53 expression

- increases apoptosis
- modifies cytokines, increasing host immune defences via thymus and T-helper cell derived opoid peptides, and enhances thymocyte proliferation.
- immuno-modulator – increases INFg, IL 1, 2, and 12
- decreases circulating cytokine interleukin 6 (IL-6) significantly
- synergistic with IL-2 therapy, increases effectiveness up to ten fold, allowing use of only 10% of the usual dose.
- NK cells have receptors for melatonin and IL-2; melatonin increases NK number and lytic activity.
- inhibits NFkB transcription factor, reducing pro-inflammatory cytokines.
- Inhibits AP-1 activator protein, decreasing cancer cell proliferation.
- down-regulates 5-lipoxygenase gene expression
- reduces TNF secretion
- reduces cachexia, along with omega 3 EPA and antioxidants R+ alpha lipoic acid, grapeseed extract OPCs, and vitamins C and E.
- increases response and survival with chemotherapy – reduces myelosuppression (bone marrow damage) and thrombocytopenia (loss of platelets needed for blood clotting).
- Melatonin levels tend to be lowest in estrogen- receptor positive breast cancer cases.
- Aromatase inhibitor/ down-regulator, blocking estrogen bio-synthesis from testosterone via CYP-19 aromatase and NADPH-CYP reductase, at serum levels of 1 nM – as seen with natural night-time synthesis of melatonin in healthy subjects.
- decreases production of estrogen receptors in breast cells, and is a primary selective ER modulator, and therefore synergistic with Tamoxifen
- increases serotonin, which has an anti-depressant effect.
- naturally increases with meditation (focused awareness exercises) or breathing exercises.
- naturally increases with aerobic exercise.
- occurs naturally in rice, corn and oats.
- inhibits telomerase,
- increases p53
- thermo-regulator

Melatonin levels and cycles can be naturally regulated by sleeping in a completely dark room between 10 pm and 6 am, for a period of at least one month. A night-mask may be used. There must be no exposure to light above 50 Lux intensity – which means no night-light, no exposure to the refrigerator light, no turning the light on in the bathroom at night, etc.

Melatonin production is said to be disrupted by electro-magnetic fields, so it is recommended that no electrical appliances or outlets be within 1 meter from your head during sleep.

If possible also get at least 20 minutes exposure to outdoor natural light in the early morning hours.

CO-ENZYME Q-10

Co-enzyme Q-10 or ubiquinone is a fat soluble antioxidant critical to cell energy production. CoQ-10 carries protons and electrons in the inner membrane of the mitochondria – the sugar-oxygen combustion chambers inside all cells – to assist energy production. It can re-activate production of ATP bio-chemical energy for repair and healing in damaged cells, tissues and organs.

- intestinal absorption is poor, and may limit effectiveness; take with some oil or fat, – olive, flax.
- essential for production of immuno-globulins
- maintains vitamin E and related tocopherols and tocotrienols in an anti-oxidant state.
- CoQ-10 is absolutely a must for any organ failure, such as congestive heart failure, liver failure or kidney failure, as may be triggered by chemotherapy drug poisoning.
- use preventatively before, during and after chemotherapy with heart-damaging drugs – for example Herceptin or the anthracyclines such as Adriamycin, Doxorubicin, Epirubicin.
- do not use CoQ-10 during radiation therapy, as it reduces effectiveness.
- strongly inhibits mitochondrial pyruvate dehydrogenase kinase enzyme. This reduces lactate, a cancer growth factor and inhibitor of apoptosis.
- CoQ-10- may improve survival in several types of cancer; early studies show dramatic regression rates in advanced breast cancer – in combination with alpha lipoic acid, selenomethionine, vitamins B1 as benfotiamine, B3 as nicotinamide, vitamin C, vitamin E, beta carotene, 3-6-9 essential fatty acids, and magnesium.

CoQ-10 with appropriate adjuncts will restore mitochondrial control over apoptosis, resulting in dramatic killing of cancer cells and clearance of tumours See the "Mitochondrial Cancer Cure."

Strongly inhibits metastasis in melanoma.

Reports describe clearance of liver metastases and pleural effusions.

I prescribe 300 mg a day, and never reduce this. At doses of 600 to 1,200 mg there can be problems with heartburn, headaches and fatigue.

ALPHA LIPOIC ACID

Alpha lipoic acid or thioctic acid is a water and fat soluble thiol anti-oxidant. It is called the universal anti-oxidant because it works in both the fatty cell plasma membranes and the aqueous interior (cytosol) of the cell It is 100 times stronger inhibitor of free radicals of oxygen than vitamins E and C combined. It protects DNA, the mitochondria energy producing part of a cell, and reduces cellular inflammation.

- increases glutathione activity

- very supportive of detoxification from drugs and poisons
- reduces fibrosis by down-regulating an iso-enzyme of transitional (transforming) growth factor beta TGFß responsible for fibroblast matrix deposition. Very important in restoring kidney filtration.
- recycles vitamin C and E
- NFkB inhibitor
- blocks heat shock proteins
- improves insulin function and decreases insulin resistance
- essential for production of immunoglobulins
- improves mitochondrial energy production by squelching oxidative stress
- inhibits pyruvate dehydrogenase kinase (synergistic with C0-Q-10), reducing lactate, increasing apoptosis.
- powerful therapy for all forms of neuropathy – from chemo drugs like the platinums or diabetes.
- Reduces angiogenesis by chelating copper.
- Chelates heavy metals
- neuroprotective
- allows toxic homocysteine to accumulate in cancer cells.

R+ is the naturally occurring form. If the product does not say R+ then it is synthetic, and 50% is in the L+ form, which is not only useless, it is toxic. Sustained release is used because it has a very brief half-life in the blood, clearing in minutes. Do not waste your time, money and health on products that do not meet this standard.

Rx 150 to 300 mg three times daily of a time-release preparation of R+ ALA. I have long used the lower dose schedule, based on human studies using it for diabetic neuropathy, but was inspired to increase it to the higher range by Keith Block, MD. Dr. Block is a medical oncologist (chemo doc) with over 30 years clinical experience. He runs an integrative cancer center in Chicago, and is editor-in-chief of the excellent peer-reviewed medical journal Integrative Cancer Therapies. He has an excellent book which is in concordance with my ideas and writings. See www.lifeovercancer.com for lots of useful resources, scientific references, and his book on cancer.

Some naturopathic physicians use Poly-MVA, a trimeric palladium lipoic complex with vitamins thiamine and B12. I do not think it worth the price, and so cannot recommend it.

R+ALA is highly synergistic with grapeseed extract OPCs, which recycle it into its active state.

R+ALA is incompatible with artemisinin therapy, and is not recommended concurrent with curcumin.

VITAMIN E

Vitamin E is a family of compounds called tocopherols and tocotrienes, which are fat-soluble anti-oxidants. Vitamin E compounds protect fats in cell membranes from oxidizing. When vitamin E levels are too low, the cell membranes get stiff and cannot pass nutrition in and wastes out.

Synthetic vitamin E is dl-alpha tocopherol, and should be avoided, Natural source vitamin E has always been considered to be d-<u>alpha</u>-tocopherol. This is what has been sold for generations as vitamin E. However, the most biologically important form of E in food is <u>gamma</u> tocopherol, Taking a lot of the alpha-E will dilute down the gamma E in cell membranes, which turns out to be unhealthy. This why many studies of synthetic E show poor outcomes, and those on alpha-E do not show benefit. I only recommend the mixed tocopherols, such as Vitazan E-10.

Especially as injected vitamin E succinate or VES, vitamin E promotes apoptosis, independent of genes p21 and p53. Stimulates cell differentiation, inhibits angiogenesis, inhibits TNF, turns off NFkB and other pro-inflammatory genes.

Vitamin E is protective against breast, colon and prostate cancer. The alpha form of tocopherol is particularly linked to reduction of risk of lung cancer – up to 53% at high doses.

Vitamin E increases the cytotoxic activity of 5-fluorouracil, doxorubicin and cisplatin by inducing p53. It reduces mucositis.

Vitamin E is highly protective of lungs, brain and other high oxygen tissues. In this regard it is a good match with grapeseed extract OPCs. Vitamin E is maintained in an anti-oxidant state by Co-enzyme Q-10, and also synergizes with selenium and vitamin C.

Vitamin E is very protective against radiation damage. High doses may reduce radiation effectiveness against cancer cells, and so are not recommended during radiotherapy.

Vitamin E is often described as a blood thinner, but it rarely actually increases bleeding. Some individuals may have an unexplained interaction with menaquinone MK-4 and vitamin K activation.

ANTI-OXIDANT SUMMARY

- Always use natural sources and forms.
- Use moderate doses, unless you intend to have a pro-oxidative effect. High doses tend to switch into pro-oxidants, particularly in high-oxygen tissues such as the lungs and brain.
- Use mixtures, as these nutrients form a complex and inter-dependent network.
- Anti-oxidants alone are never a cure for cancer (and neither is oxygen) but they help us to manage the oxidative stress which is the prime driver of apoptosis of cancer cells.
- Some cancer alternative pioneers thought some foods contained oxygen inhibitors, and thus reduced the ability to oxidize toxins: tomatoes, alcohol, coffee, lentils, beans, and meats. Certainly alcohol and coffee and other stimulants impair glucose tolerance and insulin sensitivity. Hoxsey and Koch warned against eating tomatoes. Legumes were not a staple in pre-agricultural diets; but seem healthy in the context of the Mediterranean diet.

D - LIMONENE

Limonene is found in citrus fruit and celery. D-limonene down-regulates K-ras to reduce epidermal growth factor receptor EGFR over-amplification.

MUSHROOMS

Common white button mushrooms *Agaricus bisporus* contain potent aromatase inhibitors, useful in breast and prostate cancers. Women who eat mushrooms frequently have reduced risk of breast cancer.

CURCUMIN

Curcumin is derived from the yellow curry spice, the turmeric root –*Curcuma longa* or yu jin. Dietary intake is protective against various cancers.

Induces apoptosis by altering all the Bcl-2 family of proteins. Active in many cancers, such as liver, kidney, sarcoma, colon, rectum, ovary and multiple myeloma.

Highly chemoprotective, blocks tumour induction by chemical carcinogens, inhibits cancer initiation, promotion and progression

Curcumin slows phase 1 liver detox while accelerating phase 2 detox, preventing the build-up of toxic intermediates. This makes it essential in detoxification programs, to prevent the nasty side-effects often euphemistically referred to as a "healing crisis."

- Antioxidant against superoxide, hydroxyl radicals, peroxynitrite.
- Inhibits inducible nitric oxide synthetase by reducing its mRNA transcription.
- Decreases eicosanoids such as 5-HETE and PGE-2 to strongly reduce inflammation
- Prevents activation of nuclear factor kappa B, inhibiting inflammation. It does so primarily by binding iron and copper ions which induce NFkB.
- Curcumin reduces pain, and is widely used in formulas for pain and inflammation. Look for synergies with boswellia, bromelain, ginger and picrorhiza.
- Stimulates the reticulo-endothelial immune system, activates phagocytosis by immune cells, reduces IL-6.
- Inhibits spontaneous DNA damage from lipid peroxidation
- Induces heat shock protein HSP-70 to protect cells from stress
- Reduces activity of tumour necrosis factor alpha TNFα and basic fibroblast growth factor bFGF.
- Significantly inhibits angiogenesis by blocking VEGFR and binding APN.
- Significantly inhibits number and volume of tumours
- Inhibits epidermal growth factor receptor and tyrosine kinases.
- Inhibits spread of cancer and invasiveness by blocking MMP-2 and MMP-9 matrix metallo-proteinases.
- Reverses liver damage from fungal aflatoxins and mutagens in tobacco smokers

Some naturopathic physicians like a combination of curcumin with black seed – the cumin spice seed Nigella sativa. TCM doctors may use "Canelim" tablets with curcumin, and other herbs. Curcumin combines well with genestein from soy, synergistic with EGCG from green tea. It may not work as well if mixed with high dose alpha lipoic acid.

A favourite of my colleagues at the Cancer Treatment Centers of America is Vital Nutrients brand *BCQ*. I often use the Canadian version called *Can-Arrest*. The new lecithin based *Curcumin 7X* from Albi Naturals is very potent in low doses due to superior absorption. It is able to reduce COX-2 tumour growth signalling due to inflammation. This actually slows tumour growth, reduces pain and protects the patient's quality of life in a clinically meaningful way.

The renowned Dr. Mark Gignac, ND eliminates the need for pills by giving 3 to 6 grams a day of curcumin in virgin organic coconut milk.

Curcumin absorbs poorly unless combined with an adjunct such as bromelain or bioperine. Ideally you will take the Can-Arrest formula. In some cases I will prescribe curcumin compounded by my pharmacist with bromelain. This assures it is medically useful.

Curcumin is not to be given if there is biliary duct obstruction.

Curcumin binds iron, so discontinue its use if you are diagnosed with iron-deficiency anemia or are at risk due to blood loss.

Do not take curcumin if you are getting chemotherapy with the drugs cyclophosphamide, irinotecan or campothecin. If on other chemo drugs, check with your naturopathic physician.

CABBAGE

Cabbage was prescribed for cancer by the great physician Hippocrates of Cos – he would poultice cancerous breasts with green cabbage leaves.

A particularly valuable form of the amino-acid methionine in cabbage gives us *Fare You*, a remedy for mouth sores (mucositis) in chemotherapy or radiotherapy..

Sulforaphanes are found in all the cabbage family vegetables, but especially broccoli sprouts. These prevent cancer by inhibiting histone deacetylase enzymes, opening up activity in tumour suppressor genes.

Cabbage is also rich in powerful anti-cancer indoles and isothiocyanates. Indoles regulate hormone and xenobiotic metabolism and detoxification. Isothiocyanates ITCs are thio-glucoside conjugates called glucosinolates. ITCs up-regulate anti-angiogenic factors such as IL-2 and tissue inhibitor of metalloproteinases TIMP, while down-regulating pro-angiogenic factors such as VEGF and pro-inflammatory cytokines such as IL-1β, IL-6, GM-CSF and TNFα.

INDOLE-3-CARBINOL

I3C naturally occurs in cruciferous Brassica vegetables, including broccoli, cabbage, cauliflower, Brussels sprouts, kale, bok choy, watercress, radishes, horseradish, rutabaga, turnips, collard greens and mustard greens. These foods are strongly associated with broad cancer protection.

I3C is released from these foods by chewing, then most converts to diindolylmethane (DIM) in the acid of the stomach. You can buy DIM supplements, at twice the price of I3C, but the only advantage is that DIM is less likely than I3C to spoil quickly in heatI3C converts into several anti-cancer compounds, and so performs better clinically than DIM alone.

- strongly inhibits signal transducer and activator of transcription **STAT-3** DNA copying activator protein required for proliferation and differentiation
- inhibits **beta-catenin**, a cancer trigger, i.e. of a leukemic blast crisis
- inhibits platelet-derived growth factor receptor PDGFR
- induces aryl hydrocarbon hydroxylase
- decreases "bad" 16-OH and 4-OH estrogens by 50 %
- increases "good" 2-OH estrone and estradiol by 75 %
- down-regulates estrogen receptor activity
- reduces dioxin xenohormone signalling
- inhibits breast cancer reoccurrence 90 % compared to Tamoxifen at 60 %
- induces apoptosis, regulates apoptosis genes; stimulates p53 phosphorylation and disrupts p53-MDM-2 , its ubiquitin ligase.
- Induces BRCA-1 and BRCA-2 expression, repairing DNA mutations and thus preventing as well as treating cancer.
- I3C and BRCA-1 co-inhibit estrogen receptor alpha ERα
- DIM down-regulates androgen receptors even in hormone-refractory prostate cancer
- arrests cancer cells in G1, as p53 release leads to induction of the p21 cyclin-dependent kinase CDK inhibitor.
- Down-regulates cyclin D1, CDK 2 and CDK 4
- Down-regulates phosphorylated Akt, inhibiting the mTOR signalling pathway
- Down-regulates the anti-apoptotic protein Survivin.
- strongly inducing liver phase 1 and 2 enzymes CYP 1A1 and CYP 1A2, as well as gut detox enzymes. In women it induces CYP3A2.
- increases p21 transcription, blocks ras proto-oncogene.
- regulates nuclear promoter Sp1 transcription factor
- inhibits human papilloma virus HPV
- protects PTEN functionality
- inhibits urokinase uPA, associated with breast cancer growth and metastasis.

DIM capsules may be taken at bedtime, 200 to 400 mg. Indole-3-carbinol is usually dosed at 200 mg three times daily, at meals.

I-3-C and DIM are also useful for other hormone overload problems such as acne, premenstrual tension, menstrual disorders and menopause. It helps manage sulphite sensitivity. It probably also clears out xeno-estrogens such as organo-chloride pesticides, via induction of synthesis of the cytochrome P-450 detoxification enzyme CyPA1.

I3C reliably reduces PSA in prostate cancer, is great service in breast cancer, and other hormone-dependent cancers. It is also strongly indicated for pancreatic cancer and lymphomas.

GARLIC

Allium sativa or garlic is a great health food. It is the best immune building food, and promotes longevity.
- immune tonic par excellence
- detoxifier
- anti-angiogenic because it boosts nitric oxide synthesase activity
- diallyl disulphide DADS, from the breakdown of allicin, alters protein and polyamine metabolism in cancer cells, and normalizes cell cycle and adhesion properties.
- chemoprotective, anti-proliferative anti-mitotic and tumour shrinking effects have been observed with garlic extracts.

When I was 24 years old, and in good shape, I was invited by an older local man to climb up a large hill to a ruin of an oracle temple in Greece. I could not keep up with him, which disturbed me because he appeared he could be 60 years old. After turning back several times to goad me on, he threw me a head of garlic and advised me to eat a few cloves. He said this is why he was so strong in his 80's! I will never forget how impressed I was with his vigour, and I have no doubt his advice to eat lots of garlic every day was very wise. Anyone beginning to catch a cold or other illness would do well to mince some garlic cloves up and down them with a glass of warm water. That is usually the end of the problem.

CATECHIN

Catechins are common in tea and many plant medicines. Catechins are bioflavonoids which increase activity of antioxidant enzymes which:
- inhibit formation of adhesions after surgery
- inhibit mutagenesis and carcinogenesis
- induce apoptosis in a dose-dependent fashion
- inhibit tumour growth
- arrest malignant cells in G0-G1 phase of cell cycle
- enhance wild type p53 expression
- inhibit protein kinase C activation by tumour promoter.

CARTILAGE

The famous Cuban studies by Dr. Lane with shark cartilage may have been overstated, and those who did well in his study were taking other active treatments including the Hoxsey herbal formula. I have not been convinced that it is cost-effective, and have never prescribed it. Patients I have observed taking it have had little change.

Cartilage is avascular – it contains no blood vessels, and does contain substances which inhibit angiogenesis.

Shark cartilage had a period of popularity, but quality and price issues have deterred its wide acceptance. Frozen or dried, it is proven to have little to no effect. Anti-angiogenic therapies of all types have been plagued by the ability of cancers to adapt and become resistant to these agents. There are alternative pathways to making blood vessels, and the tumours find them.

Bovine tracheal cartilage preparation Catrix has produced dramatic improvement and even remissions in human cancers given by injection and then orally at 8 of 375 mg capsules every 8 hours. It is not in use in Canada, to my knowledge.

SOY ISOFLAVONES

Soy foods are strongly associated with reduced risk of breast, prostate, and other hormone dependent cancers as well as lung cancer in smokers. Despite many good animal studies and technical papers on its mechanisms of action, there are no actual human clinical studies on its use as a therapy.

In the lab 45 mg stimulates breast cancer cell proliferation, higher doses inhibit breast cancer. In humans it appears under 60 mg daily is anti-estrogenic, but over 80 mg daily is estrogenic.

In humans the effect is consistently **inhibitory of pre-menopausal ER+ breast cancer.** Most important is the exposure to soy before menarche. Soy isoflavones competitively inhibit endogenous estrogen from entering receptors, reducing growth signalling.

- genestein is reported to inhibit angiogenesis, reduce estrogen levels, partly block estrogen receptors, reduce tumour cell nucleic acid synthesis, inhibit tumour glucose oxidation, inhibit topoisomerase II and enhance efficacy of radiotherapy.
- soy isoflavones inhibit DNA gyrase
- soy isoflavones induce apoptosis; genestein particularly promotes p53 activity.
- soy protease inhibitors help maintain cell contact inhibition and reduce tumour invasiveness.
- tofu increases sex hormone binding globulin and reduces the testosterone/estradiol ratio.
- soy intake reduces risk of ER+/PR+HER-2 breast cancers by RR 0.73

However, when endogenous estrogens are low, as in the menopause, there is a net estrogenic effect from soy isoflavones, causing a **possible increase in growth of post-menopausal ER- breast cancers**. Soy foods should be taken only a few times weekly. There is no benefit, but no risk in ER+ post-menopausal tumours. Soy foods can be used in moderation.

Soy has an excellent synergy with Tamoxifen, so anyone on this drug should eat soy foods freely. High intake with Tamoxifen adds a 60% risk reduction.

Over 5 years of high-dose isoflavone supplementation can trigger uterine hyperplasia.

Fermented soy foods are more bioavailable and safer. Unfermented soy foods can inhibit the thyroid gland.

The Chinese developed a nitrogenated low temperature fermented organic soy beverage Haelen in the early 1980's as a hospital nutrition supplement. It is extremely rich in the anti-cancer isoflavones:

- genestein 228 mcg/ml
- genistin222 mcg/ml
- daidzein 184 mcg/ml

It is also high in protease inhibitors which reduce mutation in cancer cells. It is an excellent source of bioactive free amino acids (protein). The usual dose is 8 ounces daily. It tastes terrible.

The best form to support chemo and radiation is the aglycone genestein/daidzein combination found in the Vital Nutrients product. For those with a soy allergy or sensitivity, kudzu root is rich source of these isoflavones.

BROMELAIN

A protein digesting enzyme extracted from pineapple stems. Better quality products will state a rating of their protein-busting activity from actual bioassays. For example, a GDU of 4 means 1 milligram of this bromelain product will liquefy 4 milligrams of animal gelatin.

- reduces tumour progression and metastases by modulating cell adhesion molecule CD44
- anti-inflammatory – depletes kininogen and activates series 1 prostaglandins.
- reduces platelet aggregation
- prevents clots by activating plasminogen.
- Fibrinolytic, digests fibrin to break down clots safely.
- It increases absorption to medically relevant blood levels of important water-insoluble bioflavonoids such as quercetin and curcumin.

BIOPERINE

Bioperine is a trademarked thermo-nutrient from black pepper made by Sabinsa Corp. It is put into many products to improve absorption of medicinal ingredients, such as quercetin or curcumin. The usual intake is 5 mg 1 to 2 times daily. Never exceed 15 mg per day.

KELLEY METABOLIC CURE

William Kelley, MS, DDS cured himself of pancreatic cancer in 1964 with a program based on a raw food diet, supplements (up to 160 pills a day!), coffee enemas, liver flushes and pancreatic enzymes. The combination of pancreatic enzymes is claimed to "destroy and strip away about 97% of such starch capsules, thereby enabling tumours to be recognized, digested, liquefied and removed from person's bodies via their bloodstreams." This is the rationale behind the popular Mugos Wobenzyme products.

The use of pancreatic enzymes for cancer originated in 1902 with John Beard, an embryologist at the University of Edinburgh. Later Drs. Ernst Krebs & Ernst Krebs Jr. revived the enzyme concept, combining it with laetrile. The Kelly program will trigger an initial rise in tumour markers, and the tumours may swell. The white blood cell count will rise, and as the tumours are breaking down the patient will experience flu-like achiness, fever, headache, nausea, and irritability. The program is given in 25 day cycles with 5 days rest between cycles to allow elimination of tumour wastes. High response rates are claimed in his books *Cancer Cure* and *Cancer – Curing the Incurable.*

Recall Pottenger's theory that solid tumours arise in sympathetic dominant cases which have low pancreatic enzymes. Nicholas Gonzalez practices a variant of the Kelly protocol, giving sympathetic dominant types a vegetarian diet with large doses of B-complex vitamins, magnesium and potassium; these folks need lots of vigorous aerobic exercise and pancreatic enzymes. For the parasympathetic dominant types with immune cell cancers such as leukemia and lymphoma he prescribes high intake of red meat, large doses of calcium, zinc, selenium, vitamin B12 and pantothenic acid – but avoids magnesium, potassium, thiamine, riboflavin and niacin.

Dr. Gonzalez also routinely uses coffee enemas and glandular remedies. Doses of proteolytic enzymes range to 40 capsules daily. The whole program can end up being over 160 capsules of supplements daily!

Most importantly, recent research shows enzyme-based therapy for pancreatic cancer is quite inferior to chemotherapy, with gemcitabine giving about 10 months longer survival, on average, and far better quality of life.

BUDWIG DIET

Dr. Johanna Budwig, biochemist, in 1951 devised a cancer protocol centered on flaxseed oil and sulphorated milk proteins. These are described in her books *Cancer--A Fat Problem* and *The Death of the Tumour.* She says the absence of linol-acids in the average Western diet is responsible for the production of oxidase, which induces cancer growth and is the cause of many other chronic disorders. The beneficial oxidase ferments are destroyed by heating or boiling oils in foods, and by nitrates used for preserving meat. Sulphorated oils are water-soluble and benefit oxygen and electron transfer across the cell membranes, including the mitochondria membranes.

Put in your blender or mix with an egg beater:
- 1 cup organic low-fat cottage cheese or quark.
- 2-8 Tbsp.(1.5 to 3 ounces)of organic cold-pressed flaxseed oil
- 1-3 Tbsp. of fresh ground organic flaxseed
- enough water to make it soft Acidophilus milk or buttermilk may also be used.
- if desired add a small pinch of cayenne pepper or garlic
- Minimum daily: 4 ounces low-fat cottage cheese with 1 ½ ounces flaxseed oil.

- I can also recommend some cold-pressed non-GMO canola oil, extra virgin coconut oil, and extra virgin olive oil for variety.
- When properly mixed the product has no oily taste and there will be no fatty residue around the rim of the container – the fats will be water-soluble!
- Note: **Digestive enzymes with <u>lipase</u> may be used instead of the quark/ cottage cheese**, if you are dairy intolerant or wish to take the oil straight up. I prescribe plant source digestive enzymes.
- In the case of a very ill person, the mixture may be given in champagne, which enhances absorption as well as being palatable.

Carbohydrates containing natural sugar, such as dates, figs, pears, apples and grapes, are also included in the diet, and may be blended into the preparation for flavour. Yoghurt, poppy seed, buckwheat, oats, rice millet, chives, parsley, dill, marjoram, lemon juice, sauerkraut, greens, turnips, radishes, kohlrabi, cauliflower, walnuts and natural yeast are considered beneficial. Freshly squeezed vegetable juices are fine – carrot, celery, apple, and red beet. Grape juice is fine. Teas are allowed, particularly peppermint, rosehip and green tea.

Forbidden foods on this diet: sugar, animal fats, butter, refined oils, peanuts, commercial salad dressings, margarine, shortening and preserved meats.

Try to avoid plastic wrap on fatty foods such as cheese or meat. The plasticizers are nasty "xenobiotics" which means they can mimic estrogen and other growth stimulators. The worst scenario is microwaving soft plastic. If you buy food in plastic rewrap in wax or butcher's paper or store in glass or nalgene plastic containers.

GERSON THERAPY

Dr. Max Gerson, M.D. developed a diet of primarily raw foods, with emphasis on fresh juices of vegetables, fruits. He gave his patients Lugol's iodine solution, pancreatin enzymes for digestion, thyroid extract, mineral and vitamin supplements. He prescribed raw calf liver either orally as a juice or by injection! He was often able to arrest or even regress metastases, although he less often saw clearance of the primary tumours. He published the book The Gerson Therapy, Results of Fifty Cases describing cured cases, but was labelled a quack. His clinic was forced out of the U.S.A. and now operates in Tijuana, Mexico, under the direction of his daughter Charlotte. Dr. Steve Austin, N.D. was my professor of nutrition and of oncology at National College of Naturopathic Medicine in the early 1980's. He has conducted a preliminary independent survey of the results of the Gerson approach. The diet takes great effort to make everything fresh throughout the day, and actual compliance falls off quickly once the patient returns home. However, even with excellent compliance, results are startlingly poor. Dr. Austin says about Gerson patients "All they do is the therapy, they don't have a life. It's not worth it."

I must acknowledge potassium iodide is worthwhile, that raw foods provide needed potassium and enzymes, and that raw liver is an excellent tonic for the fatigued cancer patient. However, the Gerson diet is just too cumbersome and too radical to be of practical importance to the average patient. Ditto macrobiotic diets.

NOT RECOMMENDED.

ISSELS' THERAPY

Josef Issels described cancer as a series of multiple and chronic challenges and insults. Issels combined a variety of techniques to adapt to the individual patient and their current status. For over 50 years he used Coley's toxins, a non-specific mixed bacterial vaccine. The patients for whom it provoked periodic fevers saw regression and resolution of tumours. He also used a specific autologous vaccine made from mycoplasma and related organisms found in the patient's own blood. He emphasized correction of the pro-malignant milieu, tumour debulking, and host support. He often removed tonsils and teeth as sources of focal infections and toxicity. His work is now carried on by his son Christian Issels, ND, based in Phoenix, Arizona. He has added emphasis on comprehensive immunotherapy. Treatments may include intravenous vitamin C, auto-hemotherapy, miasmatic homeopathy, Sanum pleomorphic medicines, dendritic cell vaccines, and neural therapy.

MATTHIAS RATH PROTOCOL

Dr. Mathias Rath has proposed a protocol to increase apoptosis, inhibit angiogenesis, reduce tumour growth, and regulate the extra-cellular matrix ECM integrity to control invasion and metastasis:
- green tea EGCG
- vitamin C
- N-acetyl-cysteine
- Amino acids proline, lysine and arginine
- Minerals copper, selenium and manganese

JONATHAN TREASURE PROTOCOL

Jonathan is a respected English-trained medical herbalist from Oregon. He suggests a program remarkably similar to my ideas at the time of the first edition of this book, so he is obviously a genius...
Here it is:
- Curcumin
- Green tea EGCG
- Resveratrol
- Licorice
- Rosemary
- Grapeseed extract oligomeric proanthocyanidins
- Ginger

INSPIRE HEALTH

My dear colleagues at Inspire Health **www.inspirehealth.ca** in Vancouver have been helping people I refer to them for the last 18 years or more. I have also been blessed with many referrals from them for my co-management of local cases. They are my mentors and friends. I encourage everyone to look at what they can offer anyone with a major health challenge. They offer a day and a half workshop which introduces vegetarian dietetics, complementary and alternative medicine in cancer, mind-body healing, art and music therapy, relaxation, stress management, visualization and meditation, and many other important topics. They have a very talented multidisciplinary team of practitioners for alternative medical therapies such as low dose naltrexone, targeted vaccines, intravenous vitamin C, Chinese medicine and acupuncture. They commonly prescribe two supplements they have custom made for their clients:

- Integration One: selenomethionine, glutathione, zinc citrate and Ester-C calcium ascorbate.
- Integration Two: beta carotene, vitamin A, vitamin E, Co-enzyme Q-10, vitamin D3.

AVEMAR

Avemar is a fermented wheat germ extract with documented efficacy as an aid to improving quality of life, and survival, with chemotherapy and beyond. Wheat germ fermentation yields the natural flavones 2,6-dimethoxy-p-benzoquinone (2,6-DMBQ), a redox regulator which chaperones cancer cell glucose metabolism. It impedes cancer cell growth, increases apoptosis, inhibits metastasis and has immune-modulatory effects. It also is a mild poly (ADP-Ribose) polymerase (PARP) inhibitor – mutated cancer cells use this enzyme to repair DNA damage from chemo and radiation

MEDITERRANEAN DIET

The traditional diets of populations around the Mediterranean Sea are both preventative and therapeutic, reducing the risk of all-cause mortality, including the top two – cardiovascular diseases and cancers.

The Mediterranean diet can reduce levels of fibrinogen, C-reactive protein,interleukin-6 and homocysteine. It improves endothelial function, regulates leukocytosis and oxidized low-density lipoprotein cholesterol.

The active components of the Mediterranean diet are available everywhere:
- Fresh vegetables – excluding potatoes.
- Fruits
- Nuts
- Legumes
- Grains
- Fish
- Mono-unsaturated fats such as extra virgin grade olive oil and avocado.

193

My final word is always be grateful that you have food, thank those who grow and deliver it, and bless those who make and serve it. Do not consume worry and stress about food choices, which can poison your meal. Do your best to be moderate and thoughtful, and that will be enough. You may wish to bless the food to your needs, and visualize your body taking from it that which is good, and leaving the rest.

A NUTRITION-BASED STRATEGY FOR CONTROLLING CANCER CELL ENERGETICS:

MITOCHONDRIA RESCUE HEALS CANCER

When a cancer tumour grows to be a mass of cells about 1 to 2 millimetres in diameter, it must get extra blood and lymph vessels or it can't maintain its abnormal rate of growth. Oxygen and nutrients can passively diffuse only across that magic millimetre. As malignant cells run low on oxygen, they release distress signals that recruit peripheral stem cells and immune cells to make chemicals, such as vascular endothelial growth factor VEGF, that sprout new blood and lymph vessels. This all happens long before a tumour is visible to any current diagnostic test.

In every way possible, immune cells act to support the health and growth of the tumour cells. It is the primary function of the immune system to support and repair tissues that are damaged or struggling to survive. Macrophages even provide the tools to soften the intracellular matrix and allow tumour invasion into healthy tissue, including into blood and lymph vessels.

By the time a cancer is diagnosed, at a diameter of about 1 centimetre, chaotic blood vessels in the tumour are typically so leaky they raise the fluid pressure in the tumour so high it squashes the blood flow, and the tumour develops areas of low oxygen = hypoxia. Hypoxic cells strongly resist being killed by radiation, and the poor blood supply also precludes adequate chemo drug delivery. There may even be areas that have no oxygen at all = anoxia, and parts of the tumour will die. Areas with severe anoxia die by necrosis.

The cancer cells survive in a low oxygen condition by switching to fermentation of sugars for energy, which is theoretically about 18 times less efficient than aerobic glycolysis. The lactic acid by-product of fermentation is a potent stimulant of cancer growth and spread. The induction of lactate dehydrogenase 5 drives anaerobic transformation, and LDH-5 strongly stimulates angiogenesis, through hypoxia-inducible factor one alpha HIF-1α..

When the nuclear chromosomes in a cell become mutated, or epigenetics are altered, cancer can arise. There is a built in defence mechanism called apoptosis – the off-switch for bad, old and damaged cells. This apoptosis program is innate in every human cell, and will turn off and recycle any cells found to have passed 50 doublings or having more than 50,000 to 60,000 errors or mutations in its DNA. The p53 gene runs this check on the DNA at the cell-cycle checkpoint just before copying the cell. It is like the Scandisk utility checking your computer hard-drive for errors.

Mitochondria are a key player in **the apoptosis process – the "off-switch for bad cells."**

There are about 1,000 mitochondria in every cell, the little combustion chambers in the cell where sugars are burned or oxidized to make energy. We inherit them from our mother's egg, They have their own DNA and function quite independently from the rest of the cell, including the chromosomes you got from both parents.

Mitochondria low in oxygen build up free radicals of oxygen, particularly hydrogen peroxide. Mitochondria build-up ROS doing their work, but will have excessive ROS due to hypoxia, alterations in cell membrane composition – such as DHA deficiency, and from internal genetic and epigenetic phenomena – such as acetylated/methylated mDNA. They shut down, resistance to apoptosis increases, and the cell is immortalized.

It is then a zombie that cannot die, no matter how sick and stressed.

Inducing apoptosis is the goal of radiation and chemotherapy, and is obviously a workable strategy to treat and cure cancer. We have known for years how to wake up the mitochondria in patients with chronic fatigue syndrome and fibromyalgia. We have not been keen to try this with cancers because we did not want to give the cancer more energy to grow on! Merely removing lactic acid to "alkalize" the tumour makes no sense, and will not in itself retard tumour growth. Restoring mitochondrial function as a whole, i.e.. restoring oxidative phosphorylation, has been suggested as a means to restore caspase activity and thereby apoptosis, in most cancers.

Steven Levine and group have proposed "membrane-calming" as a "neuro-bioenergetic" re-balancing for aging and cancer. Membrane hyper-excitability, particularly via inducible over-expression of voltage-gated ion channels, is linked to mitochondrial dysfunction . Hexokinase HK localizes to the outer mitochondrial membrane, suppressing the caspase cascade responsible for apoptosis.

Lactate dehydrogenase LDH is a glycolytic control enzyme. In cancer cells LDH becomes independent of oxygen status, and under both aerobic and anaerobic conditions will convert pyruvate to lactate.

Pyruvate dehydrogenase PDH moves pyruvate made by glycolysis into the mitochondria.

A rat study using the drug dichloroacetate DCA demonstrated that blocking the enzyme pyruvate dehydrogenase kinase – which makes lactate from pyruvate – wakes up the mitochondria in implanted human breast cancer cells, and the cancer cells immediately switch off. The bad news is the DCA drug is very experimental, despite the New Scientist article brazenly titled "Cheap, safe drug kills most cancers." The only cancer study with DCA is with breast cancer in rats. The only human studies testing DCA targeted acidosis advanced diabetes, and showed tremendous toxicity problems. All of the patients either died or dropped out of the studies before were supposed to end! I have read many commentaries on DCA referring to it as a safe or relatively non-toxic drug. This is truly alarming, as it is more toxic than any chemo drug I have ever seen. Within a few weeks use it takes the myelin off peripheral nerves just like in multiple sclerosis, causing pain, numbness, tremor and staggering. It can cause central nervous system damage including confusion, sedation, hallucinations and memory impairment.

It also very toxic to the liver and is known to cause cancer! It can trigger oxalate-based kidney stones and increase uric acid levels, risking gout.

After a brief flurry of self-prescribing DCA from American internet sites, the only Canadian source is now an MD in Toronto who is selling it – at quite a mark-up in price. Despite medications to control side-effects, it is not always a safe therapy, even though the tumour shrinkage we see is tantalizing.

Fortunately, there are a number of non-toxic natural medicines which inhibit this enzyme and are proven to wake up the mitochondria in cancer cells in humans. These agents are approved by Health Canada for over-the-counter sale – for other purposes. Many have been shown to arrest human cancers in published studies.

Natural inhibitor of pyruvate dehydrogenase kinase:

*R+ Alpha lipoic acid (natural form) 150 to 300 mg 3 times daily, best in a time-release carrier.

Other natural agents which evidence suggests will activate the mitochondria to turn off cancer cells:
*L-carnitine -a potent mitochondria booster, but needs ALA to regulate the ROS created. Give 3 to 10 grams daily.   If acetyl-L-carnitine is available, use 500 to 1,000 mg 3 times daily.
***Gamma tocopherol form of vitamin E, 800 IU daily.
*Omega 3 marine source oils assist in membrane repolarization and stabilization.
B1 or thiamine, especially as the fat-soluble benfotiamine 80 to 160 mg 2 times daily. At least take a B-complex containing 50 – 100 mg each of thiamine (B1), riboflavin (B2) and niacin (B3) as nicotinamide twice daily.

Further remedies for mitochondrial reactivation:

Coenzyme Q-10 – 100 mg 3 times daily – absorbs best when taken with fats or oils
Quercetin (with bromelain for absorption) – 2 capsules 2 to 3 times daily
Grapeseed extract (oligomeric proanthocyanidins) – 100 mg 3 times daily
Ganoderma lucidum (Reishi) mushroom extract – 500 to 1,000 mg 3 times daily
Indole-3-carbinol 200 mg 2 to 3 times daily
Ellagic acid – can be as 8 ounces of unsweetened pomegranate, grape or berry juices

This grouping of supplements is novel, although all are remedies I have used for many years in a practice focused in oncology. It is sufficient to get good responses in many cases of advanced cancer. There is no reason to limit care to these agents. They combine well with targeted vaccines, mistletoe injections, IV vitamin C, and other aggressive therapies. As with any generic protocol for cancer, we also would want to integrate agents known to target the specific growth factors driving the particular cancer we are treating.

Typically we have a scan or tumour-marker test to confirm a response within 4 to

6 weeks of starting this program. If they are stable, we continue. Often they are better than stable, with a partial or complete response possible in many cases.

There are many other agents which basic science research shows can support mitochondrial recovery, including curcumin, melatonin, selenium, SOD, glutathione, L-carnitine, resveratrol, coriolus, berberine and iodine.

I have no ethical compunction about prescribing a safe and rational new protocol to patients who are experiencing progression of their disease despite trials of all known effective agents. Desperate times call for desperate measures. Fortunately results have been quite gratifying in some very advanced cases of breast and colon cancer which were escaping control or never did respond to all the usual therapies. Even more exciting are the responses seen in cancers I have never had results with in the past, including lung cancer and sarcomas.

These supplements have little interaction with many common oncology drugs, including Coumadin and Dexamethasone. I would not mix this program with cytotoxic chemotherapy or radiation therapy, preferring other supports during these modalities, and for about 3 weeks after the last dose.

DICHLOROACETATE – DCA

Dichloroacetate or DCA, as discussed in the mitochondria rescue section, is a great concept but too toxic to be practical. This is how it is used.
- Rx: 15 + mg/kg/day. 5 mg /kg is needed for brain and nerve tumors
- Use for 1 to 3 weeks, then 1 week off . Some colleagues dose it 4 days on and 4 days off.
- Repeat as needed
- Thiamine or B1 prevents peripheral neuropathy
- R+ alpha lipoic acid prevents sedation, confusion, hallucinations, memory problems, hand tremor.
- Proton pump inhibitors such as Pantoprazole (Pantoloc) prevent heartburn, nausea, vomiting and indigestion.
- See www.medicorcancer.com

I urge everyone who insists on trying it to combine it with benfotiamine, co-enzyme Q-10 and R+ alpha lipoic acid to synergize its efficacy. Continue these after the drug proves intolerable, and must be stopped, to repair the damage and continue the effect.

It is thought that caffeine can improve responses to DCA, in doses of about 480 mg daily or about 12 cups daily of black tea.

DCA does shrink tumours amazingly quickly, but it also can put people in wheelchairs rapidly.

NOT RECOMMENDED for long-term unsupervised use. An interesting new concept is using it only on alternating weeks with artemisinin, as DCA is said to help the cancer cells recharge with iron. Perhaps with this synergy and reduced exposure, it may be found to be safe enough to enjoy its potential benefits.

Recently, the first human study on DCA for cancer showed some benefits, with acceptable adverse effects, in treating brain cancers. They used only 5 mg/kg BW, which is one-third of the dose that had been commonly suggested for tumors elsewhere. To get to therapeutic levels in tumors outside the nervous system, the required doses risk more harm than benefit. It is possible to administer DCA intravenously.

Chapter Six – **Botanicals And Plant Extracts In Cancer Care**

The most High hath created medicines out of the earth, and a wise man will not abhor them. –Ecclesiasticus 38:4

Many plants have shown anti-cancer properties against cancer cells in test tubes in vitro and in living creatures in vivo, but only a few have been developed further. Highly cytotoxic extracts, such as the alkaloids from periwinkle and the etoposides from Podophyllum, have occasionally been made into patented drug isolates or synthetics, crossing over into orthodox medicine. Plants are biological entities, living beings, with many survival needs in common with us. They have DNA, so cytotoxic anti-DNA compounds are uncommon. Plants have almost unimaginably varied and subtle mechanisms for modulating biochemical systems. Many traditional plant medicines are treasure troves of potent but relatively non-toxic biological modifiers.

The research gap – Whole plant extracts are not patentable as drugs, and are more difficult to fit into drug-style blinded studies. The elaborate formulae of Traditional Chinese Medicine, coupled with the TCM revulsion for placebo, has caused many time-proven cancer remedies to be ignored by Western medicine. Despite being used rationally by millions of doctors on billions of people for thousands of years, the white coat crowd still considers them completely "unproven." The "scientific" doctor can put people on long-term drug therapy with a synthetic drug which may have been given to humans for as short a time as 4 to 6 weeks in a drug trial, and they will tell you they know what it will do to you. That is quite remarkable – they must be psychic! How many drugs have been recalled or faded from use when long term harm or unexpected adverse affects show up after some years of this crude human experimentation?

Still, the same brain trust will tell you ginseng is potentially dangerous because "we don't know what it will do." I always say a physician's job is to manage risk, not just avoid risk. If they don't know it is safe after millennia of use, I say prove it isn't or step aside. The fact that drug-oriented doctors won't research my field of medicine is not a reason for me to abandon it. I just have to be patient and wait for them to catch up.

The Hoxsey Formula, and many other botanical approaches from European, Native American and Eclectic herbology are being used today without benefit of any scientific human studies. Many other promising herbs await screening. A few like Essiac have been tested and discarded as useless. I am not so naïve that I trust the government, medical institutions and scientific community to scrutinize the home-spun remedies and sort out the good from the false, and develop the good ones into cures for us. Drug company pirates are exploiting traditional knowledge bases, stealing biological organisms, patenting them to exclude those who own them by heritage from further access, and converting them to synthetic commodities for resale at inflated prices. I inherited my genetics from my ancestors, not Monsanto. Their knowledge is my culture, and I am an appointed steward to pass this knowledge onto future generations. I am free to access the God-given gifts for healing from the world around me. Medicinal plants are part of my web of life.

HOXSEY FORMULA

The Hoxsey herbal tonic is a fascinating bit of folklore, and a case study in how a valuable remedy has been marginalized and ignored by science.

Harry M. Hoxsey, ND (1901-1974) treated cancer with topical agents and an internal herbal formula. He had considerable success, and at one time ran several clinics across the United States. The formula was said to have been used in the veterinary practice of his great-grandfather since 1840. Horses with cancer were apparently cured by extracts of the herbs applied as a salve. Similar formulas are found in the textbook of Dr. Eli Jones, MD – an American homeopath and herbalist who was famous for his work in cancer at the turn of the 20th Century. A very similar formula called Syrup Trifolium Compound was developed by Parke-Davis & Company in 1890. Extract of Trifolium Compound was a variation listed in the 1898 edition of King's American Dispensatory. Compound Fluid Extract of Trifolium was a recognized remedy in the 1926 National Formulary. It was widely used by many physicians.

Harry Hoxsey was a home-spun legend, who had flamboyant style, and was controversial, yet achieved legal and peer recognition for being able to cure cancer. Two USA federal courts upheld the therapeutic value of the tonic, and the American Medical Association admitted that the external salve had merit. Harry wrote a book describing his methods titled *You Don't Have to Die*. The failed attempt by Dr. Malcolm Harris, Secretary of the AMA to buy the secret tonic formula – for his own profit – resulted in years of harassment and arrests. Harry won a major settlement in a defamation lawsuit over a description of him as a "quack feeding off the flesh of the dead and the dying" and the lie that "his father's death resulted from cancer," when in fact it the gentleman died from the infectious disease erysipelas. Through various manipulations, including making naturopathy illegal in Texas, site of Hoxsey's largest clinic, he was driven from the field, without any scientific investigation of his claims. Harry closed up his clinics in the USA in the late 1950's. His former head nurse Mildred Nelson continued his clinical style in Tijuana, Mexico as the Biomedical Clinic, since 1963. Harry died in 1974, of prostate cancer. This is quite ironic, as I find the formula particularly useful in advanced prostate cancers. His fascinating and politically charged career was documented in the 1987 film *Hoxsey – Quack Who Cures Cancer? – How Healing Becomes a Crime*.

Hoxsey stated that cancer developed as a result of -
- low cellular potassium ions
- poor thyroid function
- poor liver function
- poor elimination of toxins

Hoxsey may have had a mail-order degree, and may have been unsophisticated, but he had a clear concept of cancer as a disease resulting from a disturbance of the entire internal ecology and metabolism. He viewed his herbal extract as a **tonic** which was primarily an **alterative**, meaning it cleansed and strengthened all the vital organs. His view of cancer as a constitutional and blood disease is typical of the Eclectic viewpoint as espoused by Eli Jones, and by naturopathic physicians today.

Naturopathic physicians in oncology all agree cancer is a disorder of the physiology, psychology and ecology of the patient – that in fact cancer is a systemic disease affecting the entire person. We see that the genetic mutations thought by conventional medical thinkers to be the root problem of cancer, are readily modifiable by epigenetic factors including nutrition, exercise, relaxation, visualization, and other lifestyle choices We believe that in herbs we can find the healing wisdom of the life force, *Vis Medicatrix Naturae,* the healing power of nature..

The Hoxsey cancer clinics used a secret herbal tonic of alcohol-free fluid extracts made from fresh herbs. It was independently analyzed to contain, per 5 ml:

20 mg red clover blossom *Trifolium pratense*
20 mg licorice root *Glycyrrhiza glabra*
20 mg burdock root *Arctium lappa*
20 mg buckthorn bark *Rhamnus frangula*
10 mg queen's root *Stillingia sylvatica*
10 mg Oregon grape root *Berberis aquifolium*
10 mg poke root *Phytolacca decandra*
 5 mg Honduras bark *Cascara amarga*
 5 mg prickly ash bark *Xanthoxylum flaxineum*
150 mg potassium iodine KI
U.S.P. Aromatic elixir 14 flavouring syrup

Some speculate that may apple *Podophyllum pelatrum* may have been a constituent as well. This toxic herb later gave rise to the chemotherapy drug Etoposide, now in use in medical oncology.

The McLean variant of the formula adds chaparral, kelp, peach bark, and Jamaican sarsaparilla root. Dr. Richard Schulze has adapted the Dr. John Christopher variant of the Hoxsey formula to include red clover, chaparral, burdock root and seed, Oregon grape root, yellow dock, golden seal root, lobelia and garlic.

The tonic was diluted by putting 2 fluid ounces in 14 ounces of tap water. Adult dose was 1 to 5 teaspoonfuls 4 times daily after meals and at bedtime. For children the dose was 5 to 30 drops 4 times daily. The tonic was often prescribed for 5 years, then to be taken for 3 to 4 months every Spring and Fall. Most patients tolerate it very well. Hoxsey herb mélange is blood-purifying, laxative, anti-estrogenic and detoxifying.

The laxative effect is mild, but can cause problems with diarrhea. Any digestive upset can be countered with carminatives such as fennel, anise, caraway and mint. Reactions such as a rash on the forehead, face or neck, frontal or sinus headaches, loss of appetite, nausea, weakness, discharges and bowel intolerance may occur from the potassium iodide, necessitating a reduced dosage until cleared. Iodine at these doses is not safe in pregnancy or nursing, or in cases of hyperthyroidism. Licorice can trigger hypertension or edema, with loss of potassium.

The patient was also given dietary restrictions, including the strict avoidance of tomatoes, pork, salt, vinegar, alcohol, sugar, white flour and processed foods. Patients were advised to drink lots of pure water, and juices such as unsweetened grape juice.

Hoxsey claimed a cure rate of 25% for internal cancers, and up to 60% for breast cancer.

Hoxsey claimed a cure rate of 85% for skin and external cancers, which he treated with escharotics – salves which kill cells on contact and cause a layer of tissue to dissolve and slough off. Only the topical powders and salves applied to burn off tumours were viewed by Hoxsey as directly "anti-cancer" medications. These escharotics were very painful, and have fallen into disuse with medical advances in the field.

Hoxsey Red Paste – combined zinc chloride, antimony trisulphide, and bloodroot Sanguinaria canadensis powder. This caustic and cytotoxic paste is painful, killing all tissue it contacts. It is very useful on melanomas. This is reminiscent of the "Fell Remedy," which pre-dates Hoxsey..

Hoxsey Yellow Powder – combined USP Sulphur 2 oz, arsenic sulphide 0.5 oz, and 6 oz talc. Grind for a full hour in a mortar to solubilize. It only kills cancer cells. It is also very painful.

Open wounds were dusted with boric acid as a disinfectant. A healing ointment of Vaseline, rosin, refined camphor, beeswax, tincture of myrrh Commiphora abyssinica, and oil of spike (– spikenard or Aralia racemosa?) was used to aid any damaged non-cancerous tissue.

Red clover blossom *Trifolium* boiled down to a tarry solid extract which was applied topically, sometimes with the addition of Sanguinaria extract.

Phytolacca F.E. (fluid extract) 1:16 dilution as a compress was put on breast tumours for 4 weeks, and would promote drainage and even expulsion of the tumours through the skin. The cancer can literally come to the surface and fall right off.

Dr. Steve Austin, ND has observed that the Biomedical Center in Tijuana, Mexico is having moderate success salvaging perhaps 20% of a variety of advanced, medically terminal cases. Results of an informal and limited follow-up study were published in 1984. Mildred Nelson estimates 80% of cases respond to the therapy.

A recent so-called investigation of the Hoxsey method by the University of British Columbia was "inconclusive," citing a lack of "sufficient time, personnel and funds." Thanks for nothing! My own experience is similar to Dr. Austin's, seeing occasionally dramatic results in astrocytoma, lymphoma, breast cancer, etc.

I have often combined the Red Clover Combination from St. Francis Herb Farm in Cormack, Ontario, with homeopathic remedies such as *Conium, Carcinosum, Arsenicum* and Pascoe nosodes such as *Glioma, Lymphangitis* or *Prostata*. I prescribe one dropper-full (20 to 25 drops) three times daily, in a little water, sip slowly, take no food or drink for 15 minutes. I do not use it in all cases, and I would not stake my life on it alone, but it is a reasonable adjunct in selected cases.

ESSIAC

Essiac was named by the Canadian public health nurse Rene Caisse, who learned of the formula in 1921. Rene met a patient who attributed her survival of breast cancer to an herbal mix originating with Ojibwa First Nations. It is a decoction (water extraction) of:

- Sheep sorrel *Rumex acetosella **L***.
- Slippery elm bark *Ulmus fulva*
- Burdock root *Arctium lappa*
- Indian or Turkish rhubarb root *Rheum officinalis*

The popular brand Flor-Essence adds watercress herb, kelp, blessed thistle and red clover to the traditional, and some would say authentic Essiac formula. Respirin Corporation owns the rights to the original Essiac formula and trade name, yet others claim variations that are the "real McCoy."

Like the Hoxsey formula, this mixture is a rich source of anthraquinones emodin and rhein which stimulate PGE2 synthesis, alter calcium transport, are anti-inflammatory, antitumor and antibacterial. Caisse had many anecdotes to tell, and had some medical referrals of cases, but scientific testing on animals at the National Institutes of Health (NIH) in Bethesda, Maryland was inconclusive, and the therapy nearly passed into history on her death. It was re-popularized recently by Elaine Alexander after a CBC radio program on Rene Caisse's life. A standardized and authentic formula is made by Respirin Canada, who obtained the rights to her formula in 1978, just before Rene passed on.

This herbal formula is healthful, keeps the bowels moving, but is not in my experience and opinion a cancer therapy. The best results are said to be in patients who have not had extensive chemotherapy or radiation. Unfortunately, few patients we see in British Columbia fall into this category. A recent scientific study in Canada failed to demonstrate any benefit whatsoever to cancer patients. Frankly, I have seen thousands of people use it, with no discernible change when the go on it, or when they go off of it.

ONCOLYN

Oncolyn is a proprietary combination of polyphenols and anthocyanins developed by Dr. Arthur Djang, M.D., Ph.D., M.P.H. Dr. Djang was a prominent orthodox medical researcher who pioneered the ninhydrin technique of latent fingerprinting, the isoenzyme technique for early diagnosis of myocardial infarction, and has many scientific publications in medical and cancer research. On retiring, he travelled to China, his ancestral homeland, where he was exposed to hospitals integrating Western allopathic and Eastern TCM methods.

He returned with some ideas for natural anti-cancer formulations, which he verified with cell culture and animal research techniques.

The Oncolyn formula is not published, so I do not know what it contains. My investigation suggests green tea polyphenol extract and grapeseed extract may be present, and one source suggests it may also contain a seed extract, perhaps from apples. I wish I knew exactly. It is unethical for me to prescribe secret formulas.

Oncolyn has been shown in tissue culture and rodents to be antioxidant, dismutagenic, pro-differentiation, anti-angiogenic, and anti-metastatic. Dr. Djang says 1 tablet daily will neutralize the toxins of tobacco smoking. For cancer the prescribed dose is 1 tablet with 500 mg vitamin C, 3 times daily before each meal, and vitamin E 400 I.U. twice daily. Improvement is expected in about 2 weeks.

I have observed a number of significant responses to this product, for example two cases of advanced pleural mesothelioma which made a dramatic regression. That is a tough cancer to treat by any means, so I was impressed. It is unfortunate the formula is secret, but a conversation with Dr. Djang after a public lecture about his research did reinforce my commitment to using green tea and grapeseed extracts. A combination of bioflavonoids and polyphenols had already become a core part of my basic cancer program, based on my experience and that of other naturopathic doctors. I like to add in curcumin and other synergists. I think Oncolyn is a good product, but needs other support and refinements.

GREEN TEA and EGCG POLYPHENOL

Tea and its extracts are included under the botanicals, rather than as a food beverage, as the effective therapeutic doses are well beyond what is possible by tea consumption. It is a phyto-nutraceutical.

Unfermented green tea *Camellia sinensis* leaf is a source of polyphenols such as epigallocatechin-3-gallate EGCG, epigallocatechin EGC and epicatechin-3-gallate ECG. EGCG is an antioxidant 200 times more powerful than vitamin E. EGCG is the top contender for the most active medical principle in green tea extract.

The top leaves are steamed to inactivate enzymes which would oxidize the polyphenols into tannins. If they are not steamed, natural fermentation makes the tannins that make "black tea" more mouth-puckering than green tea.

Many large-scale epidemiology studies show a significant preventative value in green tea as a daily beverage, particularly at intakes of 5 to 10 cups of tea daily.

However, that is a lot of fluid, and too much caffeine for many people. Black tea ranges up to 80 mg of caffeine per cup, and green tea is less, but still yields at least 10 mg per cup, and may reach 40 mg per cup. Other stimulating alkaloids in the tea leaf are theobromine and theophylline.

Encapsulated standardized extracts, low in caffeine, are necessary to reach the doses needed to use EGCG and related polyphenols as a therapy. Green tea EGCG has been a core therapy in my protocols since 1996. The broad and potent effects of green tea on cancer is truly remarkable:
- inhibits many cancers by blocking cells in G0-G1 phase and arresting cells in G2-M phase of the cell cycle. This is regulated through its effects on p21 and p27 gene proteins.
- Induction of apoptosis is dose dependent. Induces apoptosis in cancer cells by down-regulating anti-apoptotic bcl-2 protein, up-regulating pro-apoptotic Bax, and activation of caspases 3, 7 and 9.
- Enhances wild type p53 expression.
- Inhibits oncogene expression, including Kirsten-ras or *K-ras* which regulates tyrosine kinases.
- Reduces expression of the multi-drug resistance gene *mdr-1.*

- Inhibits protein kinase C activation by tumour promoters. Protease inhibition reduces cellular proliferation, angiogenesis, inflammatory cytokine production, and increases apoptosis.
- Inhibits dihydrofolate reductase, reducing synthesis of cancer cell proteins and nucleic acids.
- Inhibits aryl hydrocarbon receptor by binding the receptor's chaperone protein HSP90, increasing resistance to breast cancer. Synergistic with quercetin in regulating this receptor. By suppressing transformation of the aryl hydrocarbon receptor it protects against xenobiotic carcinogens such as dioxins.
- Inhibits NFkB, controlling inflammation, apoptosis and protein degradation.
- Regulates human kallikreins, active in prostate cancer.
- Anti-angiogenic, strongly inhibits vascular endothelial growth factor VEGF induction by IGF-1 and thus VEGF over-expression..
- Inhibits IGF-1, increases IGF-BP-3, may block human growth hormone HGH or it's receptors.
- Pro-oxidant, green tea EGCG can increase hydrogen peroxide H_2O_2 stress on DNA. Therefore give vitamin E to balance.
- EGCG is a major proteasome inhibitor, modulating many regulatory proteins. For example, EGCG specifically inhibits multi-catalytic enzymes leading to accumulation of p27/Kip1 and IkBα, an inhibitor of NFkB. This arrest the cell at G1, and removes protection from apoptosis by AP-1 inhibition via inhibited phosphorylation of c-jun.
- Inhibits cyclin D1 and cyclin E.
- Inhibits tNOX in cancer cells but not in healthy cells. tNOX is a growth regulating cell surface enzyme.
- Anti-cachexic, the primary phenol catechin inhibits TNF alpha
- Promotes differentiation through modulation of transforming growth factor beta two -TGFß-II
- Tea polyphenols are matrix protease MMP-2 and MMP-9 inhibitors, controlling tumour spread.
- Inhibits topoisomerase I, an enzyme which plays a critical role in DNA metabolism and structure, making it essential for tumour cell survival. Effective drugs which inhibit this enzyme are limited by toxicity. Topoisomerase inhibitors do <u>not</u> mix with glucosamine compounds.
- Inhibits 5-alpha-reductase, reducing testosterone levels. Inhibits ornithine decarboxylase in the prostate.
- EGCG inhibits urokinase uPA, an enzyme involved in tumour invasion and metastasis, via breaking down of the basement membrane cell junctions. uPA is over-expressed in most cancers.
- Increases xanthine oxidase XO, which inhibits adenosine deaminase ADA, decreasing DNA turn-over in cancer cells.
- Catechins in green tea rapidly transfer electrons or hydrogen from ROS damage sites on DNA, preventing the development of strand breaks. Very active against hydrogen peroxide, so don't use during IV vitamin C therapy.

- Green tea polyphenols reduce DNA damage from ultraviolet radiation UV-A and UV-B, reducing the inflammation, erythema, and skin cell hyper- proliferation. Thus it prevents skin cancer and will reduce the growth of established tumours in the skin.
- It will deplete vitamin E status, particularly in the kidneys and liver.
- EGCG inhibits telomerase.
- Immune effects include strong enhancement of B-cell activity, increased IL-1α and IL-1β from monocytes, increased cytotoxic T-lymphocyte and NK activity, iodination of PMNs and monocytes.
- Reduces risk of cancer recurrence 50% in post-op stage I & II breast cancer.
- Shown to inhibit breast, colon, prostate, lung, esophageal, stomach, pancreas, urinary bladder and melanoma
- The unique amino acid theanine increases Adriamycin uptake by tumours, significantly increasing efficacy.
- Synergistic with curcumin, grapeseed extract, reishi extract and quercetin.
- Incompatible with intravenous vitamin C therapy. IVC clears the blood in a very short time, so just do not use green tea concentrates the day of the vitamin C drips.
- No known drug interactions. It only very weakly alters CYP3A4 activity in humans, at high doses.

The tea leaf contains 8 to 12% polyphenol antioxidants, and 1 to 4% caffeine. A cup of brewed green tea yields 10 to 40 mg caffeine. For therapy one would need to drink several cups daily. Brew a better tea using water at a temperature below a hard boil. The limit is what the Chinese call "crab-eyes" size bubbles in the kettle – bigger than "shrimp-eyes" but smaller than "fish-eyes" size. A cool overnight infusion of two tablespoons green tea in a litre of room temperature water is also fine for medicinal use, if the caffeine intake is tolerable.

Green tea is an excellent primary cancer remedy, operating at many functional sites and molecular targets in cancer therapy.

I like to use 2,100 mg daily of 95% polyphenol extract of green tea. – 700 mg capsule three times daily at meals.

Green tea polyphenols absorb better if taken with bioperine from black pepper, or with tartaric acid as found in grapes, wine, bananas and tamarind. Tartaric acid is a natural dihydroxy derivative of succinic acid.

Some depletion of vitamin E stores will occur from green tea therapy, and would cause liver and kidney injury if left un-checked. **Always take an extra 400 IU daily of natural source vitamin E when on high dose EGCG** medication. This applies even if you are taking a blood-thinning drug such as Warfarin (Coumadin).

High dose EGCG (over 1,000 mg) can act as a pro-oxidant, creating oxidative stress in cancer cells. This can be useful in some chemotherapy regimens. Green tea has no apparent activity on CYP1A2, CYP2D6, CYP12D6, and CYP12C9 and potentially yields a mild inhibition of CYP3A4, although one study says there is no effect from green tea catechins on CYP3A4. Some preclinical evidence suggests possible inhibition of CYP1A1, 2B1, 17, and 2E1, which are of little clinical relevance in chemotherapy.

ROIBOOS TEA

Aspalathus linearis is rooibos or red bush tea from South Africa. Rooibos is a very pleasant tasting tea which is extraordinarily anti-oxidant. It is also great to drink cold in the summer. While not proven to fight cancer, it seems healthful and adds flavour and variety. It does induce GST and UGT liver enzymes, and so may interact with some drugs which are metabolized by these pathways.

GRAPESEED EXTRACT – See <u>Nutrition Chapter</u>

BILBERRY – See <u>Nutrition Chapter</u>

BOSWELLIA

Boswellia carteri is closely related to Frankincense, a respected herb used for 5,000 years in Egypt, China and India. This gummy tree resin was a gift from the three wise men from the East (Magi) to the Christ-Child in the Christmas legend. It has always been prized as a pain reliever and natural anti-inflammatory, and was indeed a treasure of the ancient world and a gift fit for a King. Today we often use 65% extract of boswellic acid from a closely related species *Boswellia serrata* at 1,000 mg three times daily for pain and inflammation. Remember inflammation in late stage cancer is a slippery slope to disaster, so always have an anti-inflammatory component in the program.

- Inhibits 5-HETE eicosanoids and lipoxygenase LOX , notably the LOX-5 series LTB-4 leukotriene.
- Reduces activity of plasma betaglucoronidase and GAG synthesis
- Inhibits topoisomerase I & II better than camptothecin or etoposide drugs. Topo-II inhibitors do <u>not</u> mix with glucosamine compounds.
- Cytotoxic and pro-apoptotic for glial (brain) cancer, nasopharyngeal cancers and leukemia.
- Synergistic with selenomethionine
- Significantly reduces edema in brain cancers, reducing pressure inside the skull. It can allow reduced doses of steroids and in some case will replace dexamethasone for cerebral edema due to brain cancer, brain metastases, radiotherapy, chemotherapy or leukoencephalopathy.

CURCUMIN

Curcumin is derived from the yellow curry spice turmeric Curcuma longa or yu jin. The turmeric root has about 3% curcumin, and medically this is standardized to about 80 to 95% purity by weight. The active principle is diferuloylmethane. Dietary intake is protective from various cancers, but the medical dose would be 90 grams a day of the root, so obviously we use the capsulated curcumin.

- induces apoptosis in cancers e.g. liver, kidney, sarcoma & colon, via the ubiquinone-proteasome pathway.
- inhibits NFkB and its entire inflammatory cascade
- inhibits the master regulatory enzyme **phosphorylase kinase.**
- inhibits both tyrosine and serine-threonine dependent kinases*.
- powerful inhibitor of COX-2 and PGE-2 promoters of tumour growth and inflammation.
- inhibits mTOR, PKC, EGFR tyrosine kinase and TYK2.
- protects PTEN
- inhibits cancer initiation, promotion and progression
- highly chemoprotective, blocks tumour induction by chemical carcinogens
- reverses liver damage from fungal aflatoxins
- reduces mutagens in tobacco smokers
- slows phase 1 liver detox pathways while speeding up phase 2, reducing build-up of toxic intermediates.
- inhibits oncogenes c-jun, c-fos, c-myc, NIK, MAPKs, ERK, P13K, Akt, JNK, IkBa kinase, CDKs and iNOS.
- inhibits TNF, MMP-9, AP-1, EGR-1, STAT1 & 3, beta-catenin, HER-2, Bcl-2, Bcl-SL, ICAM-1, TF and cyclin D1.
- decreases interleukins to strongly reduce inflammation
- stimulates the reticulo-endothelial immune system
- activates phagocytosis
- inhibits complement pathways
- inhibits spontaneous DNA damage from lipid peroxidation
- induces heat shock protein hsp70 to protect cells from stress
- blocks cell cycle progression at G2/S phase transition.
- significantly inhibits angiogenesis
- blocks APN protein, reducing tumour blood flow and invasiveness.
- inhibits the Sonic Hedgehog signalling pathway
- significantly inhibits number and volume of tumours
- combines well with genestein from soy
- synergistic with EGCG from green tea
- Curcumin can in rare cases trigger thrombocytopenia or low platelet count.

*Only curcumin inhibits both tyrosine-dependent kinases and serine-threonine-dependent kinases, as noted above. Aggarwal, Lee, and group at MD Anderson have shown that if oncogenes are suppressed by TNF induction, with inhibition of Akt, JNK and IkBa kinase, there will be an eventual break-out of oncogene activity by the induction of a parallel pathway involving p44/42 MAPK and p38 MAPK. Only curcumin shuts down both signalling pathways long-term.

Very useful in radiation therapy, improving safety and efficacy, but curcumin is <u>not recommended with chemotherapy.</u> Curcumin radio-sensitizes by increasing ROS, and markedly increasing MAP kinases, leading to reduced oncogene MDM2 expression.

Radio-protective by reducing lipid peroxidation.

The renowned Dr. Mark Gignac, ND eliminates the need for pills by giving 3 to 6 grams a day of curcumin in virgin organic coconut milk.

Curcumin absorbs poorly unless combined with an adjunct such as bromelain, lecithin or bioperine (piperine from black pepper). Bioperine approximately doubles curcumin absorption.

The top brand now is **Curcumin 7X** from Albi Naturals. Its lecithin base and volatile oils make it significantly better absorbed, and thus clinically more potent in a lower dose. Rx 1 capsules 2 to 3 times daily at meals.

Naturopathic oncologists in the U.S.A. are using Vital Nutrients brand BCQ curcumin, bromelain, boswellia and quercetin. Canadian naturopathic physicians in oncology use BCQ or CanArrest, 2 capsules three times daily at meals. Some people develop upset stomachs, bloating, diarrhea and related complaints with long-term use. In these circumstances switch to quercetin with bromelain.

If curcumin is a powerful COX-2 inhibitor, does it cause increased risk of heart attack and stroke, like several anti-inflammatory drugs like Vioxx pulled off the market lately? Fortunately, no. The synthetic drugs strongly inhibited prostacyclin PGI-2, which interacted with thromboxane TxA-2 to trigger clots, mainly heart attacks and thrombo-embolic disease. Curcumin slightly increases prostacyclin PGI-2 levels, reducing risk of clots a bit, while very strongly inhibiting tumour promoters COX-2 ad PGE-2.

ALOE VERA

This succulent has acemannan polysaccharides in its leaf which are immune stimulating, thymus stimulating, increase antibody-dependent cytotoxicity, and inhibit angiogenesis. Aloe emodin is anti-metastatic. Aloe reduces PGE-2, inhibits kinins, histamine and platelet aggregation.

Aloe vera extract has potent anti-oxidants which augment catalase, glutathione GSH and superoxide dismutase SOD. This makes it particularly valuable in reducing lipid peroxidation during radiation therapy. Use it on the skin (but never use oils!) to treat radiation burns.

Aloe root, particularly from the South African cape aloe, has a long history of use as a healer of gastro-intestinal GI ulceration and inflammation, and it relieves constipation.

I have had a number of very dramatic responses to an old laxative formula called #42's in patients in great pain and reliant on morphine that have become constipated, with no appetite and feel gravely ill. #42's are made with two parts sweet wormwood *Artemesia vulgaris* or *Artemesia annua* tops to one part Cape aloe *Aloe capensis* root powder, and the usual dose is 2 capsules 3 times daily or as needed. It is remarkable how little pain people have when their bowels move, and how their entire health picks up. Once the bowels move and pain decreases, they can reduce the narcotic pain-killers. It breaks a vicious cycle of bowel paralysis, bowel toxins from the constipation, increased pain, and more drugs. This little herbal gem has rescued a number of patients from premature death, or death without awareness due to being mentally "snowed under" by opiates.

ARTEMESIA / WORMWOOD

Artemisia vulgaris or absinthum is a traditional medicine for parasites, including malaria. Chinese doctors call it *Qinghao*. It is very useful in cancer.
- wormwood herb relieves constipation, particularly moving the upper GI tract. It is a key component of #42 capsules for severe constipation, as seen in patients on opoid narcotic pain-killers. It also rebalances gut flora (probiotic organisms).
- increases bile flow, detoxifying the liver.
- removes many intestinal worms and parasites.
- reduces inflammatory cytokine growth promoters.

Artemesia annua or sweet wormwood is the source of Artemisinin and Artemether, new ideas in cancer treatment.

- **Artemisinin** is a hormone balancer, particularly reducing excess estrogen and prolactin. It is best studied in breast cancer.
- It is activated by iron ions, which cancer cells accumulate. Cancer cells have abnormally high numbers of surface receptors for transferrin, to uptake the excessive levels of iron they need to proliferate. Dihydro-artemisinin has a peroxide bond activated by iron to generate hydrogen peroxide. This stresses cancer cells which are always catalase deficient. The high-valent oxo-iron species create a cascade of reactive oxygen species called endoperoxides, depolarizing the mitochondrial membranes and disrupting the electron transport chain. Cancer cells are approximately 100 times more susceptible to dying from artemisinin than healthy cells.
- Induces apoptosis and slows growth in fibrosarcoma.
- Inhibits angiogenesis, disrupting the blood supply to tumours.
- Targets translationally-controlled tumour protein TCTP.
- Inhibits cysteine protease enzyme, and also a SERCA-type calcium transporter enzyme.
- It has very short period of action, clearing the bloodstream in about 2 hours.
- Common doses run between 1 to 2 mg. per kilogram body weight. i.e. 160 lb =72.7 kg = 73 to 146 mg daily. 3 -4 mg/kg can be used for a week in severe cases, but beware of heart and nerve toxicity.
- The usual dose has been 100 to 200 mg daily for 1 to 2 months, then take a break for the liver and blood cells to recover.
- There is evidence showing that the liver rapidly increases its ability to get rid of the drug, so that after a week it is difficult to achieve therapeutic blood levels. Dr. Yarnell suggests dosing it at 300 mg 3 times daily for one week, then take a week break from the drug.
- **I prescribe 300 to 600 mg, 1 to 3 times daily, for one week on, then one week off.**
- Take on an empty stomach, away from food as it interacts with dietary iron.
- Artemisinin is not water soluble, so always give with some oil such as omega 3

fish or seal oil supplement or full-fat dairy for optimum absorption.
- Anaemic patients can take iron supplements on the week off the drug, and eat red meat. We let then reload with iron, then we burn it out again. We only give iron if lab tests prove a deficiency, do not self-prescribe iron.
- Synergistic with intravenous vitamin C, amplifying the peroxide stress.
- It may synergize with butyrate, which is produced by gut bacteria acting on fibre such as psyllium husks.
- It is much more useful to **test sTfR – soluble iron tranferrin receptor. If it is greater than 28, there is a need for iron therapy.**

Contraindications:
- Sedentary lifestyle – works best in those more physically active
- Smokers – must be off tobacco at least 6 months
- Radiation therapy or surgery – wait until 2 months after – radiosensitizer and antiangiogenic.

Toxicity:
- **Mild and transient symptoms can occur, but tend to clear with continued use: cold extremities, numbness, tinnitus, dizziness, headache, GI discomfort, anorexia, nausea, vomiting, or diarrhea. If these are severe or persistent, lower the daily dose.**
- Increased liver enzymes AST and/or ALT, a sign of mild liver damage.
- Anemia due to loss of iron. Monitor hemoglobin levels and RDWs - immature replacement red blood cells.

Other forms of artemesia under investigation for use in cancer:

Artemether:1 mg /kg BW for 8 weeks. Usual adult dose is 40 mg twice daily, but it can all be taken in one dose. This is the more toxic form, and the limiting factor in using combination products. Take well away from food, with whole milk, ice cream, etc. After 8 weeks if responding, continue using it but every second day only, for another 3 to 4 months. Periodic use for up to 2 years can be considered, 5 days on and 5 days off.

Synergize with 250 mg vitamin C and 200 IU vitamin E at breakfast and lunch.

Artemix: Combines artemether, artemisinin and artesunate. Usual dose is 1 capsule twice daily, as for artemether. Said to be easier on the liver than plain artemether.

RED CLOVER BLOSSOMS

Trifolium pratense or red clover is a common ingredient in many herbal cancer formulas, including the Hoxsey Tonic.

Contains the coumarin type phyto-estrogens and tumour inhibiting compounds genestein, daidzein, biochanin and formononetin. These are the primary dietary isoflavones in Asian, Mediterranean and Latin American diets associated with lower risk of cancer.

Red clover tops contain significant levels of phytoestrogens as estriols, which are mild and can counteract the more cancer stimulating estradiols, perhaps by occupying the estrogen receptors, without triggering the same signals into the nucleus.

Iso-flavones inhibit 5-aplpha-reductase, lowering dihydro-testosterone, and sequesters DHT. They are also an aromatase inhibitor.

The National Cancer Institute tested red clover 94 times, with only one slightly positive test showing insignificant activity against cancer. If it is useful, it is as an alterative as described by the Eclectic herbalists: normalizing circulation, assisting digestion, accelerating eliminative processes, thus correcting faulty metabolism. Traditional herbalists call it a "blood purifier."

Phyto-estrogens are weak estrogens, and many have such a low affinity for the estrogen receptors that they just block up the receptor, keeping real estrogens out, and therefore block growth signalling. Only phyto-estrogens of a specific size, shape and electrical charge can distort the receptor and trigger tumour growth signals. Many phyto-estrogens such as red clover, soy and ginseng are cancer-fighters, and are safe in ER+++ breast cancer.

BIRCH / BETULINIC ACID

White birch bark and leaves are a source of betulin and betulinic acid, a traditional non-toxic inhibitor of tumours such as melanoma, lymphoma, lung and liver cancer. Betulinic acid decreases bcl-2 expression and cyclin D1 to inhibit proliferation, migration and to induce apoptosis in cancer cells. Chaga mushrooms grown on birch trees convert betulin in the bark to betulinic acid. Chaga mushroom extracts inhibit gap junctional intercellular communication via inactivation of ERK1/2 and p38 MAP kinase. JHS Naturals provides a good Chaga extract.

GINKGO BILOBA

The ancient *Ginkgo biloba* tree has survived from the time of the dinosaurs. It is an extraordinary tonic for memory and peripheral circulation. In cancer we use it for peripheral neuropathy. As it interacts with intestinal Cyp 3A4, it is not used during chemotherapy. It has been studied as a protectant against ovarian cancer.

GRAVIOLA

Annona muricata is also called graviola, soursop, and **paw paw**. It is a small evergreen tree with large glossy leaves, native to tropical America from the Caribbean to the Amazon. Its large heart shaped edible fruit is slightly sour and acid, and it is widely used in drinks and sherbets. Graviola leaves have long been used in local folk medicine for diarrhea, as a lactogogue to increase breast milk, for viral and bacterial fevers and for worms and parasites. Its seeds are crushed to make a stronger remedy for worms and parasites, and are strongly insecticidal. The leaves and bark are used indigenously for diabetes, heart disease, asthma, hypertension, in difficult childbirth, influenza and cough. In general it is cooling, sedative and antispasmodic. Among its many constituents are procyanidin, P-coumaric acid, beta-sitosterol, stigmasterol, myristic acid, HCN, malic acid, and unique acetogenins.

In 1976 the National Cancer Institute found the acetogenins to be definitely cytotoxic to cancer cells. The most potent acetogenins have adjacent bis-tetrahydrofuran rings (THF), e.g. bullatacin. The mechanism of cytotoxicity is inhibition of mitochondrial Complex I electron transport, robbing the cells of ATP energy. In tumour cells they also inhibit the NADH oxidase of plasma membranes, which with ATP depletion thwarts energy dependent resistance mechanisms.

Graviola is active against breast, colon, pancreatic, prostate and other cancer cells in vitro. One test reported its activity in such a screening test to be thousands of times more potent than the common chemotherapy drug Adriamycin. This was an extract mixed with cancer cells in a Petri dish – that is not evidence it is good for human use. No blinded human studies have been reported. Proponents claim it is immune building, antibacterial, antiviral and antiparasitic, and is tonifying. The usual dose is 2 to 5 grams twice daily of the powdered leaf, 1 to 3 ml twice daily of a 4:1 tincture, or ½ cup 1 to 3 times daily of a tea of the leaf or bark.

My experience with it indicates it is active against cancers, but by the time any response is seen, it is creating violent stomach upset and must be discontinued. It is just not tolerable enough to be useful. Furthermore, it is impractical with many protocols as it mixes poorly with many better remedies, such as Hoxsey formula, burdock root, vitamin C, vitamin E, Co-enzyme Q-10, cysteine and flaxseed oil. It would not be sensible to attempt mitochondrial rescue while reducing energy production with graviola.

NOT RECOMMENDED.

ASHWAGANDHA

Withania somnifera – ashwagandha or winter cherry is a herb from the Hindu Ayurvedic tradition. Think of it as the East Indian equivalent of ginseng. It is an adaptogen, helping the body deal with stress. It is a slightly sedative nervine, antioxidant, immune modulating, blood-building and rejuvenating. Ashwagandha prevents loss of adrenal gland function, vitamin C, and body weight when under stress. It increases function in the dopaminergic systems. Ashwagandha is anti-inflammatory, via inhibition of cyclooxygenase. It is quite non-toxic even with long-term use.

Ashwagandha is a great protectant from the damage to healthy cells by chemotherapy and radiation. It particularly protects bone marrow from damage, and stimulates stem cell proliferation to replace red blood cells, white blood cells and platelets. It also enhances therapeutic effectiveness of radiation against cancer cells because of an anti-tumour and radio-sensitizing steroidal lactone withaferin. This radio-sensitizes by dramatically reducing tumour glutathione.

Cautions: May increase testosterone, so it is not recommended in prostate cancer. Contra-indicated in hemachromatosis patients. May decrease tolerance to opiates and narcotic analgesics. May potentiate sedatives such as benzodiazepines and barbiturates.

MISTLETOE

Viscum album or sang ji sheng is a hemiparasitic plant which has subtle variations in its lectins depending on which species of tree it grows on i.e. fir, apple or pine.

White-berried European mistletoe or *Viscum album* has been a successful remedy for advanced cancer since 1917. Approximately 79% of German and Swiss medical doctors advise their cancer patients to use it. Mistletoe therapy is part of "anthroposophical medicine" founded by Dr. Ita Wegman, inspired by the anthroposophy of Rudolph Steiner, who also created Waldorf schools and Bio-Dynamic agriculture.

The two brands which are the best are Helixor and Iscador. Iscador is fermented, while Helixor is not. The mistletoe is extracted and standardized for cancer cell-killing viscotoxins and immune-stimulating viscolectins.

The primary actions are cytoxic killing of cancer cells, DNA protection and stabilization, anti-inflammatory effects, and immune modulation. This means getting the immune system to remove your cancer. Mistletoe lectins stimulate macrophages, T-cells, NK cells and cytotoxic complement. Injections increase cytokines TNFa, IL-1, Il-2, IL-5, IL-6, GM-CSF, gamma interferon and others. It is immuno-modulatory, increasing Th1 and TH2 cytokines, binding T-cells to tumour receptors, activating lymphocytes against tumour antigens, and promoting eosinophilia. It takes about 3 to 4 weeks to work up to the full dose, as we must condition the immune system to react to the medicine. The neutrophils will increase rapidly, but transiently, while the lymphocytes increase after 2 to 3 months therapy. Eosinophils increase according to the dose of lectins delivered. These immune effector cell counts are useful for monitoring response to mistletoe therapy.

Natural killer NK cells will increase in number and activity. Mistletoe will protect NK cells from damage during chemotherapy and radiation. NK cells kill cancer cells, and prevent metastasis

Other mistletoe lectins are directly cyto-static and cyto-toxic to cancer cells, down-regulating VEGF and increasing apoptosis.

Mistletoe lectins are able to protect DNA, and this is of great utility during chemotherapy and radiation.

Mistletoe therapy is commonly prescribed during radiation and chemotherapy in Europe, and is proven to reduce risk of adverse reactions by ½. Patient care costs and loss of productivity costs are reduced by ½ as well.

Mistletoe is strongly anti-viral, so is particularly indicated in hepato-cellular carcinoma, squamous cell carcinomas, lymphomas and leukemias.

The anthroposophical product **Iscador** is my favourite. I have used it for over two decades, and often see a strong response, even in very advanced cancers. After some training and supervision most patients will self-administer every 1 to 3 days as a subcutaneous injection. A small dose is placed just under the skin to form a little bubble, which should provoke a red flare like an allergic hive or welt, as the immune system reacts. Inflammatory reactions are expected, and occasionally become problematic and require desensitization procedures. We try to provoke a mild fever – about a 1° C rise on the average. A proper regulatory fever will spike in a few hours. Fever over 12 hours is not healthy, and merits review. The site of the injection will get red and itchy, within 24 hours, but should not exceed 5 cm. or 2 inches in diameter, and should vanish by about 48 hours. Large, severe or persistent rashes are an indication to reduce the frequency and dosage of the medicine.

It is common to see tumour progression decelerate or even stop, improved general health, and reduced pain. It is a good bone marrow stimulant in drug-induced myelosuppression and in primary marrow diseases. The results I have seen in managing advanced cancers has been dramatic. Increased survival time in many advanced cancers is well documented in recent well-controlled clinical trials in Europe and America. Quality of life is nearly always significantly improved. This includes reduction or elimination of pain, restoration of appetite, appropriate weight gain, and general wellness. Over time the tumours may shrink and even disappear. Over the years, some advanced cases are even cured. For example, actress Suzanne Somers attributes her success over breast cancer to mistletoe.

My experience, over more than two decades, is that we can expect a good response in about 50% of advanced cancers. Many patients go from being disabled and terribly sick to being active and functional, and this can last from months to years, even in the face of a terminal prognosis.

Because it excites an immune-response to the tumours, there can be some short-term increase in tumour size. This is particularly problematic with brain tumours, primary or metastatic.

When a good response is achieved, most other medications may be reduced or eliminated. The maximum cost at this time is approximately $260 Canadian per month, though usually it is quite a bit less than this due to my innovations. Actual cost depends on the dose required to get the biological response we are seeking.

Different species of mistletoe grow on specific species of host trees. The various species of mistletoe have subtle differences in the balance of viscotoxins and viscolectins. While still largely inter-changeable, we prefer to start with specific types of mistletoe extracts for different cancers.

Iscador brand type Qu is from oak trees – the Latin name for oak trees is *Quercus*. The Qu type mistletoe is used by men, including all digestive tract cancers from top to bottom, all uro-genital cancers including prostate, as well as thyroid, larynx and respiratory tract cancers. The unfermented Helixor brand type A (from fir trees) is used for men's cancers as well.

Helixor A is also used for children, sensitive patients who over-react to other forms of mistletoe, for leukemia and multiple myeloma.

Iscador type M and Helixor brand type M from apple trees (*Mali* is Latin for apple tree) are preferred for women.

P type from pine trees (*Pini* is Latin for pine tree) are used primarily for skin, testicular, nerve, and nasopharyngeal cancers, sarcomas, and sometimes for post-menopausal breast cancer. Use in lymphatic cancers such as B-cell lymphoma and CLL. P type is the most potent for stimulating the bone marrow.

The "Series 0" box has seven ampoules, and we give one every two days. We hope to see a red flare in the skin around the injection site, about 1 inch in diameter, arising in an hour or so, peaking at 24 hours, and gone by 48 hours. We do not give another dose until the previous reaction has vanished or at least diminished to a small red dot. Report to the doctor any reaction over 2 inches or 5 cm. in diameter. The other important rule is to never give Iscador during a fever over 38 °C or 100.4° F. We just wait until the fever is down to proceed.

Iscador will usually provoke a small increase in body temperature. A rise of core body temperature of 1°C is a sign of a good response.

Other signs of immune system activation by mistletoe can include flu-like symptoms, aching, shivering, and headache. It is rare, but in some cases these side-effects may necessitate a dose reduction or increased intervals between injections, or both. Usually they are minor and transient.

My innovative fast track to getting to the full-dose of mistletoe: If the Series 0 was well tolerated, we next give 1/2 ampoule of the "Spezial 5 mg" series. If that reacts well, the next doses are 2/3 ampoule, 3/4 ampoule, and finally the full ampoule. From then on, the dose remains 5 mg or one full ampoule. It is quite convenient to use insulin syringes, which have a fine ½" long needle, which is safe for patients to use themselves, and which are marked off in 100 units, so ½ ampoule is 50 units, ¾ ampoule is 75 units, a full ampoule is 100 units, and so forth.

For some special cancers we use type P from pine trees. For example, in lymphoma or sarcomas.

The P type starts with "Series 0," but after that we use "Series 1" and may later use "Series 2," both of which have escalating dosages in each box, and can go up to 20 mg.

Within 3 months the patient should be examined by their oncologist to confirm an objective response. This may involve a CT scan, MRI, Pet Scan, or tumour marker blood test.

A pause of 2 weeks is suggested every year in the first 2 years of use, then 4 weeks off in the next 2 years, and **8 weeks break in the 5th year and beyond.**

If the Iscador stops producing a local skin reaction, it may stop controlling the cancer. You must report this to your naturopathic doctor, who will alter the dosage to restart the therapeutic response.

The maximum recommended subcutaneous dose is 400 mg, but the usual dose should not exceed 1mg/kg/day.

Helixor brand is available in higher doses than Iscador. It is not a problem to switch from similar doses of one product to the other. The Helixor A is the best tolerated, and it is the better immuno-modulator. Therefore it is best for children, and during chemotherapy. Helixor P is harsher due to higher content of cytotoxic lectins.

During mistletoe therapy there may very occasionally be an activation of a hidden focus of infection in the body, such as an occult dental abscess with anaerobic bacteria. Other extremely rare occurrences are gallstones, colon infection and regional lymph node swelling.

Cachexic patients may not do as well with mistletoe, as the increase in cytokines aggravates their metabolic wasting syndrome. Naturopathic physicians assess the vital force of the patient before prescribing stimulatory therapies. In the right case, it can turn around the cachexia, but with supports such as reishi mushroom extract, omega 3 EPA oil, antioxidants and astragalus.

Some doctors use mistletoe extracts by intra-venous, intra-peritoneal, intra-pleural and intra-tumour injection. There is a risk of anaphylactic shock reactions by these routes of administration. A colleague uses mistletoe intravenously, starting with 100 mg in 500 ml. sterile water and 50 grams vitamin C. The mistletoe is raised in 100 mg increments to a maximum of 800 mg. or to tolerance. The usual limitations are nausea, and general aches and pains. Generalized urticaria (hives) are dose-dependent, and respond well to Benadryl. Induction of a fever of 102°F is considered an ideal reaction to IV mistletoe. Peri-lesional injection triggers a local inflammatory swelling that can be problematic if the tumours are in the lungs, spine, head or neck. Bone pain may be significantly reduced. Once the inflammation subsides, tumour shrinkage is possible.

CAT'S CLAW

Uncaria tomentosa or Una de Gato is a vine from Amazonia which indigenous tribes consider a sacred plant. Cat's claw inner bark contains pentacyclic oxindole alkaloids and carboxyl alkyl esters which are antioxidant and remarkably potent inhibitors of TNF-alpha synthesis. It may have a role in treating weight loss from cachexia and anorexia. It may reduce side effects of radiation therapy and chemotherapy – patients report less hair loss, nausea, skin problems and secondary infections. It has steroids and alkaloids with antibiotic, antifungal, antiviral and anti-allergy properties – in short, it is immune modulating. Peruvian traditional doctors are said to use it for cancers and other serious diseases, and since 1960 it has been used in some South American hospitals for cancer, with unconfirmed reports of "consistent results." Prominent medical herbalist James Duke reports it is combined with curcumin and *Dracontium loretanum*, which is related to Jack-in-the-Pulpit. In vitro studies show 5 alkaloids with activity against lymphoma and leukemia cells. Use 1 ml of tincture or up to 2 grams of dry extract three times daily. Personally, I find little use for it. Many people use it because they believe the immune system can attack and overcome cancers – but this herb is not specific to cancer, and has little impact.

LAETRILE

Various seeds of pit fruit, such as peaches and apricots, were used for cancer by ancient Chinese, Egyptians, Greeks and Romans. Laetrile was isolated from apricot pits by Ernst Krebs, MD in the 1920's. His son, Dr. Ernest Krebs, Jr., separated a cyanogenic compound from the enzyme emulsin, thought to dissolve the protein of the cancerous cell. He felt giving these two components separately at short intervals eliminated the toxicity seen with the whole kernel extract. The theory behind the use of these cyanide compounds is that normal cells have an enzyme rhodanase which dispels hydrocyanic gas formed during digestion. Cancer cells lack this enzyme, and have higher than normal levels of the enzyme betaglucoronidase, which is very susceptible to hydrocyanic poisoning. The betaglucoronidase enzyme is associated with the evolution sexual reproduction, including the penetration of sperm into an egg, and is normally only found in the early embryonic stage of human life, called a trophoblast. Cancer cells are the only mature somatic cells with this enzyme in appreciable amounts. The laetrile would therefore be non-toxic to normal cells, and selectively destroy the cancer cell, targeting its unique chemical ability to digest through barriers and spread.

Dr. Kanematsu Sugiura at Sloan-Kettering found laetrile inhibits tumour growth and significantly retards metastasic spread. Despite his reputation as a meticulous scientist, his work was denied and ignored.

The Contreras Clinic in Tijuana, Mexico used it for many years. Dr. Austin and I agree that the Contreras clinic does help cancer cases, but not noticeably better than orthodox oncology. Laetrile doesn't appear to be a miracle drug, but may be useful.

Laetrile is considered by some to be cytotoxic, presumably from the cyanide compound amygdalin. It can cause nausea, vomiting, headache and dizziness. There have been unsubstantiated reports of death from cyanide toxicity. The American Cancer Society considers it an example of the worst sort of cancer quackery. The historical record on Laetrile has been polarized and distorted. I do not know who to believe. What little science there is has been lost in a cloud of propaganda. I have never used Laetrile, out of trepidation over its reported toxicity. I always prefer to work with the least toxic approach. I cannot say I have ever met anyone who has tried authentic Laetrile. However, many cancer patients today self-medicate with 4 to 5 raw apricot pits daily, and

some claim results. This is probably the most toxic form of laetrile, and can trigger muscular weakness, respiratory distress, dizziness, nausea, vomiting, diarrhea, fever and toxaemia. Vitamin C increases cyanide absorption, so the combination of C and Laetrile is absolutely forbidden.

MILK THISTLE

Silybum marianum or milk thistle is the gentlest and most effective **healer of the liver**. The active principles include silibinin and silymarin. Silibinin is a polyphenol consisting of quercetin bound to a lignin.

Highly hepatoprotective from chemical damage, so is recommended for any patient undergoing chemotherapy. It will support liver function where there are liver mets or a primary cancer of the liver. It increases bile flow, and helps the liver conserve glutathione. Normal doses raise liver GSH about 35%, while increasing liver and small intestine GSH-S-transferase by 6 to 7 fold.
- induces Cip-1/p21 and Kip-1/p27.
- inhibits tumour necrosis factors – the TNF group.
- directly inhibits IL-1a and IL-1b production, which mediate acute phase pro-inflammation response including T and B immune cell activation.
- Inhibits IL-6
- **Strongly inhibits epidermal growth factor EGF**, and its receptor EGFR, a driver of growth in all types of carcinoma.
- Inhibits cyclin-dependent kinases cyclin-D1, CDK-2 and CDK-4.
- silibinin inhibits cancer cell growth by 48% and induces apoptosis to increase by a factor of 2.5.
- Significantly reduces phospho-mitogen-activated protein kinase/

extracellular signal-regulated protein kinase 1/2 (MAPK/ERK1/2) to inhibit growth. Up-regulates or increases stress-activated protein kinase/ jun NH(2) terminal kinase (SAPK/JNK1/2) and p38 mitogen-activated protein kinase (p38 MAPK) activation.
- inhibits angiogenic factor VEGF
- inhibits fibroblast growth factor FGF
- inhibits insulin-like growth factor receptor IGF-1R.
- slows prostate, colorectal, liver and skin cancer growth

WHEAT GRASS JUICE

Ann Wigmore, N.D. emphatically recommends this juice, made fresh several times daily, consumed within 20 minutes of extraction. Chlorophyll has been emphasized as a cancer cure by our elders such as Dr. Fred Loffler, and Dr. Allen Tyler. It is "detoxifying."

COFFEE

Coffee contains caffeine and theophyllines which block PI-3 kinase enzyme crucial to cell growth. Moderate coffee intake is linked to lowered risk of oral, GI and breast cancers. Caffeine reduces skin damage from the ultraviolet rays in sunlight, reducing risk of non-melanoma skin cancer. It may have anti-clotting properties. Intake of 4 or more cups daily is linked to depletion of B-vitamins and calcium.

It has long been used in Mexican cancer clinics as a retention enema of 4 to 6 ounces of brewed coffee to relieve pain, presumably by flushing toxins out of the liver by increasing bile flow. This seems strange to some, but it has a history of use for many generations in hospitals and medicine. It actually works. A retention enema is not just washing out the lower colon and rectal canal with a quart of more of water. A regular cup of coffee is cooled to body temperature. Insert ½ to ¾ cup into the rectum using a rubber bulb syringe, or a standard enema bag, tube and tip, and lube. Lay on your back in the bathtub, or with a towel under your bottom, somewhere near a bathroom. If the urge comes to expel some of the coffee, that is OK, but with a little practice it should be possible to hold it in for 10 to 15 minutes. By that time it should all have been absorbed by the haemorrhoidal veins, and be sent up the hepatic portal system straight into the liver, leaving nothing to expel.

TAHEEBO

Tabebuia avellanedae or Pau d'Arco inner bark and heartwood contains anthraquinones and napthoquinones such as lapochol. Taheebo has been used since 1960 at Santo Andre Hospital in South America on terminally ill cancer patients. Native folklore suggested that it might be useful for breast cancer, Hodgkin's lymphoma, leukemia, cancer pain, and to increase the blood cell counts. Taheebo is anti-neoplastic, acting directly against oncogenes.

Health Canada advises it is completely harmless as a beverage, but has "no proven merit in treating cancer." Some patients tell me it really helped them, and I have observed a few very dramatic responses to it. I would use it myself if I had cancer.

It is regarded as a treatment for overgrowth of the yeast Candida albicans, parasites, bacterial and virus infections. This would be expected to reduce inflammatory growth factors, which would slow cancer growth. The inner bark chips need to be boiled for about 15 minutes, then steeped another 15 minutes. Drink it freely. As a tincture, use 15 to 20 drop 2 to 3 times daily.

Very high doses can cause nausea, vomiting, and prolonged bleeding time.

CHAPARRAL

The creosote bush *Harrea divertica Coville* leaves and twigs contain nordihydroguaiaretic acid (NDGA). This powerful antioxidant removes glucose from the cancer cells, reducing their growth. It has a long history of use by Native American practitioners for rheumatism, arthritis, urethral complaints, lymphatic swellings, and for tissue repair. It was popularized by Jason Winters, who claims it is especially effective for melanoma. He often combined it with red clover and gotu kola. Large doses will commonly cause nausea, loss of appetite, stomach ache and vomiting.

Occasional acute toxic cholestatic hepatitis and jaundice has been reported with some species of chaparral, sometimes resulting in fulminant liver failure requiring liver transplantation, or resulting in death. Clearly a herb to use with caution, if you are not sure of the exact species and constituents you are dealing with. However, Dr. John Bastyr, ND used it freely in his arthritis formula, with no problems.

CARNIVORA

The Venus fly-trap plant *Dionea muscipula* juice is treated to remove poisonous constituents, then mixed with alcohol and water to make the patented phytonutrient Carnivora. It is an immune modulator used by some American Presidents. According to Dr. Helmut Keller, microbes, viruses, parasites and tumours are rapidly reduced by the activation of helper T-cells and inhibition of suppressor T-cells. Carnivora makes protein kinases which block the production of tumour proteins, starving the cancer cells. Carnivora also balances autoimmune disorders.

A standard protocol is 12 ml. diluted in 250 ml. normal saline given intravenously in a 4 hour drip. Doses can range from 30 to 100 ml daily in 500 ml saline by a 4 hour I.V. drip. For brain cancers dilute the product in 20% mannitol to carry it across the blood-brain barrier. The product may also be taken in water or tea 120 to 250 drops daily. For disease in the respiratory tract it may be inhaled via a cool-steam vaporizer. Sterile preparations may be injected subcutaneously 1 ml. twice daily or intramuscularly 2 ml twice daily. An extract may be encapsulated, and taken at doses of 1 to 2 of 125 mcg capsules up to four times a day.

It can cause a fever and increased white blood cell count. As we have seen with graviola, Coley's toxins, and mistletoe, the immune system is challenged, the reticuloendothelial system responds, and all manner of infections, parasites, viruses and the malignant cells are robbed of energy and forced into apoptosis. I have not used this product much clinically, and when I have the results were very disappointing. NOT RECOMMENDED.

LAMINARIA

Laminaria spp. are brown algae, which yield laminarin. Laminarin inhibits basic fibroblast growth factor BFGF, a heparin-dependent angiogenic factor that binds to the extra-cellular matrix. And cell surface receptors.

PODOPHYLLUM

Podophyllum pelatrum or Mayapple yields the irritating resin podophyllin. Tinctured to 25%, podophyllin can be used as an escharotic to remove superficial basal or squamous cell carcinoma. I use this in a formulation I developed which I call "Wart Death" to remove benign growths. An extract of this plant has been made into the synthetic chemo drug Etoposide.

FEVERFEW

Tanacetum parthenium or feverfew is rich in parthenolides which inhibit nitric oxide synthesis and 1κβ kinase-alpha, which inhibits leukemic stem cells. Rx 3 to 4 mg of parthenolides daily. It may combine well with glutathione depleters such as vitamin K3, vitamin C, L-glutamine and sage *Salvia miltiorrhiza.*

HORSE CHESTNUT TREE

Aesculus hippocastanum leaves contain active coumarins, anticoagulants, antioxidants, and the haemolytic saponin escin. Its favourable impact on vascular permeability is blocked by cyclooxygenase COX inhibitors. Escin protects the integrity of the vascular basement membrane, inhibiting invasion and metastasis. Use intermittently, for 2 to 4 weeks at a stretch, as it is slightly toxic to the kidneys. We use it extensively for varicose veins and haemorrhoids, both topically and internally.

PLANT STEROLS & STEROLINS

Beta-sitosterols and sterolins were discovered in the traditional Hottentot medicinal plants of the *Hypoxis spp.* by Dr. Patrick Bouic, Ph.D., an immunologist from South Africa. These common plant fats are extremely powerful modulators of the immune system.

I use them with marine omega 3 oils for all auto-immune diseases. Rx: 1 to 3 capsules daily of a professional quality extract such as Vitazan Ultra-Immune formula will increase the adrenal hormone building block DHEA, which reduces circulating cortisol. Plant sterols, sito-sterols and DHEA are not recommended for prostate cancer.

Sterols and sterolins will increase IL-2, IFN-gamma, activate NK and T-cytotoxic C8 cells to lyse cancer cells, reducing inflammation and immunosuppression. Interleukin six IL-6 is down-regulated.

It is to be considered in squamous cervical cancer because it is active against human papilloma virus, giving a remission rate of 50% for HPV infections.

Reduces 17-beta estradiol or E2 signalling.

Sterols appear to be most useful in breast cancer, prostate cancer, lymphomas and leukemias.

Rare adverse events can occur, namely bone marrow injury and blood dyscrasias.

SEA CUCUMBER

Sea cucumber extract is a potent anti-coagulant 4 to 8 times more powerful than heparin. The active principle is a fucosylated chondroitin sulphate glycosaminoglycan. It is blocks tumour cell selectin binding, which inhibits angiogenesis and metastasis. Health Concerns brand is a good product. It can be effective in doses that have a minimal effect on clotting time, as measured by PTT or INR testing.

BERBERINE

Oregon grape root – *Berberis* or *Mahonia aquifolium* contains the alkaloid berberine, which has a long use in Chinese and other medical traditions as a broad-spectrum antimicrobial and ant-inflammatory. Other herbs containing this alkaloid are *Coptis chinensis* or golden-thread, andrographites, barberry *Berberis vulgaris* and golden seal root *Hydrastis canadensis*. These "cold" herbs cool inflammation, including radiation injury.

- All are used for infections, including parasites. Berberine is a natural anti-biotic, immuno-stimulating, and increases leukocyte count.
- Berberine is a potent herbal cytotoxic iso-quinolone alkaloid which poisons DNA topoisomerases I and II. Its pharmacological profile is very similar to the natural drug Camptothecin, which is now being used for a variety of cancers.
- Berberine induces apoptosis in brain cancers, leukemias and carcinomas.
- Berberine is an excellent free radical scavenger of singlet oxygen and the super-oxide anion radical.
- Berberine is anti-mutagenic by modulation of DNA transcription.
- Decreases levels of adhesion molecule ICAM-1 and transforming growth factor beta TGF-β1

NETTLES

Stinging nettles or *Urtica dioca* is strongly anti-inflammatory because it blocks LOX-5 series to reduce levels of leukotriene LTB4. Nettle extract significantly suppresses TNFa. It can be eaten fresh as a steamed vegetable in the Springtime, 40 to 60 grams per serving. As a tea take 3 to 4 cups daily. Extract Rx: 500 to 850 mg twice daily, between meals.

BLOODROOT

Sanguinaria canadensis is a herb once known as "Puccoon" root. It is a somewhat toxic herb.

Sanguinaria contains about 1% iso-quinolone alkaloid sanguinarine. Small doses induce emesis, large doses can kill. We use it by hormesis – a very tiny dose of a toxin is used as a stimulant. We colloquially refer to it as a "kicker" in a herbal/homeopathic formula. Use 1 to 10 drops of the tincture per dose.

Bloodroot is part of Frank Beallie's "Another Herb" tablet, with sheep sorrel, red clover and Galencia ginger. This is also made as an ointment called "Black Salve." Traditional versions of Black Salve sometimes included chaparral herb, comfrey leaf, plantain leaf, mullein leaf, chickweed herb and pine tar.

Bloodroot is an integral part of Hoxsey's red paste escharotic. Before him it was mixed with zinc chloride in "Fell's remedy."

Note "Hoary puccoon" is completely unrelated – *Lithospermum officinalis* has an anti-thyroid hormone action.

BLACK SALVE

A traditional ointment for cancers consisted of pine tar, tallow, chaparral herb, red clover blossoms, comfrey leaf, plantain leaf, chickweed herb, mullein leaf, olive oil and soy oil.

A modern variant of this combined sheep sorrel, blood root, red clover and Galencia ginger. Cover with moist dressings of vitamin E on gauze.

BOTANICALS DESERVING FURTHER INVESTIGATION

Rattlesnake plantain: *Goodyera pubescens* is a scarce rainforest Orchid used by natives in North America for ulcers and cancers. Many interesting testimonials are on file at the B.C. Cancer Research Centre, and my inquiries into some of these cases suggests real potential for external and internal use. The plant is rare, delicate, and not foragable.

Bindweed: *Convolvulus arvensis L.* is a common field weed related to Morning-glory vines. Dr. Daniel Rubin, N.D. has found it has significant C-statin angiogenesis inhibitor properties. Farmers love to see someone pay to take the darn nuisance out of their fields!

Graviola: *Annona murica* was found to be very powerful but the active principles could not be made synthetically to produce a drug, so the research money dried up – or so the legend goes. It is too harsh on the GI tract to use orally. The active principles need to be delivered in a new posology..

Saposhnikovia divericata: rhizome has an acid arabinogalactan polysaccharide Saposhnikovan A which is a potent potentiator of the reticulo-endothelial immune system.

Pseudo-ginseng: *Panax pseudoginseng var. notoginseng* because it moves stagnant blood but prevents haemorrhage.

Violets: *Viola papillonacea* – fresh violet leaves as infusion or a compress relieves pain and inhibits tumour growth. Used by Hippocrates and often mentioned by herbalists throughout the ages.

Mountain mahogany: *Cerocarpus spp.* is a relative of the birch tree. A 106-year-old Paiute medicine man told Dr. Bill Mitchell, ND about this for prostate cancer. Rx: 60 drops tincture twice daily.

Japanese plum yew: *Cephalotaxus fortunei* bark is prescribed by Dr. Bill Mitchell, ND for lymphomas and leukemias. Rx: 30 drops tincture twice daily.

It is a fact of history that the source of many advances in orthodox medicine has been the botanical formularies of the "irregular" physicians, the homeopaths, and the herbal "wise women" and "wise men" of the world. Each time regular doctors falter, and the so-called war on cancer has indeed stalled, there are raids on the knowledge base of those on the front-lines of natural medicine. The originators of the clinical use of these valuable medicines are almost never acknowledged, for they are of course quacks for using them without the blessing of the science industry bio-pirates.

It seems as if until a God-given healing force on the planet is turned into a commodity for profit, it has no value in the current medical system. This must end. The healing power of nature has the same value as life. Without it, no medicine works.

"Today's mighty oak is just yesterday's nut that held its ground."

Chapter Seven – Traditional Chinese Medicine – TCM In Cancer

The classic Eight Principles system of TCM categorizes patient's conditions and matches up herbs in terms of hot/cold, excess/deficiency, yin/yang and interior/exterior. Further consideration is given to the state of various forms of the vital energy chi or qi, the state of the blood, the vital essences such as jingo and parameters such as stagnancy, dampness, dryness, fire, wind, toxins, phlegm and obstructions. Once the language and cultural code is cracked, these are actually quite logical and simple rationales for selecting therapies. An experienced TCM practitioner will always be able to discern a strategy to improve balance and health, and can readily monitor through pulse and tongue diagnosis whether the overall state of the patient is improving or not.

CHI DEFICIENCY – use immuno-stimulants such as *Astragalus membranaceus* or huang qi, *Ligusticum porterii*, and licorice root. *Fu zheng pei beng* nourishing formulations like Bu Zhong YI Qi Wan reinforce the body essence to build a foundation of positive chi. Ginseng and Notoginseng extracts are immune stimulating. Immune tonics work best when given early in the day, such as one dose at breakfast and another before lunch.

STAGNANT BLOOD – induce fibrinolysis and inhibit platelet aggregation with cayenne *Capsicum frutescens*, horse chestnut *Aesculus hippocastanum*, carthamus flower *Carthamus tinctorius*, corydalis rhizome *Corydalis yanhusuo*, notoginseng *Panax pseudoginseng*, myrrh, sage *Salvia miltiorrhizae*, *Sporangium simplex*, red peony root *Paeonia rubra*, and turmeric *Curcuma longa* or *Curcuma zedoaria*. Protein and tyrosine kinase inhibitors in soy miso inhibit platelet aggregation. Stagnancy from lack of chi flow makes tumours form. The Chinese use the term *huoxue huay* for enlivening the blood and dissolving stasis. Naturopathic physicians would add omega 3 marine oils, serratiopeptidase or bromelain enzymes, Sanum Mucokehl, or lumbrokinase. Stagnant blood can show up as a purplish color to the tongue – 4 times more common in cancer than in healthy patients.

YIN DEFICIENCY – nourish with ligusticum root *Ligusticum porterii*, lycium fruit *Lycium chinense*, Chinese foxglove root *Rehmannia glutinosa*. <u>Avoid</u> astragalus *Astragalus membranaceus* and atractylodes root *Atractylodes macrocephala*

CLEAR HEAT TOXINS – inflammation or fire toxin are reduced by isatis root *Isatis tinctoria*, cassia *Cassia obtusifolia* and formulae like Qing Wen Bai Dou Yin. The Chinese term is *qingri jiedu* for clearing heat and eliminating toxins. Patients with a red base to the tongue covered with a thick yellow patchy coat are very hot and toxic! My TCM training put me many years ahead of oncologists in understanding the role of inflammation (heat) in cancer. *Oldenlandia* is a wonderful TCM detoxifier.

DISPERSE MASSES – tumours accumulate when the chi or vital force fails to move matter and it stagnates and forms into hard masses. Herbs which soften and disperse these perform the function *ruanjian sanjie*.

DISPERSE CONGEALED PHLEGM – phlegm and dampness can obstruct channels and create tumours. Herbs which dissolve phlegm and disperse dampness perform the function *huatan qushi*.

POISON AGAINST POISON – toxic herbs can be used, similar to Western style cytotoxic chemotherapy, and this is called yidu gongdu. This strategy of *gong xie* means "attack the disease evil," and contrasts with the more common fuzheng supportive and corrective strategies.

Herb formulae used in cancer may have many ingredients, with groups or modules of herbs designed to serve one of these core principles of treatment, and with accessory herbs which direct the others to a particular organ or meridian. Each formula is customized to the individual condition, and not just to the disease. If one aspect of the condition improves before another, that cluster of herbs may be removed from the formula. In North America we may use pill forms of the formulae, and may use two or more different formulae together, each specific to one of the treatment principles.

MEDICINAL MUSHROOM POLYSACCHARIDES

Asian traditional medicine has long used mushrooms as immune tonics, including *Coriolus versicolor*, maitake – *Grifola frondosa*, shitake – *Lentinus edodes*, *Agaricus blazei, Cordyceps*, and reishi – *Ganoderma lucidum* or ling zhi. All can be effective, if good quality extracts are used. We prescribe <u>hot water extracts</u> only. The mushroom cell wall is cellulose, like paper or wood, it is indigestible by humans. However, ground mushroom decocted in hot water yields up its medicinal ingredients. Asians have always prepared this medicine as a tea or soup. A hot water extract is made by drying the tea made from the mushroom, and this concentrate is what is in the caps, not just ground up mushroom or its filamentous mycelia form. The brilliant cancer watch-dog Ralph Moss, PhD has recommended JHS Naturals brand single mushroom extracts, which I prescribe for my patients. A typical dose may be 500 to 1,000 mg three times daily. When I want a mixture of the mushrooms I take the recommendation of my friend Gregg Turner and give Nikken *Kenzen 14* mushroom complex. Several caps can atop a cold or flu in its tracks.

Reishi or *Ganoderma lucidum* or ling zhi mushrooms contain cytotoxic triterpenes which have been shown to inhibit DNA synthesis via DNA polymerase beta. Reishi extracts aid in cachexia because they down-regulate TNFα. This also influences apoptosis and reduces chemo-resistance. Reishi balances inflammatory Th1 and Th2 cytokines, and gamma interferon IFNγ. Reishi reduces IL-2, IL-3 and IL-4. Reishi extracts increase IL-2, IL-6, CD3, CD4, CD56 and CD+ lymphocyte counts, and mitogenic reactivity to phytohemagglutinin. Extracts inhibit transcription factors NFkB and AP-1, which in turn inhibits uro-kinase plasminogen activator uPA and its receptor uPAR. Suppresses cell adhesion and cell migration, reducing invasiveness in breast and prostate cancers. Reishi is an adaptogen, and is very synergistic with ginseng and coriolus. I have been greatly inspired by Dr. Steven Aung, MD who uses wild reishi, and reishi formulated with pollen, pearl, *Gynostemma pentaphylla, Coriolus versicolor* or *Panax ginseng*.

Coriolus versicolor extracts PSP and PSK are proprietary hot water extracts from fungal mycelia that run about 30% high molecular weight polysaccharides (HMWPS). It is the highest of all in beta-glucans. They are proven immunomodulators via inhibition of cytokines IL-8 and TNFα. Coriolus PSK stimulates natural killer cells, and lymphocytes to increase IL-2 by 2.5 fold. Trials with 1,500 mg twice daily have shown increased survival in patients undergoing chemotherapy with cisplatin for many cancers. Coriolus induces apoptosis in leukemia cells, raising IL-6 and IL-1β, while reducing IL-8.

Shiitake lentinan corrects ovarian cancer resistance to cisplatin or 5-FU.

Agaricus blazei is very high in beta-glucans. Highly synergistic with Rituximab, the R in CHOP-R chemo for non-Hodgkin's lymphoma.

Chaga mushrooms grown on birch trees convert betulin in the bark to betulinic acid; JHS Naturals has a good Chaga extract. Chaga mushrooms inhibit gap junctional intercellular communication via inactivation of ERK1/2 and p38 MAP kinase.

AHCC – active hexose correlated compound is a proprietary Japanese low molecular weight compound from fermented shiitake and other medicinal mushrooms grown in rice bran, which has been found to prevent many chemo side-effects and increase the effectiveness of methotrexate, 5-fluorouracil and cyclophosphamide when used at doses of 3 grams daily. It may also protect from radiation damage and reduce stress from surgery. It is particularly useful in protecting chemo patients from damage to bone marrow, preventing hair loss, and has demonstrated it can reduce nausea, vomiting, pain and can improve appetite. 1 in 3 patients show a complete or partial response in terms of improved quality of life at dose of 3 to 6 grams daily.

In British Columbia we have many beautiful conk mushrooms which are very similar to the Asian medical mushrooms. The Chaga conk *Inonotus obliquus* grows on birch, alder, cottonwood, beech and hickory trees. The coriolus relative growing here is known as Turkey tails, and one look at the colourful ring pattern informs why.

They are considered useful as anti-virals, disinfectants and for gastro-intestinal cancers.

BU ZHONG YI QI TANG

Rich in high molecular weight polysaccharides HMWPS from *Lycium barbarum*, *Gynostemma pentaphyllum* or Jiao gu lan, *Acanthopanax senticosus* or Siberian ginseng, and *Astragalus membranaceus*. Increases IL-2 and may be synergistic with melatonin and glutathione.

SIBERIAN GINSENG

Eleutherococcus senticosus or *Acanthopanax senticosus* is a wonderful herb for fatigue and stress. It is not a true ginseng, but is an adaptogen herb from Northern China and Siberia which was used for purposes similar to the ginseng of Southern China. It balances blood sugar and is strengthening. I have taken it daily for many years. Siberian ginseng may inhibit sarcomas. Use *Wu Cha Seng* brand wild-crafted root 4 tablets twice daily.

GINSENG

Panax ginseng or ren shen contains ginsenosides which are known to be antineoplastic-cytotoxic

- cause G1 arrest similar to p53 protein
- induce redifferentiation
- induce apoptosis.
- activate and modulate the reticulo-endothelial immune system
- activate p21 gene transcription, and expression of p27 protein.
- suppress Bcl-2, caspase 3, 5-alpha-reductase, androgen receptors, cell adhesion, invasion and metastasis.

Traditionally ginseng is used as a tonic for digestion and fatigue in the elderly, and as a panacea for longevity. It is proven to lower blood sugar by increasing insulin receptors, reduce stress reaction, and enhance immunity. It is believed to improve lassitude, pain tolerance, mental concentration, memory, physical vitality and appetite.

The traditional style of use is a tea of ginseng root. This is a warming and digestive stimulating beverage. The root is made into the more yang energy "red" ginseng by repeated steaming. This neutralizes certain enzymes.

Women are often given the "white" or unprocessed root, which is more yin. I put an inch or two of a stout root in a ceramic Chinese herb pot full of water, set inside a large double-boiler pot, at a low boil for a few hours.

Ginseng alone or with royal jelly and other herbs is energizing and tonifying for yang and chi deficient patients. It particularly tonifies the digestion in the elderly. In China ginseng is usually used for treatment of inflamed stomach and stomach ulcer.

Ginseng may be synergistic with vitamin C for leukemia.

The patented natural product Careseng is an enriched extract with 8% Rh2 and 75% related aglycan ginsenosides which are synergistic. It is said to be very potent, and strongly synergistic with cytotoxic compounds, activating execution caspases. It is claimed it can overcome multidrug resistance (MDR gene) to restore tumour sensitivity in late-stage disease. It may block angiogenesis, and may block cancer cell entry into G1 growth phase, arresting tumour growth. A synthetic form of these ginsenosides is being developed as a drug under the designation PBD-2131. While many of my colleagues use it, I have yet to be convinced it has any value at all. It is very expensive, running into thousands of dollars a month for many patients. I spoke with an MD from China who did these infusions on cancer patients for 4 years, without seeing any significant responses. NOT RECOMMENDED for first-line therapy due to high cost and low response rate.

FARE YOU

"Fare-You Vitamin U complex" is a pharmaceutical grade extract of green cabbage, with a few adjuncts.

Vitamin U is S-methyl-L-methionine – $C_6H_{15}NO_2S$, aka Methylmethioninesulfonium Chloride, aka Cabagin-U.

Vitamin U is a gastric mucosa regenerator prescribed for peptic ulcers: gastric and duodenal ulcers, achylia gastrica, hyperacidity, chronic gastritis, and regurgitation or gastro-esophageal reflux disorder GERD.

I have found it to be an excellent remedy for diverticulitis, colitis, proctitis and mucositis.

This compound is also found in egg yolks, alfalfa and various green leafy vegetables. The historic Nature Cure for stomach ulcers was a quart of fresh green cabbage juice daily.

Hippocrates used cabbage for cancer. Cabbage also contains indoles, sulphoranes and iso-thiocyanates.

I began to use it for mucositis in chemo patients and the results are just amazing. The Leukemia Bone-Marrow Transplant Unit in Vancouver has seen it work – and would love to get funds to research it.

Rx: 1 to 4 tablets three times daily.

JINGLI NEIXAO

This traditional Chinese medicine (TCM) herbal formula is scientifically formulated, clinically tested, and found effective in the treatment of a variety of tumours. It is a herbal chemotherapy which relieves pain, detoxifies and is anti-inflammatory. Jingli is a good example of the TCM strategy of *Fu Zheng Pai Beng* which strives to tonify and nourish the vitality of the patient rather than attack the cancer. In TCM terms it cools heat, disperses phlegm and sweeps away toxins; it relieves stagnation of phlegm – primarily by soothing and cooling the liver. Jingli will be prescribed along with other naturopathic and TCM herbs which will modify its various qualities to better fit the individuals we treat. Jingli is prepared for my patients by a local compounding pharmacist. The ingredients and their rationale for use are:

Lonicera: Honeysuckle flowers or *chi yin hua* purge blood of heat and toxins due to their antimicrobial and anti-inflammatory properties. Softens lymphatic swellings and relieves fevers.

Ginseng: Ginseng root or *ren shen* improves appetite, is a tonic to the digestive organs and supplements energy by normalizing sugar metabolism.

Angelica: Japanese Angelica or *tang kuei* both builds and moves the blood.

Atractylodes: Atractylodes or *tsang shu* is a digestive tonic, relieves nausea, purges dampness, and is rich in vitamin A.

Prunella: All-heal or *xia ku cao* is used worldwide for liver inflammation, or stagnant inner heat. It relieves congestion of fluid and lymph.

Pinellia: Pinellia or *ban xia* strengthens digestion, relieves inflammation in the liver and pancreas, treats nausea, and strongly resolves phlegm.

Sargassum: Sargassum seaweed or *hai tsao* cols fevers, resolves phlegm, relieves congestion and softens tumours.

Laminaria: Ecklonia kelp or *kun pu* decongests lymph nodes, moves fluid and softens masses.

Paeoniae: Peony or *Bai shao* builds blood, purifies or detoxifies the blood, relieves pain, stops diarrhea, promotes liver function. Supports yin and ying chi.

Bupleurum: Bupleurum or *Chai Hu* is the premier liver support herb, and relieves pain. It detoxifies, cools, decongests and dispels wind.

Poria: Polyporus mushroom or *fu ling* tonifies the digestion, relieving nausea or diarrhea. It resolves dampness and edema. It is calming and supports good sleep.

Rx: 1 to 2 capsules, three times daily with meals.

LIAN BI ANTI-CANCER TABLETS

Lian bi is a formula made of rare and strange traditional Chinese medicine (TCM) products and used in major Chinese hospitals for malignant tumours. It is used in support of surgery, radiation and chemotherapy to enhance tumour shrinkage and shorten treatment time. It also relieves pain and arrests bleeding. Among the cancers it treats are lung, nasopharyngeal, lung, cervix, stomach and epithelioma villosum.

The ingredients and the rationale for their use:

Rock arborvitae: Tree of life cedar or *Thuja* is antibacterial, antifungal and antiviral.

Gecko: Gecko lizard skin for lung and adrenal vitality.

Ophidia: Serpent grass

Seven leaf flower:

Prunella: All-heal or *xia ku cao* is antibiotic and resolves stagnant internal heat.

Bezoar: Cow gallstone powder is anti-inflammatory and cooling.

Musk: Musk gland essence is a circulatory stimulant, benefits the heart and lungs.

Rx: 6 tablets three to four times daily, for courses of 15 days.
Keep dry with the lid tightly closed.

LOTUS KANG LIU WAN

Traditional Chinese medicine (TCM) herbs processed by modern scientific methods give us a gentle but effective formula for pain, inflammation and toxicity due to cancerous tumours. It is a gift from the wise men of the East.

This formula contains no undisclosed ingredients, no animal parts, no heavy metals, and no toxic herbs. It is not experimental or risky. The ingredients and their rationale for use are:

Selaginella: Life-saver king or *shi xiang bai* astringes and arrests bleeding. In rare instances Selaginella products may provoke pancytopenia. Watch for itching, bleeding gums and joint pains.

Schefflera: Goosefoot shrub or *chi yeh lien* relieves pain, relaxes muscles and reduces swelling.

Paris: Single-footed lotus cools fever, detoxifies, reduces swelling and disperses bruising.

Tribulus: Tribulus fruit or *chi li* dispels stagnant moisture and relieves liver heat and wind due to yin deficiency.

Prunella: All-heal or *xia ku cao* is antibiotic and resolves stagnant internal heat.

Boswellia: Frankincense or *ru xiang* is strongly anti-inflammatory, relieves pain by invigorating blood circulation, and promotes tissue repair.

Myrrh: Myrrh or *mo yao* relieves pain and swelling by eliminating blood stasis. It is antiseptic and promotes wound healing.

Rx: 2 capsules three times daily after a meal.

ANTICANCERLIN

A TCM tablet for post-surgical long term management of carcinomas of the pancreas, stomach, rectum, liver and esophagus. It may also have a role in lung, urinary bladder, nasopharyngeal and thyroid cancers, as well as leukemia. It can shrink tumours, increase appetite and strength, relieve pain and reduce complications such as jaundice. In advanced pancreatic cancer the average remission is over 18 months.

Dose is 4 tablets (0.25 gram extract per tablet) 3 times daily. It is mild, safe, and cannot to be expected to do what some more aggressive formulas do. Add synergists.

PING XIAO PIAN

For solid tumours. Alumen, Lacca Sinica Exsiccata and Guano Trogopterorum disperse stagnation, activate the blood, which is anti-inflammatory, analgesic and promotes tissue regeneration. Strychni seed stimulates the heart and nervous system to promote vital energy. Agrimoniae herb and Aurantii fruit are dispersive, cardiotonic, and stimulate digestion. Sal Nitri and Curcumae root complete the formula. A favourite of my colleague Dr. Geoff Szymanski, RAc, NDA variation was sold to practitioners by Eden Herbs as Can-Z.

LIU WEI DI HUANG WAN

A classical formula for kidney yin deficiency. For "false-fire" yin deficient patients, who show various inflammatory signs and symptoms. The key herb Rehmannia glutinosa tonifies the adrenal glands, prolongs the action of cortisol or the drug cortisone and antagonizes depression caused by steroid hormones. I have seen some wonderful remissions of cancer of the esophagus and stomach with this simple old formula. It heals and restores damaged kidneys too. For small cell lung cancer patients undergoing radiotherapy or chemotherapy it is shown to increase the proportion having a complete response, lengthen survival and reduce toxicity to blood elements. I give it in doses of 12 pellets twice daily of the patent medicine "Rehmannia Six."

LIU WEI HUA JIE TANG

This formula supplements qi, dramatically increasing long term survival in stomach cancer.

SHIH CHUAN DA BU WAN

Shiquan or "Ginseng & Tang kuei Ten Herb Formula" is a TCM formula containing astragalus and ligusticum. It has a long history of use to build the qi, blood, yin and yang – and since it builds all four of the vital elements, it is rightly called a supertonic. Many large and high quality research studies from Asian universities and hospitals prove to the highest standard that this formula significantly improves responses to chemotherapy while dramatically reducing side-effects. Shih Chuan Da Bu Wan is used in China for leukemia, stomach and uterine cancers. It has been shown to stimulate hemopoietic (blood-building) factors, and interleukin production. It can potentiate the effectiveness of chemotherapy drugs and reduce their toxicity, especially leukopenia, thrombocytopenia, weight loss and fatigue.

JIN GUI SHEN QI WAN

Supplements the kidney yang. Small cell lung cancer patients undergoing radiotherapy or chemotherapy have been given this formula with a positive increase in complete remissions, lengthened survival and reduced haematological toxicity. Also called Rehmannia Eight Herb Formula, or Ba Wei Di Huang Wan. This is very good for reviving failing kidneys, in concert with CoQ-10 and R+ alpha lipoic acid..

SHO-SAIKO-TO

A Japanese formulation of 7 Chinese herbs being tested at the Memorial Sloan-Kettering Cancer Center for ablation of non-resectable liver cancer (hepatocellular carcinoma). Phase 1 trials in Japan showed hepatoprotective, antiproliferative and immune-stimulating effects. This is a Kampo style standardized extraction of raw traditional herbs, prepared by Honso Pharmaceutical Co.

LING ZHI FENG WANG JIANG

The reishi mushroom Ganoderma lucidum, "poor-man's ginseng" Codonopsis pilosulae, lychee fruit Lycii chinensis, and Royal jelly, the food of the Queen bee, and honey made up this pleasant and effective nutritive general tonic for the qi and blood. It greatly strengthens and invigorates the fatigued cachexic patient. It can restore appetite, nutrient and medication absorption and body weight. This was a real treasure, but is no longer being manufactured. We now use reishi, ginseng and royal jelly together for a similar effect. .

CHING WAN HUNG OINTMENT

"Capital City Many Red Color" ointment treats radiation burns. It relieves pain promptly, decreases inflammation, reduces swelling, and detoxifies. It promotes regeneration and healing of burned tissue. The TCM mechanism is to Detoxify Fire Poison. Myrrh, frankincense and carthamus are precious ingredients.

DANG GUI LU HUI

Effective formula for chronic myelocytic leukemia. The active principle appears to be indirubin in the Qing dai or Isatis tinctoria, which is immune stimulating and inhibits DNA synthesis specifically in immature leukemic cells in the bone marrow. Synthetic indirubin is used at oral doses of 150-200 mg, is less toxic than the drug Myleran, but similar to Hydroxyurea in GI toxicity, thrombocytopenia and marrow suppression.

YUN NAN BAI YAO

Yunnan Baiyao is an excellent formula of Panax pseudoginseng var. notoginseng. Called san qi in TCM, it may also be spelled Bai yao. It contains ginsenosides and also the unique saponin notoginsenosides or pseudoginsenosides protopanaxadiol and protopanaxatriol which distinguish it from ginseng. Extracts will scavenge superoxide radicals, contain antitumor polysaccharides, and are anticarcinogenic – but the herb is best known as a fantastic haemostatic.
- stops bleeding on contact or when taken internally. It will stop internal bleeding in the lungs, GI tract and nasopharynx from local cancers or from leukemia.
- relieves pain and stops swelling from blood stagnation
- corrects thrombocytopenia rapidly – platelets can double in just two weeks.
- Notoginseng has arabinogalactan polysaccharides which are potent stimulators of the reticulo-endothelial immune system.
- Notoginseng is a radiosensitizer, and has an anti-leukemic effect.

Use the powder directly on bleeding tissue. Take internally with water, 1 or 2 capsules or 0.25 to 0.50 grams (1/16 to 1/8 of the little glass bottle) of the loose powder. This powder was claimed to be a potent secret weapon of the Viet Cong because it saved many an isolated guerrilla soldier by staunching bleeding from gunshot wounds or other trauma, when no medical assistance was available.

The Chinese use notoginseng unstintingly in many cancer formulations. It moves blood stagnation, or "cracks stagnant blood." This stagnancy causes the formation of all tumours. Stagnant blood also is said to be the cause of pain. This is what we naturopaths call a "crackerjack" herb for cancer.

PC SPES

A proprietary Chinese herbal formula for prostate cancer was manufactured by NovaSpes, Inc. Spes is Latin for "hope." Declared constituents included Chrysanthemum rebescens, Isatis indigotica, Glycyrrhiza glabra, Ganoderma lucidum, Panax ginseng, Seronea repens, Scutellaria baicalensis, Panax notoginseng (pseudoginseng). This formula was extremely potent, and had significant side-effects, as well as being very successful in treating prostate cancer. It would suppress androgen receptor expression as well as 5-alpha reductase. It induced apoptosis by down-regulating the genes bcl-2 and bcl-6, suppresses cell proliferation in a number of cancers in vitro, and acted as a radiosensitizer.

Health Canada recently banned this product due to contamination with the drug Coumadin, a potent blood thinner, at doses equal to a low maintenance dose. Some batches also have been laced with diethylstilbestrol (DES) a very potent estrogen known to produce effects in users and in their offspring. I never used this product, as the side-effects were no better than the orthodox hormone blockade medications, and at much more cost. I had been burned before by Chinese products that looked "too good to be true." They usually turn out to be laced with drugs, as in this case. I have other Chinese herbs I trust which are quite a bit safer.

SALVIA

Sage Salvia miltiorrhiza or dan shen regulates the blood. It is synergistic with the COP chemotherapy protocol used in lymphoma.

POLYGONUM

Polygonum cuspidatum or Hu chang is an herb rich in the anthraquinone emodin. It has been shown to significantly increase leukocyte counts in patients made leukopenic by radiotherapy.

BURDOCK ROOT

Burdock root *Arctium lappa* or niu bang zi contains lignans which reduce sex hormone bioavailability, induce differentiation, and inhibit tumour cell proliferation. John Boik suggests burdock seed tincture would be a useful synergist with the Hoxsey herbal formula. The Japanese eat it as "Gobi root."

SCUTE

Scutellaria baicalensis or huang qin normalizes platelet-induced haemostasis, associated with metastasis and tumour advancement. Baicalensis a COX-2 and LOX-12 inhibitor, which can assist in narcotic reduction and is also strongly anti-inflammatory. Several cytotoxic flavones have been identified which arrest cells in G1. It has DNA binding activity, is anti-mutagenic, anti-angiogenic, stimulates lymphocytes and white blood cells in general, inhibits conversion of fibrinogen to fibrin by thrombin, inhibits proliferation, inhibits protein tyrosine kinase, inhibits topoisomerase II, inhibits cAMP phosphodiesterase, decreases androgen receptor expression, inhibits MMP enzymes and activates caspase-3 apoptotic enzymes. It is likely most useful in prostate, breast and vaginal cancers.

BUPLEURUM

Bupleurum chinense, Bupleurum falcatum or Chai Hu is a cooling herb used to treat liver qi stagnation. Its saikosaponins are strongly anti-inflammatory, inhibit angiogenesis and induce apoptosis in liver cancer cells. The anti-inflammatory effect is due to stimulation of adrenal cortical trophic hormone (ACTH) from the pituitary gland, which in turn stimulates the adrenal gland to make more cortisol. The adrenal gland will actually increase in weight. Licorice is synergistic by reducing the breakdown of the cortisol produced.

The ancient formula Xiao Chai Hu Tang or "Minor Bupleurum Combination" is a classic for improving liver blood flow and function caused by the gut reaction to stress.

ISATIS

Isatis tinctoria or "dyer's woad" is the source of royal indigo purple dye. It is in the Brassica family and so contains anti-cancer indoles. It has beta-sitosterols which modulate the immune system. The leaves have an alkaloid tryptanthrin which is a strong COX-2 inhibitor, making it anti-inflammatory and anti-allergic. The root has traditionally been used for solid tumours and modern studies with the purified compound indirubin at 150 to 200 mg daily show responses in leukemia.

RUBIA

Rubia cordifolia or qian cao gen contains a peptide which strongly inhibits tumours in vivo.

ANDROGRAPHITES

Andrographites paniculata is a rich source of berberine and other factors which increase interleukin two IL-2 and interferon gamma INFγ. The sugar-coated TCM tablets *Kang Yan* are a pleasant herbal medicine.

TELOMERASE FORMULA

A novel patented formula with Hoelen, Angelicae root, Scutellariae root and Glycyrrhizae root suppresses the expression of the full length of human telomerase reverse transcriptase (hTERT), in cell lines resistant to chemotherapy and hormone therapies.

CHINESE DIETETICS

Avoid beef, fatty meats, wine, goose, salt, excess sweets, and foods that are smoked, sour, fried, spicy, very rich or stimulating.

Mung bean sprouts and royal jelly are protective.

Foods are classified as hot, cold, yin, yang, and so forth, allowing diets to be formulated which balance and harmonize according to the Eight Principles diagnosis obtained by pulse and tongue assessment on each contact with the patient.

Chapter Eight – Energy Healing & Other Remedies

ACUPUNCTURE

Most people know acupuncture can relieve pain, even to the point where surgery can be done with little or no other anaesthesia. However, when done in its proper context of traditional Chinese medicine TCM diagnosis and prescription, it can balance the parasympathetic and sympathetic branches of the autonomic system, reset the command and control centers in the central nervous system, and rebalance the entire organism. It reminds the various parts to reconnect and work together for the common good. This is so important in a disease such as cancer, which is all about a loss of control.

Parasympathetic stimulation with acupuncture, for example to the Vagus nerve branches in the ear, will control inflammation by down-regulating synthesis of cytokines TNF, IL-1β, IL-6, IL-18, and inducing homeostasis in the cholinergic anti-inflammatory pathway. This effect is achieved via the tyrosine kinase Jak2 and STAT-3 transcription activator. The modulation of parasympathetic tone can be assessed by looking for improved heart rate variability.

Acupuncture needling causes the local release of platelet aggregation factor PAF and kinins which set off a healing response. There is an increase in cellular immunity, IL-2 production, NK cell activity, and macrophage phagocytosis. It can modulate cortisol and other hormones.

The special point Pee Gun can be used for all masses; it is located 3 ½ cun lateral to the inferior tip of the spinous process of the twelfth thoracic vertebra. Burn 14 red bean size moxa every 7 days, on the side of the body affected by cancer. A cun is an "inch" – but the actual length varies from patient to patient and from one area on the body to another – it is proportional to various anatomical parts in the region. For example on the face it is the width of the eye, but on the scalp it is 1/12th the distance from the front hairline to the back hairline. Moxa is made from the leaf of the mugwort plant Artemesia vulgaris, and when lit it slowly smoulders, warming the acupuncture point. Moxibustion is an alternative to needling or can be used with needles. While its smoke is relatively non-toxic, I usually would rather needle the point and then put an infrared heat lamp over the area to warm the needles gently, which has the same effect of increasing the Yang and dispersing the stagnant qi.

Turtle technique on a mass involves needles from 3 directions towards the center, and ginger moxibustion to a fourth needle into the center of a tumour. The moxa is burned in little cones set on a thin slice of fresh ginger root, which has several holes punched through it with a toothpick; this is even more Yang than plain moxa.

Primary points to consider, in the context of 8 Principles or 5 Element balancing would include PC-6 and HT-7, GV 12 and 13 coupled with BL-38.

Secondary points which activate chi and blood with LI-4 and LV-3 (the Four Gates) plus ST-36, SP-6, GV-4and 6, CV-4 & 6, LU-9, LV-2. CV-6 is special for regeneration and stabilization.

The classic Yin-Yang fortifying pair GV-4 and CV-14 can be treated with moxibustion to improve blood counts in chemotherapy.

Tertiary cancer points include SP-3, PC-6, LI-4, ST-36, CV-12, GV-20; Hwato jiagi 17 pairs.

Stimulate the Yang to invigorate the chi and dissolve stagnant blood with the master and coupled points of the Du channel SI-3 and BL-62, and consider also GV-4, 14, 20 & 26, BL-23 and GB-20. Needle and moxa BL-17 and 43 and GV-9 and 14 to strengthen a Yang deficient patient.

Tonify qi with CV-12; ST-36 and 44; LI 4, 10 and 11.

Prosperity treatment uses 4 points: 1 cun above, below and lateral to the umbilicus. Insert and turn clockwise starting from CV 7 for constipation. Insert and turn counter-clockwise starting with ST-25 Left for diarrhea. Supplemental constipation points include GB-34 & ST-36.

For vomiting consider CV-12 & 22, ST-12, PC-6, ST-36 and HT-1.

To support the bone marrow use the Sea of Marrow points GV-15, 16, 19 & 20. Other anemia points to needle are BL-14 & 17 & 20, GV-4 & 14, CV-4 & 12, LV-13, SP-8 & 10, LI-11; moxibustion may be used on ST 36, SP-6 & 10, CV-4 and GV-4. For blood deficiency use Chong Mo master and control points PC-6 with contralateral SP-4.

Ascites can be moderated with ST-22 and CV-9

Acute leukemia treatment – BL-18 & 23, GB-39.

Immune support: SP-6, KI 3 & 6.

QI GONG

Qi gong is a traditional Chinese practice cultivating a balance of yi -intention or consciousness, with qi – vital energy – to balance mind and body. Qi gong exercises are thought to move energy through the organs, and qi gong masters are said to be able to move the energy in patients by the force of their own will. I have seen demonstrations of qi gong which are very dramatic. I have experienced the movement of palpable energy from a distance by a qi gong master. Chinese research points to improved immune function – macrophage phagocytosis, white blood cell counts, CD-20, IL-2 and NK cell activity. Cancer patients undergoing self-control qi gong therapy also demonstrated decreased inflammation, improved appetite, regularized bowel function, normalized liver function, increased self-healing, and weight gain. Late-stage cancer patients gain increased survival time. It is interesting that qi gong training is said to return the person to their "original self," releasing them from their "socialized self." This mirrors the concept of reinforcing the inner direction of psychic energy versus the outward directed energy, which is a focus of the psychotherapeutic approach of LeShan and Simonton. The chi energy of qi gong healing is the same universal healing energy used in Reiki and Healing Touch.

HOMEOPATHY

Homeopathy is a 200 year old system of using very dilute substances to provoke the healing systems of the body to higher function. Vaccination is a crude form of homeopathy, using a tiny dose of a specially processed substance that in a full dose of the active substance would have provoked the actual disease in a healthy patient. It is "like-cures-like," using a triggering dose to get the body to work on the problem by giving it a dose of information about the disease. Homeopathy reinforces correct functioning of the innate regulatory mechanisms for defence and repair. It is very gentle, and results can be very gratifying. It is highly individualized, and a good homeopathic prescription takes some time and thought by an experienced practitioner.

George Vithoulkas defines health as "Freedom from physical and emotional pain, freedom from selfishness, increased adaptability and creativity." This very holistic view is well served by homeopathy, as a true *simillimum*

or well-matched remedy will act on the physical, mental, emotional and even spiritual dimensions of life. With it we strive to optimize the dynamic expression of the person's unique and essential nature, and bring out the most healthy variant of self that is possible.

In all cases consider *Scirrhus* 30 – 200 CH or *Carcinosum* 30 – 200 CH weekly. This does not mean give it slavishly to every patient though!

Other leading remedies are

Arnica montana , Carbo vegetalis, Euphorbium for pain

Arsenicum album for drug toxicity and in palliation

Arsenicum iodatum for cachexia.

Hydrastis canadensis for constipation and lethargy

Conium maculatum for hard masses.

Dr. Robin Murphy, N.D. has written an excellent alphabetical repertory with a good section on cancer under "Generals."

Dr. Ivo Bianchi, M.D. uses Heel brand "homotoxicology" products such as *Gallium-Heel* 20 drops morning and night for 2 months, to be repeated 3 to 4 times a year, for prevention – to halt oncogenesis, in cancer therapy, and to promote detoxification; *Lymphomyosot* for lymphatic drainage; *Glyoxal-compositum* to neutralize toxins released by damaged cellular processes – do not repeat too often, allow time for it to work; Traumeel to ease pain and speed healing of mucositis induced by chemotherapy. *Zeel* functions as a COX-2 inhibitor on par with prescription drugs.

There are many self-help books available, and progressive pharmacies are once again carrying over-the-counter homeopathic remedies. Homeopathic physicians such as naturopathic doctors are essential for best results in treating serious illness, and for advice on combining homeopathic products with other medicines. Homoeopathy both for drainage, immunity and for removing inherited taints is invaluable. It also has an important role in neutralizing industrial toxins. Medicines indicated below have special affinity on particular organs:

Naturopathic Oncology

Acidum aceticum – stomach cancer
Acidum hydrocyanicum – lung and skin cancer
Acidum lacticum – breast cancer
Aloe socotrina – colorectal cancer
Arsenic (Metal) album 30 – Eases passing into spirit, breathlessness
Arsenicum iodatum – cancers of the skin and urinary tract. Radiation burns.
Arsenicum bromatum – melanoma and squamous skin cancers
Asteris rubra – breast cancer
Aurum muriaticum – oral cancer – cheeks, tongue, palate. Cancers of the ovaries, uterus and cervix.
Aurum muriaticum natronatum – cancer of the ovaries, uterus and cervix.
Baryta carbonicum and *Baryta iodatum* – cancer of the brain and of the lymph glands
Bismitum – pharyngeal, esophageal and stomach cancer.
Cadmium sulphuratum. – cancer of the stomach or pancreas
Calcarea carbonica – constitutional for the bones
Carcinosum 200/1M – cancerous history in the family
Ceanothus americanus – cancer of the spleen, pancreas, liver, and leukemia
Chelidonium majus – cancer of the liver or gallbladder
Cobaltum metallicum 30 – cancer of the lungs.
Cholesterinum – liver cancer
Condurango – cancers of the stomach, axilla, esophagus; painful cracks in corner of the mouth.
Conium maculatum – breast cancer.
Gallium aparense – tongue cancer
Graphites – duodenal and pylorus cancer
Hekla lava – cancer of bones
Hydrastis canadensis – cancers of stomach, pancreas, and upper GI tract.
Kalium chloratum – kidney damage from chemo
Kreosotum – cancer of the larynx, stomach, uterus and vulva. Clears toxins.
Lachesis mutans – cancers of the ovary, uterus and cervix. Hot flashes.
Leptandra – cancer of the head of the pancreas
Lilium tigrum – cancers of the ovary, uterus and cervix.
Lycopodium – leukaemia, lung and liver cancer.
Nitricum acidum – rectal cancer
Ornithogalum umbellatum – stomach cancer
Phosphorous – cancer of pancreas and of the bones, especially the lower jaw and tibia. Adverse reactions to surgical anaesthesia. Hemorrhage.
Phytolacca decandra – cancers of the breast and parotid gland.
Plumbum iodatum – brain cancer
Pulsatilla nigricans – cancers of the breast, ovaries, uterus and cervix.
Ruta graveolens – rectal cancer
Sabal serrulata – prostate cancer
Sanguinaria canadensis – bleeding from tumours
Scrophularia n.- breast cancer, Hodgkin's lymphoma

Sepia – cancers of the breast, ovaries, uterus and cervix.

Silicea 30 – to expel poison from the affected lesion. Immune system support.

Sulphur – detoxification support

Symphytum offinalis – bone and blood cancers

Taurox – carbobenzoxy beta-alanyl taurine, homaccord of 3X, 6X 9X potencies – dose morning and noon. Down-regulates IL-6 and Th2 says Lise Alschuler & Dan Rubin, in 3-6 weeks of use.

Terebintha – bladder cancer

Thuja occidentalis -. Cancers of the skin, brain, kidney, stomach, colorectal, testicular, breast, prostate and leukemia; especially good for cancer of head and neck, especially squamous carcinomas or papilloma warts.

PSYCHOLOGY

"…not one single person has ever truly healed from cancer without undergoing a transformation and healing of their inner self." Jeremy Geffen, MD *The Journey through Cancer*

Every experienced physician knows that a lot of patients in their practice are expressing physical illness related to psychological and emotional factors. These are aspects of the mind, which is seated in the brain, but is most likely non-local. Everybody has complex thoughts and feelings based on prior learning, imagination, hormonal balance, nutritional status and culture. These can become imprinted into the physical body – we say "Issues get into the tissues."

There are scientific studies that deny the connection of mind and body, but patients know this is trash science. It is perfectly obvious to all lay people that we are what we think. The best news neuroscience has to tell us is that the brain is highly plastic, and can adapt and restructure to great challenges, is only we overcome its tendency to rigid pre-learned responses.

Depression has been found to increase risk of breast cancer by 42%. In turn, cancer often elevates levels of interleukin six IL-6, triggering cognitive dysfunction and depression.

The stress hormone adrenaline (epinephrine) protects cancer cells from dying by apoptosis. Adrenaline activates PKA and BAD phosphorylation, increasing tumorigenesis. This also blunts the efficacy of chemo and radiation therapies induction of apoptosis. Learning to relax is a *bona fide* cancer therapy.

Social roles are altered by cancer symptoms, treatment side-effects, disfigurement, fatigue, worries about reoccurrence, financial stress, anxiety about becoming a burden to loved ones, and changing roles such as formerly gender-defined household duties. We can easily become conflicted about the desire to self-sacrifice versus the drive for self-care. We are all selves, yet we get squeamish about being "Selfish."

Grieving starts the moment the patient hears the word "cancer" from their doctor. People tend to go into denial, then anger, bargaining, depression and helplessness, before they can emerge with some resolution. It is normal to fear death, loss of control, pain, weakness, medicalization of one's life, social ostracism, financial loss, and so on. It is important to address these concerns, give stress-busting techniques to relieve anxiety, and clarify a person's self-image.

Studies show what people really want from their care-givers:

- Non-hierarchical, integrative and collaborative relationships, particularly with doctors
- To have their expectations, goals and treatment priorities heard
- Flexible scheduling of care
- Value for treatment cost
- Holistic patient-centered care

Being in the dying process tends to obscure the fact they still have living to do. All living persons should be working towards emotional and mental health, through self-effort and professional therapy. Personally, I like neuro-linguistic (NLP) psychology and Time-Line therapy, forms of cognitive therapy proven to relieve clinical anxiety. Good psychotherapy opens up a person to new expression of their physical, psychological and spiritual selves.

Patients who become ENGAGED with their own healing take responsibility for their lifestyle, emotions, and spirit. They change the things they can, and accept what they cannot. This creates serenity, and from this place all challenges can be seen as opportunities to grow and do better at extracting a meaningful life from their existence. It matters not how long we live, but how.

The rational and scientific evaluation of psychosocial interventions in cancer is in its infancy. Clearly measures which will be useful will have to have potent psychogenicity, the ability to stimulate lasting and major change in the thoughts, moods, habits and lifestyle of these cases. The response to the threat of cancer should be a realization of a need for significant change, a willingness to act, an application to self-help strategies, and achievement of quality experiences in the new modes of being.

Carl O. Simonton and others have shown there is real survival value in positive affirmations, meditation, creative visualization, peer support, professional psychological facilitation, and therapy. Other de-stressing techniques may include yogic belly breathing, skin temperature biofeedback, and autogenic progressive relaxation. It is an absolute Law of Nature that IF YOU CAN WORRY, YOU CAN DO IMAGERY!

My favourite tool is a CD of relaxation and visualization exercises called *Remembered Wellness* by my dear colleague Dr. Theresa Clarke, MD, Chief Medical Officer of Inspire Health clinic www.inspirehealth.ca .

I also freely refer for psychotherapy, hypnotherapy, Time-line Therapy and counselling.

Feelings of loneliness, worthlessness, and fear are common inner conflicts. Increasing self-worth attitudes can improve self-caring and create an indomitable will to live. Poor outcomes are associated with a helplessness or hopelessness response to the cancer diagnosis and treatment plan. Unmitigated stress flattens the daily diurnal peaks of the adrenal stress hormone cortisol.

LeShan, Booth, Thomas and others have described a cancer personality profile. There is a tendency to value and live through others, with most thoughts and activities being outwardly directed. **"Type C" behaviour pattern** is associated with higher risk of developing cancer, and a less favourable course of the disease. Patients with this coping style:

- rarely express anger, anxiety, hostility, fear, resentment or sadness
- inwardly experience despair, hopelessness, self-loathing, and a loss of reason to live, goals and dreams.
- are unassertive, appeasing, yielding and very cooperative
- tend to be overly concerned with meeting the needs of others, and do not put their own needs forward.
- suffer fear of rejection which creates isolation
- fear emotional relationships are dangerous and doomed
- feel they can be themselves, or be loved, but never both
- cancer may be provoked by the loss of a crucial relationship (brittle object relationship)
- may often feel the only way out is Death

Gabor Mate has written a brilliant book entitled *When the Body Says No – understanding the connection between stress and health.* His position is that if we do not know our own needs and identity, we cannot discern when to say no, to avoid being exploited or hurt. We unfortunately do not have to consciously perceive stress and emotionality for it to hurt us physically.

A wise man once said "Fear is faith in evil." Even in the face of great losses, people with hope and faith will find comfort and protection from the fact they fear no evil.

Hope is faith that what is good will triumph.

The keys to recovery from afflictions of mind and soul are:

- the proper perception and expression of anger
- the ability to forgive
- reaching out for social support
- practicing an attitude of gratitude
- cultivating laughter, joy and hope.

Empathy, emotional contact and respect from peers can improve a person's self-understanding, self-acceptance and self-approval. With the will to live, to fight for life, comes restoration of emotional outlets, and inner growth, even in the face of physical catastrophe. This sets the stage for healing of anxiety, despair and disappointment. As Gotthard Booth says in *The Cancer Epidemic*, "Illness is a reminder of the purpose of life." Rabbi Zusia said it best: "When I die, God will not ask me why I was not Moses.

He will ask me why I was not Zusia." We all have a chance here to let our little light shine, every day. That is all we actually should be concerned with.

Lawrence LeShan has had tremendous success with advanced cancer using positive psychology. Rather than looking for psychological defects and trying to fix them, he advocates restoration of emotional and creative expression. He finds cancer victims often have lost a main emotional focus in their lives, and have lost hope of finding any satisfactory substitute. He has cured cases by helping them design a re-vitalized life providing meaning, enthusiasm, zest and fulfillment. Cancer patients need to learn how to live fully – as LeShan says "love, laugh, play, learn, sing praises and exercise."

Social roles are majorly impacted by cancer and cancer treatment related symptoms such as fatigue, hair loss, disfigurement, and sexual dysfunction. Gender-roles, family ranking, and household duties are altered, and financial stress adds to the burden. There are worries about reoccurrence, anxiety about becoming a burden to loved ones, and nameless fears.

There really is a silver lining in every cloud. There is an opportunity for growth in every challenge. People who embrace and feel good about their cancer therapy tend to have far less side-effects than those who fear it and have morbid expectations. Anxiety and depression set a patient up for a poorer response and more harm from chemotherapy.

Pain is much more easily borne by a patient who feels hopeful in facing a challenge than one whose thoughts dwell on what is lost and what is threatened by their disease. Hope is not something to avoid arousing, it is essential, for the physical therapeutic value as well as for psychological well-being. As Buddha said, pain is inevitable, but suffering is optional.

A weekly support group and self-hypnosis for pain was associated with doubling of life-span in advanced stage IV breast cancer, ovarian cancer and melanoma. This work by Spiegel from 1989 has not been confirmed in subsequent studies, but certainly quality of life improves, if survival does not.

Particularly vulnerable are patients who lack a significant social support network. Patients who report a poor level of social well-being show higher pre-surgical levels of the angiogenesis cytokine VEGF.

To be filled with **joy, gratitude and love** is to be healed, whatever the circumstances of the physical body.

Love is all there is. Love is the only true meaning in life and death. The old term "placebo response" is now being called a "meaning response." People heal when they find meaning in their life. When they express their inner selves, they can remember love, speak their truth, and move into a still and sacred place where they co-create a reality where they are kind to themselves and all others.

The Ten Tools of Triumph for Survivors

1. <u>Stay 100% present</u>. We must not let our minds race ahead of us, imagining all manner of horrific outcomes. We must remain as calm, composed and lucid as we possibly can. That may be extremely difficult under the circumstances, but we cannot afford to waste priceless energy and time falling into fear. We may have little time left. We must make that time count – to its maximum. That means staying completely in the here and now.

2. <u>Ignore all predictions of doom.</u> No one can predict the future. When we hear frightening news from a reputable source such as a doctor, we are conditioned to believe what we hear. But health forecasts, like all forecasts, can prove to be inaccurate. The first thing we must do is decide what we are going to believe. If we choose life, we must see the cup as half full rather than half empty. We must believe there is still the potential for survival. This is not denial, it is determination. And it is the first manifestation of a survivor's greatest single asset: hope.

3. <u>Silence your mind.</u> Cancer treatment and recovery is emotionally and physically gruelling. The psychological stress of living on the edge is intense. It is essential that we regularly escape, re-energize and rekindle our resolve. That way, we can return to the climb stronger and more effective. But because we cannot always physically change our surroundings, we need to be mentally able to change locations. Retreat into silence.

4. <u>Take charge.</u> Every moment that follows disappointing news offers an opportunity to take control. We can arm ourselves with valuable information, decide what treatment we wish, who is going to deliver it, how and when. We can commit to taking charge of ourselves and our care. An effective plan can lead to effective action, which can lead to an effective outcome – but only if we first think rationally and act decisively to develop that plan. Action is the greatest antidote to fear. Take it.

5. <u>Focus all your energy on getting better.</u> It has been said that "Where focus goes, energy flows." As energy is the most precious resource survivors have, we must be absolutely militant in our use of it. We must dispense it with the greatest discretion. That means balancing outside commitments and personal health in a whole new way. It also means learning to temporarily say no to the needs and wants of some others and putting our needs and wants first. Our lives depend on it.

6. <u>Decide to be a survivor.</u> We are not cancer patients. If we are alive and living with cancer, we are survivors. We must say it, and keep saying it. And we must do everything in our power to think, act and live like a survivor every day. This will not guarantee we will survive, but it will maximize our chances of doing so. To become who we are capable of becoming, we must live like we already are that person. We are survivors, period.

7. Patch into the power of your personal purpose. The German philosopher, Nietzsche, wrote that human beings can endure almost any how if they have a why for which to live. In other words, the greater our reason to live, the greater our chance of survival. The strength of our will to live is directly proportional to the strength of our personal purpose. Aside from hope, that purpose is the single greatest asset we have. It can become a beacon that guides us back from the edge. We must know why we want to live – and always remember it.

8. Measure success by effort, not outcome. Cancer is not about winning or losing. Death is not defeat. Dishonour may be. The only way to dishonour ourselves is to fail to make one hundred percent effort. Giving it everything we have means maximizing our quality of life for whatever time we have left. Quality of life, and just as importantly, quality of effort, is more important than quantity of life. If our effort is absolute, we will be triumphant no matter what the outcome.

9. Can/Will yourself to move. Treatment can be physically debilitating. It can steal away your energy and leave us devoid of life and enthusiasm. But if we are to climb back, we must move. We must overcome our own inertia and sometimes, even our desire to rest. Time does not heal all wounds – we must heal our own by forcing our bodies into motion. The first step takes place in our minds.

10. Make essential changes in your life. Cancer is not a death sentence. It is a call to life – a wake-up call. It demands we re-examine our lives and make vital changes. If we do not, we risk returning to illness. There is no guarantee we can prevent cancer from recurring. But for whatever time we have left, we must decide what matters and what does not, what is crucial and what is optional. Change after cancer is not optional. It is essential.

The Ten Tools of Triumph for Caregivers:

Care for yourself first. If we do not care for ourselves we cannot be there to care for our loved one. Caring for ourselves can be as simple as taking a five-minute rest break, going for a walk, making sure we eat properly and sleeping in our own bed each night. Do it – every day.

Put your fears aside. We will be given statistics and a prognosis that may not be encouraging. We must decide that we are going to be on the positive side of the numbers. If there is no positive side, decide we are going to be the exception. Visualize a positive outcome. Look to other survivors. Read success stories. We must surround ourselves with hope.

Manage your mind. Beware the "What-ifs" our minds can endlessly imagine. They will drain our energy and clutter our minds so we will be unable to process all the information coming at us. We must stop our minds from spinning by using whatever technique works for us – meditation, music, playing with our children, reading a book. A quiet mind is a clear mind. It is also a more productive and effective one.

Expect the unexpected. Change is challenging. The new drugs, treatment methods, tests, unexpected setbacks and continuous uncertainty can wear us down. We must embrace this uncertainty and adapt to it as best we can. It is part of the experience. Concentrate only on what we can control and let everything else go.

Celebrate what you have. At the end of each day, we must think of something for which we can be grateful. It could be something as simple as a smile from a friend or a snowflake on our tongue. Whatever it is, celebrate it – and remember it.

Pace yourself for the long run. Cancer is a long-term illness. The caregiver has to conserve energy to endure the journey. If we give too much too early, we will not have enough left later. So we must find our own pace and stick to it. If we put in a very long day, we must try to make the next one shorter.

Ask for assistance. Asking for help is not a sign of weakness. It is a sign of strength. It allows us to manage a demanding situation and build a support team around us. Ask for help from friends and family, but most importantly, seek psychological assistance from professionals. We cannot do it all if we ant to be effective.

Insulate yourself against anger. Anger is part of the experience – for both caregiver and survivor. If it is directed at us, remember it can be a by-product of medications, sleeplessness, frustration and fear. Deflect it by understanding that its true target is the illness, not us. Stand tall.

Adapt to your changing role. Most of us define ourselves by what we do, and we are comfortable in those roles. But when our roles suddenly change, we can be thrown off balance and struggle to find our equilibrium. Our new role as caregiver must take priority.

Support, don't smother. We will want to do everything we can for our loved ones, but it is possible to do too much. If they feel they are losing independence, resentment can build. Know when to back off. Ask them if they want help before giving them any. Allow them to do what they can for themselves. Stand strong apart and together.

From: *Climb Back from Cancer – A Survivor and Caregiver's Inspirational Journey.* Cecilia and Alan Hobson – Everest summiteer and cancer survivor and his partner. See www.alanhobson.com "Ten Tools of Triumph" is a trademark phrase and this excerpt from his book is copyrighted material. Not to be reproduced without the author's permission.

SPIRITUALITY

"Everything is connected, in a discontinuous sort of way" – Dr. Zucchini, explaining quantum mechanics
"We are all one – but not the same one, I am telling you!" – Guru Paul
"There are more things in heaven and earth than are dreamed of in your philosophy..." – Hamlet, by William Shakespeare

Because it is a life-and-death struggle to overcome cancer, it is a spiritual process. Treating this "ghost in the machine" is not an area of expertise of most medical practitioners.

I do not believe there can be "false hope." I believe despair and fear to be false emotions. Remember fear is faith in evil. Place your faith in something positive. Hope is life-enhancing on a daily level, and many people also have hope concerning a possible eternity.

A diagnosis of an incurable disease can create false hopelessness.

A patient does not have to accept pain, abandonment, suffering or giving up being productive only because the future is uncertain.

Stress is lessened by reasserting personal control. Doing "everything that can be done" just feels better than giving up.

A reminder of our mortality can bring profound meaning back into the lives of patients and their families.

A terminal diagnosis means a person has time to prepare for their death. Resolution of conflicts and the giving and receiving of forgiveness are possible gifts.

Expressive therapies such as music or art help modulate neuro-endocrine-immune parameters.

Religious faith, prayers, rituals and spiritual practices are coping mechanisms positively associated with better outcomes. People who have faith in a higher power, and particularly those who attend church or practice their religion actively have measurably lower rates of complications, less need for medications, and tend to survive longer with more quality of life. People of faith tend to feel peace, assurance, meaning and well-being which allows them to embrace life. Faith in an afterlife or spiritual survival does correlate with an increased fighting spirit seen in cancer survivors. They fear death less, yet fight to survive more.

Prayer is easy. You don't have to have any particular faith, just a willingness to express your heart-felt desires. You can ask for or just reflect on love, gratitude, protection, guidance, surrender, forgiveness, inspiration, peace, and blessings. You can also ask for these blessings for anyone you can imagine! By practicing the Buddhist art of Loving Kindness you can enter into a mindfulness that engenders compassion and a natural equanimity.

Simple mind-body techniques may include compassionate heart-focussed meditation, journaling, or breathing exercises.

REIKI HEALING

Reiki is the laying on of hands in a traditional manner to provide the receiver with the healing life energy as the practitioner directs healing energy to a specific part of the body or the entire body.

It allows you to go within, to accept this Universal Life Energy as a partner in your healing process.

Reiki is compatible with all other modalities of healing – traditional and alternative.

Reiki is safe, gentle and easy for all ages. You need only to relax and accept the healing energy. Your clothes remain on during your treatment.

Usually the whole body is treated, front and back while laying on your back, by placing the healer's hands on major organs, endocrine glands and chakras. The energy offered is a universal energy which flows through a practitioners body and out through their hands. It is not a personal energy from the reiki practitioner.

All you need to do as the receiver is feel the relaxation, experience peace, safety, well being, feel your body accepting the non invasive healing energy and balanced wellness.

A Reiki session is about one hour. Your session will support you body's natural ability to heal. Many times emotions are released with the treatment which is quite normal and very beneficial. Often you will find a very restful place within where you will relax totally, allowing this intelligent energy to work within you body, where it is needed.

This ancient respected practice accelerates healing, and the re-balancing of body, mind and spirit.

The laying on of Reiki hands is a natural, powerful and effective healing tool and one of the easiest to include into life. It can activate the inherent healing power that is in all of us.

I have experienced and witnessed many profound healings with Reiki, and recommend it for every cancer patient.

OXYGEN THERAPIES

Ozone (O3) is a highly reactive form of oxygen which increases tissue oxygen levels. On contact with ozone the red blood cells release 2,3-DPG, which shifts the oxygen disassociation of hemoglobin. Usually the hemoglobin protein will give up 1, and only rarely 2 of the 4 oxygen O2 molecules it carries. The ozone-DPG reaction releases all 4 oxygen molecules. High tissue oxygen improves tissue healing and immune response to infections..

Ozone up-regulates the immune system if given in low doses, increases superoxide dismutase (SOD), increases catalase, and detoxifies the liver. Ozone is radio-sensitizing.

Ozone gas may be insufflated into the rectum. It may also be bubbled through 50 to 100 ml of blood which is then returned to the body (autohemotherapy). Another popular method withdraws up to 80 ml. of blood and irradiates it with ultraviolet-B light, then returns it to the vein oxygenated, charged and activated.

I think the effectiveness of ozone for most cancers is minimal, and I attribute its being over-rated to the wide-spread myth that oxygen somehow kills cancer cells on contact. I have yet to clearly observe ozone helping a cancer patient, but will refer for this therapy if the patient insists and their cancer is associated with any virus. Ozone is known to help with viral hepatitis. Immune cells fight viruses better when well-oxygenated. Viral associated cancers include cervical, lymphoma, leukemia, prostate, nasopharyngeal, head and neck.

Hydrogen peroxide (H2O2) is used orally, or intravenously at 0.03%, and has significant risks. Hydrogen peroxide, even that produced by our own macrophage immune cells, permanently inactivates our NK immune cells – which we need to kill cancer cells. Dark field microscopy suggests peroxide may trigger very dangerous changes in the blood. I do NOT recommend H2O2 in any form for cancer.

I do recommend oral food grade hydrogen peroxide for gut infections with anaerobic bacteria such as *Clostridium difficile*, responsible for antibiotic-induced pseudo-membranous colitis.

We can get hydrogen peroxide to selectively form in cancer cells, but not in healthy cells, with intravenous vitamin C drips. This is the sensible way to use hydrogen peroxide in oncology.

Hyperbaric oxygen therapy (HBO2T) is breathing of 100% pure oxygen at elevated pressure to super-saturate the body with oxygen, and force it deep into cells. Ordinary air is about 21% oxygen, but it is the pressure, not just the concentration of oxygen, that makes this therapy so powerful. Tumours do use fermentation to make energy without oxygen, but also burn fats and carbohydrates with oxygen. They are NOT poisoned by oxygen as some people suggest. Some have also suggested HBO2T would increase tumour growth due to its power to stimulate increased angiogenesis. HBO2T has no net benefit in treating cancer, but may safely be given if needed for other medical reasons. Some practitioners suggest HBO2T must never be used within 4 weeks of radiation therapy for safety concerns. Nonetheless, some of my colleagues are using it during radiation therapy to increase its potency in killing cancer cells. Oxygen fixes the radiant energy into chemical energy, creating compounds which break up big molecules, including cancerous DNA.

DMSO

Di-methyl sulfoxide is a powerful solvent with analgesic, vulnerary (wound healing) and anti-inflammatory properties. It is useful also as a carrier to move medications through cell membranes. Intravenous use is more risky than orally or by enema. It can cause halitosis or bad breath – in this case a garlic oyster smell and taste, headache, dizziness, nausea and sedation. It may be a useful adjunct in leukemia, uterine and cervical cancers.

Methyl sulfonyl methane (MSM) in capsule form may provide many similar benefits, and may be better in bladder cancer. MSM is great for arthritic pain, hay fever, strengthens hair and nails, and has many other beneficial side-effects.

EDTA CHELATION

Chelation is an intravenous treatment which removes toxic heavy metals such as lead. EDTA chelation has been used, amid some controversy, for cardiovascular disease. It may not actually remove arterial plaque or atherosclerosis, but it does have an anti-aging effect. It is documented to disrupt bacterial biofilms, which may be a factor in cardiovascular diseases. Unanticipated benefits in cancer status have been reported. Chelation may inhibit free radicals and enhance immune defences. Some now think the usual adjuncts of vitamin C, magnesium and B-vitamins in the drips may be more active than the disodium EDTA itself. It is safe when administered by a physician certified by the American College for the Advancement of Medicine (ACAM). Take it 1 to 3 times per week, supplementing all the while with oral vitamin C, B complex, zinc, selenium, and anything else the routine blood analyses indicate to be imbalanced.

714X

Gaston Naessens argues that this chemical source of nitrogen for the body will stop the cancer cells from producing "co-carcinogenic K factor" (CKF) which protects them from immune cells. It contains camphor, organic salts, ethanol and water. 714X is injected into the lymph nodes for 3 series of 21 days each, spaced by three days off, then boosters as needed. Do not combine with vitamin E or vitamin B12 supplementation, which decrease its effectiveness. It is also incompatible with anti-angiogenics. I do not think this is any sort of major breakthrough in cancer care, and am not troubled by its lapse into obscurity.

SHORT-WAVE DIATHERMY

Dr. John Bastyr, ND said that passing 13 meter short-wave radiation through a tumour will dissolve it. The patient needs to be fit to handle the toxic debris from rapid tumour lysis (break-up). Consider also diathermy to the pituitary gland. Unfortunately these machines are rare these days, and operating one can disrupt computers and cell-phones in the clinic and vicinity. The magnetic field these things put out is truly extraordinary. A patient with a cardiac pace-maker walking into a clinic when a diathermy machine is on might faint, or worse.

RIFE RAY MACHINE

Royal Rife in San Diego in 1934 demonstrated an electromagnetic therapy termed the Rife Ray which could be tuned to specific frequencies to destroy specific disease organisms, including viruses, within living tissue. Rife build a uniquely powerful light microscope and observed a viral size organism he associated with cancer cells, and observed his ray killing them. He then treated human tumours, and claimed great success, but was stopped from the practice by the American Medical Association by 1939.

Some of my patients and colleagues have Rife devices and I do not believe they cause any harm. However, I have seen many patients sit around wasting many hours of the last months of their lives waiting for this contraption to do something for them. It never has. NOT RECOMMENDED

HYPERTHERMIA

Cells with a low pH (high in acid) or with nutritional deficiencies, such as hypoxic tumour cells, are more sensitive to heat damage than healthy cells. Rapidly proliferating cells are also slower to develop a tolerance to heat over 42°C. Cancer cells are generally deficient in "chaperone proteins," including heat shock proteins HSP.

HSP cover the hydrophobic portions of amino acid chains emerging from the cell's endoplasmic reticulum, and later assist new proteins to achieving the proper tertiary structure (shape). Heat induces apoptosis via intracellular triggers and branched chain polysaccharide alterations, and can also induce necrosis. Core body temperature elevation may be safely tolerated to about 42 to 42.5 degrees Celsius. Core body hyperthermia is not recommended in cases of liver injury or disease. Destruction of malignant tissue is expected in the range of 42 to 44°C. For each degree above 41°C half the amount of time is needed to kill the same number of cells. At 44° a malignant tumour may be destroyed in about 30 minutes. Dr. George Crile Jr. of Cleveland estimates cancerous cells are destroyed at temperatures about 3°C lower than that which will destroy adjacent normal tissue, at any given duration of exposure.

Hyperthermia in the range of 41 to 42°C for 30 to 40 minutes, or 2°C. above their baseline for 30 to 60 minutes, produces an anti-neoplastic immune response. There is up-regulation of NK cell activity and mitogenesis, increased interleukins IL-1 and IL-2, increased circulating CD4/CD8 cell ratios, and increased circulating peripheral mononuclear cells. Diaphoresis is also detoxifying. Hyperthermia is radio-sensitizing, by inhibition of repair of chromosome aberrations and single strand DNA breaks, which results in apoptosis of radiation injured cells.

In 1891 Dr. William Coley began injecting a mixture of streptococcal bacteria endotoxins into 140 patients with advanced sarcomas to induce an artificial fever. His "metabolic hyperthermia" had positive responses directly related to the temperature reached and the duration of the fever. Dr. Issels carried on the practice with bacterial lysates. Cancer patients are often Th-2 dominant, with an immune system unresponsive to cancer. The lymphocytes just end up enslaved by the tumour making growth factors and angiogenic factors. When the Th-1 reactive state is restored, fever marks the attack of immune cells on the tumour with antigen processing, antibody, complement and cytotoxic modes of attack. This is the basis of targeted vaccine therapy with Polyvaccinum and the mistletoe lectin injection therapies.

At the turn of the 20th Century Dr. Westermarck developed whole body hyperthermia in hot baths. Others worked with short wave diathermy, microwave, infrared and ultrasound heating. In 1976 Dr. Leon Parks, a cardiothoracic surgeon introduced hyperthermia by extracorporeal circulation using computerized perfusion technology. This method results in pain palliation and effective reversal of tumour growth in a significant number of patients. One of my esteemed colleagues, Dr. Garrett Swetlikoff, ND, who for many years was my personal physician, uses hyperthermia in his practice. The Heckel HT2000 whole body hyperthermia unit uses infrared A and a thermal insulation blanket to reach a core body temperature over 43° Centigrade in sessions of 1 to 2 hours.

Ashwagandha herb is an excellent adjunct during hyperthermia.

ANTINEOPLASTINS

Dr. Stanislaw Burzynski, MD, PhD developed two synthetic peptide (amino acid chain) formulations he named "antineoplastons," which switch off oncogenes and switch on tumour suppressor genes. He found these naturally occurring peptides and organic acids tend to be low in the urine of cancer patients. They are not toxic. The average dose of A10 fraction is 7.7 g/kg/day, and the As2-1 fraction is given at 0.36 g/kg/day. After 20 years of harassment by the USA Food and Drug Administration FDA, he is now conducting approved trials through his Houston, Texas clinic. He appears to have the most success with brain and prostate cancers. I have seen a distinct response in a pancreatic cancer case I attended. It costs thousands of dollars per month.

ELECTRICAL THERAPY

A small electrical current applied to a tumour has an antineoplastic effect, by normalizing cell proliferation rates. Cancer cells tend to have an abnormally low trans-membrane potential (TMP) which will increase with direct current (DC) application of less than 10 volts. Cancer cells have a low voltage of about 15 – 20 millivolts. Normal cells average 75 – 90 millivolts. Normal non-dividing cells will respond to DC with a lowering of their TMP.

The effect is greatest when the anode electrode is applied to the tumour. Acid and chlorine forms at the anode, alkali plus hydrogen forms at the cathode, and the cancer in the middle depolarizes, then dies.

The optimum current is 7.5 volts DC, 20 milliamperes, to a level of 35 -100 coulombs per cubic centimetre of tumour. Pads may be applied to superficial tumours for percutaneous stimulation, or electrodes can be applied to acupuncture needles for deeper tumours. Stimulation is applied for 15 to 30 minutes. Large tumours may take 100 milliamperes of current for up to 4 hours, for a dose of up to 100 coulombs of electrical energy. The treatment stings, so local anaesthetic medication may be used.

The ideal tumour for this therapy is superficial and under 5 cm. in diameter. The lysis products provoke a favourable immune response. The fragments are ideal for processing by the macrophage immune cells.

The short-term response rate may be 85%. Long-term survival is higher with this adjunctive therapy in lung, esophageal, liver and kidney cancers. In China this treatment is used in hundreds of hospitals, with galvanic current applied to platinum electrodes inserted into the tumour under ultrasound guidance. Incisions may be made under local anaesthetic. In Europe this has been pioneered by Nobel laureate Professor Bjorn Nordenstrom of Sweden and Dr. Rudolf Pekar of Austria. Dr. Pekar claims a 3 year remission rate of 73%. Chinese reports indicate about 35% complete remissions, 43% partial remissions, 15% unchanged, and only 7% experiencing progression of their disease. The Chinese say they see about 70% 3 year survival in total, for a wide variety of cancers.

After galvanotherapy the tumour cells may be seen to re-differentiate into fibroblasts and repair the area.

Electrotherapy has little effect in advanced disease with metastases, and does not inhibit the tendency to metastasize.

MAGNETICS

Magnets of 650 gauss static field strength may be used for 1 to 2 hours daily. Magnetic therapy dates back to the discovery of natural magnets in the earth in ancient China, balls of crude iron called "lode stones." The Chinese were the first to discover the magnetic compass, using a sliver of magnetized iron. The earth has a strong magnetic field, and every cell and most large molecules in them has some electrical charge, which tends to line up with the magnetic field. When we live in artificial environments with electrical wires in the walls and concrete with iron rebar grids in the floors, and so on, we are blocked from our natural magnetic field, and may have strong and disorganized fields all around us. It is recommended that we not have electrical appliances such as clock radios near our heads when we sleep.

Nikken of Japan is the world leader in medical and health magnetic products, to wear, sleep on, and use therapeutically. They make the **Pi-Mag water** treatment system which makes water thinner, by breaking down the clumping of water into smaller "micro-clusters." This water is a super solvent for better detoxification. Microcluster water forms a 3 molecule deep blanket around regulatory and structural proteins, supporting them, helping them fold correctly, and stabilizing their functional shape. Magnets of appropriate strength and configuration can relieve pain, improve sleep and speed healing processes.

SHARK CARTILAGE

Shark cartilage was a fad I never went in for, observing no responses in those treated by other doctors. A thoroughly negative study was presented June 2, 2007 at the American Society of Clinical Oncology 43 rd Annual Meeting, Abstract 7527 by Dr. Charles Lu of the MD Anderson Cancer Center. Bovine cartilage is a little better, but still not very useful. NOT RECOMMENDED. Do not confuse this product with shark liver oil alkylglycerols, which are useful for low blood cell counts.

LOW DOSE NALTREXONE

Cancer cells have receptors for opiates. The mu opiate receptor is particularly involved in cell proliferation and angiogenesis. Morphine and related narcotic drugs actually increase cancer cell growth, invasion and metastasis.

Methyl-naltrexone is an opoid antagonist, used to detox alcohol and drug addicts in doses of 50 mg and up. In very small doses of 3 to 4.5 mg at bedtime, it is a strong immune-modulator. Dr. Bernard Biharis was using it for AIDS when he observed a remission from lymphoma. Night-time dosing increases met-enkephalins, beta-endorphins, NK cell number and activity, cytotoxic CD8+ T-cell number in circulation, and may induce apoptosis via increased number and density of tumour cell endorphin receptors.

LDN is particularly useful in cancers such as breast, prostate, ovary, uterus, bladder, lung, throat, liver, pancreas, colon, rectum, carcinoids, kidney, glioblastoma, chronic lymphocytic leukemia, lymphoma, multiple myeloma, and melanoma.

About 2% of cases will suffer sleep disturbance, and will do better at a dose of 1 to 2 mg. Good responses are seen in about 25% of cases. Improvement may be seen by a month, and remission within 6 months. See www.lowdosenaltrexone.org and www.LDN-help.com

It can only be used orally if the patient is on narcotics such as codeine or morphine for pain. An injectable form from Wyeth called *Relistor* cannot cross the blood-brain-barrier, and so can be used on patients who are on opiate narcotics. It will allow analgesia but abolish the opiate-induced constipation. The standard dose of Relistor is 8 0.4 ml yielding 8 mg, but in the cancer therapy context the dose is reduced to 0.05 ml or 1 mg.

Dr. Berkson, MD suggests combining LDN with alpha lipoic acid for dermatomyositis.

UKRAIN

I do NOT recommend Ukrain, as it is too expensive for the meagre results it gives. However, for your information, Ukrain or NSC-631570 is a semi-synthetic compound of the chemotherapy drug Thiotepa and a botanical extract - thiophosphoric acid triaziridide and an alkaloid chelidonine from the traditional liver herb Chelidonium majus. It has been used for about 20 years in Austria. The National Cancer Institute in the USA has found it active against many cancer cell types, including adenocarcinomas, epithelial carcinomas, sarcomas, melanoma and lymphomas.

Ukrain selectively accumulates in tumour cells, where it is directly cytolytic and cytostatic, inhibits topoisomerases I and II, inhibits synthesis of DNA, RNA and proteins. Ukrain induces apoptosis by activation of endodesoxyribonucleases. Ukrain initially increases oxygen consumption in cells, but later it returns to normal in healthy cells but stops completely in the cancer cells!

Ukrain in small doses is a biological response modifier (BRM) which means it is immune-stimulating. It can activate NK cells, improve the CD4/CD8 ratios, and increase phagocytosis by white blood cells.

The dose is commonly 5 to 20mg daily to weekly, intravenously or intramuscularly, usually 2 or 3 times a week. It is best to avoid mixing it directly with other products, and to inject each 5 ml x 5 mg ampoule slowly over a minute or more. A common strategy is to use 5 mg once a week as a BMR, alternating with 20 mg later in the week for a cancer cytolytic effect. Do not mix with cortisone, digitalis, sulphonamide antibiotics or sulfonyl urea antidiabetic drugs.

Ukrain is well-tolerated, with only moderate toxicity. There is no cumulative toxicity or late effects. Allergic or anaphylactic reactions are not seen. Ukrain is not recommended in pregnancy, breastfeeding, in growing children, or during high fever. Tumour markers may fluctuate early in therapy. Tumours may swell reversibly early in therapy, so be cautious with cancers within the skull.

Ukrain may cause some nausea, tumour swelling, dizziness, depression, insomnia, drowsiness, fatigue, apathy, restlessness, sweats, shivering, itching, increased urination, stabbing pains, tingling sensations, burning feeling in the tumour, and tumour hardening. These are due to tumour lysis releasing toxic matter, and will disappear as the tumour is removed.

Consider Ukrain in cancer of the breast, pancreas, colon, bladder, prostate, ovary, cervix, endometrium (uterus), lung, testes, head and neck, lymphoma and melanoma. Phase II studies show a doubling of median survival time in advanced pancreatic cancer, used alone or with chemotherapy.

Having seen all this research, I was quite disappointed to see no highly significant response in anyone I know who has actually used it. It is not something I administer to my patients. NOT RECOMMENDED.

IMMUNE THERAPIES

Cancer cells form all the time, and the immune system removes them safely almost all of the time. There is always some element of immune compromise when cancer becomes a disease. The immune cells actually get drawn in by inflammation, set up a repair process, it becomes chronic – "the wound that never heals"- and the immune cells end up working for the tumour.

Macrophages and other lymphocytes secrete growth factors, assist angiogenesis and contribute to invasion and tumour cell migration. Tumour-associated macrophages TAMs, always phenotype M2, migrate to hypoxic zones in tumours, remodel the matrix, and release vascular endothelial growth factor VEGF, as well as angiopoietins ANG-1 and ANG-2

Macrophages can be made highly tumoricidal by activation with macrophage activating factor GcMAF. Gc protein is serum vitamin D3 binding protein. Cancer cells secrete **nagalase**, also called serum alpha-N-acetylgalactosaminidase, which deglycosylates Gc, the principle precursor of MAF. Nagalase activity in blood is normally in the range of 038 to 0.63 nM/min/mg protein, but in breast cancer this can rise to 2.38 to 6.28. inhibiting nagalase reverses immune-suppression and can lead to tumour eradication.

Tumour cells, peripheral stem cells, and immune cells release inflammatory mediators including:

chemokines – such as CCL-2 and CCL-5 which promote migration of monocytes into tumours, where they differentiate into macrophages.

cytokines – such as transforming growth factor beta TGFß, tumour necrosis factor TNF, colony stimulating factor CSF, and the immune-suppressant interleukin ten IL-10. TGF is a potent immunosuppressor, making it harder for immune cells to find and kill cancer cells. TGFß stops differentiation of T-cells into active cytotoxic or helper cells. TGFß blocks production of IL-2 needed to proliferate T-cells. It is supported in blocking immune function by interleukins IL-4, IL-5 and IL-10. TGFß inhibits secretion of tumour necrosis factors TNFa and TNFß, inactivating cytotoxic NK cells and lymphokine-activated killer cells. When activated by stromal cell thrombospondin-1 TGFß suppresses T-cell effectors activated against tumour antigens, creating local immune tolerance. TNFa is an acute pro-inflammatory cytokine which stimulates the immune system. TNFa is made by macrophages, proliferating T-lymphocytes, B-cells and NK cells. It is supported in immune stimulation by interferon INF and interleukins IL-2, IL-6 and IL-12. IL-6 is also called B-cell stimulatory factor BSF-2, and is produced by peripheral lymphocytes and monocytes. Modulate with EGCG, mushroom extracts, ALA, Vitamin C.

IL-8 is modulated by black seed *Nigella sativa* thymoquinone.

Prostaglandins – such as PGE-2, synthesized by COX-1 and COX-2 enzymes, promoter of inflammation and an immune suppressant.

Regulatory T-cells within tumours are co-opted to suppress cytotoxic T-cells directed against tumour antigens. Tumours induce regulator CD4+ and CD25+ T-cells to block immune recognition of tumour antigens. Effector T-cells may be activated peripherally to tumours, but stromal cells mask the tumour cells. Fibroblasts activated and induced by cancer cells release thrombospondin-1 which activates TGFß to create immune tolerance and immune suppression. Tumour cells also down-regulate dendritic cell processing of tumour antigens. Without antigen recognition there is no response to the cancer by cytotoxic T-lymphocytes, natural killer NK cells, monocytes, macrophages or B-cells.

Immune therapies are limited by the fact that most cancer cells are able to disguise their abnormality until they are very well established. Common epithelial cancers – carcinomas – show a very late immune response, and often their mutation rate exceeds the plasticity of the immune system to adapt. Without immune modifiers, the immune system hasn't a chance of picking up on the abnormalities until the patient is very sick. The cancer gets a big lead off, and the immune system can rarely catch up in time to prevent severe damage or death.

Recall from Chapter One that a huge volume of the DNA genetic code in every cell is made up of virus information, virus promoter sequences, and cancer-provoking oncogenes and proto-oncogenes. When cancer gets mature, and highly mutated, the viral overload can express and be the final step which destroys life.

Any inflammation, infection, parasite or other immune stressor can tip the balance in a very ill cancer patient. There are many cancer fighting immune therapies that have been used, and more in active development. This is potentially the most promising new direction for contemporary cancer research. Until we can get reliable and specific anti-cancer vaccines, the general immune status of our cancer patients remains a central concern for naturopathic physicians.

The modern level of cleanliness and the use of vaccinations and immunizations to avoid childhood and infectious diseases have been linked to the modern epidemics of immune disorders (Greave's hypothesis). Kids who are exposed to more germs and dirt have less allergies, less asthma, and so on. It is possible our drive to have a safe and sterile environment is making our immune systems weak, and contributing to our inability to deal with cancer cells as they form. We need an active reticulo-endothelial system, hardened by exposure to infections, to create immunity to the next disease we encounter.

Cancer patients are often Th-2 dominant, with an immune system unresponsive to cancer. The lymphocytes just end up enslaved by the tumour making growth factors and angiogenic factors. When the Th-1 reactive state is restored, fever marks the attack of immune cells on the tumour with antigen processing, antibody, complement and cytotoxic modes of attack. This is the basis of targeted vaccine therapy with Polyvaccinum and the mistletoe lectin injection therapies.

Cimetidine has been found to be an immune-modulator. It is a H2 histamine receptor blocker, and histamine negatively regulates T-helper responses. This Th1 -c Th2 regulation is particularly helpful in colon cancer.

Many patients are seduced to try therapies which increase the natural killer NK cell number or activity. Unfortunately, they fail to understand that raising NK number and activity is not an indicator of anti-cancer effect.

NK cells only effectively remove single cells or small nests or clusters of cancer cells. They will only attack large tumour masses and have a significant effect if directed by lymphocytes activated against the tumour, and supported by nutrients such as selenium, zinc, beta-carotene and reishi mushroom extract.

T-cell balance and immune function can be restored by omega 3 oils, vitamin E and plant sterols and sterolins.

Natural immunity can be raised by using cross-reacting antigens. The first immunization success was the introduction of cowpox inoculation to make antibodies effective against smallpox. Jenner introduced this in 1796, and in 180 years smallpox was extinct. This is the very principle on which the great medical art and science of homeopathy is based – the use of "Similars" to provoke the body to heal itself.

DR. GUNN'S TARGETED VACCINE HYPOTHESIS

Dr. Hal Gunn, MD is a noted General Practitioner in Oncology, and a founder of the Centre for Integrated Healing, now known as Inspire Health www.inspirehealth. caInspired by Dr. Roger Roger's work with the Petard Protocol including Staphylococcal lysate vaccine, he has proposed and patented a brilliant idea. It appears bacterial and viral vaccines will only work if the vaccine represents a specific infectious pathogen to which the cancer-bearing organ is primed to respond to. Once the embedded immune cells in the organ respond to the vaccine pathogen they are evolved to deal with, the immune response turns on the cancer. Not only are growth and invasion factors being produced by the tumour-associated immune cells now withdrawn, the immune cells turn and attack the tumour cells. This concept of targeting the organ-based immune response rather than the specific type of cancer, is really unique.

Therefore a cancer in the lung, whether it is a primary lung cancer or a metastasis from a totally different type of cancer, will only respond to a vaccine made from a lung pathogen, such as *Streptococcus pyogenes*. Other cancers which respond to *Streptococcus pyogenes* would in tissues which this bacteria infects commonly, namely lymphoma, sarcoma, melanoma, stomach and breast.

A cancer in the liver, whether a primary hepatocellular carcinoma or a metastasis to the liver from an entirely different cancer, will only respond to a vaccine made from a liver pathogen, such as *Escherichia coli* or *Hepatitis B* virus.. Colorectal and pancreatic cancer would be expected to respond to a vaccine containing *Escherichia coli*, such as *Polyvaccinum Forte* PVF. BCG would be useful for bladder, colon, and stomach. Mixed respiratory virus MRV vaccine would be useful for lung cancer, as would vaccines from bacterial lung pathogens such as *Klebsiella pneumoniae, Nocardia rubra, Haemophilus influenzae*, and *Moraxella catarhalis*. *Pseudomonas aeruginosa* should be useful for cancers of the lung, lymphoma and soft tissue cancers. Cervical cancer should respond to vaccines with *Lactobacillus casei* or human papilloma virus HPV. Multiple myeloma should respond to a vaccines for viral hepatitis. Brain cancer should respond to herpes varicella zoster or chicken pox virus, as this virus can cause encephalitis. The same should be true for meningococcal and measles vaccines. *Staphylococcus aureus* lysate should work anywhere staph infections are common, including skin, breast and rectum.

The Polish **Polyvaccinum** preparation has long been used by doctors in British Columbia, and has induced remissions in advanced cancer cases. A typical protocol would be 3 ampoules of *Polyvaccinum Forte* in a 10 ml rubber-topped multi-dose vial, and with a 100 unit insulin syringe, give 0.05 ml or 5 units of vaccine injected subcutaneously. Typical sites are the thighs or abdomen. Inject about three times a week, gradually increasing the dose by 0.01 to 0.02 cc. until it is sufficient to evoke a red flare (erythema) up to a maximum of 5 cm. in diameter within 24 hours. This is the same response we look for from mistletoe injections, i.e. Iscador or Helixor therapy. A good response is often accompanied by a mild fever, though on occasion it may be a high fever. The usual top dose is about 0.40 cc or 40 units on the insulin syringe. Occasionally we get up to 75 units per injection without a response, in which case we continue at that dose; within a few months a response should be evident. Best results are seen in lung cancer, lymphoma and melanoma.

BCG VACCINE

Bacillus Calmette-Guerin BCG immunization is a non-specific immune enhancer from a form of tuberculosis bacteria common in cattle. A suspension of 75 mg live bacillus per ml. is smeared into a 5 cm square of 20 skin scratches every four days for a month, then once weekly, for courses of ten to sixteen applications. BCG may also be injected into tumours such as melanoma at doses of 0.05 to 0.20 ml of the suspension per nodules. It is often used for bladder cancer, where it is instilled by a catheter directly into the bladder. Therapy starts with a course of 6X weekly injections. Dosing may then be in 3 week courses every 3 to 6 months, for about 3 years. It outperforms chemotherapy for transitional cell cancer. BCG therapy can be supported with vitamins A, B6, C E and zinc.

Corynebacterium parvum bacteria preparation is superior to BCG for stimulating macrophages. It is given intravenously, intra-tumour, or subcutaneous by two to four injections in the lymphatic drainage field around tumours, totalling 2 mg for the first treatment, then at 2 to 4 mg per treatment. For fever, hydrothorax, cor pulmonale, thrombocytopenia, liver disorder or severe weakness consider raising the dose up to 8 mg.

Coley's toxins from the bacteria Streptococcus pyogenes and Serratia marcescens; preparations from Corynebacterium parvum or Corynebacterium pseudodipthericum; staphage lysates from Staphylococcus aureus or Staphylococcus epidermidis; vaccines from Escherichia coli, Klebsiella pneumoniae, Haemophilus influenzae, Moraxella catarhalis, Streptococcus pneumoniae, Streptococcus salivarius, and Streptococcus pyogenes induce a cytokine APO-2 ligand, which is like tumour necrosis factor TNF, but even more active in killing cancer cells.

Also used are DNCB extract or MBV mixed bacterial vaccine. Any viral vaccine can also provoke increased non-specific immunity. An example is the common MRV – mixed respiratory virus vaccine

MTH-68/N – a promising immune response modifier using paramyxovirus from chickens, weakened and modified, and given by a nasal spray. This attenuated Newcastle disease virus is harmless to humans, only occasionally provoking a "pink-eye" sort of conjunctivitis. Advanced cancer patients frequently experience disease stabilization, reduction in pain, improved performance status, and sometimes get full remissions after several months. Developed and used in Budapest, Hungary by Laszlo and Eva Csatary.

A newly discovered native picornavirus Seneca Valley Virus 001 selectively infects small cell lung caner cells and retinoblastoma cells, taking out 10,000 bad cells for every healthy cell killed. Picornaviruses include common-cold type rhinoviruses and stomach flu enteroviruses.

Reolysin is a patented reovirus product which infects and kills cancer cells and cancer stem cells when the intrinsic viral defence system is inactivated by up-regulation of the ras pathway.

Bee venom therapy is an excellent way of stimulating immune-arousing inflammation around a tumour.

Uric acid may increase the immune response to vaccines by up-regulating B-cell activated cytokines and amplifying immunoglobulin IgG-1. Uric acid is released by dying cells as a danger signal, and the immune system is programmed to respond vigorously to it.

Naturopathic physicians for generations have used immune gland extracts of animal origin. Thymus gland has been given as capsules or by injection to activate or modulate T-cells. Thymosin 8 mg may be injected every two to three days for one to two months, including during chemo or radiation therapies. If thymic factor is substituted, the dose is about 30 mg. Polyerga is a pig spleen peptide extract which at 300 to 500 mg daily can increase white blood cells and their output of gamma interferon. This inhibits metastasis, improves appetite, reduces pain, improves overall vitality, and increases survival time.

Some of my American naturopathic colleagues are collecting dendritic cells from their patient's blood and exposing them to peptide proteins derived from the surgical samples of the patient's own tumour. The dendritic cells are the immune cells responsible for processing a foreign protein and handing it off to another immune cell to make an antibody. The dendritic cells process the tumour lysate peptides, and when returned to the patient's bloodstream, begin to activate the host's immune system against the cancer. The vaccine is administered three times at two week intervals, and results in increased interferon gamma INFγ as well as increased CD8+ cancer antigen-specific T-cell clones. Unfortunately it is very expensive. Mistletoe therapy can often activate the same response inside your body, at a reasonable price.

Dr. Leanna Standish, ND, PhD recommends the following for immune support:

- melatonin 20 – 40 mg
- coriolus PSK 600 to 1,200 mg. twice daily
- aerobic exercise 20 minutes daily

Remember surgery is very immunosuppressive, as are many chemotherapy drugs.

Isopathic preparations have been made from the patient's own blood, urine or tissue. Tumour biopsy tissue or anything at risk of carrying live tumour cells must of course first be reliably inactivated. Tissue is pulverized into a suspension, inactivated, then injected in the deltoid muscle of the upper arm at doses of 0.2 to 0.3 ml. every five to seven days, for a total of five to seven treatments. This may be repeated after two to four months.

Liver flukes are not "The Cause of All Cancers" as Hulda Clarke claims, but they are associated with cholangio-carcinoma in the bile ducts. Parasites in general are very common, and while the healthy patient need not fear about a few critters in the bowels, a very ill patient may benefit from removing an infestation that is robbing them of nutrition.

Histamine via H2 receptors mediates natural killer cell anticancer activity. Histamine blocks macrophage and monocyte respiratory burst of hydrogen peroxide and other ROS compounds which would otherwise irreversibly inhibit NK cell cytotoxicity and induce apoptosis in NK cells. Histamine has been shown to synergize with IL-2 and IFNa in treatment of melanoma and leukemia.

The strength of the immune system can be degraded by stress, whether physical, psychological and emotional. The immune cells have receptors on their surface and respond to neurotransmitters, the chemicals of thought and mood. This relatively new field of study is called psychoneuroimmunology. In the 1920's the nutrition genius

Naturopathic Oncology

Francis Pottenger studied the nutrition and health of many Stone Age hunter -gatherer remnant societies from Africa to the Arctic. He proposed a theory that immune system cancers such as leukemia, lymphoma and multiple myeloma arose in persons who are parasympathetic dominant. The Autonomic nervous system has 2 parts, the Sympathetic which turns on the stress arousal reaction of "fight or flight," and the Parasympathetic which turns it off.

Lymphocytes in the spleen and thymus gland have receptors for parasympathetic neurotransmitters. These people tend to be somewhat lethargic or laid back types, susceptible to viruses, and over-reactive to infections and inflammation triggers.

Conversely, Pottenger thought solid tumours occurred with sympathetic dominance, that is in people who are highly stressed, with low immune reactivity and low digestive function, including low pancreatic enzymes.

Determining the relative dominance of these two arms of this primitive and subconscious part of our nervous system may give a new strategy to heal the whole person. Acupuncture is one method to rapidly balance these two arms of the autonomic nervous system.

The Krebiozen therapy espoused by Professor Andrew C. Ivy was never properly tested, and remains the most interesting innovation in cancer immunology history. Made by injecting horses with the *Actinomyces* fungus from a non-cancerous tumour in cattle called "lumpy-jaw," the resulting serum yielded an "anti-growth hormone" and would stimulate reticuloendothelial immunity in human cancer patients. Modern naturopathic physicians and homeopaths using Sanum pleomorphic remedies from Actinomyces should find this a clue for further research.

Dr. Enderlein has professed that small microbes living in the blood can assemble into this Actinomycetes fungus in the metabolic ruin of advanced systemic cancer.

Gruner, Glover, Hatsumi, Issels and others have identified a filterable creature in human blood they call a cancer virus, or a bacterium of the size of a virus.

Virginia Livingstone in California makes a vaccine against an organism she calls *Progenitor crytocides* which she feels is a cause of cancer.

Enderlein, Gaston Naessens, Royal Rife, and others claim to see these critters in human blood under dark field microscopes fitted with proper condensers. Pleomorphic commensal organisms are said to be capable of spontaneously generating germs of disease in our blood. This is very unsettling to those who try to make a Universal Law out of the Germ Theory of Louis Pasteur. Pasteur recognized the milieu was "everything" just before he died, giving up the notion that the microbes were more important than the host environment.

Do we not have the "germs" of disease in every cell in the form of virus DNA fused right into our own chromosomes? Is it possible this mass of viral material, including oncogenes, in our DNA might "spontaneously generate" germs under conditions seen in an advanced malignant tumour? I believe immune-suppression might trigger super-infections, inflammation and ultimately cause cancer to flourish. The pleomorphic theories of Gaston Naessens and Professor Enderlein suggest we carry pre-viral elements in our cells, which can assemble into viruses from within our bodies, when we are toxic and metabolically disordered. If Enderlein is correct, there may also be fungal

262

pathogens or their pre-cursors latent in the blood or deeper inside the cells.

We do not merely give antifungal and antiviral medication – we work on the biochemical terrain, the nutritional and physical environment of the cells. Naturopathic immune therapies rebalance the entire ecology to regulate inflammation, enhance immune cell surveillance for cancer cells, and control bacteria, parasites, and viruses.

Naturopathic approaches to immune support include thymus products, mushroom polysaccharides, chlorophyll, plant sterols and sterolins, and psychoneuroimmunology.

Vitamin A derivative retinoic acid will decrease viral DNA such as the human papilloma virus (HPV) inside cells.

Homeopathics such as *Thymuline and Engystol* are excellent for viral control. I use them in cancer, but also to prevent or treat influenza and other viral illness. The Sanum homeopathic remedies based on Enderlein's fungal pathology concepts are remarkably strong and effective medicines.

Immune tonics work best when given early in the day, such as one dose at breakfast and another before lunch.

CANCER STEM CELL STRATEGY

Stem cells are able to replace any cell that dies of old age, commits suicide because it is damaged or mutated, or is killed by injury, toxicity or disease. They can open any part of the genetic code in the chromosomes of the cell, and create a cell specialized to do the job its place in a tissue or organ requires of it. All cells have the DNA library, but most of it is locked down and unusable except very specific parts. So the stem cells wait quietly for the signal to make a replacement, pull out the blueprints, and make exactly what was lost whole again.

When a cancer gets to be a mass of cells about 1 millimetre in diameter, they must get extra blood and lymph vessels to maintain the abnormal rate of growth. They do this by engaging local (peripheral) stem cells, muscle cells, stromal cells, platelets and immune cells such as macrophages to make chemicals that sprout new vessels. If they cannot get this increase in blood and drainage, the cancer will not continue to be a disease. Note that this all happens long before a tumour is visible to any current diagnostic test.

By the time the cancer is usually diagnosed, at a diameter of about 1 centimetre, the chaotic blood vessels in the tumour are typically so leaky they cause the fluid pressure to be so high it squashes the blood flow, and the tumour develops areas of low oxygen (hypoxia). There may even be areas that have no oxygen at all (anoxia) and parts of the tumour will die. The cancer cells survive by switching to fermentation of sugars for energy, which is less efficient. Unfortunately they do not slow down for long, because the lactate by-product of fermentation is a major growth trigger that accelerates the doubling of the cancer cells. Also, low oxygen in the tumour results in another wave of new blood vessel growth (angiogenesis) into the tumour.

The conditions inside the tumour at this point are very abnormal, so the immune cells enter to try to heal the inflammation and damage, just as they would enter any damaged tissue that has lost blood flow and chemical balance. When they cannot fix the problem – and we often refer to cancer as "the wound that will not heal" – they recruit stem cells from the bone marrow. Stem cells, under conditions found in tumours, can activate oncogenes and become malignant, i.e. possess the power of self-renewal and essentially unlimited replicative potential.

As many as 1 in 4 cells in a melanoma tumour are tumorigenic and stem-cell-like. Perhaps this is why these tumours spread early and aggressively. These cancerized stem cells are trained to produce chemicals that maintain the tumour. The abnormal cell-to-cell contacts in the tumour and the wash of growth factors convert the stem cells into malignant cells. The stem cells make actually fuse into some cancer cells, making a hybrid with the power to grow wildly. They are then able to make new full-blown tumour cells. These daughters of the stem cells are complete with all the DNA mutations and problems that make them grow too fast and behave badly towards normal tissues. Now tumour cells are doubling, while stem cells are making new tumour cells, and the tumour grows fast again.

Stem cells in tumours resist therapy by agents which target rapidly dividing cells, such as the most used cancer treatments: cytotoxic chemotherapy and radiation therapy. They grow very slowly, and are relatively inert. They resist normal cell programs that allow a cell to kill itself if it is mutated or damaged (apoptosis). They are given to generating new mutations. Killing off the bulk of differentiated cancer cells is like cutting the head off a dandelion – as long as the stem cells remain, like the root of the dandelion in the ground, the tumour will be back.

Tumour stem cells are capable of self-renewal, moving freely through the body and of forming new tumours. A cluster of about 100 cells can generate an entire new tumour in a new location.

Cancer stem cells are more like bone-marrow derived (BMD) stem cells than peripheral stem cells. For example they express surface CD44 cell adhesion molecule, the ABC transporter Bcrp/ABCG2, and use similar pathways for invasion (chemotaxis) and spread (metastasis). The ABC transporters are ATP-binding cassette transporter proteins such as Multi-drug resistance protein 1 MDR-1 or the P-glycoprotein "porter system" which pump toxins rapidly out of the cells, like bailing out a sinking boat. The stem cells seem to prefer to hide out in crevices in blood vessels, feeding off special nutrients made by the lining of the vessels (endothelium).

BMD stem cells may make up about 0.2 to 0.8 % of tumours, are 100 fold more aggressive than the "normal" cancer cells – and those are able to kill people!

Curcumin has the ability to prevent the rapid proliferation of stem cells triggered by chemotherapy. It keeps the stem cells in asymmetrical mitosis, doubling into a progenitor cell and a replacement stem cell, rather than symmetrical mitosis into 2 stem cells.

To improve therapeutic responses and to prevent reoccurrence of cancers we need to target the BMD stem cell populations in tumours. The strategies which have shown promise are:

- **inhibit NFkB,** the critical regulator of growth promoting genes in stem cells
- **P13-kinase –mTOR/Akt inhibition** selectively blocks growth of cancer stem

264

cells
- **promote PTEN** tumour suppressor gene activity.
- TGF-B1 inhibition – cut off transforming growth factor beta one, an epithelial cell growth factor.
- inhibit beta-catenin, disrupting stem cell signalling pathways Hedgehog, Notch, Wnt and Bmi.
- block the ABC transporters such as the P-glycoprotein porter.
- block IL-8 from dying cells, which causes cancer stem cells to replicate.
- force differentiation, induce apoptosis, anti-angiogenesis.
- Antioxidants to control reactive oxygen species ROS, which are driving the transition of epithelial cells to mesenchymal phenotypes, with stem-cell-like properties including invasiveness and ability to metastasize.

Most promising agents for stem cell modulation:

- Curcumin
- Quercetin – may be as *Can-Arrest* with added curcumin, boswellia & bromelain
- Green tea EGCG 95% polyphenol concentrate plus vitamin E
- Iscador mistletoe
- Grapeseed extract OPCs
- Melatonin
- Ellagic acid
- Reishi mushroom (*Ganoderma lucidum*) extract
- R+ alpha lipoic acid
- Indole-3-carbinol
- Vitamins A,C, and D3
- Omega 3 EPA oil
- Ginkgo biloba extract
- Black seed *Nigella sativa* thymoquinone

MISCELLANEOUS

There are an infinite number of weird and wacky cancer "cures" out there, most of decidedly uncertain benefit. I have no direct experience or knowledge to recommend trying or referring patients for these approaches, some of which may be valuable – but I cannot say which. Please get advice from a practitioner experienced with a therapy before trusting your life to:

- Bestatin UBX from Streptomyces olivereticuli
- Thymus glandular injections
- Amino acids such as Jinlong capsules
- Laetrile, also known as amygdalin, sarcarcinase, nitriloside or Vitamin B17
- Insulin shock therapy

- Wobenzyme N – pancreatin , bromelain and rutin
- Radiofrequency devices such as the Rife machine.
- Electrotherapy for parasites such as the Beck Zapper device
- MGN-3 with shiitake enzymes and modified arabinoxylan.
- Macrobiotic diet
- Gerson diet
- Sun Soup – a patented herbal food with shiitake
- Blue scorpion venom drops
- Carnivora extract
- Laminaria extract

Absolutely without merit: NOT EVER RECOMMENDED

- *Morinda citrifolia* or Noni juice.
- Hulda Clark's parasite treatment – this pseudo-science is textbook cancer quackery.
- Chondriana crystals
- Colostrum transfer factors
- Immuno-Augmentative Therapy (IAT)
- Germanium sesquioxide supplementation
- Cesium salts to alter cellular acidity
- Live cell therapy with foetal cells or stem cells

PART FIVE – NATUROPATHIC FOCUS ON SPECIFIC CANCERS

Chapter Nine – Key Compounds For Key Targets Of Therapy

"The universe is full of magical things patiently waiting for our wits to grow sharper."
–Eden Phillpotts, essayist

We begin to create a specific program for a specific cancer by first considering the welfare of the patient as a whole. Melded into the decision are a host of factors such as co-morbid medical conditions, medications, organ function, nutritional status, psychological condition, financial security, and social supports

We then consider the **foundation protocols** which have given reasonably consistent responses:

1. Mitochondria Rescue – using natural agents which wake up dormant mitochondria to restore the off-switch in cancer cells:
- Alpha lipoic acid (R+ form only) 150 to 300 mg 3 times daily, best in time-release form – a potent inhibitor of pyruvate dehydrogenase kinase PDHK. Do not combine with curcumin.
- Mixed tocopherols for gamma E - 800 IU daily.
- B1 or thiamine, especially as benfotiamine 80 to 160 mg 2 times daily. Also inhibits PDHK
- L-carnitine – 2 to 6 capsules 2 to 3 times daily. Energizes, but makes masses of ROS.
- Marine omega 3 oil–distilled sardine and anchovy 3,000 – 4,000 mg, or seal oil 2 caps twice daily.
- Coenzyme Q-10 – 100 mg 3 times daily – absorbs best when taken with fats or oils
- Grapeseed extract (oligomeric proanthocyanidins) – 100 mg 3 times daily
- *Ganoderma lucidum* (Reishi) mushroom extract – 500 to 1,000 mg 3 times daily
- Indole-3-carbinol – 200 mg 2 to 3 times daily
- Quercetin – 2 capsules 2 to 3 times daily
- Ellagic acid –8 ounces of unsweetened pomegranate, grape or berry juices.
- B-vitamins riboflavin (B2) and niacin (B3) as nicotinamide – 50 to 100 mg 2 to 3 times daily

2. Inflammation and Toxicity Rescue – The core group of therapies I advised in my first book *Naturally There's Hope*, in adequate doses and with supporting agents:

- Curcumin – as in CanArrest – with bromelain for absorption – 2 capsules 3 times daily
- Green tea EGCG – 700 mg 3 times daily – with vitamin E 400 IU once a day to prevent kidney toxicity.
- Grapeseed extract OPCs – NASOBIH *Nutra-Caps* with added resveratrol, 2 caps 3 times daily.

That is still a good combination, and I might commonly add the following to make a basic protocol:
- Indole-3-carbinol – 200 mg 3 times daily
- Modified citrus pectin – 4 capsules 2 times daily.
- Jingli neixao – 2 capsules 3 times daily.
- Whole foods, clean protein, low glycemic load diet.
- Reiki healing – weekly

3. **Palliative and Tonic Care** –
- Mistletoe injections – 2 to 3 times weekly.
- Intravenous vitamin C – 2 times weekly, 50 to 75 grams.
- Myer's intravenous vitamins – as needed.
- Jingli Neixao – 2 capsules 3 times daily.
- Greens, whey or rice protein and multivitamin smoothies – 1 scoop of each twice daily

On these foundations one can develop a complete program of diet, supplements, exercise, mind-body healing, stress management, self-expression, detoxification and all the elements that create real healing conditions.

We match natural agents up to the **specific growth factors** known to drive a specific type of cancer to construct rational protocols for their naturopathic management.

♦ Key natural compounds which address the biology of cancer and target critical growth factors ♦

APOPTOSIS PROMOTERS – (trigger cancer cells to enter a death/recycling program – **the primary goal of all cancer care, including chemotherapy and radiation**.) -quercetin, curcumin, **mistletoe**, green tea **EGCG**, betulinic acid, caffeine, genestein, berberine, vitamin E succinate, catechin, cayenne, poppy *Papaver somniferum* noscapine, *baicalein* from *Scutellaria, Bupleurum,* vitamin C, melatonin, ellagic acid, limonenes, indole-3-carbinol, inositol-6-phosphate, feverfew, ginger, garlic, R+ alpha lipoic acid, taheebo, reishi, EPA oils, grapeseed extract OPCs, trans-resveratrol, vitamin D, lemon grass.

MITOCHONDRIAL ACTIVATION (restores control over the apoptosis kill switch by sparking up the oxygen-sugar combustion chambers in cancer cells) – **R+ alpha lipoic acid,** coenzyme Q-10, riboflavin, niacin, magnesium malate, taurine, vitamin

A, selenium, iodine, vitamin E succinate, gamma tocopherol, melatonin, L-carnitine, palmitoylcarnitine, quercetin, & methylated flavones, ellagic acid, curcumin, olives and olive oil, resveratrol, grapeseed extract, *Coriolus, Ganoderma,* milk thistle silibinin, white peony root, oleic acid, berberine, isothiocyanates, indole-3-carbinol, ashwagandha, dichloroacetate. Support with IV vitamin C, IV alpha lipoic acid, oral or IV vitamins K2 and/or K3.

ANTI-METASTATICS- (halt the spread to other organs) – **fractionated citrus pectin, green tea EGCG**, heparin, Co-enzyme Q-10, larch arabinogalactan, aloe vera juice, EPA omega 3 oils, CLA, bromelain, beta carotene, vitamins A and C, melatonin, indole-3-carbinol, R+ alpha lipoic acid, beta-sitosterol, maitake, catechin, quercetin, rutin, curcumin, mistletoe, sea cucumber extract, calcium-D-glucarate, melanin (echinacea, black cumin, tea), resveratrol, alpha linolenic acid, apigenin, ursolic acid.

ANTI-ANGIOGENICS – (cut off blood supply to tumours, inhibit vascular endothelial growth factor VEGF) – catechin, **green tea EGCG**, curcumin, **quercetin**, vitamins A, D & E, ellagic acid, pomegranate and grapeseed anthocyanidins and proanthocyanidins, resveratrol, sea cucumber extract, beta carotene, mistletoe, shikonin, coriolus PSK, CAPE, apigenin, genestein, EPA oils, shark liver oil, selenium, zinc, luteolin, lysine, proline, vitamin C, modified citrus pectin, milk thistle, bupleurum, sanguinaria, rabdosia, ginseng, wormwood, scutellaria, magnolia, poria, ginkgo, angelica and polygonum. See also COX-2 inhibitors.

COX-2 INHIBITORS – (control inflammation to reduce growth signals) – **curcumin, boswellia**, **quercetin**, ginger, isatis tinctoria, , vitamin A, resveratrol, grapeseed proanthocyanidin OPCs, green tea EGCG, bilberry, reishi, licorice, garlic, scutellaria, feverfew, rosemary, bromelain, salicylates, green-lipped mussel extract, omega 3 oils –EPA, DHA, DPA, aloe vera, Zeel, propolis, CAPE, black seed *Nigella sativa* thymoquinone.

NUCLEAR TRANSCRIPTION FACTOR NFkB INHIBITORS – (control cell doubling at the DNA level and regulate inflammation) – **reishi**, ginger, silibinin, curcumin, indole-3-carbinol, green tea EGCG, beta carotene, apigenin, melatonin, feverfew parthenolides, organic selenium, zinc, alpha lipoic acid, vitamin C, vitamin D, calcium, vitamin E, N-acetyl-cysteine, quercetin, proanthocyanidins, resveratrol, emodin, genestein, guggulsterone, zerumbone, evodiamine, aspirin, salicylic acid, holy basil ursolic acid, melanin (echinacea, black cumin, tea), black seed *Nigella sativa* thymoquinone, ginkgo biloba.

p53 GENE MODULATORS – (turn on the apoptosis switch, which is blocked in cancer cells) – **quercetin**, genestein, selenomethionine, melatonin, catechin, green tea EGCG, grapeseed OPCs, trans-resveratrol, vitamin E succinate, curcumin, folate, N-acetyl-cysteine, retinoic acid, milk thistle, garlic.

mTOR PATHWAY INHIBITORS – (regulate kinases involved in proliferation and angiogenesis) – curcumin, green tea EGCG, indole-3-carbinol. Synergistic with anti-apoptotics, HSP inhibitors and IGF-1 inhibitors.

BETA-CATENIN INHIBITORS – (self-renewal factor necessary for tumour progression) – vitamin A as retinol palmitate or as retinoic acid, omega 3 DHA, indole-3-carbinol, curcumin. Casein kinase inhibitors support BC modulation.

EPIDERMAL GROWTH FACTOR EGF and EPIDERMAL GROWTH FACTOR RECEPTOR EGFR INHIBITORS – (control growth of carcinomas) – **silibinin** from **milk thistle**, curcumin, grapeseed extract OPCs, resveratrol, green tea EGCG, quercetin, genestein.

STAT TRANSCRIPTION FACTOR INHIBITORS – (to block production of anti-apoptotic proteins)

STAT-1: green tea EGCG; STAT-3: **indole-3-carbinol**, curcumin, cucurbitacin Q.

INSULIN-LIKE GROWTH FACTOR ONE IGF-1 INHIBITORS – (stop sugar from feeding rapid cancer cell growth) – **green tea EGCG**, vitamin D3, lycopene, exercise, low fat whole food or vegan diet. Binding protein IGFBP3 is increased by OPCs, flaxseed, CLA, dandelion root, burdock root, chicory, vitamin D3, R+ alpha lipoic acid, and vanadyl sulphate. Milk thistle extract inhibits the receptor IGF-1R. Avoid sugar, colostrum, estrogen, growth hormone.

ACTIVATION PROTEIN ONE AP-1 INHIBITORS – (control doubling in fast-growing tumours with low oxygen) – curcumin, green tea EGCG, quercetin, genestein, selenium, PTK inhibitors.

PLATELET-DERIVED GROWTH FACTOR RECEPTOR PDGFR INHIBITOR – green tea EGCG, and tyrosine kinase inhibitors such as vitamin K and milk thistle silymarin/silibinin. Consider MMP inhibitors i.e. curcumin, EGCG.

PROTEIN TYROSINE KINASE PTK SIGNAL INHIBITORS – (control growth signalling between the cell surface and nucleus) – curcumin, genestein, green tea EGCG, milk thistle, reishi, resveratrol, pomegranate anthocyanidins, shark liver alkylglycerols, *Scutellaria*, licorice, vitamin E .

MATRIX METALLOPROTEINASE MMP INHIBITORS – (stop invasion into other tissues) – Scutellaria baicalein, **green tea EGCG** polyphenols, resveratrol, Zeel, Hormeel, digestive enzymes, curcumin, bovine cartilage. See also AP-1 and COX-2 inhibitors

COLLAGENASE INHIBITORS – (stop invasion into other tissues) – green tea EGCG and EPCG, , grapeseed oligomeric proanthocyanidins, anthocyanidins, resveratrol, curcumin, quercetin, mushroom polysaccharides such as coriolus PSK, luteolin, emodin, genestein, vitamin A, vitamin C, PSK extract., melatonin, and omega 3 oils EPA and DPA. Hyaluronidase inhibitors include apigenin, boswellia, gotu kola *Centella asiatica*, horse chestnut escin *Aesculus hippocastanum*, luteolin, resveratrol, proanthocyanidins, ruscogenin from Butcher's Broom herb *Ruscus aculeatus*, and vitamin C.

STEM CELL REGULATORS- (control bone marrow derived stem cells which resist therapy and create new cancer cells) – Curcumin, quercetin, green tea EGCG, grapeseed extract, ellagic acid, reishi mushroom, R+ alpha lipoic acid, indole-3-carbinol, omega 3 oils, melatonin, Iscador mistletoe, selenomethionine, vitamins A, C, D & E.

INDUCERS OF DIFFERENTIATION – (make tumours act more normal, including tumour stem cells) –boswellia, butyrate, berberine, bromelain, retinoids, vitamins A & D, quercetin, calcium, soy, inositol-6-phosphate, poly-MVA, melatonin, and burdock root.

TRANSFORMING (TRANSITIONAL) GROWTH FACTOR BETA TGFß

INHIBITORS – (to control angiogenesis, metastasis, immune suppression and oxidative stress) – R+ alpha lipoic acid, ginkgo biloba.

PROTEASOMAL REGULATORS – (control expression of genes at the protein transcription level) – green tea EGCG, curcumin.

DNA REPAIR PROMOTERS – (heal the mutations that make cancer cells dangerous) – butyrates, vitamin A, poly-MVA, vitamins B3 & B12, garlic, tea, folic acid. Parsley inhibits mutations.

BCL-2 INHIBITORS – (regulate apoptosis) – green tea extract, curcumin, birch betulinic acid.

HEAT SHOCK PROTEIN HSP BLOCKERS – (makes cancer cells vulnerable to stress) – quercetin, alpha lipoic acid.

CELL-TO-CELL COMMUNICATION MODIFIERS – (make cancer cells better neighbours) -GLA, CLA, bromelain, green tea catechins, melatonin, integrins, vitamin D, curcumin, grapeseed OPCs, milk thistle.

TUMOUR NECROSIS FACTOR TNF INHIBITORS – (reduce inflammation and growth signals) – EPA oils, reishi, melatonin, melanin (echinacea, black cumin, tea), black seed *Nigella sativa* thymoquinone, milk thistle, cat's claw, vitamin E succinate, vitamin A, vitamin D3, soy genestein, green tea EGCG, primrose oil, curcumin, quercetin, emodin, resveratrol, hypericin, luteolin, caffeic acid.

CYTOTOXICS – (kill cancer cells directly) – berberine, mistletoe, graviola, carnivora, isatis, yew bark.

TOPOISOMERASE INHIBITORS – (reduce DNA copying needed for cells to double) – green tea (I), boswellia (I & II), berberine (I & II), camptothecin, etoposide, scutellaria (II), genestein. Topo-II inhibitors do <u>not</u> mix with glucosamine compounds.

HORMONE MODULATORS – (cut off hormone growth signalling) – flaxseed, melatonin, indole-3-carbinol (I3C), diindolylmethane (DIM), resveratrol, quercetin, potassium iodide.

AROMATASE INHIBITORS AIs – quercetin, grapeseed procyanidin B dimers, white button mushrooms *Agaricus bisporus*, melatonin, reishi, green tea EGCG, pomegranate, progesterone, iodine.

IMMUNE MODULATORS – (help the immune cells recognize cancer cells as abnormal and remove them) – astragalus, ligusticum, maitake, shiitake, reishi, Shih Chuan Da Bu Wan, ashwagandha, andrographites. *Polyerga* spleen peptides and thymus extracts. Alkylglycerols from shark liver oil, plant sterols & sterolins. Larch arabinogalactan, Echinacea, Panax ginseng, Panax notoginseng, curcumin, cat's claw and Saposhnikovia divericata, Cimetidine, Carnivora, *Iscador* or *Viscum Comp* injectable mistletoe lectin extracts. Vaccines – Coley's toxins, HAS, MRV, MBV and BCG.

ANTI-VIRALS – (stop viruses that cause some cancers) – *Engystol*, *Thymuline*, echinacea, lomatia, graviola, vitamin A, vitamin C, glutathione, Newcastle paramyxovirus nasal spray, sterols & sterolins, garlic, tea EGCG.

ANTI-PARASITICS – (reduce immune stress) – Flaxseed, psyllium husks, graviola, berberine, wormwood, oil of oregano, garlic, golden seal, cloves, black walnut, male fern, grapefruit seed extract.

MAST CELL DEGRANULATION INHIBITORS – (control histamine to slow growth) – quercetin, green tea EGCG, grapeseed proanthocyanidins, genestein, luteolin, apigenin, vitamin C, *Eleutherococcus senticosus.*

ANTI-COAGULANTS – (blood stasis due to fibrin accumulation leads to inflammation) – omega 3 seal oil, fish EPA oils, garlic, bromelain, resveratrol, anthocyanidins, curcumin, vitamin. E, *Coriolus* PSK, *Ganoderma* (reishi), astragalus, genestein, quercetin, emodin, luteolin, *Panax ginseng*, *Ginkgo biloba*, lumbrokinase, nattokinase, *Salix alba*

ANTI-CACHEXICS – (stop metabolic wasting syndrome) – EPA omega 3 oils, CLA, melatonin, vitamin E, vitamin C, carnitine, green tea EGCG, cat's claw, milk thistle, Ukrain.

PTEN PROTECTOR – (tumour suppressor gene) – indole-3-carbinol, curcumin, quercetin, isoflavones.

Chapter Ten – Integrative Care Of Breast Cancer

EPIDEMIOLOGY

The most common cancer of women in North America is breast cancer. 1% of breast cancer cases are male. Approximately one woman in 7 in North America will develop this disease in her lifetime. Before 1971 the risk was 1 in 20! It is the second leading cause of death in American women, and the leading cause of death in the age group 40 to 55 years. The death rate had been unchanged from 1920 to 1990, but has reduced slightly in recent years. Fortunately 5-year survival is about 84%, partly because it is reasonably treatable, often curable. Risk in Asia and Africa is 4 to 5 times less, indicating the strong role of lifestyle choices, and the opportunity for prevention.

Breast cancer cells have an average doubling time of about 100 days, which is relatively slow. There is time to reflect and decide among the various treatment options.

There tends to be a slightly increased risk of reoccurrence some months after surgery, related to angiogenesis and immune dysregulation from surgical trauma. Mortality rates for breast cancer do not fall off over time, as seen with most types of cancer. The steady occurrence of relapses over the years suggests the persistence of micro-metastatic disease, even after what is now considered definitive curative treatment.

RISK FACTORS FOR DEVELOPING BREAST CANCER

- Family history in first degree relative – mother or sister
- Early menarche (start of menstruation)
- Late onset of menopause
- Estrogen excess such as estrogen replacement therapy in menopause or use of birth control pills before age 35 or longer than
- 5 years. Estrogen and progesterone combination hormone replacement therapy (HRT) is also linked to increased risk of gallbladder cancer, stroke, heart attack, blood clots and Alzheimer's
- Obesity – fat cells make estrogen via aromatase enzyme
- High fat diet, especially those high in arachidonic acid and saturated fat.
- Moderate to high alcohol consumption increases risk 50 to 100% Risk is entirely dose-dependent – for example, risk increases 45 to 50% with consumption of more than half of a glass of wine daily! Steven Bowlin of Case Western Reserve University states that 25% of breast cancers can be attributed to alcohol. The cancer risk from alcohol consumption is slightly reduced by supplementing folate and MMP-2 inhibitors such as green tea.
- Excess iron load increases risk. Measure serum ferritin.
- Nulliparous – never having a child – risk up 30%

- Child-bearing after age 30. First full term pregnancy after 25 puts up risk 40% over those having a child before 20.
- Excess exposure to xenobiotics with estrogenic properties such as pesticides and herbicides. For example organo-chlorine pesticides increase risk of larger and more aggressive cancers.
- Plasticizer bis-phenol A (BPA) accumulates in breast fat and is a potent xeno-estrogen found in soft plastics such as Saran wrap, food containers and water bottles. The FDA safety limit is two parts per million – 2 ppm – but it is clinically estrogenic at two parts per billion – 2 ppb.
- Exposure to air fresheners, paint fumes, household cleaning agents, chemicals in cosmetics.
- Exposure to anti-psychotic drugs which are dopamine antagonists, and anti-emetic dopamine antagonists for vomiting, because they elevate prolactin. Depression has been found to increase risk of breast cancer by 42%.
- Low intake of calcium, vitamin D and other bone health factors promotes metastasis into the bones. Calcium build-up inside cells (cellular hypercalcinosis) is a powerful trigger of carcinogenesis, and ironically is due to a lack of proper calcium intake and utilization. If you are going to stay out of the sun and use sunscreens, you had better be taking a supplement of 1,000 to 2,000 IU vitamin D3 daily.
- MMTV-like virus, a relative of the mouse mammary tumour virus, is found in 40% of USA female breast cancers, with a 5-fold increased risk of aggressive disease, and a strong link to inflammatory breast cancer. The viral genome splices into the Notch-4 locus, activating cancer stem cells.
- A high glycemic diet – high in sugar and refined starches is associated with higher risk of breast cancer and more rapid progression of the disease.
- Insulin, prolactin, insulin-like growth factors and growth hormone are breast cancer promoters. Even slightly elevated IGF-1 and IGFBP-3 indicate significant risk for breast cancer in the Harvard Nurses Study. A major prognostic indicator for breast cancer patients is the blood insulin level at the time of diagnosis.
- Stress hormone adrenaline (epinephrine) blocks cancer cells throwing the apoptosis death switch. Stress reduces the effectiveness of cancer therapies. The psycho-neuro-immunological system or hypothalamic-pituitary axis regulates a number of chemicals which breast cells carry receptors for: insulin, prolactin, vitamin D, estrogen, progesterone, testosterone and other androgens.
- Silicone breast implants increase risk 18X of a rare anaplastic large T-cell lymphoma, to 0.2 cases per year per 100,000 women with implants.
- Breast cancer metastases preferentially target the lung when they express tumour necrosis factor TNF-related apoptosis-inducing ligand TRAIL.
- Transforming growth factor beta TGFß may be responsible for single cells metastasizing from breast tumours. Without it, only clumps tend to break off, which tend to lodge in regional lymph nodes.
- Counting circulating tumour cells predicts risk in breast cancers. Best is ≤ 5, worst is ≥ 50.

GENETIC FACTORS IN BREAST CANCER

Genetic factors may only cause 5% of cases. Jewish people have slightly higher risk than other ethnicities.

The DNA mutations that create and sustain cancers begin with genomic instability, marked by shortened telomere content, and allelic imbalance. These genetically aberrant cells will look normal when stained and examined under a microscope by a pathologist. They are not yet cancer, but are in the process of clonal evolution which can over time result in grossly cancerous cell behaviour and appearance. Breast cancers have been shown to have marked genomic instability in the cells up to a full centimetre out from the visible tumour margins. This is referred to as a "field of cancerization," tissue at risk of becoming cancer, even if the gross tumour is removed. This is why we like to see "wide surgical margins." It is likely the tumour is enslaving immune cells and stem cells to alter the intracellular matrix to promote conditions favourable to the tumours, namely abnormal control over growth and differentiation of the cells in the region.

BRCA-1 or **BRAC-2** gene on chromosome 17 normally repairs DNA tangles, independent of p53. Female carriers of mutated BRAC-1 have an 85% lifetime risk of breast and up to 50% risk of ovarian cancers. Male carriers have 4 times increased risk of developing colon cancer, and 3 times increased risk of developing prostate cancer.

BRAC-1 deficient cells cannot repair DNA. If this leads to mutations and small chromosomal rearrangements in the PTEN gene, then a potent tumour suppressor is inactivated, and tumour cell growth will be strongly stimulated.

BRAC-1 normally docks onto estrogen receptor alpha, acting as a cancer inhibitor. This protective role can be disrupted by cyclin D1, which disrupts the BRAC-1 to ERα interaction.

BRAC-1 mutation positive breast tumours are very sensitive to chemotherapy, with extremely high rates of tumour and axillary (lymph nodes in the armpit) clearance, particularly with anthracycline drugs such as Epirubicin. However, for ER+ breast cancer survival at 5 years is about 20% less than for BRAC-2 mutation carriers, or those with no mutation of the BRAC genes. So, they are easier to knock down, but harder to keep down.

BRAC-2 gene can mutate, resulting in impaired DNA repair and therefore increased risk of cancerous mutations taking hold. Usually the mutation is a deletion at site 33291 on chromosome 13. is associated with increased risk of early onset breast cancer, and 4 times increased risk of uterine cancer. Carriers of BRAC mutations tend to have tumours with higher grades, more necrosis, and more proliferative activity. Male carriers have 15 times increased risk of breast cancer and 4 times increased risk of early prostate cancer.

Both BRAC-1 and BRAC-2 mutation carriers are less able to repair radiation damage, and have abnormally high risk of cancer induction from exposure to common diagnostic X-ray and CT-scan imaging. BRAC 1 and 2 mutations only account for less than 25% of familial risk of breast cancer. Also involved in breast cancer development are genes which relate to the control of cell growth and cell signalling such as MAP3K1, FGFR2, LSP1 and TNRC9.

Naturopathic Oncology

Inhibiting the DNA repair enzyme Poly (ADP-Ribose) polymerase or PARP slows growth in BRAC-1 and BRAC-2 mutants by increasing apoptosis. PARP is a key DNA repair mechanism up-regulated in triple-negative breast cancer in response to reduction in other critical pathways of DNA repair, such as BRCA1.

BRAC mutations can be normalized with epigenetic regulators such as **selenomethionine**. BRAC-1 mutant cells normalize with **resveratrol** inhibition of Survivin expression.

The **p53** tumour suppressor gene is altered in about 50% of cases of advanced metastatic disease.

Reduced **p27** levels in the nucleus correlate with tumour aggressiveness and poor survival. p27 is a direct inhibitor of cyclin-dependent kinase 2 (cdk2) responsible for transcription factors that promote DNA replication. In advanced breast cancer a protein kinase Akt bars p27 from the nucleus by phosphorylating p27 in its nuclear localization signal sector. Phosphorylated p27 ends up sequestered in the cytoplasm, unable to bind up and inhibit the nuclear protein cdk2 involved in cell regulation. Akt also fosters cell proliferation, survival and motility through P13K kinase which is activated by the HER-2 and epidermal growth factor receptors.

HER-2/neu gene overexpression or amplification results in increased HER-2/neu protein. Too much of this transmembrane glycoprotein results in overexpression of EGFRs – epitheliod growth factor receptors. EGFR is always important in any carcinoma.

HER-2/neu + status is associated with increased NFkB activity, and therefore inflammation and all its associated growth factors. This is particularly problematic in rapidly proliferating tumours.

There is also speculation this gene may reduce estrogen and progesterone hormone receptors on the surface of the breast cancer cells, making them harder to cure. Even tumours under 1 cm in diameter and found before axillary spread high-risk for aggressive growth and spread, and they tend to go into the brain.

HER-2 positive breast cancer may respond to anthracycline chemo drugs including Doxorubicin, Epirubicin, Adriamycin, Daunorubicin, Idarubicin and Mitoxantrone. However, HER-2 negative cases do not respond to anthracyclines, and they no longer represent the standard of care for these patients.

Quercetin is able to reduce HER-2 signalling and therefore reduces activity in the EGFR. Emodin in herbs such as *Aloe vera* also modulate HER-2 expression.

In HER-2/neu + cases we also target STAT-3, mTOR and YB-1, for example with curcumin, indole-3-carbinol and green tea EGCG.

Inflammatory breast cancer may be linked to the presence of MMTV-like gene sequences from the mouse mammary tumour virus. These genetic taints are seen in 40% of breast cancers and correspond to a 5 times increased risk of aggressive disease. The MMTV virus can be carried by dogs.

Once breast cancer has occurred, the risk of a second occurrence goes up 5 fold. The five year relapse risk is 10 to 20%. A person with breast cancer is also at higher than average risk of developing cancer of the colon, ovaries or endometrium of the uterus (lining of the womb).

REDUCING RISK OF BREAST CANCER

High intake of dietary fibre, vitamin C, beta-carotene, lycopenes, legumes, cruciferous vegetables, green tea.

Dietary phytoestrogens such as soy foods modulate estrogen receptors. The dietary target for isoflavones is 40 mg daily, from foods such as miso, tofu and soy milk.

Even ¼ grapefruit daily inhibits the estrogen-clearing cytochrome P-450 CYP3A4 enzyme in the liver enough to increase risk of breast cancer by as much as 30%. DO NOT EAT GRAPEFRUIT.

Low fat diet, down to 20% of calories as fat. Monosaturates such as oleic acid in canola oil and olive oil are protective. Omega 3 fatty acids are protective, as found in wild salmon, tuna, halibut, mackerel, sardines and herring; also in nuts and seeds. This is a big issue for those with estrogen-receptor negative ER- cancers. Fish oils prevent ductal carcinoma, but not lobular carcinoma.

Risk is lower in those with high HDL – the "good cholesterol," and is better in those with high total cholesterol versus low cholesterol. Low triglycerides and low VLDL "bad cholesterol" predict a better response to treatment.

Low glycemic diet – and this is especially vital if you are sedentary, or overweight, or have been on hormone replacement therapy. A low-glycemic diet reduces risk about 22%, by controlling insulin and insulin-like growth factors.

Beans and lentils twice weekly are protective. In general vegan or plant-based diets are the lowest risk. I do insist that all animal foods be free of herbicides, pesticides, hormones and drugs. Red meat finished with grains – usually corn silage – are pro-inflammatory, whereas grass or pasture fed animals are safer, due to a more favourable omega 3 to omega 6 fat ratio.

Regular physical exercise, at least 30 minutes aerobic exercise three times a week. The ideal is to work up to 60 minutes up to 5 times per week. Hypoxia-inducible factor alpha HIFα is associated with reduced survival and increased risk of metastases. Aerobic exercise increases circulation, and also controls blood sugar and thus insulin and insulin-like growth factors.

Sunshine and vitamin D. So many people are avoiding sun exposure and using sunscreens to reduce risk of skin cancers, but now many Canadians are showing up with vitamin D deficiency, particularly in winter. In the winter take up to 2,000 IU of vitamin D3 daily.

Breastfeeding helps – the longer the better, for you and for your baby. The breast tissue completes its differentiation and carcinogens are eliminated in the breast milk. The months during pregnancy without periods also are risk reducers, so more kids and more nursing in the past may have helped keep rates lower.

Maintain good bowel bacteria with enteric-coated probiotics.

Maintain your thyroid gland. A subtle and pre-clinical hypothyroid state is a risk factor for breast cysts, fibrosis, and cancer. Iodine, exercise and immune balance are the foundation of thyroid health.

Stress management to moderate cortisol and blood sugar fluctuations.

Avoid use of antiperspirants. I like to use natural grapefruit seed extract (GSE) deodorants.

Avoid alcohol, but if you must drink, take folate or folic acid and vitamin B6.

Breast cancer resistance protein BCRP is increased by intake of quercetin, resveratrol, indole-3-carbinol, green tea EGCG, and other proteasome inhibitors. Therefore eat fruits and vegetables such as apples, onions, grapes, cabbage, broccoli, and drink green tea.

Urokinase deficiency increases the spread of breast cancer. This can be controlled with green tea EGCG.

Metastasis of breast cancer to the bones is regulated by TGFß, RANKL, and Src tyrosine kinases.

Detoxify your body of xenobiotics with an annual body cleanse. Many chemicals in plastics, pesticides, herbicides, flame retardants, etc. are hormone mimics or hormone disruptors. Health Canada and the Canadian Cancer Society claim only about 1 to 2 % of cancers can be blamed on these chemicals, but I think they are deluded or lying. The "Israeli Breast Cancer Anomaly" demonstrated that cutting 3 pesticides out of the food chain resulted in a dramatic drop of **over 30%** in the age-specific breast cancer mortality rate in a decade. This was after a 25 year period of continually increasing rates for breast cancer in Israel, and which continued in all other modern societies.

A naturopathic physician can guide you as to diet and herbs appropriate for your health. We can avoid a lot of risk by eating organic food, choosing natural personal hygiene and home cleaning products, and generally reducing our reliance on synthetic chemical products. Be aware that even a perfect lifestyle will not keep toxins out of your body. The environment is so contaminated with government-approved toxins that we all are at risk.

DIAGNOSIS & SCREENING

BLOOD TEST – Epidermal growth factor receptor EGFR proteins may be elevated in the blood long before breast cancer is otherwise detectable.

BREAST SELF EXAM – recent studies suggest BSE may not be able to detect cancer early enough to alter the clinical outcome. Breast self exam BSE is no longer endorsed by many professionals, yet most breast cancer cases I see found the lump themselves – so I refuse to discourage the practice. Also, many women prefer to be proactive, and recognize that 7 to 10% of palpable masses will be missed by a mammogram. The smallest palpable mass is about 8 millimetres in diameter, which would contain about a billion cancer cells at about three fourths of their lifespan in age. Perform BSE 5 to 7 days after menses, every month. Cancer may be detected soon after a "normal" mammogram. Watch for a persistent rash on the nipple, which may be the only warning of Paget's disease.

PHYSICAL EXAM – professional PE by a physician or nurse should be done every 3 years between ages 20-40, and every 2 years thereafter. All palpable lesions should be biopsied. Most will not be malignant.

MAMMOGRAPHY – expert opinion about the value of mammograms has changed several times in living memory. About 0.3% of asymptomatic Canadian adult women may harbour breast cancer. The current consensus is that they are probably helpful at early detection for women over age 50. Swedish studies on women ages 48-69 showed up to 45% reduced mortality from breast cancer. Modern mammograms use a very low dose of radiation, in the standard two view bilateral test. There is a potential to detect masses under 5 mm diameter. The pathognomonic (characteristic) lesion is a high attenuation mass with spiculated margins. There is a false negative rate of 10 to 30%! This can be from the mass being hidden in dense breast tissue, interpretive error, and because the entire breast is not imaged. One in three masses now labelled breast cancer by screening mammography is a non-lethal "pseudo-cancer." To avoid being over-diagnosed and over-treated, a more definitive *diagnostic mammogram* must be performed. Mammography can detect about 69% of cancers (sensitivity) and misdiagnose about 16% of cases (specificity). 95% of masses found by screening mammography are benign, but all should be carefully evaluated. In return for scaring the wits out of 19 out of 20 women who get a positive mammogram finding, there has been a gratifying reduction of about 15% in breast cancer deaths attributed to this screening tool. It is a fact that early detection means a better chance of a cure. Mammograms detect about 23% of breast cancers. Even those with a firm mammographic diagnosis of invasive breast cancer have a 22% chance it will spontaneously regress without treatment.

SCINTIGRAPHY – MIBI scans are widely used in coronary disease assessment, and have been adapted for use in breast cancer diagnosis. Miraluma scans are particularly valuable if the breast tissue is quite dense, making a conventional mammogram difficult to read. The MIBI scan uses an IV injection of approximately 1000 MBq of sestamibi isotope (technectium-99m hexakis 2-methoxyisonitrile) into a fasting patient who has avoided caffeine and other vasoconstrictors. The patient rests prone, breasts hanging down through openings in the table, so there is no compression applied to the breast. The MIBI isotope accumulates in mitochondria, and measures metabolic activity. The procedure takes about 50 minutes. The original protocol called a Miraluma scan had approximately the same utility as mammograms. However, recently the BEST scan system has added high-dose dipyridamole (HDD) to vasodilate and enhance isotope uptake. This produces accurate discrimination of normal breast tissue from inflammation, and detects early cancers as small as 4mm diameter.

ULTRASOUND – Diagnostic ultrasound is not useful for screening, but will determine with 100% accuracy if a lesion is a cyst or a solid mass. Ultrasound can augment mammography when breast tissue is very dense. Ultrasound can detect about 42% of breast cancers.

MAGNETIC RESONANCE IMAGING: MRI's will not show calcifications, but will show vascularity and can therefore discriminate a local recurrence in a surgical scar. Also it is a more sensitive test for bone metastases than a bone scan. MRI can detect 96% of breast cancers!

THERMOGRAPHY – very sensitive infrared cameras are being used to detect hot spots in the body, especially in the breast, which can indicate malignant changes in tissue including angiogenesis, as well as inflammation. Thermal scans easily discriminate fibrocystic lumps, as they have no thermal signature. Hot areas can be found as much as 3 years before a cancer is diagnosable, making preventative care a reality.

Naturopathic Oncology

The Bales Scientific thermal image processor is a refinement which allows images to be taken in a room that is not cold, as required for earlier scanners. Not only is this more comfortable, but after a baseline image is taken, cold air may be blown onto the breast, provoking a sympathetic nervous system response to cold stress. Normal tissue will undergo vasoconstriction and show up as cooler, but areas of new blood vessel growth will not cool.

Our clinic has thermography done through www.medthermonline.com

BIOPSY

FINE NEEDLE ASPIRATION – is frequently employed, although the technique has a 5% failure rate. Ultrasound or computerized stereotactic (3D) guidance is sometimes used, mainly for non-palpable lesions. Needle biopsy techniques can create micro-metastases into sentinel lymph nodes, skewing the sense of risk the patient faces, and triggering more aggressive and damaging therapies.

CORE BIOPSY – A larger needle removes a string of tissue for pathological analysis.

EXCISIONAL BIOPSY – a more invasive procedure, but more reliable. Invasion of the tumour into the margins of the biopsy sample indicates it has not been completely removed, and indicates a more aggressive tumour type.

LYMPHATIC or VENOUS INVASION: LVI or invasion of vessels by tumour cells in a biopsy sample or surgical sample indicates the cancer has had the opportunity to metastasize, and so is an ominous finding. These cases need aggressive care and close monitoring for some years after treatment. The blood and lymph vessels in tumours are thin-walled and leaky. High vascularity activates endothelial cell production of fibrin and IL-6 creating coagulation and inflammation. This fosters growth and movement of cancer cells into the circulation, and often they will end up in the bone marrow. Micrometastases in the bone marrow are seen in a majority of breast cancer cases even years after presumably curative medical therapies. We know half of breast cancer cases have no spread into the lymph nodes, but half of these will still suffer a distant spread of their cancer. These vessels are their path out of the tumour area.

LYMPH NODE DISSECTION – samples the lymph nodes, such as those in the armpit, for cancer spreading from the lateral breast through the tail of the breast. Breast tumours of approximately 1 cm diameter can produce cancer cells able to live in the lymphatic nodes. Lymph node positive status indicates the spread of the cancer regionally in the body, which increases the risk the cancer, can form metastatic colonies in distant sites. Removing these cancerous lymph nodes reduces the risk of a local reoccurrence of the cancer in the nodes, but it does not reduce the risk of reoccurrence of the cancer in the breast or at distant metastatic sites. The latter are generally aggressive, treatment resistant, and often fatal. Unfortunately, local control achieved by lymph node dissection does not increase life expectancy. Lymph node dissection is not recommended for women over age 60 that do not have any signs of lymph node involvement by physical examination by a physician.

Lymph node involvement is not as ominous as distant metastases, and women who are node-positive frequently can live out a full lifespan. Node positive premenopausal women clearly benefit from chemotherapy. Node negative premenopausal women benefit less from chemotherapy.

Breast carcinoma cells in a lymph node are stimulated to grow – independent of anchorage – by stromal cells production of the major mitogens IGF-1 and EGF.

SENTINEL NODE BIOPSY – A more conservative approach to node status, it involves the injection of a blue dye or a radioactive tracer at the tumour, and removal of the first lymph node the dye or tracer drains to. This can eliminate "strip-mining" the whole lymphatic chain, which has a high incidence of lymphedema and other morbidity. Removing lymph nodes does not improve the length of time patient will survive.

MAMMASTATIN – mammastatin serum assay (MSA) is a screening blood test for breast cancer risk developed in 1998 at the University of Michigan. It has application similar to PSA testing for prostate cancer. Overall accuracy is about 85%. High levels of the protein marker would normally be followed with a mammogram and/or genetic screening.

GRADING and PROGNOSTIC INDICATORS

Scarff-Bloom-Richardson (SBR) classification – scores the mitotic rate, nuclear pleomorphism and tubule formation seen by microscope.

Grade I: 3 – 5 points = well differentiated
Grade II: 6 – 7 points = moderately differentiated
Grade III: 8 – 9 points = poorly differentiated.

Histological grade – rates the tissue on how much normal cellular architecture such as ductal structures are preserved.

Grade I: well differentiated – still behaving like breast cells
Grade II: moderately differentiated
Grade III: poorly differentiated – very disturbed growth pattern, often capable of colonizing in new places to create a successful metastasis.

STAGING

Staging may be based on the *TNM surgical rating* system (see page 23), or on the *clinical* staging system:

Stage 0 = intraductal cancer in situ. Mortality is only 3 to 10%.
Stage I = small tumour under 2 cm with no + nodes
Stage II = medium tumour 2 - 5 cm with + axillary lymph node
Stage IIIA = large tumour over 5 cm with palpable axillary node
Stage IIIB = tumour of any size with extension into the chest wall, skin or internal mammary lymphatic chain
Stage IV = distant metastases and invasion into the chest wall. The presence of distant disease gives a 70 to 85% probability the patient will die from the cancer.

OTHER PROGNOSTIC FACTORS

MENOPAUSAL STATUS: #1 prognostic factor, breast cancer occurring before menopause is exposed to more estrogen, and tends to be much more dangerous.

LYMPH NODE STATUS: #2 prognostic factor, +/ - for metastasis. Tumours in the medial breast spread into the thoracic and mediastinal lymph nodes, while from the lateral breast they spread into the axillary lymph chains. Negative lymph node patients have a 70% cure rate with surgery and radiation. Only 1 in 3 of those who will have a recurrence will be helped with subsequent chemotherapy. Women with positive lymph node status will have under 50% survival with surgery and radiation alone.

S-PHASE: cell cycle analysis, looks at the proportion of cells in S-phase where new DNA is being synthesized in preparation for the division of a tumour cell into two cells. Higher values mean the tumour is growing more rapidly. In breast cancer the S-phase count can range from 1 to 20%; values over 7% give a poorer prognosis.

ESTROGEN RECEPTOR STATUS: ER+ or ER- determines the tumour sensitivity to hormone therapy. ER+ has a better prognosis, as the cells are more normal. ER-/PR- tumours express more COX-2 mRNA. Note that even weak receptor staining indicates the clinical utility of hormone-directed therapies. Low-positive is 1 to 10% staining while some labs have a cut-off of 10%+ staining to qualify as positive. ERβ + with node + status indicates risk of more aggressive disease. ER- status is linked to higher risk of metastasis into the lungs, via disruption of endothelial contacts by TGFß up-regulation of angiopoietin-like protein four ANGPLP4. ERα + breast cancers derive IL-6 from fibroblasts to up-regulate STAT-3 acute phase protein, allowing invasion and spreads to lungs and especially to bones. ERα+ breast cancer often gives rise to stem-cell-like phenotypes in the bone marrow or disseminated elsewhere. These increase risk of reoccurrence, and often these are resistant to the therapies that controlled the primary cancer, because they are transformed into ERα-/ERβ+/HER-2+ or EGFR2+ cells. ER+ status doubles risk of bone mets relative to ER- tumours.

PROGESTERONE RECEPTOR STATUS: PR+ or PR-. PR+ may have a significantly better prognosis, as PR inhibits aromatase, Her2/neu and COX-2 expression. It is believed that ER-/PR+ represents a false negative ER result and that ER+/PR- represents a false positive ER result, because PR is a product of an intact estrogen-ER pathway, thus PR+ is only possible if ER is also expressed. These samples should be retested to confirm the result. ER-/PR+ cases have sometimes been prescribed progestins to reduce growth and metastases. ER+/PR- cases are relatively resistant to Tamoxifen. About 50% of PR- cases will express HER-2. Male breast cancers tend to be ER- /PR- and these are relatively treatment resistant.

HER-2/neu STATUS: HER-2 receptors, also called C-erb-B2 receptors, act for both epidermal and platelet-derived growth factors EGF and PDGF. These receptors are over-expressed in some breast comedo type ductal carcinoma in situ (DCIS), ovarian, lung, prostate, and stomach cancers. Associated with earlier relapses and poorer prognosis. HER-2 – breast cancers have a 5 year survival of 96%, but HER-2 + cancers have just a 68% 5- year survival, with 2.68 X increased risk of reoccurrence, and 5.5 X risk of distant reoccurrence. HER-2/neu + status is associated with activation, overexpression and mutation in the P13K / Akt / mTOR pathway. Since PTEN gene normally opposes activation of this pathway, this status implies a loss of functionality PTEN; quercetin should always be considered to control this growth signalling. HER-2+ with ER+/PR- is high risk for relapse with brain metastases. Treatment with targeted therapies such as Herceptin or trastuzumab is essential.

Relapsed breast cancers can have ER / PR / HER-2 status different from the primary tumour of origin.

TRIPLE NEGATIVE: Some African-Americans and Hispanics show up "Triple negative" or ER- / PR- / HER-2. These cancers appear similar to basal skin cancer. Assume BRAC-1 mutation is inactivating PTEN tumour suppressor gene. VEGF is highly over-expressed in these tumours. *Iressa* or Gefitinib is an EGFR tyrosine kinase inhibitor which blocks the over-expression of EGFR in these tumours. Also target YB-1, STAT-3, mTOR, PTKs. Y-box binding protein YB-1 is a transcription/translational factor associated with poor survival, as it protects cancer cells from apoptosis. A sample protocol would be green tea EGCG, indole-3-carbinol, curcumin, Co-enzyme Q-10, selenomethionine, and grapeseed extract OPCs.

TESTOSTERONE LEVEL: Women produce the male hormone testosterone, and related androgens, in the adrenal glands. The enzyme aromatase converts it into estrogen in fatty tissue and the bones. Levels over the medial value of 0.40 ng/ml of blood are associated with reduced survival time.

EPIDERMAL GROWTH FACTOR RECEPTOR STATUS: EGFR+ is associated with local spread and reduced survival time.

DNA PLOIDY: uses flow cytometry techniques to look for multiple sets of chromosomes representing cells in mitotic division, giving an average value for the amount of DNA in the tumour cells. Abnormal DNA content strongly correlates with the aggressiveness of the tumour. Aneuploidy corresponds to poorly differentiated tumours.

E-CADHERIN: high levels of E-cadherin predict risk of metastasis and reoccurrence.

TUMOUR MARKERS: CEA, CA-125, CA 15-3, CA 19-9, CA 549, CA M26, CA M29, CA 27.29, MCA, PSA, isoferritin, tissue polypeptide antigen (TPA), mammary tumour-associated glycoprotein, kappa casein.

CYCLINS: Cyclin D1 is often over expressed in breast cancer. Cyclin E in truncated isoforms in high amounts in tumours, as measured by the Western blot test, predicts high risk of reoccurrence and poorer survival. Australian doctors say over-expression of this regulator of the transition from G1 to S phase in the cell cycle is the most powerful predictor of breast cancer outcome.

SKIN LESIONS – breast cancer forming skin lesions are very high risk – relative risk is over fifteen times normal for systemic reoccurrence.

CIRCULATING TUMOUR CELLS – Over 5 CTCs per 7.5 ml. of blood gives a poor prognosis. If they carry CK-19 mRNA the survival time is further reduced. Even a count of 3 is worrisome. Control inflammation to prevent re-seeding the site of origin.

BREAST CANCER TYPES

DUCTAL CARCINOMA IN SITU (DCIS) – is the proliferation of cancer within the milk ducts without any invasion through the basement membrane. The cancer is unicentric within a segment, and is found in occult form in about 30% of females autopsied. On mammograms DCIS will typically show microcalcifications (spicules).

Pure ductal carcinoma in situ rarely metastasizes, so if the lesion is removed with the margins of the sample free of disease, sentinel node biopsy is optional. The most common form is non-comedo cribriform type.

Mastectomy results in only a 2% risk of local reoccurrence. Lumpectomy has up to 60% failure rate, with half of the recurrences being invasive carcinoma. Even low-grade DCIS with poor margins can gradually progress to invasive forms of breast cancer. Radiation may improve control after lumpectomy.

COMEDO type ductal carcinoma in situ (DCIS) tends to present with high nuclear grade (80% are aneuploid) and necrosis, ER-, and highly over-expressing HER/neu+. HER-2 receptors, also called C-erb-B2 receptors, act for both epidermal and platelet-derived growth factors EGF and PDGF. The comedo type is more aggressive, has a worse prognosis, and warrants prompt and aggressive treatment.

LOBULAR CARCINOMA IN SITU (LCIS) – is multicentric cancer within multiple breast lobules, which never produces a mass that can be detected by mammography. Risk of occurrence in the other breast is 10 to 25%. About 37% will develop invasive cancer in either breast, with risk increasing by about 1% per year. Risk triples with just 3 years use of hormone replacement therapy with estrogen and progestins. The standard approach is bilateral mastectomy with immediate reconstructive surgery, never chemo or radiation.

INFILTRATING DUCTAL CARCINOMA (IDC) – represents 75% of all breast tumours. More frequently metastatic to bone, lung and liver.

INFILTRATING LOBULAR CARCINOMA (ILC) – up to 10% of breast cancers are ILC, with a tendency to metastasize to the meninges causing carcinomatous meningitis, to the eyes, ovaries, retroperitoneum and serosal surfaces, causing intestinal or urethral obstruction.

TUBULAR CARCINOMA (TC) – About 2% of breast cancers, tend to be well differentiated, rarely metastasize to the axilla, and typically ER+ and PR+.

MEDULLARY CARCINOMA (MC) – About 6% of breast cancers, occurring at younger ages, often metastasizing locally, producing large axillary nodes, and typically ER+, PR-, p53+

INFLAMMATORY BREAST CANCER (IBC) – Accounts for 1% of breast cancers, and is the most aggressive type, with the poorest prognosis. Five year survival is only about 18%, though some aggressive new combination protocols claim about 40% 5-year disease-free survival. The skin on the breast becomes red and dimpled due to lymphatic blockade by tumour emboli– not from inflammation! Inflammatory breast cancer cells have increased RhoC GTPase, which activates NFkB and increases motility. There is florid invasion and metastasis, particularly lymphatic spread.

1 in 4 cases will have pain in the breast or nipple. There is rapid onset of symptoms,

90% probability of axillary lymph node involvement, progression to stage III-B, typically ER- and PR-, and up to 50% risk of contralateral breast cancer.

It could be triggered by a relative of the mouse mammary tumour virus, the MMTV-like virus. Inflammatory breast cancer cells have a stem-cell-like phenotype.

There is a prolific expression of HER-2, C-myc proto-oncogene, E-cadherin and angiogenesis.

MALE BREAST CANCER – Usually ER- /PR- and treatment resistant, but may respond to Tamoxifen and aromatase inhibitors.

SURGERY

Breast cancer survival is only about 12% without surgery. **The best hope of a cure of any cancer is surgery.**

I have known several brave souls who went without surgery, and some have survived many years in good health.

I do not recommend that course of action, despite the risk of persistent post-surgical pain and other complications. You need to learn the importance of timing your surgery, supporting recovery with nutrition and preventing reoccurrence and metastasis with supplements such as green tea EGCG and modified citrus pectin through the surgical period of care.

LUMPECTOMY – tumour removed with at least a 1 cm margin of healthy tissue.

QUADRANTECTOMY – tumour removed with a 3 cm margin plus the overlying skin and underlying fascia.

MODIFIED RADICAL MASTECTOMY – removal of the entire breast

RADICAL MASTECTOMY – removal of the breast and underlying muscle and associated tissues. Radical mastectomy is not associated with better long-term survival than less extensive surgery, and so has been largely abandoned. NSABP in Pittsburgh published 5 and 10 year follow-up results, and now 25 year follow-up shows the same result.

Mastectomy is generally contra-indicated if there are distant metastases. Removing the larger tumour can de-inhibit growth of smaller satellite metastases. How tumours maximize their access to nutrients while choking off their distant competitors is not known. Vigorous angiogenesis in the other tumours follows the removal of the primary tumour. This is why we prescribe anti-angiogenic **green tea EGCG** after surgery.

In premenopausal women it is critical to do the surgery during the luteal phase of the menstrual cycle. The high progesterone levels at this time lower the potent angiogenesis stimulator vascular endothelial growth factor VEGF, and are associated with much longer survival times. For example, serum progesterone at least 4 mcg/ml corresponded to 65% survival at 18 years post-surgery versus 35% for those with lower progesterone.

Angiogenin also cycles with the proliferative and the secretory phases of the menstrual cycle. It is very productive to give anti-angiogenics such as **green tea EGCG** post-surgery in pre-menopausal women. This can distinctly reduce risk of reoccurrence of the breast cancer in the peak of tumour dormancy escape typically seen at 8 to 10 months post-surgery.

For small cancers under 1 cm. the standard of care is lumpectomy followed by radiation, and if ER+ Tamoxifen may be considered. The radiation doubles the chances of avoiding a relapse (local radiation after lumpectomy or breast-conserving surgery for early stage primary breast cancer will decrease 20 year rates of recurrence of cancer in that breast to about 14%, compared to about 39% with the surgery alone, regardless of node status.

Breast surgery, node biopsies and radiation therapy can ablate and scar lymphatic drainage of the arm via the axilla, causing lymphedema.

OVARIAN ABLATION

Removal of the ovaries by surgery (oophorectomy), or their destruction by Lupron chemotherapy or radiation, removes estrogen stimulation and is associated with improved survival. Survival increases 6% in pre-menopausal and 3% in peri-menopausal ER+ breast cancers. Premenopausal women with highly ER positive (score over 20) tumours may benefit from ovarian ablation more than they can benefit from chemotherapy.

RADIATION

Radiotherapy after lumpectomy surgery for DCIS cuts risk of local reoccurrence by approximately one half, although with minimal impact on overall survival. About 3% will see a survival benefit at 5 years, and 6% at 10 years.

The most benefit is seen in cases with lymphatic and venous invasion LVI+. Also clearly benefits cases with tumours over 3 cm, node + disease, or ER-/PR-.

The least benefit is seen in cases over 70 years of age.

After mastectomy and chemotherapy, locoregional radiation increases overall survival about 10%.

50 Gy therapy in 25 fractions, plus a boost dose of 18 Gy will lower risk of reoccurrence about 50%, which is identical to endocrine therapies such as Tamoxifen, aromatase inhibitors and fulvestrant.

RADIO-FREQUENCY ABLATION

Radio-frequency ablation RFA uses the heating effect of radio waves to bring the lumpectomy cavity to 100° C for 15 minutes. This gives clean margins and replaces radiation therapy for some cases.

HORMONE BLOCKADE

In general, all growth signal controllers in breast cancer are analogues of estradiol or testosterone hormones. Hormone blockade will starve tumours of promoting factors but resistance commonly develops in 5 to 6 years.

General side-effects can include hot flashes, impotence, reduced libido, breast enlargement, accelerated bone loss & osteoporosis, muscle weakness, muscle wasting, liver damage, reduced night vision, nausea, diarrhea, alcohol intolerance. Patients also show increased rates of death from cardiovascular disease, stroke, and infection.

Hot flashes are a particularly significant problem for many on hormone therapy, especially when they interrupt sleep, or are of a drenching nature. We may prescribe grapeseed extract, evening primrose oil, homeopathic *Sepia*, Da Bu Yin Wan, Xiao Yao Wan, Xiao Chai Hu Tang; reduce caffeine and alcohol intake.

The effects on bone health are particularly acute, and require therapy. Poor calcium status and poor bone density increases risk of metastasis of breast cancer to the bones. Micrometastases into bone marrow are common and persistent. Hardening the bones will resist spread and even inhibit tumours already in the bones. I prescribe microcrystalline hydroxyapatite calcium with vitamin D3, vitamin C and magnesium citrate.

TAMOXIFEN

Tamoxifen is a selective estrogen receptor modulator SERM with estrogen antagonist and partial estrogen agonist effects.

Tamoxifen will typically reduce risk of re-occurrence of breast cancer by about one-third. It is commonly given for up to 5 years, at which point its benefits will persist for several years after it is discontinued.

It is widely used for any breast cancer with ER+ status, for those with spread into the lymph nodes and especially for post-menopausal women. It may also benefit ER-cases, but at 3 to 10 fold less benefit than ER+ cases.

It is not well indicated in pre-menopausal breast cancer. It is used for male breast cancers.

The estrogen receptor co-activator AIB-1 gene product amplifies estrogen and Tamoxifen's estrogen agonist effect. AIB-1 is in turn amplified by HER-2. It has been found that AIB-1 positive / HER-2 positive patients seem not to be helped by adjuvant tamoxifen, and in fact may be harmed by it. HER-1 and HER-2 are related to epidermal growth factor receptors as well as modulating estrogen receptors.

Tamoxifen also increases sex hormone binding globulins (SHBG), decreases IGF, and can reduce TGF alpha. Other benefits: increased bone mass, reduced risk of heart disease, and slightly reduced risk of contralateral breast cancer (the usual 8% occurrence is brought down to 5%).

However, the contralateral tumours that do occur tend to be ER- (27% with Tamoxifen vs. 4% without the drug) which are harder to treat. Side-effects include blood clots, hot flashes, vaginal dryness or discharge, irregular menses, toxicity to the eyes with visual impairment, depression, poor concentration, asthma, and increased risk of liver cancer. The risk of endometrial cancer is increased by 2 to 3 fold, and requires annual screening tests. Report any changes in your health to your physician and get annual eye and physical exams as a minimum.

Contraindications include macular degeneration or a history of thrombo-embolic disease.

Do not take Tamoxifen with birth control pills, anti-depressant drugs of the SSRI type, Hoxsey herbal formula, grapefruit, St. John's Wort, black cohosh root, red clover blossoms, tangeritin, or high-dose vitamin D therapy. It is not recommended to use tobacco products or alcohol while on Tamoxifen.

Tamoxifen combined with Goserlin is superior in safety and in reducing reoccurrence compared to standard chemotherapy drugs like cyclophosphamide, methotrexate and fluorouracil in stage I or II premenopausal hormone responsive breast cancer. These patients first have surgery to reduce the tumour burden.

Poor metabolism by CYP 2D6 reduces responses to Tamoxifen. Resistance to Tamoxifen therapy develops from ERα activation by phosphorylated receptor proteins made by p21-activated kinase Pak-1.Activation of SRC-3 – the A1B1 oncogene – can create resistance to Tamoxifen therapy.

Breast cancer cells can also become resistant to Tamoxifen by up-regulating nuclear and cytosolic estrogen receptors, which the drug cannot reach.

Tamoxifen effectiveness can be enhanced with adjuncts such as acetyl-L-carnitine, melatonin, Coenzyme Q-10, quercetin, indole-3-carbinol and vitamin A. Soy is highly synergistic with Tamoxifen – high soy food intake adds a 60% reduction in risk of a reoccurrence of cancer – but only use soy if pre-menopausal.

Other hormone blocker drugs include Lupron and Zoladex, analogues of luteinizing hormone releasing hormone (LHRH). These have significant risks of thrombo-embolism and pulmonary embolism. LHRH agonists can cause a flare reaction as hormones spike up, then fall. This aggravation can be spared by taking an anti-androgen for one week prior to this therapy. Soy isoflavones may ameliorate many of the adverse effects of these drugs, such as bone loss.

Megace is synthetic progestin, antagonistic to estrogen. Mainly used in ER-/PR+ cases.

Casodex and Eulixen are anti-androgens.

Fulvestrant is an anti-estrogen, completely free of agonist activity. When breast cancer progresses despite Tamoxifen and aromatase inhibitors, this second-line drug will stabilize the disease and provide partial responses. Side effects can include fatigue, nausea and vomiting, chills, constipation, hot flashes and stomatitis. Tamoxifen and fulvestrant can increase invasiveness of ER+ cancers if they are deficient in E-cadherin intercellular adhesion.

AROMATASE INHIBITORS

Aromatase inhibitors block the enzyme *estrogen synthetase* which converts the androgen or masculine hormones into estrogens or female hormones. This enzyme is found in the liver, fatty tissue, muscle, skin, breast and breast tumours. Adrostenedione is converted into estrone, and testosterone is converted into estradiol. Estrone estrogen is moderately growth stimulating, but estradiol is the most potent form of estrogen for promoting breast cancer cell growth. Men have this enzyme to make estrogen from testosterone in their bones.

288

<u>Aromatase inhibitors are not effective in pre-menopausal women</u>, as they cannot overcome other hormone sources such as the ovaries. To qualify, the patient must be at least 12 months since the last menstrual period, and have estradiol in the post-menopausal range < 59 pg/ml.

AI's are effective for post-menopausal breast cancer, reducing circulating estrogen about 80-95%. AI's are now approved as first-line therapy in post-menopausal ER+ metastatic breast cancer. They can achieve a 40% reduction in metastases, 43-50% reduction in local reoccurrences, and an 18% reduction in deaths from breast cancer.

The third generation oral aromatase inhibitors include the reversible nonsteroidal agents Anastrozole and Letrozole, and the irreversible steroidal inhibitor Exemestane. They are becoming popular for patients with ER+ tamoxifen-refractory metastatic breast cancer.

Time to disease progression is similar to tamoxifen therapy, and so is overall survival, but AIs cut breast cancer reoccurrence about 3% more that does Tamoxifen. Menopausal symptoms occur, but are less severe than with tamoxifen, other than increased bone loss. There is also a significant reduction in the incidence of contralateral breast cancer, and a small reduction in distant metastases and endometrial cancer.

Aromatase inhibitors may be used in ER+ early stage postmenopausal breast cancer, especially in those intolerant of Tamoxifen, or concerned about thromboembolic risk.

96% of those prescribed AI's report some reactions.

Steroidal type AI's such as Exemestane promote less bone loss, and inhibit late bone reoccurrences in the bones, but do not inhibit early reoccurrences as well as the non-steroidal AI drugs. Exemestane is atherogenic, raising the LDL/HDL cholesterol ration and ApoB/ApoA lipoprotein ratios. This translates to a 1% increased risk of severe cardiac events. Letrozole or *Femara* is an aromatase inhibitor capable of reducing estrogen and estrone twice as much as Anastazole. When Letrozole fails, about 15% of cases can be rescued by the related drug Exemastane or *Aromasin*. Letrozole increases triglycerides in the blood, but Anastrozole has little impact on blood lipids.

Joint pains and stiffness can occur from AI's, particularly if the patient has been on Taxane chemotherapy prior to use. About 20-30% of women will get joint pain, carpal tunnel syndrome or tendon and synovium effusions, and about 5% quit the therapy because of pain. Omega 3 oils, vitamin D3 (50,000 IU/month), devil's claw root extract and melatonin can be quite helpful in these cases. Consider *Ruta graveolens* and vitamin B6 therapy for tendon and synovium effusions, and homeopathic remedies such as *Bryonia alba,* and *Rhus toxicodendron.* Exercise definitely helps too. Arthralgias tend to ease up after about 6 months of intake.

Other possible side effects are limb swelling, anxiety, flu-like symptoms, cough, vaginal dryness, vaginal atrophy, generalized pain, acute hepatitis, chest pain, and stroke.

About 70% of breast cancer cells produce aromatase, and levels directly correspond to COX-2 expression.

COX-2 creates prostaglandins, which promote the expression of the aromatase gene CYP19. COX-2 inhibitors may well produce a nice synergy with quercetin. My clinical experience with such combinations has been positive.

Paradoxically, if resistance to these drugs develops, a brief prescription of estradiol will induce apoptosis via increased bcl-2 proteins. Once the tumour/s shrink a bit, anti-hormone therapy can be resumed.

Quercetin, reishi, resveratrol, grapeseed procyanidin B dimers, flaxseed, zinc, passion flower chrysin, soy genestein, natural progesterone, melatonin and white button mushrooms *Agaricus bisporus* are natural aromatase inhibitors.

Quercetin and grapeseed extract procyanidin dimers appear to be the strongest natural AI's. Grapeseed is able to reduce estrogens by about 80%, equivalent to early AI drugs.

Indole-3-carbinol supports AIs in preventing relapse of hormone-sensitive breast cancer.

Non-steroidal AI's such as Letrozole or Anastrozole markedly effect bone loss in the first 6 months of therapy. This translates to a 1 – 2% increased risk for osteoporosis. AI's significantly degrade bone health – so it is mandatory to support bone density, mass and strength. For example Irimidex increases risk of fracture 40% in 5 years use, reducing bone mineral density 5 to 7%, enough to push an osteopenic patient into frank osteoporosis. It is now a standard to prescribe bisphosphonate drugs such as Clodronate, Pamidronate and Fossamax to maintain bone mineral density.

Naturopathic medicines can outperform these bone protectant drugs, and can be combined with them for the best results. Microcrystalline hydroxyapatite ossein complex is a bone meal product with actual bone growth factors which build bone density and mass far faster than bisphosphonates, increasing new bone, not just reducing bone loss. This means increased strength, therefore better protection from fractures. Vitamin D3 or 25(OH)D is also useful to build bone, although we do not want to give high doses, as it is a potent stimulator of the P-450 gene responsible for metabolizing aromatase drugs. Since you are asked to take calcium and D with these drugs, choose MCHA calcium complex with a modest dose of D3. I add vitamin C to the mix for bone building and bone strength, and magnesium citrate.

[Strontium is a mineral which definitely reduces fractures, but it is taken well away from calcium supplements as they compete for absorption. There is about a 30% increased risk of stroke in women taking strontium supplements. NOT RECOMMENDED]

Exercise is an essential requirement for bone health.

TESTOSTERONE

Testosterone drives libido in men and women. Women who lose their sex drive -both interest and arousal, during anti-estrogen therapy, can ask for a testosterone patch or cream. The patch usually delivers 300 mcg daily. 50% of women get reactions at the site of application, 20% get unwanted hair growth, about 8% get acne, balding and deepening of the voice. 50% will drop out of this therapy in the first year, despite more satisfying sexual events. There is a potential increased risk of cardiac events, due to alterations in lipoprotein metabolism. Some experts believe it increases risk of breast cancer.

HERCEPTIN

Herceptin or trastuzumab is a humanized anti-HER-2 monoclonal antibody which binds to trans-membrane growth factor receptors. These receptors bind to EGF and PDGF and activate tyrosine kinase activity inside the cells.

Herceptin also inactivates breast cancer stem cells.

Herceptin is effective against HER-2 / neu positive breast cancer.

Unfortunately, it creates significant heart damage and a risk of heart failure. Before it will be given the doctors will do a MUGA scan to determine your ejection fraction EF. The EF is the percentage of the blood inside the heart chambers which can be pushed out with a single beat of the heart. EF is normally over 60%, and Herceptin will typically not be given if you start at an ejection fraction under 55%. During treatment, if the EF falls below 50% the treatment may be suspended.

Naturopathic physicians can improve heart function rapidly and safely to qualify patients for this therapy, keep them in it long enough to be curative, and to repair the damage afterwards. We use herbs such as *Convallaria majus* and *Crataegus oxyacantha*, homeopathic remedies such as *Naja tripudians* and nutraceuticals such as Coenzyme Q-10 and vitamin E. Please, do not enter into Herceptin therapy unprotected!

CHEMOTHERAPY IN BREAST CANCER

Chemotherapy or Chemo uses toxic drugs to kill rapidly-dividing cells. This takes out cancer cells, but also strongly damages the lining of the gut, bone marrow, hair follicles and other healthy tissues. Most do not kill cancer cells better than healthy cells, and in fact some do far more harm to the healthy tissues. They are very indiscriminate toxins. Use of chemo is a serious life-and-death choice, so do your homework.

Every therapy "casts a shadow" – there are risks from treatment and risks with no treatment. I recommend reading Dr. Ralph Moss's book "*Questioning Chemotherapy*" for an objective review of the issues.

Chemotherapy is NOT justified for patients who are node negative and also have:
- tumours 1 cm or smaller
- tumours 1 to 2 cm with favourable indicators like ER+ status and a good histological grade.
- tumours with a low fatality rate such as tubular, colloid, mucinous or papillary forms
- only 3% of those treated will have a survival advantage

Chemotherapy gives a survival advantage to about 7% of node-positive women treated. It is only fair to note that chemotherapy does often give a significant disease-free remission or other positive response.

Naturopathic Oncology

Examples of common protocols :

- CMF – cytoxan, methotrexate and 5-fluorouracil
- FAC or CAF– cyclophosphamide orally for 14 days, adriamycin and 5-FU intravenously on days 1 and 8
- CEF or FEC– cyclophosphamide orally 14 days, epirubicin and 5-fluorouracil IV days 1 and 8
- EC- cyclophosphamide and epirubicin
- CMF – cyclophosphamide, methotrexate and 5-fluorouracil.
- TAC – docetaxel, adriamycin and cyclophosphamide
- AC – adriamycin and cytoxan/cyclophosphamide
- BRAJACTT – Adriamycin and cyclophosphamide AC every 3 weeks for 4 cycles,
  - followed by Taxol and Herceptin every 3 weeks for 4 cycles
  - followed by Herceptin every 3 weeks, for up to 13 cycles, depending on cardiac tolerance.
  - followed by adjuvant radiation
  - followed by long-term Tamoxifen hormone therapy.

High dose taxanes, bone marrow autologous transplantation and extended courses of high-dose chemotherapy have not yielded improved survival. It is best to use combinations of drugs to reduce toxicities, and not space the treatments out – a "dose-dense" approach is preferred. This is where naturopathic physicians in oncology can really help. We can often keep up the patient's health to tolerate the full dose full-course therapy. I also often find my role is to make patients medically fit enough to qualify for chemotherapy or surgery. Of course, we are there to restore health and reinforce remissions after the medical therapies are finished.

Multi-drug resistance to chemo depends on the status of the multi-drug transporter MDR-1. Its expression is induced by p13 kinase, which in turn is mediated by the pericellular polysaccharide hyaluronan. This matrix compound also interacts with Erb-B2 and cell adhesion molecule CD-44. Reishi mushroom hot water extracts overcome chemo-resistance, inhibiting NFkB, increasing apoptosis.

ZOLEDRONIC ACID

Zometa or zoledronic acid is a bisphosphonate bone-building drug which has been found to synergize with chemotherapy drugs for breast cancer. It serendipitously increases expression of genes and proteins involved in apoptosis and cell-cycle regulation.

PHYTOESTROGENS

Phytoestrogens are plant compounds which mimic estrogen. They are analogous to estriols, the weakest of the human forms of estrogen, and are never as powerful growth stimulants as estradiol, the strongest ovarian estrogen.

It is critically important to recognize that many phytoestrogens actually block up the estrogen receptors and prevent real estrogen from getting in there and making a growth signal. Therefore many plant estrogens actually stop breast cancer cell proliferation, and are valuable therapies. The tendency of oncologists and their pharmacists to lump all phytoestrogens together shows a complete ignorance of the biochemistry of plants and foods and their medical application.

The critical factor is the <u>relative binding affinity</u> or RBA of the estrogen.

- Estradiol is 100%, by definition.
- Tamoxifen has a RBA of 80%.
- Many plant estrogens have a RBA hundreds, even thousands of times weaker. The shape, size and electrical charge on these weak estrogens is not sufficient for the receptor to close around them. Unless it can bind and alter the receptor shape, it can't trigger a growth signal to the nucleus of the cell.

An excellent example is flaxseed. It is shown to be as effective as Tamoxifen in reducing breast cancer reoccurrence, yet many oncologists and the BC Cancer Agency pharmacists discourage its use and make women with ER+ tumours terrified to take it. Similarly, the weight of quality scientific evidence supports ER+ women taking soy foods, but this is still discouraged by doctors untrained in nutritional medicine.

Soy is fine with pre-menopausal ER+ breast cancer, but moderation is advised if it is ER- post-menopausal cancer, and soy food intake should be minimal in ER+ post-menopausal cases. Some colleagues say soy is highly synergistic with Tamoxifen – high intake adds a 60% reduction in risk of a reoccurrence of cancer.

Apigenin flavone from celery is anti-angiogenic and inhibits nuclear factor kappa B – NFkB.

A diet rich in plant foods provides a balance of phyto-estrogens and botanical hormone regulators.

INTEGRATIVE REMEDIES FOR BREAST CANCER

Targets of therapy: Estrogen and its receptors, aromatase, insulin, insulin-like growth factor IGF-1, NFkB, COX-2, EGFR, DNA hypermethylation, microsatellite instability, angiogenesis, P13K/Akt, YB-1, STAT-3, IL-6, TNF, Survivin, SRC-3.

ACUPUNCTURE –
- Open the breast channels: LU-1, CV-17, ST-18
- Purge stagnation: LU-9, PC-7, HT-7
- Purge toxic chi: ST-36, GB-34, LV-3

- Subdue rebellious chi & return it to its origin: PC-6, CV-3
- Tonify: LU-7, SP-4, KI-6

Acupuncture produces durable results that can outperform drugs for hot flashes, libido, energy and well-being.

ANTI-MASTOPLASIA – TCM herb formula for early stage breast disease.

ARTEMESININ – extract of wormwood uses cellular iron to create endo-peroxides inside cancer cells. It can have side-effects. Use under medical supervision.

BROMELAIN – a protein-digesting enzyme from pineapple stems that destroys fibrin, which controls inflammation, and thus growth and angiogenesis. It also modulates CD-44 cell adhesion molecule, which controls metastasis and progression.

CAN-ARREST – anti-inflammatory formula with boswellia, bromelain, curcumin and quercetin. This is a major weapon against breast cancer. BCQ is the American version of CanArrest formula.

*CO-ENZYME Q-10 – Ubiquinone supports the mitochondria in regulating apoptosis. Human trials are limited, but early indications are very encouraging. The minimum therapeutic dose is 300 mg daily.

*CURCUMIN – from turmeric root is a major repressor of inflammation and growth factors. It must have either bromelain or bioperine from black pepper as an adjunct to allow enough to be absorbed to give a significant response.

DIET – A low-fat diet particularly benefits estrogen receptor negative ER- cases. High intake of monosaturates such as olive oil and polyunsaturated fats primarily affects post-menopausal cancer cases. The breast is mainly fatty tissue, and will accumulate fat-soluble toxins such as xenobiotic pesticides and other hormone-disrupting or hormone mimicking toxins. A good rate of turn-over of healthy fats can support better health, but remember fats need anti-oxidant support or they can turn on you. A balance of omega 3 to omega 6 fats is vital to regulate inflammation and its growth factors. Folic acid from green leafy vegetables is protective. Coloured fruits and vegetables provide antioxidant mixed natural carotenoids. One valuable example is lycopene from stewed tomatoes. Fish provide needed omega 3 oils. Rice provides melatonin. Rosemary is a delightful spice which harmonizes hormones.

ELLAGIC ACID – as found in pomegranates, grapes, and all berries. Anti-angiogenic and more.

EXERCISE – improves outcomes by a variety of mechanisms.

*FLAXSEED LIGNANS – 2 tablespoons ground flaxseed daily has been shown to reduce the rate of growth of breast tumours, and is significantly effective at preventing the spread of breast cancer. It reduces invasiveness and spread into the lymph nodes. Flaxseed binds estrogen in the bowel, preventing re-uptake, and stimulates production of sex hormone binding globulins SHBGs, removing hormones from the bloodstream. Flaxseed works best with a low fat diet high in other lignan fibre from fruit, berries, vegetables, legumes, and whole grains.

GAMMA LINOLENIC ACID GLA – 2.8 grams or 8 capsules of evening primrose oil EPO daily gives a faster clinical response to Tamoxifen. It is synergistic with Paclitaxel. GLA produces anti-inflammatory prostaglandins, and inhibits the pro-inflammatory PGE-2. It decreases ornithine carboxylase activity in breast tumours, and reduces estrogen receptor expression.

*GRAPESEED EXTRACT – the oligomeric proanthocyanidins OPCs in grapeseed extract have a profound effect on breast cancer, as a cytoxic, aromatase inhibitor, and antiangiogenic. Similar anthocyanidins are found in red or purple grapes, pomegranate, bilberry, raspberry, cranberry, blackberry and blueberry.

*GREEN TEA EGCG – green tea epi-gallo catechin gallate EGCG polyphenols induce apoptosis in breast cancer cells. EGCG inhibits urokinase and matrix metallo-proteinase enzyme MMP-2, enzymes involved in tumour invasion and metastasis. Urokinase regulation inhibits insulin-like growth factor and reduces 17-beta estradiol. EGCG inhibits angiogenesis by decreasing VEGF. It is a mild anti-oxidant, and in higher doses is pro-oxidant. Give with vitamin E to prevent liver and kidney oxidative stress.

HOXSEY – herbal tonic can cure some cases. It far outshines Essiac. I like to mix the Hoxsey as a tincture with low potency homeopathics such as *Asteris*, *Conium* or *Phytolacca* 6C to 30C.

*INDOLES – indole-3-carbinol I3C, from the cabbage family of vegetables, converts 16-hydroxyestrogens to 2-hydroxy forms. 16-OH-estrone is highly estrogenic and initiates carcinogenic DNA damage. It is associated with obesity. The safer 2-OH forms of estrone and estradiol are increased by aerobic exercise, green tea, licorice root, and the entire cabbage family of vegetables. It is interesting to note that the famous physician Galen prescribed cabbage leaf poultices for breast cancer 2,000 years ago. I3C is anti-estrogenic, negatively modulates estrogen receptor transcription, and suppresses breast cancer invasion and migration. Use in triple-negative and HER-2/neu+ cancers as well as ER+. Regulates Survivin, Akt, NFkB, uPA, MMP-9, VEGF, ERα, and BRAC-1. I3C is activated in the stomach primarily to diindolylmethane DIM.

JINGLI NEIXAO – is a tremendous TCM formula for advanced disease and the seriously ill patient.

MCHA CALCIUM– Microcrystalline hydroxyapatite ossein calcium complex with vitamin C, vitamin. D3, and magnesium citrate is essential to preserve and even increase bone mass in all patients. Breast cancer therapies and menopause mean higher risk of brittle bones. Microcrystalline hydroxyapatite MCHA calcium will rapidly harden the bones. It has bone growth factors which lay strong new bone in where it is needed, as well as preserving old bone. It increases bone density, bone mass and bone strength by building the flexible protein scaffolding to which the brittle minerals attach. This will reduce risk of metastases to the bones from breast tumours. If bone mets have already occurred, this calcium can reduce or arrest the spread of cancer within bone, and generally reduces bone pain rapidly and significantly. MCHA calcium with vitamin D3 is essential to protect your bones and arrest bone cancer, even if your medical doctor has prescribed a bisphosphonate drug for your bones, such as Fossamax, Pamidronate, or Didrocal. It is best to integrate both into your treatment plan.

*MELATONIN – is highly synergistic with Tamoxifen, at doses of 10 to 20 mg at bedtime. Melatonin down-regulates estrogen receptors, reduces circulating estrogen and prolactin, suppresses tumour fatty acid uptake, and blocks estrogen and epidermal growth factors. Doses prescribed may range from 3 to 20 mg; usually I will prescribe 12mg, to be taken at bedtime only.

*MILK THISTLE – Silibinin from milk thistle extract inhibits or modulates epidermal growth factor EGF, active in all carcinomas. Regulating EGF may be useful in modulating related estrogen receptors. This wonderful herb protects and detoxifies the liver.

MISTLETOE – Injectable mistletoe is a fabulous remedy at all stages of cancer, and for support of chemo and radiation. Iscador or Helixor type M is used for pre-menopausal breast cancer, and type P is suggested for post-menopausal breast cancers.

MODIFIED CITRUS PECTIN – fractionated citrus pectins of about 10 Kilo-Daltons molecular weight can arrest metastasis, retard growth and slow angiogenesis.

OMEGA 3 OILS – flaxseed and other omega 3 oils, such as fish, marine and walnut oils, reduce rates of metastasis. These also thin the blood, and must be used with caution around surgery or with blood thinning medications. Evening primrose oil gamma linolenic acid GLA is a hormone modulator.

PING XIAO PIAN – also called Can-Z, it is a classic anti-tumour TCM formula.

PLANT STEROLS & STEROLINS – decrease 17- beta estradiol E-2 signalling. However they also increase DHEA and can rarely cause pancytopenias.

POMEGRANATE – Pomegranate flavonoids inhibit aromatase, preventing synthesis of estrogen from adrostenedione and testosterone. They also strongly inhibit 17-estradiol growth signalling in breast cancer cells.

*QUERCETIN – this bioflavonoid is an aromatase inhibitor, reducing estrogen production from testosterone in fat cells. Use with bromelain for better absorption. Consider adding COX-2 inhibitors.

*REISHI – Ganoderma mushroom hot water extract suppresses transcription factors and reduces invasiveness. It very significantly reduces nuclear factor kappa-B NFkB, which markedly increases apoptosis. Reishi extract reduces invasiveness of tumours, and inhibits DNA transcription factors. Reishi can overcome chemo-resistance in old cancers. Related mushrooms include maitake and coriolus.

*RESVERATROL – a MMP inhibitor, anti-angiogenic, NFkB inhibitor, COX-2 inhibitor, EGFR inhibitor, etc.

SOY FOODS – This is highly controversial, but highly protective diets yield about 150 mg daily of soy isoflavones. Compounds such as **genestein** and daidzein in soy are anti-angiogenic, antioxidant, induce cell differentiation, decrease luteinizing hormone LH and follicle stimulating hormone FSH. Dietary phytoestrogens can be anti-estrogenic, competing with estradiol for the type II estrogen binding sites. Phytoestrogens usually have a relative binding affinity to the estrogen receptor under 0.1% of the receptor binding strength of estradiol. 60 grams of soy foods can yield 45 mg of isoflavones, which could match the effects of Tamoxifen. <u>Best used in pre-menopausal ER+ breast cancer. Best avoided in post-menopausal cases</u>

VITAMIN A – as found in vegetables. A natural regulator of cell growth. Supplement as retinol palmitate.

VITAMIN B6 – pyridoxine 150 mg daily reduces prolactin levels. The ideal form is pyridoxal-5-phosphate.

VITAMIN D3 – 1, 25-dihydroxy D3, a fat-soluble vitamin activated by the kidneys and sunlight on the skin, inhibits IGF-signalling and associated growth stimulation of breast cancer cells, promotes apoptosis, and may have anti-estrogenic activity.D3 is especially important in estrogen receptor negative ER- breast cancer, because it regulates growth and apoptosis mechanisms which are not estrogen-dependent, such as the AR gene erbB and epidermal growth factor. <u>D</u> induces <u>D</u>ifferentiation. Good intake of vitamin D and calcium reduces risk of aggressive premenopausal breast cancer. Vitamin D binding protein derived macrophage activating factor strongly activates macrophages to destroy tumours. Compared to normal levels, low vitamin D status is associated with poorer outcomes, including 94% increased chance of metastases, and 73% increased chance of dying! A recent survey showed 76% of Canadian women with breast cancer were deficient in vitamin D.

VITAMIN E – antioxidant for fatty tissue, regulates hormones, heals damaged tissue. The injectable vitamin E succinate VES form is the most potent and the most researched, but we just use oral mixed tocopherols.

VITEX – *Vitex agnes castus* or chaste tree berry lowers prolactin PL levels, increases progesterone, decreases estrogen, lowers follicle-stimulating hormone FSH and raises luteinizing hormone LH.

ZINC – to regulate angiogenesis and growth. Found in all in raw fruits and vegetables

Avoid in Breast Cancer

DHEA – Dihydro- epiandrosterone or DHEA supplements boost IGF-1 and sex hormones. IGF-1 production in the liver is increased by DHEA and also its biological activity rises due to induced changes in IGF-binding proteins. Ashwagandha herb significantly elevates DHEA. Maca root can increase DHEA. Sterols and sterolins can increase DHEA levels and reduce cortisol levels.

EMOTIONAL HEALTH

Constrained liver chi is the start of a causal chain which leads to all tumours and lumps. Its cause is often in the emotions, such as frustration, resentment, anger –

especially when these are repressed and internalized.

Learning to express what you really feel is a key to true health. I have seen advanced cancer cured by forgiveness and loving resolution of conflicts, both external and internal.

You have a tremendous pharmacy between your ears you can use through faith, spirituality, psychology, and just plain fun. The stress arousal system regulates or secretes estrogen, progesterone, testosterone, androgens, prolactin, insulin, insulin-like growth factor, vitamin D which all have receptors on breast cancer cells. The stress arousal system also releases cortisol and other regulators of the psychoneuro-immunological system, the mind-body connection to immune regulation of breast cancer. We know that immune cells have receptors for all the brain chemicals (neurotransmitters) associated with every emotional state possible. This must have a purpose. In fact the ability of immune cells to function is linked to the balance of "mood" chemicals bound to them. Furthermore, the stress arousal chemical adrenaline (epinephrine) directly impairs the apoptosis "off-switch" in cancer cells.

Lawrence LeShan has had tremendous success with advanced cancer using positive psychology. Rather than looking for psychological defects and trying to fix them, he advocates restoration of emotional and creative expression. He finds cancer victims often have lost a main emotional focus in their lives, and have lost hope of finding any satisfactory substitute. He has cured cases by helping them design a re-vitalized life providing meaning, enthusiasm, zest and fulfillment.

The Emotional Freedom technique developed by Gary Flint is a useful tool one can learn to move through emotional traps and fixations.

A weekly support group and self-hypnosis for pain was associated with doubling of life-span in advanced stage IV breast cancer, ovarian cancer and melanoma. This work by Spiegel from 1989 has not been confirmed in subsequent studies, but certainly quality of life improves, if survival does not.

Particularly vulnerable are patients who lack a significant social support network. Patients who report a poor level of social well-being show higher pre-surgical levels of the angiogenesis cytokine VEGF.

Social roles are majorly impacted by cancer and cancer treatment related symptoms such as fatigue, hair loss, disfigurement, and sexual dysfunction. Gender-roles, family ranking, and household duties are altered, and financial stress adds to the burden. There are worries about reoccurrence, anxiety about becoming a burden to loved ones, and nameless fears.

LYMPHEDEMA

Lymphedema is a swelling caused by obstruction or loss of the lymphatic drainage. There is about 15 litres of lymph in the human body, about 3 times the volume of blood in circulation. It leaks out of cells and percolates in very diffuse networks, eventually collecting in simple ducts and channels that direct it to flow through lymph nodes. The nodes contain immune cells which scan for damaged cells, bacteria, viruses, and clean up a lot of the wastes. Eventually it all re-enters the bloodstream at the thoracic duct, in the upper chest.

Lymph channels anywhere can be blocked by tumours, as well as by cutting or post-surgical and post-radiation scarring. Lymphedema is an accumulation of fluid and protein. This protein acts as a colloid or gel matrix, holding fluid by osmosis.

Lymphedema is most common in an arm after mastectomy, surgery to remove a cancerous breast, and particularly if the lymph nodes of the armpit have been disturbed. There are about 24 lymph nodes in an average woman's armpit (axilla), and removing more than a couple can severely disrupt the flow of lymph. Even removal of a sentinel lymph node carries a 3% risk of lymphedema. Onset can be quite gradual and delayed.

Radiation often seals the deal, with up to 34% of cases experiencing lymphedema. Onset may be delayed by years.

Symptoms include arm or adjacent trunk swelling, a feeling of tightness or heaviness, aching pain, tenderness and loss of mobility. Look for Stemmer's sign – difficulty lifting the skin at the dorsum of the digits of the hands or feet. Swelling beyond a 10% increase in limb girth confirms the diagnosis.

Lymphedema is also associated with skin changes such as fibrosis, hyperkeratosis, cysts, fistulas and papillomas.

Even small injuries can precipitate inflammation (lymphangitis) and infection (cellulitis). Scrupulous skin and nail care is important.

The limb can completely lose functionality in advanced cases. Severe cases are treated with lymph-venous anastamosis micro-surgery.

Strong Xiao Xin Tan capsules are a TCM herb formula which moves the lymph. Rx 1 to 2 capsules twice daily.

A Juzo compression sleeve can help, as can pneumatic pumps or manual drainage massage. Registered massage therapists with advanced training in lymphology should be treating all cases. Self-wrapping with a compression bandage at bedtime is also helpful. Compression garments need to be replaced every six months to remain effective.

Physiotherapists may offer low-level laser therapy.

Naturopathic physicians may utilize German complex homeopathics such as *Lymphomyosot* from Heel and botanical/homeopathics such as *Lymphdiaral* from Pascoe Pharmacies. Fresh *Ceanothus spp.* "red root" removes waste from the lymphatic system. ***Gingko biloba*** extract and selenomethionine are also thought to help.

American-trained naturopathic physicians use high dose protease (protein dissolving) and lipase (fat dissolving) enzymes.

Exercise is critical to move lymph. The contraction and expansion of moving muscle pumps the lymph vessels, which have no elastic or pumping action of their own. Resistive exercise does not appear to be harmful. Nordic style pole-walking is recommended.

The best therapy I know is the beautiful marigold flower, ***Calendula officinalis***. Ferlow Brothers makes a fine organic cream to rub into congested and painful areas. Calendula makes a very pleasant tea as well, for oral intake or topical use as a poultice. It can also be taken orally as a tincture – an alcohol-water extract. Support this with at least 400 mg daily of **grapeseed extract OPCs**.

VAGINAL DRYNESS

Vaginal dryness can cause dyspareunia – pain on intercourse, and even painful cracking of labial tissues from friction by clothing. Med Oncs prescribe *Replens,* a patented lubricant provided in pre-filled applicators. Each packet is good for about 3 days, and is not estrogenic. NDs may prescribe EPA rich marine oils orally to increase production of natural lubrication.

HOT FLASHES

Hot flashes are often increased by hormone manipulations, and we are usually reluctant to use phyto-estrogenic plant medicines. Grapeseed extract OPCs can be helpful at 200 mg twice daily. Acupuncture can be very useful – for example the acupoint LV-2. Acupuncture also helps libido, mental clarity, and general balance.
A professor of naturopathic oncology tells me Maca root decreases hot flashes and increases libido, without any measureable effect on sex hormones. It is a potato-like tuber from South America.

Chapter Eleven – Integrative Care Of Prostate Cancer

EPIDEMIOLOGY

Prostate cancer is very common in developed countries. In the United States, one man in six will develop invasive prostate cancer in his lifetime. 1 in 4 African-Americans will develop prostate cancer, a rate of 137 per 100,000 in the general population. In Europe and South America the rate of incidence is 20 to 50 per 100,000. In China the rate is only 2.3 per 100,000. The 5-year survival rate is almost 99%. Clearly this is typically a slow moving cancer, but it tends to become very aggressive about 15 years into its course. It spreads into the seminal vesicles, lymphatics, liver and bones. Once it gets loose, it is as dangerous as any cancer. Survival statistics are looking better in the last several years, primarily due to earlier detection. At least half of those treated with curative intent will have their disease progress. Eighty percent live over 5 years, 61% live over 10 years and 49% live over 15 years from time of diagnosis.

KEY RISK FACTORS:
- high fat diet, especially saturated fats.
- trans-fats as found in hydrogenated margarine and shortening promote the formation of catechol estrogen-3,4-quinone from estradiol and estrone, and this destroys DNA purine bases.
- red meat, processed meats and organ meats. Blood from vegetarians actually inhibits prostate cancer cells.
- high sugar and glycemic load, such as refined grains and soft drinks Insulin-like growth factor one IGF-1 is a major growth factor for prostate cancer.
- low intake of antioxidants, vitamins C, A, E, selenium and zinc.
- being married – presumably from being over fed.
- xenobiotics such as pesticides, herbicides and fertilizers.
- estrogens promote inflammation in the prostate, increasing cellular proliferation.
- heavy metals such as cadmium
- smoking tobacco
- shift work – perhaps through altered melatonin cycling.
- family history of prostate cancer
- inflammation – elevated prostaglandin PGE-2 is strongly associated with prostate cancer. COX-1 and COX-2 create PGE2, which induces aromatase.
- mutation on gene HPC1 which codes for an antiviral protein allows chronic inflammation from a virus XMRV (causes leukemia in mice).
- cancer gene bcl-2 is active in maintaining prostate cancers.
- gene bcl-6 also plays a role in prostate cancer.
- BRAC-2 gene carriers have 2.5 times increased risk.

- serum HER-2 / neu is linked to progression, metastasis and resistance to hormone blockade. This is associated with PTEN loss and thus activation of the P13K / Akt / mTOR pathway.
- LDL hypercholesterolemia
- exposure to estrogen. Estrogen receptors (ER) in prostate tissue control expression of the telomerase gene hTERT. Increased telomerase activity marks the early stages of prostate cancer. Telomerase mRNA increases 2 to 3 fold with induction of estrogen receptors alpha & beta, up-regulating gene transcription and thus cell growth. ER alpha expression increases during the progression of prostate cancer. Risk increases with increased serum estrogen to testosterone ratio and increased 16-hydroxy to 2-hydroxy estrogen ratio.
- exposure to estrogenic *xenohormones*. Clean organic food, non-toxic personal care products and household cleaners and proper handling of chemicals in the home environment are a key to controlling risk. The role of pesticides remains controversial – to apologists for the chemical industry. Recent evidence points to many pesticides and herbicides acting like estrogen in the body. A Danish study showed the highest incidence among farmers – but the lowest incidence was among organic farmers.
- Bis-phenol-A BPA in epoxy resins, polycarbonate plastics, water pipes and as a liner in beverage cans, is a *xenoestrogen*. It is a hormone sensitizer capable of stimulating prostate cancer growth. It can enhance transcriptional efficacy in prostate cancers with androgen receptor mutations, at low, environmentally relevant doses.
- Prolactin hormone is associated with high-grade aggressive prostate cancer. Inhibitors of STAT-5 a/b mediate prolactin stimulation of prostate cells, reducing growth and reoccurrence of cancer.
- Low intake of antioxidants. A very large study is now underway to determine the role of vitamin E and selenium in preventing prostate cancer. The SELECT study by the National Cancer Institute (NCI) and Southwest Oncology Group will run for 12 years, follow 32,400 patients in Canada, USA and Puerto Rico. Participants must have no sign of prostate cancer at the start of the study.
- Seasonal variation in survival that is tentatively linked to sun exposure and activation of vitamin D. Several studies show that men who are diagnosed with prostate cancer in the summer-autumn seasons are more likely to survive than men diagnosed in the winter-spring season.
- A history of vasectomy is no longer considered a risk for prostate cancer

Most men over age 70 will have evidence of localized, indolent prostate cancer *in situ* at autopsy. Fortunately, it is usually very slow growing (indolent). Survival in localized disease without treatment is similar to age-matched controls. However, if the cancer begins to press on surrounding tissues, symptoms can arise such as urinary urgency, urinary hesitancy, urinary obstruction, terminal hematuria, nocturia, and pain in the pelvis or spine. Thrombo-embolism (clot in a vein) occurs in about 10% of cases. While early prostate cancer is relatively benign, once it is advanced and hormone-refractory it is likely to metastasize and median survival is only 6 to 12 months.

Screening should begin by age 40 in high-risk patients, and by age 50 in others. An annual digital rectal exam (DRE) by a physician can detect hard asymptomatic nodules in accessible areas of the gland. DRE and PSA tests have reduced the number of deaths from prostate cancer.

Prostatic intraepithelial neoplasia PIN has a 50 -70% risk of progressing to prostate cancer. Treat with PGE-2, COX-2 and IGF-1 inhibitors.

SIGNS & SYMPTOMS

Prostate cancer does not usually cause any symptoms in the early stages. Symptoms may mimic prostatitis or benign prostatic hypertrophy, including:
- weak or interrupted flow of urine
- frequent urination, including night-time frequency (nocturia)
- difficult urination or difficulty holding urine
- inability to urinate (anuria)
- pain or burning while urinating
- blood in the urine or semen.
- nagging pain in the low back, hips or pelvis
- loss of the lateral sulcus by digital rectal exam.
- seminal vesicle swelling
- lower extremity edema
- local adenopathy
- loss of external anal sphincter tone
- bone pains
- risk of clots is markedly elevated in prostate cancer, up to 30 times normal. Anti-coagulation therapy reduces risk of metastasis from 5% to 1%, and improves the efficacy of radiation therapy.

PSA TESTS

The prostate epithelium and periurethral glands make a protein digesting or proteolytic enzyme called prostate specific antigen PSA. It is a 27 kilo-Dalton glycoprotein. Its primary function is to liquefy the seminal clot post-ejaculation, allowing the sperm to roam free to find an egg to fertilize.

PSA dissolves the seminal proteins fibronectin and seminogelin, but is also known to activate insulin-like growth factor one IGF-1 by splitting off binding protein IGF-BP. IGF is a critical stimulus of the overgrowth of the prostate in benign prostatic hypertrophy and in prostate cancer. IGF interacts with estrogen generated by aromatase enzyme from testosterone, and related xenohormones.

PSA is an androgen-regulated serine protease. PSA varies seasonally, presumably from phytoestrogen and xenobiotic fluctuations in the diet.

Prostate specific antigen PSA reflects the total amount of prostate tissue, and is a good screen for abnormal growth of the gland. The gland usually makes 0.07 ng/ml tissue, so a 30 ml gland will yield a PSA of 2.1.

Normal range is 0 - 4. The ideal range is below 2.5. Benign prostatic hypertrophy BPH will not put PSA above 4.

Total PSA measured at age 44 to 50 predicts risk of prostate cancer occurring in the next 15 to 25 years:

≤ 0.5 risk 7.5 %
0.51 – 1.0   risk increases 2.5 fold
2.0 – 3.0   risk increases 19 fold

35% of men with early cancer and 15% with clinically significant and possibly high-grade prostate cancer will show normal range PSA values, i.e. under 4.

< 0.5 ng/ml: 7% have cancer
0.6 – 1.0:   10% have cancer
1.1 – 2.0:   17% have cancer
2.1 – 3.0:   24% have cancer
3.1 – 4.0:   27% have cancer

Probability of cancer with a non-suspicious DRE and a PSA of:
0 – 2 :   1%
2 – 4 :   15%
4 – 10:   25%
≥ 10 :   50%

Proposed new cut-offs for a biopsy to rule-out cancer:
2.5 for those aged 40 to 50
3.5 for those aged 50 to 60
4.5 for those aged 60 to 70
6.5 for those aged over 70

PSA above "normal" i.e. over 4.0 indicates risk for prostate cancer, with a selectivity or sensitivity of only 70 to 80%, and a specificity of 60 to 70%. There are false positives, and in fact only about 35 to 45 % of cases in this range represent a serious prostate cancer. Most detected in this range are indolent and non-life-threatening cancers.

PSA greater than 7 predicts high risk of eventually developing aggressive disease, and a PSA over 10 predicts 50% chance of extracapsular spread of the disease.

When PSA is in the range of 4-10, check free PSA or unbound antigen. If over 25% is in the free form, the chances of cancer are only 5-8%. When free PSA is under 14% there is a 59 % chance there is cancer. Free PSA ≤ 2.5 ng/ml predicts cancer will be found by biopsy.

Proenzyme PSA or pPSA is a 7 amino acid precursor or leader sequence, which is cleaved from the PSA to differentiate cancer from benign prostatic hypertrophy. In prostate cancer there is less efficient cleavage of the 261 amino acid pre-protein to its 244 amino acid inert pro-PSA and finally into the 237 amino acid mature protein, so the ratio of free to bound PSA is reduced in the blood of prostate cancer cases. pPSA is more sensitive than free PSA. If the percentage of pPSA exceeds the PSA level it is a strong indicator of cancer.

PSA is also called human glandular kallikrein KLK-3 or hK-3. In borderline cases a similar protein human kallikrein hK2 can verify cancer, and it is associated with increased risk of de-differentiation and lymphatic metastasis.

Urinary PCA-3 assay helps clarify the situation if there is an elevated PSA but the biopsy was negative. It is 72% specific for cancer, and 58% sensitive. A score of 35 or more is positive for cancer

A new screening test looks for Early Prostate Cancer Antigen EPCA, with a value over 1.7 indicating a 92% likelihood of cancer

The **PSA density** is calculated from an ultrasound measurement of the volume of the gland. A high density means rapid output, and such increased metabolism can be a sign of transition to cancer. PSAD over 0.15 should suggest a need for a trans-rectal ultrasound TRUS exam to rule out cancer.

PSA Velocity is the rate of change of the PSA score. The velocity is more important than the absolute number. A PSA velocity of over 0.75 ng/ml/year is suspicious for cancer in men over age 70; 0.50/yr for men age 60 to 70; and 0.25 /yr. for men age 40 to 50.

Test every 6 months if the PSA increases by a value of 1 or doubles within one year. A rise of over 2 ng/ml in one year prior to diagnosis predicts a relatively high risk of death even with radical prostatectomy surgery.

Doubling in less than 3 months is high risk, with a median survival of 3 years. Doubling in under 8 months increases risk of metastasis and shorter survival. Doubling in over 15 months is low risk, with good survival rates.

PSA velocity measurements can be biased downwards by low calorie intake, weight gain and high calcium intake, and biased upwards in black men.

After effective treatment of prostate cancer the PSA will often drop into the normal range. Further monitoring should employ the "ultra-sensitive PSA" test.

If the PSA does not rise for 3 years post-surgery, the prognosis is good.

PSA is lowered in men taking stain drugs for cholesterol, NSAIDs for inflammation, and Acetaminophen.

LAB TESTS

Standard work-up:
- CBC, Chem. screen and U/A – complete blood cell count, blood chemistry, urinalysis
- alkaline phosphatase – detects bone mets
- prostatic acid phosphatase – PAP – suggests bone mets if elevated
- IGF-1 – a 4 times stronger stimulator of prostate cancer than the male hormone testosterone!
- testosterone – free and dihydrotestosterone
- insulin, prolactin, and DHEA hormones

- blood clotting factors

Less common lab tests:
- urinary DpD – if high along with high PAP = metastasis into the bones
- urinary prostate cancer antigen three PCA-3 is prostate-cancer-specific gene product detectable in urine. PCA3 is more accurate than PSA in detecting early prostate cancers. If ≥ 35 PCA3 mRNA there is likely clinically significant (aggressive) disease.
- PSMA
- p-27- marker for aggressiveness, risk of mets and mortality
- CEA – correlates with aggressive disease
- E-cadherin
- p-53
- human kallikrein 2
- DNA ploidy analysis
- Microvessel density analysis
- Increased GOLPH-2, SPINK-1, and TMPRSS-2: ERG fusion proteins are significant predictors of prostate cancer. Urine panels of these biomarkers may turn out to be more specific than PSA testing.
- Blood levels of endoglin can detect spread into lymph nodes. Endoglin is a co-receptor of TGFβ1 and β3.
- A panel of biomarkers that predicts risk is comprised of TGFβ1, IL-6, IL-6 soluble receptor, VEGF, vascular adhesion molecule 1, endoglin and urokinase plasminogen activator.
- Counting circulating tumour cells predicts risk in prostate, cancers. Best is ≤ 5, worst is ≥50.
- Dr. Lemmo follows CRP, ferritin and zinc/copper ratio.

TESTOSTERONE

Surgical castration should result in a serum testosterone of less than 15 ng/dl.

Medical castration or androgen deprivation therapy ADT results in a testosterone level of about 20 to 50 ng/dl.

It is clear that the lower this is driven, the better the control of the cancer.

There are patients who present with abnormally high testosterone, whose prostate cancer cannot readily be controlled with naturopathic remedies. These are often presenting with a Gleason of 8 or more. If the PSA is rising despite our best efforts, ADT must be considered.

IMAGING & SCANS

Trans-rectal ultrasound TRUS of the prostate locates lesions and measures the volume of the gland, useful to calculate the PSA density PSAD. Prostate cancer cells make more PSA than normal prostate cells, so high output from a small gland confirms the presence of cancer.

Endorectal magnetic resonance imaging MRI rules out capsule penetration. Cancer outside the prostatic capsule is very dangerous. MRI can also be used to find occult cancers, where PSA is suspicious, but biopsies are negative.

Chest X-ray CXR, computerized tomography CT scan, bone scan and ProstaScint scans rule out mets to bone, lymph and lung

Positron emission tomography PET scans detect tissue that is hyper-metabolic. Cancer lights up with a hot glow from radioactive sugar.

Three dimensional contrast-enhanced power Doppler ultrasonography provides color images with great sensitivity and specificity for detecting prostate cancer. It is sensitive to increased microvessel density, and so can find cancers missed by digital rectal exam and grey-scale ultrasound imaging.

GLEASON SCORE

Scores the degree of abnormality in the biopsied cells, with high numbers indicating a worse prognosis:

2 to 4= well differentiated

5 to 7= moderately differentiated

8 to 10 = poorly differentiated

Gleason 6 is considered low risk, particularly if low tumour volume i.e. ≤ 0.5 ml.

Gleason 7 =48% 5 year survival, high risk of dying from prostate cancer.

Gleason 8 =25% 5 year survival

The Partin tables are a nomogram which uses the Gleason score, PSA and clinical assessment to determine if patients are likely to benefit from surgery. The 3 variables are combined in a multinomial log-linear regression to give a percent predictive probability, with 95% confidence that the patient will progress to a given final pathological stage. See http://urology.jhu.edu/prostate/partintables.php

STAGING

The Jewett system designates stages A & B as local disease, C is invasive, and D is widespread. The TNM system is also used.

Stage A or T1: clinically undetectable by DRE or imaging, found at surgery.

Stage A1 or T1a: well-differentiated focal tumour.

Stage A2 or T1b: moderately or poorly differentiated tumour, may have multiple foci.

Stage T1c: elevated PSA, needle biopsy positive.

Stage A: up to 98% live 5 years or more.

Stage B or T2: tumour confined to prostate, detectable by palpation or imaging.

Stage B0 or T2a: non-palpable, detected by PSA, involves less than ½ of one lobe of the gland.

Stage B1 or T2b: single nodule in over ½ of one lobe.

Stage B2 or T2c: more extensive tumour in one or both lobes.

Stage B: up to 65% live 5 years or more from the time of diagnosis.

Stage C or T3: disease extends through the prostate capsule and may involve the seminal vesicles.

Stage C1 or T3a: clinical unilateral extra-capsular extension.

Stage T3b: bilateral extra-capsular extension.

Stage T3c: extends to the seminal vesicles.

Stage C2: extension causing bladder outlet or urethral obstruction.

Stage C about 60% will live 5 years or more from time of diagnosis.

Stage D or T4: metastatic beyond the seminal vesicles. This represents about 20 to 30% of cases.

Stage D0: persistently elevated serum acid phosphatase.

Stage D1: invades regional lymph nodes.

Stage T4a: involves bladder neck, external sphincter or rectum.

Stage D2: distant lymph nodes positive, mets to bone or visceral organs.

Stage T4b: fixed to pelvic wall or involving levator muscles.

Stage D3: relapse of prostate cancer after adequate endocrine therapy.

Stage D: 30 % live 5 years. Most get 12 to 18 months remission from treatments and then live an average of another two years.

HIGH RISK CASES

The patients at high risk for reoccurrence after primary therapy:
- small cell or ductal types – uncommon histologies.
- Initial PSA greater than 10. At this level there is a 20 – 30% risk of spread beyond the gland.
- Gleason score over 8. However, prognosis is better if the PSA is still under 10.
- PSA reoccurs within 2 years of primary therapy
- PSA doubling in less than 6 months with a slope > 0.15 ng/ml
- Reoccurrence in the axial skeleton shows a median survival of 53 months, while reoccurrence in the appendicular skeleton has a median survival of 29 months.
- STAT-5 activation is linked to early reoccurrence, loss of cell surface E-cadherin expression, invasion and spread.
- Abnormal p53 gene expression significantly increases risk of recurrence
- Advanced metastatic prostate cancers can over-express EZH-2 messenger RNA and EZH-2 protein, which mediates cell proliferation, cellular memory, and transcriptional repression. Higher levels of this biomarker in tissue samples indicates an aggressive and advanced cancer.
- 4 times risk of reoccurrence and aggressive disease progression after radical surgery if elevated levels of B7-H3 protein, a cell-surface protein ligand which bind to receptors on lymphocytes which regulate immune response.

- A virus previously linked to sarcomas and leukemias, xenotropic murine leukemia virus-related virus XMRV, is now linked to more aggressive prostate cancer. It was found in 27% of cases in one study.

SURGERY

BIOPSY – increases 120 day mortality to 1.3% versus 0.3% without biopsy. Infection is the main risk.

CRYOSURGERY – freezing off tissue layers is technically demanding, but equals or exceeds other surgical and radiotherapy techniques in efficacy, and has a relatively low rate of complications.

SYSTEMATIC SEXTANT BIOPSY – provides a Gleason grade. In localized prostate disease it can be used to predict risk of lymphatic spread by calculating it in a formula called the "Hamburg algorithm."

PROSTATECTOMY – radical surgery has the potential to cure as long as the disease is within the gland capsule. Surgery is the preferred therapy for younger men in stage A or B. Radical prostatectomy causes urinary incontinence in 54% of patients and erectile difficulties in 75% of cases. Early complications include rectal injury, thromboembolism, heart attacks, sepsis, anastomotic urinary leakage; mortality rate is 1 - 2%. Late complications include impotence, incontinence and cancer relapse. Impotence rates used to be about 95%. Recent trends to nerve-sparing surgery have reduced post-op impotence problems to about 60% for the short term – but still up to 75% long term. At the time of this writing the best nerve-sparing surgeon in my area is Dr. Larry Goldenberg in Vancouver, phone 604-875-5003.

LYMPHADENECTOMY – surgical resection of lymph nodes.

ORCHIECTOMY – surgical castration or resection of the testes to remove testosterone hormone stimulation in stage D prostate cancer.

RADIATION

Radiation can be an effective treatment for prostate cancer. It is safer than surgery for early stage cancer of the prostate, particularly for the elderly. Impotence risk is similar to surgery, but with radiation injury, it develops months to years after treatment.

Organs close to the prostate that may also be injured are the bladder and rectum. The morbidity- lingering side-effects – include bowel adhesions, urinary urgency, frequency or incontinence, bladder pain, diarrhea, proctitis and rectal bleeding.

The statin drugs appear to slow the spread of aggressive forms of prostate cancer, and to radio-sensitize tumours.

Red rice yeast extract contains a naturally occurring form of the drug Lovastatin.

Anti-coagulation therapy increases the efficacy of radiation therapy to the prostate, probably by reducing iron levels.

EXTERNAL BEAM – using conventional X-ray and gamma ray sources; 3-D conformational style using leaflets to limit the treatment area.

PROTON BEAM – This is similar to what I worked on in my research years, except we busted up the protons and just used the pi-mesons. I have seen benefit in some fellows who went to the accelerator at Loma Linda in San Diego. Proton boosts to conventional stereotactic radiation reduces reoccurrences, though the overall survival benefit is equivocal.

BRACHYTHERAPY – pellets of radioactive material such as Cesium are threaded into the gland in a catheter, and left there permanently. It yields a very high dose, over a long time period. Usually the peak dose has occurred in 3 to 4 months, but significant radiation often remains for two years, and diminishes slowly thereafter. It affects the entire pelvic region. Brachytherapy is used in all stages from A to palliation in late D. It produces less urinary and sexual problems than nerve-sparing surgery, but creates slightly more bowel issues. Radiotherapy may provoke less incontinence and impotence than surgery, but will make later surgery more difficult, and has a lower cure rate than surgery alone. The perineum is highly innervated, and is very reactive to both surgery and radiation. Radiotherapy complications can include radio-enteritis, radio-cystitis, impotence in 75%, urinary incontinence in 38%. Fecal incontinence, loose stools and stool leakage occur after radiotherapy at rates 3.6 times higher than seen from radical prostatectomy surgery.

Iodine-125 brachytherapy delivering a total dose of at least 140 Gy yields 90% disease-free survival at 10 years for low-risk cases, and 78% 10 year disease-free survival for T2 stage disease.

ULTRASOUND – High intensity focused ultrasound (Ablatherm HIFU) is reported to yield 93% biopsy negative and stable PSA under 1.0 ng/ml at five years.

HORMONE BLOCKADE

Hormone blockade starves the cancer of growth promoting factors on a systemic or body-wide basis. It is useful in advanced disease or as an alternative to radiation and surgery. However, resistance commonly occurs in 5 to 6 years, and there can be increased risk of death from infections, diabetes mellitus, bone fractures and cardiovascular diseases.

Primary androgen deprivation therapy ADT is not of benefit to elderly men with localized disease.

In node+ high-risk localized cancer it is of benefit when combined post-op with radiation therapy. When androgen deprivation and radiation therapy are combined, the PSA will rise slowly and plateau by 2 years. If it continues to rise past two years, it indicates cancer recurrence.

Lupron is a synthetic analogue of gonadotropin-releasing hormone, which shuts off testicular output of testosterone, but not adrenal production. Lupron can cause hot flashes, reduce bone mineral density, raise triglycerides, and increase bad LDL cholesterol – but the adjunct use of soy ipriflavones counteracts these effects.

Lupron is commonly combined with Flutamide, which blocks receptor access by all testosterones, regardless of tissue of origin. Note that drugs like Flutamide which specifically block cell nucleus testosterone receptors give no survival benefit over surgical castration, and can cause depression, diarrhea and dementia.

Other complications may include impotence, reduced libido, breast enlargement, muscle wasting, muscular weakness, weight gain, increased fasting blood sugar, anemia, increased serum cholesterol, increased blood urea nitrogen, acceleration of osteoporotic bone loss, and hot flashes.

Androgen-deprivation therapy lowers the red blood cell count, hemoglobin and hematocrit to female levels.

The anemia typically shows up as a significant drop in hemoglobin and clinically manifests symptoms such as fatigue, coldness, dry skin, and possibly increased breathlessness on exertion. Muscle wasting usually is a slow erosion of endurance, strength and power. Regular exercise, both cardio and weight-training can maintain muscle and bone health, as well as improve sugar metabolism.

Androgen-deprivation therapy encourages metastasis of prostate cancer cells that remain. Suppress this risk with anti-angiogenics such as green tea **EGCG** and vitamin E.

Androgen-deprivation therapy triggers bone loss. Always support bone density, bone mass and bone strength with **MCHA calcium** with boron, magnesium citrate, vitamin C and vitamin D3.

In advanced prostate cancer intermittent pulsing of the therapy prevents treatment resistance and testosterone independence. Testosterone lowering drugs are used for a while to lower the PSA and testosterone, then they may be stopped until the PSA returns to the baseline. Intermittent therapy with Goserlin and Biclutamide is just as effective as continuous, so take a break when PSA level is down by 90% or under 4 mg/dl. Resume when it rises by over 10 mg/dl. Intermittent therapy is safer and delays onset of androgen-independence and disease progression.

Studies show hot flashes from prostate cancer therapy may respond well to acupuncture treatment twice a week, and also the newer anti-depressant drugs of the SSRI type (selective serotonin re-uptake inhibitors) such as Effexor (Venlafaxine). Grapeseed extract, evening primrose oil, Da Bu Yin Wan, Sepia may also be tried.

Recently we have seen the introduction of the anti-fungal drug Ketoconazole in relapsed and androgen-deprivation therapy resistant prostate cancer. This drug happens to weakly inhibit Cyp-11A and Cyp-17A, involved in the synthesis of precursors to dihydro epiandrosterone DHEA and androstenedione AED. These are the building blocks for intracrine testosterone synthesis – the making of this androgen hormone inside the prostate cancer cells. The prostate cancer cell genes for androgen synthesis are up-regulated by interleukin IL-6, which we can inhibit with green tea EGCG and curcumin.

Conventional wisdom says testosterone must be eradicated – by chemical or surgical castration. However, prostate cancer occurs at a time in a man's life when testosterone and progesterone production has sharply declined – and estradiol has risen. Remember testosterone and progesterone are estradiol antagonists, are far weaker carcinogens than estradiol, and stimulate p53 gene activity. The prostate gland has the same embryonic origin as endometrial tissue lining the womb – and endometrial cancer is clearly estrogen dependent. Estrogen stimulates the Bcl-2 oncogene, linked to prostate cancer as well as breast and endometrial cancers.

Prostate cancer is also linked to exposure to estrogenic xenobiotics. For example, Bisphenol-A BPA in epoxy resins and polycarbonate plastics is a xeno-estrogen. This hormone sensitizer stimulates prostate cancer cell growth. During hormonal therapy some prostate cancers develop androgen receptor mutations which allow estrogens and xeno-estrogens such as BPA to enhance transcriptional efficacy at low, environmentally relevant levels.

Boron can increase estradiol levels in the blood, so keep dietary and supplemental intake low.

However, high enough doses of estradiol, such as from 100 mcg/d transdermal patches, can reduce testosterone to castrate levels ($\leq$ 1.7 nMol/L or $\leq$ 50 ng/dL) with minimal side-effects. Thrombo-embolic risk rises, but can be managed.

On the other hand, ERβ activity antagonizes ERα activity, reducing inflammation in the prostate. Encourage ERβ activity with quercetin and phytoestrogens such as red-clover.

Other hormone therapies:

- Luteinizing hormone releasing-hormone analogues: Zoladex.
- Anti-androgens: Megace, Casodex, Eulixen, Chlormadinone.
- Aromatase inhibitors: Arimidex
- Proscar
- Tamoxifen

Prolactin is associated with high-grade prostate cancer. This effect can be mediated by inhibitors of STAT-5a/b, to reduce tumour growth and reoccurrence.

Progesterone does somewhat inhibit prostate cancer. Synthetic progestins such as medroxyprogesterone bind to androgen receptors better than natural progesterones. Progesterone suppresses Bcl-2 and increases p53, increasing apoptosis. Therapeutic doses are about 6 to 8 mg daily.

There is a monoclonal antibody Ipilimumab in trials now, showing some promise in prostate cancer.

Asymptomatic men with PSA $\leq$ 3.0, who receive regular screening, may take as a preventative a 5-alpha-reductase inhibitor, such linolenic acid, saw palmetto, pygeum and small-flowered willow.

NATUROPATHIC TREATMENT OPTIONS IN PROSTATE CANCER

Targets of Therapy: IGF-1, IGFBP, testosterone, estrogens, NFkB, COX-2, PGE-2, EGFR, TGFß, p53, mTOR/P13K/Akt, IL-6, SRC-3, TNFa, FGF, VEGF, IL-6, anti-coagulation.

*ALPHA LIPOIC ACID – R+ ALA regulates insulin-like growth factor one IGF-1, and mitochondrial control of apoptosis.

*ARTEMESININ – creates massive oxidative stress via endoperoxides on contact with iron in the cancer cells.

BORON – reduces cleavage of IGF from its binding protein IGFBP by PSA.

Estrogenic.

*BOSWELLIA – inhibits tumour growth by inhibition of 5-lipoxygenase, DNA synthesis, and topoisomerases I & II.

CIMICIFUGA – Black cohosh modulates hormones via the aryl hydrocarbon receptor and induces apoptosis in prostate cancer cells.

*CO-ENZYME Q-10 – Helps mitochondrial function and upregulates superoxide dismutase SOD.

*CURCUMIN – blocks formation of inflammatory cytokines PGE-2 and HETE; significantly inhibits proliferation of prostate cancer cells; inhibits volume and number of prostate tumours by inhibition of angiogenesis and induction of apoptosis; may prevent progression of prostate cancer to a hormone refractory (resistant) state. LOX 5-HETE eicosanoid from arachidonic acid is as strong a growth stimulator for prostate cells.

DELPHINIDINS – anthocyanidins from pigmented fruit such as blueberry and bilberry increase apoptosis and inhibit NFkB, Bcl-2, Ki-67 and PCNA.

*DIETETICS – diet may not cure the disease, but it heals the patient. Men with prostate cancer are most likely to die from some other disease, such as heart attack or stroke. Therefore it is essential to address the general health of the patient with lifestyle modifications such as weight reduction, calorie restriction – sugars and fats in particular, and regular vigorous exercise. Avoid red meat, eggs, poultry fat, fried foods, dairy, alcohol and sugar. Avoiding red meat, and using only low-fat white meats, low-fat dairy and emphasizing fish, fruit and vegetables will modulate and stabilize PSA, especially if weight loss is achieved. Dr. Dean Ornish has shown vegetarian diet with exercise and meditation will slow prostate cancer progression. Saturated fat promotes metastases to bones. Trans-fatty acids as found in hydrogenated fats, margarine and shortening promote the formation of catechol estrogen-3, 4-quinone from estradiol and estrone, which destroys DNA purine bases. Omega-3 fatty acids from fish and nuts protect from these toxic estrogens. Also involved in these reactions are sulphur-containing amino acids, which we can get from eating beans, garlic, onions and leeks. Reduce high omega 6 foods such as silage or grain-fed red meat, corn, grains. Dean Ornish has shown vegetarian diet plus exercise and meditation will slow the rise in PSA and the progression of prostate cancer. Blood serum from vegetarians inhibits prostate cancer sell growth *in vitro* 8-fold more than from cancer-free meat eaters. Control insulin levels, as with the Schwarzbein Principle diet or the Matsen glycemic index diet. Regulate IGF-1 and IGFBP with vitamin D and lycopene foods, green tea and grapeseed oil.

EXPECTANCY – watchful waiting is often appropriate in localized prostate cancer in elderly patients, as it is can be very slow-growing or indolent. This indolent phase can typically go on for 15 to 20 years before becoming and aggressive cancer. Radical surgery and radiation frequently cause harsh side-effects, and since prostate cancer often occurs at an age where there are competing threats to mortality such as heart disease. Candidates for waiting with expectancy have:

- total sum Gleason score under 4 (some say up to 3+3 and stage T2A)
- PSA less than 10 ng/ml

- diploid chromosomes = in normal pairs
- slow PSA rise (velocity) = under 1 ng/ml increase per year; stable or declining
- doubling time over 10 years.
- a life expectancy shorter than the natural course of prostate cancer, i.e. over age 60.

*FLAXSEED – mice bred to develop prostate cancer who were fed diets rich in flaxseeds (5% of their food intake) had half the number of tumours, and the tumours were far less aggressive and had a higher rate of apoptosis. The lignans in flax inhibit the development and the growth of prostate tumours. The lignans bind hormones and xenobiotics in the stool and increase sex hormone binding globulins in the blood. I have taken it for several years to prevent development of hormone dependent cancer.

*GENISTEIN – see SOY

GINGER – inhibits 5-HETE; synergistic with capsicum/cayenne.

*GRAPESEED EXTRACT – Oligomeric proanthocyanidins OPCs increase apoptosis, reduce angiogenesis, and increase insulin-like growth factor binding protein three – IGFBP-3. Reduces proliferation, especially in synergy with green tea EGCG and curcumin.

**GREEN TEA EGCG – inhibits growth of prostate cancer by a variety of mechanisms including inhibition of 5-alpha reductase, anti-angiogenesis, arrest of cell cycle at G2-M and by inducing apoptosis. Prevents progression of PIN. Angiogenesis and VEGF-A expression needs to be suppressed after prostatectomy.

*HOMEOPATHY – *Sabal serrulata, Conium maculatum, Thuja occidentalis, Carcinosum, Scirrhinum, Lycopodium.* Use in 30C to 200C potencies to start.

HOXSEY – herbal tonic. I use St. Francis herb farm *Red Clover Combination* and add homeopathic remedies, usually in 6C potencies. Contains iodine, an aromatase inhibitor, so use with caution.

**INDOLE-3-CARBINOL – diindolylmethane DIM is the activated form of indole-3-carbinol, which converts hormones like estrogen, progesterone and testosterone into less aggressive, less growth stimulating forms. DIM down-regulates the androgen receptor, even in hormone-refractory prostate cancer. I have seen it reduce PSA scores reliably. It also induces arrest of growth at G1 of the cell cycle, inducing apoptosis genes. It inhibits STAT-3 DNA transcription activator. Inhibits matrix metallo-proteinase MMP-9, which inhibits metastasis and growth of prostate cancer in the bones. Inhibits human papilloma virus HPV.

LYCOPENE – reduces growth and proliferation by up-regulating direct intercellular gap junction communication, and by reducing serum IGF-1 levels. Increases liver glutathione GSH. Use 6 mg for prevention, 30 mg for therapy (10-15 mg 2 times daily). This is not a very powerful remedy.

MAITAKE – mushroom polysaccharides such as maitake D or MD fractions prolong survival.

**MELATONIN – this pineal gland hormone down-regulates 5-lipoxygenase gene expression, prevents DNA oxidation, blocks the mitogenic effects of prostate cancer promoting hormones and growth factors, and reverses LHRH resistance. It will prolong life in late stage palliative care.

MILK THISTLE – silibinin slows prostate cancer growth, inhibits epidermal growth factor EGF.

MISTLETOE – Use type Qu Iscador or type A Helixor.

MODIFIED CITRUS PECTIN – reduces growth, angiogenesis and metastasis.

MUSHROOMS – White button mushrooms suppress production of 5-alpha reductase enzyme.

NALTREXONE – low doses (up to 3 mg hs) are excellent, if the patient is not on any opiates. This is a prescription drug used in higher doses for heroin and morphine addiction.

OLIVE OIL – the best inhibitor of PGE2 synthesis by prostate cancer cells, which are able to convert AA to PGE2 at a rate 10 times higher than benign prostatic hypertrophy (BPH) cells. Inhibition of 5-HETE induces massive apoptosis in prostate cancer cells.

**OMEGA 3 OIL – marine omega 3 oils are popular among naturopathic oncologists in the USA, to control inflammation. Anti-coagulation reduces risk of metastasis.

*POMEGRANATE – the fruit, juice, fermented juice and seed oil yield a variety of inhibitors, including ellagic acid. Its polyphenols increase cell cycle arrest and apoptosis, while reducing androgen receptors and growth. Pomegranate down-regulates pro-inflammatory eicosanoids.

QUERCETIN – inhibits 5-HETE to reduce inflammation, as does curcumin and melatonin.

RED WINE – reduces risk of prostate cancer by 6% per glass, per day! Resveratrol, anthocyanidins and proanthocyanidins are thought to be the active principles.

REISHI – *Ganoderma* mushroom reduces transcription factors and invasiveness; regulates nuclear factor NFkB to increase apoptosis. An immune balancer *par excellence.*

* RESVERATROL – a dietary stilbene, 5-10% of the mass of grape skins. Inhibits carcinogens, disrupts epidermal growth factor receptor, antagonizes androgen receptors, and scavenges prostate cancer cells.

RUTIN – polyphenols in red wine induce apoptosis in prostate cancer cells. The inhibition of tumour growth was highest from the rutin, gallic acid and tannic acid, and less from the quercetin and Morin polyphenols.

SAW PALMETTO – this herb is fine for slowing benign enlargement of the gland. It inhibits 5-α-reductase. It does <u>not</u> falsely lower the PSA readings, as was once claimed. Do not mix with hormone blockade therapies.

SELENIUM – no longer strongly recommended for prevention, and it may actually increase the growth of some prostate cancers.

*SOY – soy foods are the most important dietary protectant from prostate cancer risk. Soy is rich in genestein, an isoflavone which inhibits growth of prostate cancer. **Genestein** competitively inhibits hormones at receptors, increases sex hormone blocking gonadotropin, reduces growth signalling by tyrosine protein kinases, and is anti-angiogenic. Protein as found in soy foods helps maintain metabolic balance and immune competence. Give with vitamin D3.

VITAMIN C – high doses inhibit growth and spread.

VITAMIN D – slows the rise of PSA, inhibits cell cycle progression and may induce apoptosis. Inhibits IGF-1 which is a very strong growth stimulator for prostate cancer cells, even more stimulating than testosterone! Take as activated vitamin D3. Get sun on your skin in moderation. Use shade and mild aloe sunscreens to prevent sunburn. Vitamin D has a powerful synergy with soy genestein, says a notable FABNO.

VITAMIN E – VES inhibits prostate cancer cell growth and induces apoptosis in a dose-dependent manner. It significantly reduces mortality from prostate cancer. Alpha and gamma tocopherols are very active. Vitamin E is synergistic with lycopene and selenium.

ZINC – the prostate collects high concentrations of zinc. Zinc is useful for prevention and treatment of benign prostate enlargement (BPH). Zinc inhibits prostate cancer growth by increasing activity in gene p21, increasing apoptosis, inhibiting 5-alpha reductase, and binding prolactin and dihydrotestosterone.

ZYFLAMEND – a patented anti-inflammatory herb extract with ginger, rosemary, holy basil, green tea, barberry, oregano, skullcap, turmeric, goldthread and Hu zhang.

Avoid in Prostate Cancer
- DHEA supplements as they boost IGF-1 and sex hormones. The IGF-1 production in the liver is increased by DHEA and also its biological activity rises due to induced changes in IGF-binding proteins. The exception to this rule is a brief trial of DHEA to restore responsiveness to androgen deprivation in treatment refractory advanced prostate cancer.
- Sterols and sterolins can increase DHEA levels and reduce cortisol levels. Maca root can increase DHEA. Ashwagandha herb can significantly increase DHEA and so its use is limited to short-term radiation or chemotherapy support.
- Chondroitin supplements used for arthritis may increase the spread of prostate cancer.

An example of a successful protocol:
- Melatonin
- Flaxseed
- Milk thistle extract
- Indole-3-carbinol
- Can-Arrest

FABNOs also recommend:
- Green tea EGCG
- Omega 3 marine oil
- Curcumin
- Modified citrus pectin
- Homeopathic *Scirrhinum/Carcinosum* in the morning alternating with an evening dose of *Lycopodium*.
- Botanicals *Cephalotaxus, Annona, Mahonia, Trichosanthus, Catharanthus, Taxus*

Chapter Twelve – Integrative Care Of Colorectal Cancer

EPIDEMIOLOGY

Colorectal carcinoma (CRC) is of course linked to the food passed through these organs. A high-fat, low fibre diet, alcohol and low intake of vitamin C, folate, calcium, selenium, flavones and indoles are all risk factors. 94% of cases are over 50 years old. Risk goes up the more red meat and processed meats you eat, and down with eating more vegetables, including tomatoes.

- Sedentary habits put you at risk.
- A history of breast or endometrial cancer increases risk.
- People with a history of inflammatory bowel diseases such as Crohn's regional enteritis or ulcerative colitis (UC) have increased risk of CRC.
- *Cryptosporidium parvum*, usually an opportunistic organism only infecting the immuno-suppressed, can trigger colon adenocarcinoma.
- *Bacteroides fragilis* bacteria can overgrow in the colon, creating chronic inflammation and risk of cancer.
- Central adiposity (fat around the waist and viscera of the belly) is a risk factor, and is associated with insulin resistance, high insulin and IGF growth factors, especially IGF-2 over-expression.
- Most colorectal cancers start as benign polyps in the colon. Familial polyposis syndrome puts some people at higher risk. The stem cells in the colonic crypt produce enterocytes which mature, migrate to the top of the crypt and are shed into the lumen of the colon. Polyps are hyperplastic growths which can become inflamed and degenerate into neoplastic adenomas, followed by invasion through the crypt walls, and metastasis. Prevent cancerous conversion by folate, calcium D-glucarate, fibre, pectin, probiotic and antioxidant supplementation.
- Calcium reduces polyp formation and progression of hyperplastic polyps to tubular adenomas and carcinomas. Best results are seen with supplementation over 1,200 mg, added vitamin D, and combined with a low fat, high fibre diet.
- Neuro-endocrine tumours are common, and the primary treatment target is VEGF and angiogenesis.
- Colorectal cancers exhibit MET oncogene amplification or the erb-B3 pathway. Target EGFR.
- K-ras mutations are linked to polypoma and adenoma progression to colorectal cancer. D-limonene down-regulates k-ras, correcting over-amplification of EGFR. K-ras controls the PKCi oncogene.
- COX-2 inhibitors reduce polyp conversion to neoplasia.
- Once CRC has occurred, there is a 20% chance another will occur within 5 years.
- Hypomethylation leads to loss of imprinting of the IGF-1 gene.

317

- Anal and rectal cancers have estrogen and other hormone receptors.
- Counting circulating tumour cells predicts risk in colon cancers. Best is ≤ 5, worst is ≥50.

SYMPTOMS & SCREENING

Patients may have vague abdominal pains, sometimes mimicking peptic ulcers.

There may be alteration in the bowel habit and tenesmus (urging but nothing will pass). There is often a low grade chronic but intermittent blood loss detectable by stool testing for occult blood.

Carcinoembryonic antigen (CEA) may be elevated, in direct relation to the size and extent of the tumour. Normal is under 4. When the CEA is > 5 at diagnosis, the prognosis is poorer. CEA will also be elevated from alcoholic cirrhosis, ulcerative colitis, pancreatitis, and cancers of the breast, ovary, bladder and prostate.

Lymph nodes can be screened for CEA mRNA and cytokeratin twenty CK-20 produced by disseminated CRC cells.

Feces can be screened for COX-2 mRNA, which is more sensitive than serum CEA screening.

Tumour dimeric pyruvate kinase M2PK, a marker of anaerobic glycolysis measured in feces or EDTA plasma, is more accurate as a screening tool than CEA. However, it is elevated in inflammatory bowel diseases IBD.

Colonoscopy is preferred to sigmoidoscopy, to detect adenomatous polyps and colonic carcinomas high up in the bowel. 3 to 5% of small polyps are carcinomas.

A new light test uses a 700 nanometre wavelength light source to inspect the color of the oral mucosa. Reflectance under 47.9% is a 100% sensitive indicator of risk of hereditary non-polyposis CRC. There is an alteration of the gingival extracellular matrix in these persons.

FIVE YEAR SURVIVAL RATES

Colon: localized – 88% spreading – 58%average – 62%
Rectal: localized – 80%spreading – 47% average – 63%

INDICATORS OF HIGH RISK COLORECTAL CANCER

- Lactate dehydrogenase LDH or LD elevation in the blood indicates risk of 50% shorter survival time.
- More than 2 mets.
- ECOG performance status 2
- Alkaline phosphatase > 3 times the upper limit of normal

TUBULAR ADENOMA

75% of neoplastic polyps are tubular adenomas.
Invasiveness varies with size:
- under 1 cm diameter = 1% chance of invasive tumour
- 1 to 2 cm diameter = 10% chance
- over 2 cm diameter = 45% chance

VILLOUS ADENOMA

The larger and less common polyp, occurring in the recto-sigmoid area, or on the right in the cecum or ascending colon. 30% are invasive cancers, and they metastasize freely. Frequently associated with bleeding and a protein-rich mucus secretion. This leads to frank blood and mucus from the rectum, fatigue, and malnutrition. Blood tests may show low protein, low albumin and low potassium.

LEFT-SIDED CRC

62% of CRC is left-sided. In situ CRC develops in 1 to 2 years into annular lesions encircling the bowel. The infiltrated gut wall is flattened and may show mucosal ulceration. These produce characteristic "napkin-ring" constrictions, seen with X-rays taken with a barium contrast enema. The early warning signs are a change in bowel habit to diarrhea or constipation, and melena (blood in the stool).

RIGHT-SIDED CRC

38% of CRC is right-sided. These lesions tend to be clinically silent until quite large, as the cecum is spacious. Bulky, fungating, cauliflower-like tumour protrudes into the lumen. There may be weakness and malaise, anemia and weight loss.

METASTASIS

Any CRC can dissect the gut wall and invade by direct extension into adjacent tissues. Metastasis is via lymphatics and blood vessels to the regional lymph nodes, liver, lungs, bone, brain and the peritoneal serosal membrane. CRC mets are linked to over-expression of the WNT/TCF pathway.

MODIFIED DUKE'S CLASSIFICATION

A – limited to mucosa
B – invading deeper layers, 1 in 4 will be fatal
B1 – into muscle layer, nodes clear
B2 – through the entire gut wall, nodes clear
C – regional spread, more than ½ of cases will die from it

C1 – in gut wall and node positive
C2 – through the entire wall and node positive
D – distant metastatic spread

MEDICAL TREATMENT OF COLORECTAL CANCER

SURGERY

If under 3 cm. diameter (just over an inch), local resection to remove the tumour plus adjacent mesenteric lymph nodes can be curative.

Larger rectal lesions may result in a temporary colostomy, only 15% will have to have a permanent colostomy.

Large or obstructive tumours may be debulked with radiation before surgery. Check CEA before surgery. 2% may die from the surgery.

RADIATION

Patients with higher levels of p53 mutations are unresponsive to radiotherapy and have reduced survival.

Pre-operative radiotherapy at just 5 fractions in 1 week may do more than chemotherapy or post-operative radiotherapy.

Post-op adjuvant radiation in about 28 fractions over 6 weeks can improve survival where the tumour has penetrated the gut wall, involves the regional lymph nodes, is within 15 cm. of the anal verge, or has invaded the small intestine, bladder, ovaries or uterus.

Palliative radiation for inoperable tumours, for pain or excess bleeding gives 90% of cases relief within 6 weeks. Dukes stage B2 or C rectal cancers do better with radiation plus chemotherapy.

Surgery and radiation for anal cancers can have significant morbidities, such as loss of sexual function and chronic diarrhea or fecal incontinence.

CHEMOTHERAPY

The chemo drug of choice is 5-fluorouracil. Adjunctive chemo agents include levamisole or leucovorin (calcium folinic acid). Vitamins C & E synergize with 5-FU.

The response rate is poor at 20%. Adjuvant chemo does not help the 20 % of cases with high levels of microsatellite instability in their tumour DNA. These cases have deficient mismatch gene repair, making them very vulnerable to ahrm from chemo drugs, and unlikely to benefit. Nausea and diarrhea can be severe, and will benefit from L-glutamine supplementation. Myelosuppression is also a risk – the bone marrow is injured, so blood cells cannot be created.

Irinotecan is a topoisomerase inhibitor which inhibits cell division by inducing single strand DNA breaks. It can be useful with or after 5-FU with leucovorin rescue.

Oxaliplatin is a third generation platinum compound which cross-links DNA, inducing apoptosis. It is synergistic with 5-FU.

Taxanes work better combined with vitamin D Calcitriol. Follow chemo with curcumin to prevent stem cell proliferation by symmetrical mitosis. This reduces rates of relapse and inhibits the development of chemo-resistant cells.

IMMUNOTHERAPY

CRC produces antigens recognizable by T-cells. Monoclonal antibodies are useful after surgery, and repair post-surgical immunosuppression. Edrecolomab is monoclonal Ig2A antibody to human CRC Ep-CAM antigen.

NATUROPATHIC TREATMENT OPTIONS IN COLORECTAL CANCER

Targets of therapy: NFkB, EGFR, erb-B3, IGF-1, VEGF, DNA hypomethylation, STAT-5.

*ALPHA LIPOIC ACID – increases apoptosis of CRC cells, inhibits IGF and NFkB.

AVEMAR – fermented extract of wheat germ improves survival times.

BLACK SEED – *Nigella sativa* or black cumin seed contains thymoquinone which is an antioxidant synergistic with green tea EGCG. The combination is similar in effectiveness to 5-FU chemotherapy.

CALCIUM – inhibits proliferation, increases differentiation in human colonic cells. This strongly prevents polyps and subsequent cancers. Use 1,200 mg daily. Calcium-D-glucarate is more costly but is the ideal detoxifier – use 1,500 mg..

CORIOLUS – PSK very significantly increases survival at doses of 3 to 6 grams daily of 25-38% HMWPS hot water extract.

*CURCUMIN – highly chemo preventative in CRC, and protection lasts years after stopping supplementation. Induces heat shock protein HSP70, and apoptosis. Reduces inflammation. COX-2 inhibitors such as curcumin and aspirin reduce risk of development or reoccurrence of dysplastic polyps and adenomas by 50%. Curcumin is safer. Reduces lipid peroxidation, always high in advanced CRC. Use after chemotherapy.

DIET: Colorectal cancer is very much a consequence of the modern agricultural diet with high glycemic carbohydrates, low fibre, low calcium, and damaged fats. Traditional hunter-gatherer dietary ingredients such as nuts and oil seeds and fish help prevent CRC. As Dr. Diana Schwarzbein, MD says, food is best if it could be hunted, fished, milked, picked or gathered. Identify, avoid or desensitize for food allergies or sensitivities.

FARE YOU – cabbage extract heals ulceration and inflammation, regulates apoptosis.

FIBRE – Eat lots of dietary fibre as organic vegetables and fruits, and whole grains. Fibre binds cytotoxic unconjugated bile acids, steroid hormones and xenobiotics; provides media for good bacterial flora and fauna to produce short chain fatty acids, such as butyrates which strongly regulate the DNA; lowers insulin levels, lowers gut pH (increases acidity); lignans slow cell division and inhibit angiogenesis.

*FISH OILS – omega-3 oil dihexanoic acid DHA reduces polyps, especially larger ones, lowers risk of conversion to CRC. Eicosapentaenoic acid EPA induces cAMP to re-differentiate CRC. Seal oil may also be used.

FOLATE – folic acid or its salt folate are B vitamins highly protective against colorectal cancer. It methylates and silences DNA, decreasing mucosal cell proliferation in the luminal aspect of colonic crypts. Folate is very high in green leafy vegetables, such as salad greens.

*GRAPESEED EXTRACT – proanthocyanins improve survival in poly-metastatic CRC with some restoration of body weight and quality of life. Inhibits EGF, VEGF and NFkB.

*GREEN TEA EGCG – regulates insulin-like-growth factor IGF-1, NFkB and angiogenesis.

HOMEOPATHY – *Aloe socotrina, Cadmium, Carcinosum* for the bowel; *Nitricum acidum, Ruta graveolens* for the rectum.

*INDOLE-3-CARBINOL – inhibits NFkB, induces apoptosis, cell cycle arrest, detoxifies hormones, etc.

LDN – Low dose Naltrexone at 3 – 4.5 mg at bedtime can be very useful, but the patient cannot be on any opiate or narcotic pain-killers.

LYCOPENE – and related carotenes control inflammation and progression.

MELATONIN – extends life expectancy.

*MILK THISTLE – Inhibits EGFR and related TGFα, MMP's, NFkB transcription, sequesters IGF-1 while increasing IGFBP-3; modulates VEGF and cell cyclins.

MISTLETOE – injectable mistletoe Qu for males and M type for females.

PROBIOTICS – Replacing good gut bacteria such as *Lactobacillus casei* creates healing fatty acids such as butyrates from dietary fibre, reducing atypia and risk of cancer. Reduces invasiveness factors created from dairy foods by bad gut bacteria such as *Listeria*.

PROTEIN – support protein status with sugar-free whey protein powder, and L-glutamine.

PSYCHOLOGY – physicians will find CRC patients are often poorly compliant and treatment resistant. They tend to internalize stress. Empower them with control. They need creativity, art and self-expression.

*QUERCETIN – inhibits EGF receptor kinase to induce apoptosis in CRC, inhibits expression of p21-ras mutations, inhibits growth by binding to ER-II receptors, inhibits NFkB and VEGF, etc.

*REISHI – *Ganoderma* mushroom extract strongly inhibits NFkB.

*RESVERATROL – increases apoptosis, inhibits NFkB and EGF.

RETINOL – see vitamin A.

SELENOMETHIONINE – antioxidant, preventative.

*VITAMIN A – as retinol palmitate suppresses CRC, increases survival by inhibiting lipid peroxidation.

*VITAMIN D – Inhibits CRC cell proliferation by regulating DNA transcription in well-differentiated tumours expressing the cytoplasmic vitamin D receptor. Can reduce mortality by a whopping 39%. Rx: up to 5000 I.U. 3 to 7 days a week. *Serum calcium must be monitored if on high dose therapy*. Calcitriol increases efficacy of Taxane chemotherapy.

VITAMIN E – Vitamin E succinate VES arrests CRC tumour cells in G1 phase, leading to apoptosis. It is associated with increased survival time in terminal CRC, combined with omega 3 oils. If injectable VES is not available, choose mixed tocopherols with gamma and delta forms.

CARCINOID (GI NEUROENDOCRINE) TUMOUR

Carcinoids are neuro-endocrine GI tumours. Symptoms may mimic irritable bowel syndrome IBS.

Diarrhea and flushing suggest metastasis into the liver.

Test for high Chromogranin-A (Crom-A), urinary 5-HIAA and neuron-specific endolase.

Carcinoids respond well to octreotide LAR – long-acting somatostatin analogue.

Targets: IGF-1, TGFα, TGFβ1, fibrosis and EGFR.

Rx:
- R+ alpha lipoic acid
- nattokinase
- ginkgo biloba extract
- artemisinin and lactoferrin
- Cortisol may be moderated with niacinamide, B-complex, Vitamin C, rhodiola, tryptophan, licorice root, and formulas such as ITT brand *Cortisol Manager* or Thorne brand *Cortrex*.
- vitamin D3
- curcumin.
- green tea EGCG extract
- grapeseed extract OPCs
- rhodiola
- plant source digestive enzymes
- milk thistle extract

Chapter Thirteen – Integrative Care Of Lung Cancer

EPIDEMIOLOGY

Lung cancer is a very common cancer, with high mortality. Regional and distant spread is common. More than half of cases will have widespread metastases at the time of first diagnosis and will not survive for a year.

The most significant causative factor is tobacco smoking. 30 pack years of cigarettes increases risk 20 times over non-smokers. Risk for a non-smoking spouse of a smoker is up 30%. Risk falls back near normal about 10 years after quitting smoking. Tobacco also increases risk of leukemia, as well as cancer of the mouth, esophagus, stomach, pancreas, pharynx, larynx, kidney, ureter, bladder, and cervix. It increases risk of cardiovascular disease (CVD) such as heart attack and stroke, and of course causes chronic lung diseases (COPD) such as emphysema.

Even second-hand smoke dramatically increases free radicals of oxygen ROS in the lungs.

Synthetic beta carotene is associated with a higher risk of lung cancer in smokers. Beta carotene is not effective as an antioxidant in high oxygen tissues such as the lungs, and is likely converted to a pro-oxidant by tobacco poisons. The naturopathic profession concluded from these beta carotene studies that antioxidants must be natural source, moderate doses, and most important – all the antioxidants need to be taken at the same time to provide a synergistic network. Food provides antioxidants in combinations which allow them to recycle each other and support each other in managing oxidative stress on the DNA and other large bio-molecules. We know vitamin C, E (alpha tocopherol especially) and selenium work as a team, and that all dietary antioxidants require intrinsic R+ alpha lipoic acid and glutathione to neutralize the extra energy they pick up from ROS. The best single antioxidant of all for the lungs is grapeseed extract OPCs. Dr. Arthur DeJong, MD PhD, creator of Oncolyn, claims grapeseed extract OPCs inhibit tobacco damage to the lungs.

Approximately 15% of all lung cancers are diagnosed in people who have never smoked. Non-smokers who develop lung cancer may have an abnormally high expression of p58 and cJUN N-terminal kinase.

Exposure to radon gas, entering a home from the soil and rock below, can more than double risk of lung cancer. This can occur even at levels well below the official guidelines. Particularly susceptible to radon gas are persons with a genetic variant causing reduced glutathione-S-transferase M-1. Radon injury is additive and synergistic with tobacco smoke.

Other independent and additive risk factors include tuberculosis, and toxic petrochemical, arsenic, asbestos, uranium or other radiation exposure.

Low intake of vegetables and lack of exercise increases risk of lung cancers. A diet high in the cabbage family of vegetables, the cruciferae, is highly protective, reducing risk of lung cancer by about a factor of 3. Tea and wine are also protective.

Red and processed meat intakes are associated with increased risk of cancers of the lung. Iron content may be an active principle. Increasing fish and vegetables while reducing red meat is protective.

Inorganic phosphates from fertilizers, and in soda pop and meats are linked to higher risk.

Bronchogenic cancers arising from the bronchial endothelial lining constitute 90% of lung cancers – squamous cell, large cell, small cell, broncho-alveolar and adenocarcinoma. 5 year survival is about 15%.

Metastasis is linked to over-expression of the WNT/TCF pathway.

Small cell cancers have a 5-year survival rates are about 5 to 10%, making this one of the most deadly cancers, deserving very aggressive therapy. Survival time can be just a few months from diagnosis, in a majority of cases.

Surgery is the best hope for a cure. I recommend the mitochondrial rescue strategy for lung cancers.

SIGNS & SYMPTOMS

Cough, sputum, haemoptysis (coughing up blood), respiratory stridor (breathing with great effort), frequent or persistent upper respiratory infections URI, weight loss, and fatigue.

Paraneoplastic manifestations include ACTH and HGH irregularities.

Dogs can detect 11 specific exhaled volatile organic compounds VOCs on the breath of those with lung cancer. An electronic "nose" has been developed which also reliably detects these aromatics in the breath.

STAGING NSCLC PRIMARIES

T-X: positive sputum or washings, no tumour

T-is: carcinoma in situ

T-1: tumour under 3 cm diameter

T-2: tumour 3 cm or more, or involving mainstem bronchus or visceral pleura, or subtotal atelectasis, or subtotal obstructive pneumonitis.

T-3: tumour invading the chest wall, diaphragm, mediastinal pleura, or atelectasis or obstructive pneumonitis of the entire lung.

T-4: tumour invading the mediastinum, esophagus, heart, great vessels of vertebral body. Malignant pleural effusion.

N-0: no regional lymph node metastases

N-1: in hilar or peribronchial ipsilateral nodes.

N-2: in mediastinal or subcarinal ipsilateral nodes

N-3: in any scalene or supraclavicular nodes or contralateral hilar or mediastinal nodes

M-0: no distant metastases

M-1: distant metastases

Occult: T-X N-0M-0
Stage 0: T-is N-0M-0
Stage I: T-1,2N-0M-05 year survival is about 45%
Stage II: T-1,2N-1M-05 year survival is 20 - 25%
Stage IIIA: T-3 N-0,1 M-0can be treated surgically in some cases T-1,3 N-2 M-0
Stage IIIB: T-4N-0,2 M-0 cannot be cured with surgery.
Stage IV: any T any N M-1+ cannot be cured with surgery.

NON-SMALL CELL LUNG CANCER – NSCLC

75% of lung cancers, the non-small cell category includes 4 subtypes with clinically similar behaviour -squamous epidermoid, adenocarcinoma, large cell and undifferentiated.

Slow growth is common, with no rapid impact on quality of life. Often these tumours are diagnosed after 5 to 8 years of silent growth. Typically they are found as a space-occupying lesion on a routine chest X-ray or CT.

The lesion may be directly biopsied, or sputum cytology, fibre optic bronchoscopy washings or brushings, aspiration of pleural effusions, biopsy of nodes or metastatic tumours can provide a diagnosis.

Proteomic analysis of protein expression and post-translational modifications reflects the biochemical pathology and assists in making a prognosis of node involvement and of mortality risk.

A rise in the C-reactive protein CRP marker of inflammation > 0.5 mg/L is associated with progression of dysplasia to frank cancer.

Non-small cell lung cancer has a low response rate to chemotherapy, but there is potential for surgical cure if it is found while still localized.

Risk of brain metastases is 14 times higher from tumours over 3.9 cm in diameter. Overall 5 year survival is 15%.

Significantly poorer survival and relapse-free survival is seen in tumours expressing the cell adhesion molecule CEA CAM-1--also called AE1 / AE3. Such cases warrant aggressive adjuvant treatment.

Monoclonal antibodies targeting the epidermal growth factor receptor EGFR can cause regression of adenocarcinoma and squamous cell carcinoma of the lung, with symptomatic improvement. The natural alternative is milk thistle.

RADIATION FOR NSCLC

Radiation is sometimes given after surgery, or in late disease, but the lungs are very sensitive to radiation, and when they scar up they cannot move air. Radiotherapy actually increases early deaths about 21% in early NSCLC

Acute radiation pneumonitis may follow 1 to 6 months after therapy, with bloody cough, chest pain and breathing distress.

Drugs which support recovery are prednisone, azathioprine or cyclosporine A.

Consider anti-oxidants vitamin E and grapeseed extract. N-acetyl-cysteine is a lung protectant and anti-oxidant, but may be anti-apoptotic.

Taxol is radio-sensitizing for lung tissue, as are taxanes in yew bark tea.

Coriolus PSK significantly improves survival in NSCLC treated with radiation.

Proton beam radiation is used in stage 1 cases that decline or cannot take surgery. It is available at Loma Linda in San Diego, California, and several other American clinics.

RADIO-FREQUENCY ABLATION

Radio-frequency ablation RFA can be considered for those patients not medically fit for surgery or radiation therapy.

Tumours must be under 3.5 cm diameter, and cannot be adjacent to major blood vessels or other vital structures. The ideal tumour size for this procedure is under 2 cm. diameter.

Probes are inserted and radio-waves heat and destroy the tumour tissue.

Two year survival is over 91%. Dr. Halkier at the Royal Columbian Hospital in New Westminster is currently providing this therapy.

Standard RFA devices can ablate a zone of about 5 cm. diameter, and so allowing for a 1 cm. margin, the absolute maximum tumour size treatable is 4 cm. at its largest diameter. Recent experimental multi-polar devices ablate up to 8 cm, so can theoretically it can treat well-selected tumours to a maximum diameter of 8 cm.

CHEMOTHERAPY FOR NSCLC

Cisplatin, carboplatin, mitomycin, vinblastine, ifosfamide, gemcitabine, and paclitaxel.

NSCLC up-regulates COX-2, increasing levels of prostaglandin PGE-2. COX-2 inhibitor Celecoxib has been shown to improve responses to pre-op or neo-adjuvant chemo with paclitaxel and carboplatin.

Iressa (gefitinib) is an epidermal growth factor receptor EGFR inhibitor (receptor specific tyrosine kinase inhibitor) showing some efficacy, but it is linked to deaths from interstitial pneumonia. The most common problem with it is diarrhea. *Tarceva* (erlotinib) is proving to be quite useful, inhibiting EGFR tyrosine kinases and therefore cell proliferation, angiogenesis, invasion, and metastasis.

Chemotherapy for metastatic NSCLC is always palliative. In general, whole-brain radiation of cancer metastases will only add about 2 months increased survival.

SMALL CELL LUNG CANCER (SCLC)

Small or oat cell carcinoma (SCLC) accounts for about 25% of lung cancers. It follows a very rapid clinical course, with survival of only 1 to 2 months in extensive disease. Survival is only 4 to 5 months in limited stage disease, which is defined as tumour in one hemi-thorax and regional lymph nodes, including ipsilateral (same-side) supraclavicular adenopathy (swollen nodes above the collarbone) and pleural effusion.

A primary driver of SCLC is fibroblast growth factor receptor FGFR.

RADIATION FOR SCLC

Hemi-body radiation outperforms chemo for small cell lung cancer.

CHEMOTHERAPY FOR SCLC

Small cell lung cancer usually responds rapidly and vigorously to chemotherapy, but if reoccurrence occurs within 3 months, then secondary chemo has no impact on survival and only a 5% response rate. If reoccurrence is more than 3 months post-primary chemo, then a 20% response rate is expected.

Limited stage disease will respond 80-90% of the time, with 12 to 18 months until reoccurrence.

Extensive stage disease will respond 60-80% of the time with 7 to 10 months until reoccurrence.

A platinum drug is usually combined with a second chemo drug i.e. cisplatin + etoposide (from podophyllotoxin) is often the treatment of choice.

Variations include the less toxic carboplatin, plus doxorubicin, cyclophosphamide, gemcitabine or taxol (as docetaxel or paclitaxel)

Anti-angiogenic Avastin or bevacizumab combined with chemotherapy improves median survival by 2 to 2 ½ months, and increases one year median survival by 10%. There is an increased risk of haemorrhage, haemoptysis, GI perforation, hypertension and congestive heart failure.

MESOTHELIOMA

Mesothelioma is cancer of the pleural membranes, which lie between the lungs and the chest wall.

Exposure to asbestos fibres is the leading cause. Brake mechanics are high risk, as are pipe-fitters working with asbestos insulation, etc.

Mesothelioma can have an indolent course, but when it grows rapidly, it is commonly fatal.

In mesothelioma the standard of care is cisplatin with pemetrexed. Pemetrexed is a multi-target (3 enzymes) anti-folate drug which inhibits DNA synthesis. This drug combination has a 41% response rate, with an average survival of 12 months.

Targets of therapy: NFkB, COX-2, P13K/Akt, PTEN.

I have seen good responses in mesothelioma with the product Oncolyn, presumably due to COX-2 inhibition, increasing apoptosis and reducing cell proliferation. I prefer to substitute green tea EGCG, omega 3 oils, curcumin and grapeseed extract. Indole-3-carbinol, quercetin and isoflavones help support the PTEN tumour suppressor gene.

NATUROPATHIC TREATMENT OPTIONS IN LUNG CANCER

Targets of therapy: mitochondrial rescue, EGFR, HER-1 and HER-2, MAPK, P13K/Akt, VEGF and angiogenesis, tyrosine kinase receptor inhibitors, COX-2, NFkB, IL-6, IGF-1, FGFR, retinoid receptor and farnesyl transferase (ras) inhibitors.

Special attention is paid to control of inflammation and the correct anti-oxidants. Emphasize COX-2 inhibitors, angiogenesis inhibitors, and inhibitors of NFkB.

*ALKYLGLYCEROLS – from shark liver oil inhibit angiogenesis and protein tyrosine kinases.

*ALPHA LIPOIC ACID – R+ ALA inhibits NFkB, anti-oxidant, detoxifier, induces apoptosis.

ARTEMESININ – to control tumour iron. Also avoid red meat. Support with DHA, lactoferrin and black tea (with no milk), at meals.

*ASTRAGALUS – a TCM chi tonic herb, often found in liquid extracts with ginseng, significantly enhances survival with small cell lung cancer. Astragalus-based herbal formulas improve survival and reduce harm when combined with platinum-based chemotherapy .

*CAN-ARREST – COX-2 inflammation inhibitors. Curcumin inhibits COX-2 and mTOR.

*CO-ENZYME Q-10 – restores apoptosis via mitochondria rescue, and more.

CORIOLUS – mushroom extract PSP or PSK slows progression of NSCLC, especially in combination with radiation and chemotherapy. Maitake is NOT useful in lung cancers.

ELLAGIC ACID – from berries, pomegranate juice.

GENISTEIN – soy genestein inhibits protein tyrosine kinases and topoisomerases.

**GRAPESEED EXTRACT – antioxidant in the high oxygen environments of the lungs and brain. In cancers the OPCs and resveratrol increase apoptosis, decrease angiogenesis, and inhibit tumour DNA synthesis. Also a robust anti-inflammatory.

*GREEN TEA EGCG – anti-angiogenic, mTOR inhibitor, and much more.

HOMEOPATHY – *Acidum hydrocyanicum, Argentum nitricum, Carcinosum, Cobaltum, Kalium bichromatum, Lachesis mutus, Lycopodium, Oxalic acidum, Scirrhinum, Tuberculinum.*

*INDOLE-3-CARBINOL – causes tumour cell cycle arrest via cyclin kinases, mTOR inhibitor.

L-CARNITINE – is used by FABNOs for bio-energetic regulation.

LIU WEI DI HUANG WAN – for deficient lung yin, as in small cell cancer. Enhances chemotherapy and radiation therapy outcomes. Cools the fires of inflammation.

*MELATONIN – stabilizes cases with no liver mets and not more than one brain met. Significantly increases survival and time until progression. Tumour response rate and one year survival doubles by combining melatonin with chemotherapy.

*MILK THISTLE – anti-angiogenic plus it strongly inhibits epidermal growth factor EGF and its receptor EGFR.

*MISTLETOE – Iscador or Helixor mistletoe lectins stabilize disease, improve quality of life, and extend survival.

Use Iscador Qu or Helixor A for men, and M type for women

MITOCHONDRIAL RESCUE – R+ alpha lipoic acid, thiamine, L-carnitine, D-ribose, CoQ-10 and omega 3 oils.

N-ACETYL-CYSTEINE – NAC is mucolytic and a lung protectant antioxidant, but it can act against pro-apoptotic therapies. NOT RECOMMENDED

OMEGA 3 OILS – Rx 1,200 mg each of EPA and DHA, while cutting all omega 6 fats such as red meat and corn oil.

POMEGRANATE – anthocyanidins and tannins in pomegranate fruit and juice inhibit tumour progression.

*REISHI – mushroom extract inhibits NFkB and thus COX-2, especially raised in small cell lung cancer SCLC.

*RESVERATROL – inhibitor of NFkB, antioxidant which modulates MnSOD, anti-angiogenic, pro-apoptotic and regulator of cyclin-dependent kinases.

SHIH CHUAN DA BU WAN – reduces metastasis.

SMOKING CESSATION – to quit smoking take L-glutamine or Thorne research Sulfonil to reduce cravings. Take grapeseed extract OPCs and N-acetyl-cysteine to neutralize toxins. Homeopathic *Tabacum* 6C is detoxifying, and may be included in the calming tincture of oat straw *Avena sativa*. Be nice to yourself.

I like to "staple" the ear acupuncture points Shen men, Liver and Lung, or for the weaker patient I may apply silver magrain pellets, which do not break the skin. TCM acupuncture points include LI-4, LI-20, ST-36, LV-3, PC-6, and the great trilogy at the radial wrist: LU-7, extra point Tim Mee, and a delicate puncture of "Dr. Cheung's Secret Point" which enters above LI-5 and is directed down to the Lung meridian to LU-9 at the wrist crease.

THYMUS – Thymuline, Thymosin, thymus extracts oral or intravenous.

VACCINES – Lung targeted viral or bacterial vaccines; for example Pneumovax.

VITAMIN C – pro-oxidant and pro-apoptotic when used in high intravenous doses.

*VITAMIN D3 – regulates differentiation, stem cell remediation. High intake gives four times better survival in NSCLC. It improves immune function and reduces risk of death "from all causes."

* VITAMIN E – lung protectant, anti-oxidant in high oxygen tissues. Alpha-tocopherol is the most active form.

A successful protocol for NSCLC from Dr. Mark Gignac, ND, FABNO and attributed to Jeanne Drisco, MD.

This illustrates the American style of integrative care, using the best of naturopathic and medical oncology:

- Taxol with Carboplatin chemo every 1 to 3 weeks
- IV Vitamin C – 25 to 50 grams concurrent with the chemo infusions.
- curcumin – 3 to 6 grams daily
- melatonin- 20 mg twice daily
- genestein – 125 mg 4 times daily

- resveratrol – 125 mg 4 times daily
- vitamin D3 – 5000 IU twice daily
- green tea extract – 2 capsules twice daily

Chapter Fourteen – Integrative Care Of Ovarian Cancer

EPIDEMIOLOGY

The cause is unknown, but ovarian cancer is associated with cancers of the breast, colon, or uterus; p53 gene over-expression; obesity, hypertension, diabetes; nulliparity or low parity, infertility, ovarian cysts, ovulatory drugs; exposure to talcum powder in the perineal area, antihistamines, antidepressant drugs, benzodiazepine tranquilizers, hair dyes; sedentary lifestyle, and lack of sunlight.

5 to 10% of cases are familial.BRAC-1 and BRAC-2 mutations account for about 15% of cases, with 2 in 3 showing serous type tumours.

Age at onset is typically 55 to 59.

Prolonged unopposed estrogen replacement therapy (without progesterone) increases risk 80% after 10 to 19 years of use. Risk is reduced after taking oral contraceptives more than 5 years, tubal ligation, breast feeding, pregnancy and early menopause.

Non-steroidal anti-inflammatory drugs NSAIDs such as acetaminophen, taken long term, reduce risk by 22- 28%

Aspirin 3 times per week reduces risk 40%, possibly by cyclooxygenase inhibition.

Statin drugs decrease risk and increase survival time.

Alcohol intake raises risk, but this can be reduced by intake of high-folate foods such as green leafy vegetables, or a folate supplement.

Diets high in saturated fat, eggs, milk and cholesterol raise risk, while legumes and vegetables are protective. Vitamin E and C at low doses reduce risk by 60%. Tea drinking lowers risk in a dose-dependent manner, about 18% per daily cup

Ginkgo biloba extract taken for at least 6 months reduces risk of non-mucinous ovarian cancer by 60% .Ginkgo has been shown to reduce OC cell growth rate *in vitro*.

Metastasis into the abdominal cavity is common even with small tumours, so most ovarian cancers are at an advanced stage when diagnosed. There is a 75% reoccurrence rate, and recurrent tumours tend to be very drug-resistant.

Prognosis is improved when the tumour is debulked before chemo, often by surgery, sometimes by radiation.

5-year survival is about 33 - 55%. Surgery and chemo often produce a remission, but relapses are common by

1½-2 years. Relapse within 6 months shows a very dangerous tumour.

Advanced, aggressive and metastatic disease usually involves increased cytoplasmic clusterin, which is anti-apoptotic. Anti-apoptotic protein Bcl-2 is elevated about 10-fold in cases of ovarian cancer.

SIGNS & SYMPTOMS

Symptoms are non-specific, and include vague pelvic or abdominal discomfort, abdominal swelling or bloating, indigestion, urinary frequency, urinary urgency, irregular menses, abnormal vaginal bleeding, blood clots, ascites, diarrhea, constipation, appetite changes, weight loss, shortness of breath, fatigue, back pain. Palpable abdominal masses under 8 cm. in premenopausal women are usually benign. If a lumpy mass persists over 2 months, appears to grow, or develops after menopause, it should be investigated as ovarian cancer.

SCREENING & DIAGNOSIS

Pelvic exam may be followed by abdominal or transvaginal ultrasound. CT or PET scans are sometimes done.

Tumour markers include **Ca-125**, alpha feto-protein AFP, human chorionic gonadotropin HCG, lysophosphatidic acid LPA, serum glycoprotein YLK-40, apo-lipoprotein A-1, truncated transthyretin, and cleavage fragment 4 from inter-alpha-trypsin inhibitory heavy chain H4, interleukin eighteen IL-18, and fibroblast growth factor two FGF-2.

The risk of malignancy index RMI is calculated as a product of CA-125 level, an ultrasound score, and a score for the patient's menopausal status.

An experimental screening test for early detection developed at Yale achieved 95% specificity by combining tests for four serum proteins : prolactin, leptin, osteopontin and IGF-2. Now two more protein biomarkers – macrophage inhibitory factor MIF and Ca-125 have been added, improving specificity of the 6 marker test to 99.4%.

HISTOLOGICAL TYPES

80 to 90% of ovarian cancers are epithelial adenocarcinomas. Stromal tumours are rare.

Clear cell variant has the poorest prognosis

Germ cell tumours account for less than 5%, arise in teens to early 20's, aggressive but amenable to chemotherapy

Low malignant potential tumours – rare indolent low-grade serous carcinomas have a 5 year survival rate of over 60%, but are unresponsive to chemotherapy. Generally these are fatal by about 10 years. Most of these tumours have mutations in BRAF or KRAS genes associated with kinase signalling cascades.

STAGING

Stage I – 15% of cases, disease is limited to ovaries. Survival is 70 – 90%

Stage II – 15% of cases, there is extension of disease into pelvic tissues

Stage III – 65% of cases, peritoneal implants, which spread by local extension into the omentum, diaphragm and the liver. 5 year survival is about 20-30%.

Stage IV – 5% of cases, distant metastases. Stage IV median survival time is 13.4 months, median progression free survival is 7.1 months. Overall survival to 5 years is about 8%.

SURGERY

Debulking, oophorectomy or total abdominal hysterectomy (TAH). After a second-look laparoscopy, check CBC, chemscreen and CA-125 quarterly for at least 2 years.

RADIATION

External beam sources or local radioactive phosphorus. Seldom used due to complications like GI enteritis, liver function changes, pulmonary fibrosis, and loss of haematogenous marrow. Can be considered for palliation of metastatic disease.

CHEMOTHERAPY

Commonly used agents are cisplatin, taxol, carboplatin, adriamycin, cyclophosphamide, and Topotecan. Liposomal doxorubicin (Adriamycin) is also used. About 20% of cases fail to respond to primary chemotherapy. 40 to 50% relapse within 2 years of primary therapy. Cancers which relapse within 6 months are generally unresponsive to further chemotherapy. Only 15 to 20% respond to second-line chemo, and none are cured. Naturopathic integrative supports can improve these dismal statistics.

Intavenous cisplatin is sometimes augmented with intraperitoneal cisplatin, put directly into the tummy, which penetrates right into the cancerous tissue about 1 - 2 mm or 6 - 8 cell layers.

Post-chemo Ca-125 predicts risk of relapse:

≤ 10 predicts 24 months median progression-free survival
11 to 20   17 months MPFS
21 to 35   7 months MPFS

HORMONAL THERAPY

Anti-estrogens, anti-androgens, gonadal releasing hormone GNRH analogues are palliative treatments of last resort for patients who have failed cytotoxic chemotherapy. Response rates are only 4 -15%. .

IMMUNOTHERAPIES

IL-2, IP LAK cells, interferon, BCG, monoclonal antibodies. Mouse studies show good responses to a combination of EGFR antibody with photodynamic therapy.

I consider mistletoe therapy to be a potent immune modulator in ovarian cancer.

Dendritic cell processing of ovarian cancer antigens is blocked by tumour production of the immuno-suppressive interleukin ten IL-10.

NATUROPATHIC TREATMENT OPTIONS IN OVARIAN CANCER

Targets of therapy: HER-2 and EGFR, VEGF and angiogenesis, Bcl-2, MMP-2, P13K /Akt /mTOR pathway, IL-8, MYC oncogene, NFkB, aromatase, TGFβ-1.

BROMELAIN – a proteolytic enzyme from pineapple stems which targets CD44 tumour cell receptor, EGFR, Ras and filamin to control tumour growth, progression, and metastasis.

CLA – conjugated linoleic acid; preferably <u>not</u> derived from dairy foods.

*CURCUMIN – dose-dependent toxicity to OC cells, induces apoptosis by decreasing anti-apoptotic protein Bcl-2.

FLAXSEED – lectins modulate hormones through sex hormone binding globulins.

*GENESTEIN – see SOY

GINGKO BILOBA – prevents occurrence, regulates circulation.

GINSENG – dose-dependent inhibition of growth of OC cells by RH2 ginsenosides. Enhances response to cisplatin.

GLUTHIONE – reduces cisplatin neurotoxicity, improves chemo responses. Give intravenous glutathione or oral precursors such as N-acetyl cysteine, HMS 90 whey extract or milk thistle extract.

*GRAPESEED EXTRACT – grapeseed oligomeric proanthocyanidins are an aromatase inhibitor, COX-2 inhibitor, epidermal growth factor EGF inhibitor, and more.

*GREEN TEA EGCG – enhances Adriamycin uptake by OC cells, improving chemo response while inhibiting metastases. MMP-2 inhibitor, anti-angiogenic, and much more.

HOMEOPATHY – Aurum muriaticum natronatum, Lachesis mutus, Lilium tigrum, Pulsatilla anemone.

*INDOLE-3-CARBINOL – a component of the cabbage family of vegetables which converts estrogens into mild forms which cannot stimulate tumour growth. Induces cell cycle arrest, apoptosis, and growth inhibition.

LYCOPENE – 6 to 30 mg prevents and treats OC.

*MELATONIN – enhances IL-2 and chemotherapy responses. Reduces chemo toxicity. Improves quality of life and control in cases where no standard treatment is available.

*MILK THISTLE – dose-dependent inhibition of OC; potentiates cisplatin and Adriamycin responses.

MISTLETOE – Iscador or Helixor M type injectable mistletoe lectins are a vital biological response modifier BRM. Supports chemo and radiation.

MORINDA OLEIFERA – the "drumstick tree" yields isothiocyanates and glucosinolates.

MUSHROOM POLYSACCHARIDES – shitake lentinan corrects OC resistance to cisplatin or 5-FU. Coriolus PSK increases IL-2 by 2.5 fold, and also augments cisplatin therapy.

OMEGA 3 OILS – anti-inflammatory.

*QUERCETIN – dose-dependent inhibition of OC, down-regulates OC cell signal transduction, binds to type II estrogen receptors, aromatase inhibitor, inhibits high aerobic glycolysis, arrests OC cells in G0-G1 phase, inhibits development of heat shock proteins. Synergistic with both cisplatin and genestein.

RED RICE YEAST- extract contains a natural statin drug. Statins are associated with increased survival in epithelial ovarian cancers.

*RESVERATROL – as an MMP-2 inhibitor, reduces invasion and spread.

SELENIUM – is cytotoxic to ovarian cancer cells. Improves Taxol and Adriamycin responses by managing oxidative stress.

*SOY – inhibits hormone responsive tumours; enhances actions of chemo drugs, radiation, and quercetin; protease inhibitors block OC cell urokinase, inhibiting invasiveness. Soy isoflavones block IL-6 production and promote transforming growth factor beta TGFß which reduces ovarian cancer cell proliferation and viability by an estrogen dependent pathway. Protein supports metabolism and repair. Genestein reduces Cisplatin chemotherapy resistance, increases the cytotoxic effect 33 to 43%.

VITAMIN A – vitamin A and retinoic acids induce differentiation, apoptosis and control cell proliferation, including stem cells.

VITAMIN D3 – synergistic with vitamin A. Many ovarian tumours are rich in vitamin D receptors, and OC is more common in areas with less sunlight.

VITAMIN E SUCCINATE – by injection only, this non-antioxidant (redox neutral) form of d-alpha vitamin E is active against cancers, possibly via mitochondrial rescue.

ZEEL – as an MMP-2 inhibitor and anti-inflammatory, *Zeel* homeopathic combination, or *Hormeel*.

Chapter Fifteen – Integrative Care Of Uterine, Cervical & Vulvar Cancers

CERVICAL CANCER

The widespread use of the Pap smear has reduced the death rate in North America from cancer of the cervix of the uterus. This valuable screening test was developed by Dr. George Papanicolaou in the 1930's.

Squamous cell disease appears to be triggered by the sexually transmitted human papilloma virus HPV, particularly strains HPV-16 and HPV-18. This virus causes "genital warts" – cauliflower-like warts on any body part used sexually. The disease process does not stop with spontaneous clearance of the warts.

The virus is particularly carcinogenic in association with an impaired tumour-specific T-cell response and an increase in immune suppressor cells.

It now appears that HPV screening tests, at 96% sensitivity, outperforms the PAP cytology test, at 56% sensitivity, for detecting risk of cervical intra-epithelial neoplasia CIN and cervical cancer.

A new bivalent L-1 virus-like-particle VLP vaccine against strains HPV 16 and 18 is now available. This is expected to prevent up to 70% of cervical cancers. It appears reasonably safe and effective, and is being administered to pre-pubescent girls. I can reduce cancer incidence by 92%. It can also eradicate chronic infections in 95% of cases. It is possible to get cervical cancer from HPV strains 31, 33, 45, 52 and 58, which are not covered by this vaccine. It is also possible to get other life-threatening or life-damaging sexual diseases if one is not practicing safe-sex techniques.

There is a strong association with smoking tobacco, as the cervical mucus can secrete concentrates of cigarette carcinogens 10 to 20 times higher than seen in the blood. Risk of activation of cancer from HPV rises sharply in smokers.

Birth control pills in a person with folate deficiency is a risk. Always take a B-vitamin complex if on birth control pills.

The presence of E-cadherin predicts higher risk of re-occurrence and metastasis.

5-year survival is about 70.5% This disease is quite rugged when advanced, so please treat it aggressively. Use the preventative, screening and early intervention techniques that are available!

SIGNS & SYMPTOMS

Warning signs include:
- abnormal bleeding – which may only be on contact, i.e. provoked by intercourse or medical examination..
- A foul or bloody vaginal discharge.
- Ulceration of the cervix.

- Pain in the back or pelvis.
- Unexplained weight loss.

A Pap smear of grade IV is severe dysplasia, strongly suspicious for carcinoma in situ. Pre-invasive stages are slow-growing and usually asymptomatic. A Pap grade of V is invasive squamous cell carcinoma. 95% of biopsies will have human papilloma virus.

Polyps on the cervix are rarely (1%) cancerous.

ALLOPATHIC TREATMENT OF CERVICAL CANCER

Allopathic treatment may follow a Pap test or biopsy guided by colposcopy. The conal biopsy technique removes localized cancer, and the cervical stump remains satisfactory for childbearing. Invasive cancer requires more radical surgery. Early treatment by surgery can be curative. However, it is resistant to cure once it has spread.

Radiation may be by implants, brachytherapy or external beam. The adjacent vagina, bladder and bowels are susceptible to inflammation and fibrosis from radiotherapy.

NATUROPATHIC CARE OF CERVICAL CANCER

Targets of Therapy: HPV, E-cadherin, EGFR, immune imbalance.

DHEA – Dehydroepiandrosterone DHEA strongly inhibits the proliferation and induces the death of HPV-positive and HPV-negative cervical cancer cells through an androgen- and estrogen-receptor independent mechanism.

ESCHAROTICS – "Vaginal depletion packs" made by Eclectic Institute are professional naturopathic escharotics which can cure squamous cell carcinoma in situ. Active principles are vitamin A, oil of *bitter orange*, tea tree oil *Melaleuca cajeputi*, *Thuja occidentalis, Hydrastis, Phytolacca*, and magnesium salts. Dr. Tori Hudson, N.D. adds zinc chloride and *Sanguinaria*. The cervix may be cleaned with hydrogen peroxide and pre-treated with proteolytic enzymes before using the Vag-Pack paste. Repeat the Pap smear 3 months after treatment. Clinical studies have demonstrated a very high rate of remission. Dr. John Bastyr, ND used an escharotic of 1 part saturated zinc chloride (ZnCl) to 3 parts tincture of *Sanguinaria*. The cervix is prepared with bromelain or chymotrypsin enzymes, rinsed with *Calendula* succus (marigold juice), painted with escharotic, including the endocervical canal, then rinsed with *Calendula* succus after the abnormal tissue has blanched (turned white).

FLAXSEED – lectins modulate hormones through sex hormone binding globulins.

FOLATE – or folic acid from green leafy vegetables donates methyl groups to silence oncogene mutations such as Ras or BRAC2. 5 to 10 milligrams daily can reverse early cervical dysplasia, and reduces carcinogenesis risk from human papilloma virus HPV types 16 and 18.

*GRAPESEED EXTRACT – grapeseed oligomeric proanthocyanidins are aromatase inhibitor, and modulate cell adhesion molecule signalling.

*GREEN TEA EGCG – enhances Adriamycin uptake by OC cells, improving chemo response while inhibiting metastases. MMP-2 inhibitor, anti-angiogenic, and much more. Green tea extract can be applied directly onto cervical lesions.

*HOMEOPATHY – *Aurum muriaticum natronatum, Lachesis mutus, Lilium tigrum, Engystol.*

*INDOLE-3-CARBINOL – a component of the cabbage family of vegetables which converts estrogens into mild forms which cannot stimulate tumour growth. Also has several other anti-cancer effects such as cell cycle arrest, apoptosis, and growth inhibition. Dr. Maria Bell, M.D. an oncologist at the University of South Dakota Medical Center has reported dramatic results with indole-3-carbinol I3C – in 12 weeks complete regression of stage 2 and 3 cervical cancer in 4 of 8 women dosed at 200 mg. daily, and 4 of 9 dosed at 400 mg daily. Those receiving placebo had no improvement.

*MELATONIN – enhances IL-2 and chemotherapy responses. Reduces chemo toxicity. Improves quality of life and control in cases where no standard treatment is available.

MISTLETOE – injectable M type mistletoe lectins activate the immune response and destroy viruses.

PSYCHOLOGY – Dr. Christiane Northrup, M.D., author of *Women's Bodies, Women's Wisdom* suggests that low self-esteem, religious shame about sexuality, and passive or pessimistic reactions to stress can set the stage for more severe disease.

*QUERCETIN – down-regulates cell signal transduction: e-cadherins predict risk of metastasis and reoccurrence. Aromatase inhibitor, binds to type II estrogen receptors, inhibits high aerobic glycolysis, arrests cells in G0-G1 phase, inhibits development of heat shock proteins.

*REISHI – *Ganoderma* mushroom extracts support immune control of HPV. Quality mushroom products such as Aloha Medicinals *Immune Assist* can also be used.

SELENOMETHIONINE – is cytotoxic to cancer cells. Improves Taxol and Adriamycin responses by managing oxidative stress.

*STEROLS & STEROLINS – suppress human papilloma virus HPV. This immune modulator balances the helper-suppressor T-cell ratio and thus the tumour-specific response. Most persistent HPV infections are associated with concurrent exposure to *Chlamydia trachomatis*. I prescribe Vitazan brand *Ultra-Immune*.

*VITAMIN A – Vitamin A palmitate, retinoic acids and beta carotene in very high doses strongly re-differentiate these cancers. To support apoptosis and control cell proliferation, including tumorigenic stem cells. Carotenes may be given to 200,000 units daily, and vitamin A at 50,000 I.U. or more daily, under close supervision by a physician.

VITAMIN B6 and B12 – manage energy production and cell growth. Supportive of folate biochemistry.

*VITAMIN C – for all viral dependent cancers. IVC, or oral doses to 12 grams daily or to bowel tolerance.

VITAMIN D3 – synergistic with vitamin A to control stem cell differentiation.

*ZINC – zinc citrate helps regulate squamous cell cancers, inhibits COX-2.

Oral HPV Protocol from NCNM:

- Folic acid -10 mg
- Vitamin C – 6 grams
- Carotenoids – 150,000 IU
- Green tea extract 500 mg
- Indole-3-carbinol or DIM – 200 to 300 mg
- 60 drops 3 times daily of tinctures of:
    Echinacea – 2 parts
    Hypericum – 2 parts
    Mahonia – 1 part
    Lomatium – 1 part
    Thuja – 1 part
    Thymus – 1 part

UTERINE CANCER

Often an adenocarcinoma of the glandular epithelium of the corpus uteri – the endometrium. It is linked to exposure to unopposed estrogen. Early onset and late end of menses is a risk, as is obesity, polycystic ovary syndrome, birth control pills, hypertension and diabetes. Progesterone is protective, and can be used to reverse simple hyperplasia without atypia.

Genetic mutations include PTEN loss with resultant activation of the P13K / Akt / mTOR pathway.

Early warning signs include spotting of blood between menses (metrorrhagia), any post-menopausal vaginal bleeding, colicky abdominal pains, backache, leg edema, weight loss, and there can be a cough with bloody phlegm (haemoptysis).

5-year survival is about 84%.

NATUROPATHIC CARE OF UTERINE CANCER

Targets of therapy: P13K / Akt / mTOR pathway, e-cadherins, angiogenesis, aromatase, inflammation.

*ALPHA LIPOIC ACID – R+ ALA inhibits heat shock protein and induces apoptosis.

BETA-CAROTENE – Pro-vitamin A, supports redifferentiation, pro-apoptotic.

*CURCUMIN – mTOR inhibitor, anti-inflammatory.

FLAXSEED – lectins modulate hormones through sex hormone binding globulins.

FOLATE – or folic acid from green leafy vegetables donates methyl groups to silence oncogene mutations such as Ras or BRAC2. 5 to 10 milligrams daily can reverse early cervical dysplasia, and reduces carcinogenesis risk from human papilloma virus HPV types 16 & 18.

*GREEN TEA EGCG – enhances Adriamycin uptake by OC cells, improving chemo response while inhibiting metastases. MMP2 inhibitor, anti-angiogenic, mTOR inhibitor, and much more.

HOMEOPATHY – Aurum muriaticum natronatum, Lachesis mutus, Lilium tigrum.

*INDOLE-3-CARBINOL – a component of the cabbage family of vegetables which converts estrogens into mild forms which cannot stimulate tumour growth. Also has several other anti-cancer effects such as cell cycle arrest, apoptosis, growth inhibition and mTOR signalling pathway inhibitor. Dr. Maria Bell, M.D. an oncologist at the University of South Dakota Medical Center has reported dramatic results with indole-3-carbinol (I3C), seeing in 12 weeks complete regression of stage 2 and 3 cervical cancer in 4 of 8 women dosed at 200 mg. daily, and 4 of 9 dosed at 400 mg daily. Those receiving placebo had no improvement.

*MELATONIN – enhances IL-2 and chemotherapy responses. Reduces chemo toxicity. Improves quality of life and control in cases where no standard treatment is available.

MISTLETOE – M type lectins are potent immune modulators.

PSYCHOLOGY – Dr. Christiane Northrup, M.D., author of *Women's Bodies, Women's Wisdom* suggests that low self-esteem, religious shame about sexuality, and passive or pessimistic reactions to stress can set the stage for more severe disease.

*QUERCETIN – down-regulates cell signal transduction and e-cadherins to reduce risk of metastasis and reoccurrence. Aromatase inhibitor, binds to type II estrogen receptors, inhibits high aerobic glycolysis, arrests cells in G0-G1 phase, inhibits development of heat shock proteins and is anti-angiogenic.

REISHI – *Ganoderma* mushroom extracts support immune control of HPV.

SELENOMETHIONINE – is cytotoxic to cancer cells. Improves Taxol and Adriamycin responses by managing oxidative stress.

STEROLS & STEROLINS – suppress human papilloma virus HPV. Most persistent HPV infections are associated with concurrent exposure to *Chlamydia trachomatis*. Target inflammation and angiogenesis in all squamous cell cancers.

VITAMIN A – Vitamin A palmitate, retinoic acids and beta carotene in very high doses strongly re-differentiate these cancers. To support apoptosis and control cell proliferation, including tumorigenic stem cells. Carotenes may be given to 200,000 units daily, and vitamin A at 50,000 I.U. or more daily, under close supervision by a physician.

VITAMIN B6 and B12 – manage energy production and cell growth, and support folate metabolism.

VITAMIN C – supports healing.

VITAMIN D3 – synergistic with vitamin A to control stem cell differentiation.

ZINC – zinc citrate helps regulate squamous cell cancers, inhibits COX-2.

An American colleague suggests this protocol for atypical endometrial hyperplasia:

- One week juice fast
- Vegan diet, supplemented with MediClear protein
- Vitamin A 50,000 IU daily
- Mixed tocopherols
- DHEA 10 mg twice daily
- Progesterone cream 2 weeks per month, 25 mg dose applied to the inner labia

VULVAR CANCER

Associated with human papilloma virus HPV and smoking. Survival rates are good if the tumour is under 4.0 cm. and there is no nodal involvement.

NATUROPATHIC CARE OF VULVAR CANCER

Survival rates are good if the tumour is under 4.0 cm and there is no nodal involvement.
Quit smoking!
Adjuncts to strengthen the immune system and suppress the HPV:

- sterols & sterolins
- vitamin A
- *Ganoderma lucidum* reishi mushroom extract
- *Una de Gato* or cat's claw vine
- Mistletoe M type lectins

Chapter Sixteen – Integrative Care Of Upper Digestive Tract Cancers

ESOPHAGUS

Risk factors for esophageal cancer include alcohol, tobacco, fungal toxins, pickled and preserved foods, red meat, and deficiencies of vitamins and minerals.

Asians and some others are known to often get a very red and flushed face from drinking alcohol. This is linked to aldehyde dehydrogenase ALDH-2 deficiency. It is now linked to increased risk for esophageal cancer. This risk can be moderated with selenomethionine.

p63 gene expression is elevated early in squamous cell esophageal cancer. This homologue of the tumour suppressor gene p53 probably plays a role in the development of this cancer.

Squamous cell cancers are frequently associated with the human papilloma virus HPV.

Early detection is rare, lateral invasion and metastasis can occur very early, so most are diagnosed with disseminated disease. Metastasis is usually to the lungs, liver, bones and kidneys.

First signs may be dysphagia, substernal pain, hoarse voice, coughing provoked by eating or drinking, haemorrhage and anemia.

Allopathic treatment begins with surgery, and may add adjunctive or palliative chemotherapy with 5-fluorouracil, cisplatin and mitomycin.

Radiation is often used in palliation.

5-year survival is about 14%, making this one of the deadliest types of cancer.

NATUROPATHIC and INTEGRATIVE CARE OF ESOPHAGEAL CANCER

Targets of therapy: IGF-1, EGFR, PTKs, HPV, IL-10, IL-16, SRC-3, p53 repair and p63 modulation.

ACUPUNCTURE – for dysphagia needle LV 3, LI 4, CV 21, 23 and 24.

ALOE – Aloe vera leaf gel mixed into juice is a vulnerary, healing wounds and inflammation. It mildly inhibits tumour growth. Take up to 2 ounces daily. Aloe juice and root are more laxative.

ALKYLGLYCEROLS – from shark liver oil will inhibit protein tyrosine kinases.

*ALPHA LIPOIC ACID – R+ ALA inhibits IGF-1, promotes apoptosis.

CORIOLUS – PSK or PSP mushroom extract significantly extends survival and improves quality of life.

*CURCUMIN – COX-2 and MMP-3 inhibitor, blocks growth and invasion.

FARE YOU – cabbage extract heals ulceration and inflammation, regulates apoptosis.

*GRAPESEED EXTRACT – grapeseed OPCs inhibit IGF-1, EGF, and angiogenesis, regulates p53.

*GREEN TEA EGCG – Blocks the insulin-like growth factor IGF-1 receptor, inhibits MMP-3, anti-angiogenic, protein tyrosine kinase inhibitor, and much more.

HOMEOPATHY –*Aurum muriaticum, Condurango, Gallium aparense, Hydrastis canadensis.*

INDOLE-3-CARBINOL – regulates transcription factors, induces cell cycle arrest and apoptosis.

*LIU WEI DI HUANG WAN – benefits yin, significantly improves survival. Yi Qi Yang Yin Wan can also be used, as indicated by TCM diagnosis.

*MILK THISTLE – Silibinin inhibits EGFR and PTKs responsible for esophageal cancer growth.

MISTLETOE – Use Iscador Qu or Helixor A for males and M type for females.

QUERCETIN – induces apoptosis via mitochondria, controls tumorigenic stem cells, modulates hormone signals.

REISHI – mushroom extract inhibits protein tyrosine kinase signals, inhibits NFkB.

SELENOMETHIONINE – improves survival.

*STEROLS and STEROLINS – inhibit human papilloma virus HPV.

*VITAMIN A – regulates differentiation, anti-viral.

*ZINC CITRATE – inhibits COX-2, prevents and treats oral and esophageal cancer.

STOMACH CANCER

Gastric cancer is a non-polyposis colorectal spectrum disease. Stomach cancer is usually an adenocarcinoma.

Risk factors include low intake of fruit and vegetables, high intake of dietary nitrites, pickled and preserved food; a history of pernicious anemia, atrophic gastritis, gastric ulcer, adenomas and family history of cancer of the stomach.

Early signs can include anorexia, early satiety, nausea, vomiting, epigastric discomfort mimicking peptic ulcer, anemia, and disseminated intravascular coagulation with consequent bruising and bleeding.

Surgery is followed by radiation, or chemotherapy with 5-fluorouracil, doxorubicin, methotrexate, cisplatin and etoposide.

5-year survival is only about 24% with allopathic care alone.

Signal transducers and activators or transcription STAT-3 expression indicates a poorer prognosis.

There is an increased risk of reoccurrence in those with CD44 polymorphisms. High CD44 expression increase resistance to chemo and radiation, and poorer prognosis, as this protein confers stem cell-like properties.

A new treatment has increased median survival from 3.8 months to 10.3 months, using a vaccination with diphtheria toxoid and gastrin-17 peptide. This mirrors Dr. Hal

Gunn's concept of tissue-targeted vaccines.

NATUROPATHIC CARE OF STOMACH CANCER

Targets of therapy: EGF, EGFR, AP-1, FGF, Keratinocyte-GF, TGFß, STAT-3, SRC-3, CD44.

ALOE – *Aloe vera* leaf gel mixed into juice is a vulnerary, healing wounds and inflammation. It mildly inhibits tumour growth. Take up to 2 ounces daily. Aloe juice and root are more laxative.

*ALPHA LIPOIC ACID – R+ ALA inhibits TGFß, regulates apoptosis via mitochondria.

BERBERINE – antimicrobial & cytostatic alkaloid found in Barberry, Oregon Grape root, Coptis and Scute.

CORIOLUS – PSK or PSP mushroom extract significantly extends survival and improves quality of life.

*CURCUMIN – COX-2 and MMP-3 inhibitor, blocks growth and invasion. Inhibits EGF and AP-1.

ELLAGIC ACID – Pomegranate, berries, grapes – detoxifies nitrosamines and fungal toxins.

FARE YOU – cabbage extract heals ulceration and inflammation, regulates apoptosis.

*GRAPESEED – Grapeseed extract OPCs: inhibit EGF.

**GREEN TEA EGCG – Blocks the insulin-like growth factor IGF-1 receptor, inhibits MMP-3, anti-angiogenic, inhibits AP-1, and inhibits DNA turn-over enzymes ADA and XO.

HOMEOPATHY – *Aceticum acidum, Aurum muriaticum, Cadmium metallicum, Cadmium sulphate, Condurango, Hydrastis canadensis.*

INDOLE-3-CARBINOL – regulates transcription factors, induces cell cycle arrest and apoptosis, regulates mucins.

LICORICE ROOT – *Glycyrrhiza uralensis* extract induces apoptosis in gastric carcinoma cells, and strongly inhibits inflammation.

LIU WEI HUA JIE TANG – benefits yin and qi to significantly improve survival. Liu Wei Di Huang Wan can also be used.

*MILK THISTLE – inhibits NFkB transcription, EGFR and related TGF-α, MMP's, and IGF-1 while increasing IGFBP-3; modulates VEGF and cell cyclins.

MISTLETOE – Use Iscador Qu or Helixor A for males and M type for females.

*QUERCETIN – induces apoptosis via mitochondria, controls tumorigenic stem cells, modulates hormone signals. Inhibits EGF and AP-1.

*RESVERATROL – MMP-3 and EGF inhibitor.

SELENOMETHIONINE – inhibits AP-1.

SHIH CHUAN DA BU WAN – herbal tonic which supports blood cells and organs.

*SOY – Genestein inhibits AP-1.

VITAMIN C – inhibits *Helicobacter pylori* possessing Cag-A virulence factor, a powerful source of inflammatory growth signals.

LIVER & GALLBLADDER CANCER

Hepatic cancer is associated with hepatitis B and C viruses, cirrhosis, alcohol, red meat intake, fungal aflatoxins, anabolic steroids, and xenobiotics.

90% are hepatocellular cancers. Biopsy of hepatocellular carcinoma can trigger needle-track seeding of the cancer in about 2.7% of cases.

Biopsy or surgery on cholangiocarcinoma has a risk of provoking cancer spread of 16% or 1 in 6 cases.

The true gross pathological size of hepatomas tends to be over-estimated by CT or MRI imaging techniques.

A drop in insulin-like growth factor one IGF-1 correlates with development of hepatocellular carcinoma in cases of hepatitis-C or HCV cirrhosis.

Serum alpha-fetoprotein AFP may be elevated, and is a useful marker to follow during treatment.

Early signs can include obstructive jaundice, hepatomegaly, splenomegaly, anorexia, fatigue, belly pain, ascites, weight loss and elevated liver enzymes

Survival rates are very low – 5-year survival is only about 7.5%.

The favoured chemotherapy is doxorubicin.

Radiofrequency ablation is sometimes possible for inoperable tumours under 4 cm in diameter. They cannot be too near major blood vessels.. An umbrella-like needle array is put into the tumour, and radio waves heat the tissue to 80 -100 + degrees Celsius, causing coagulation. The killing zone is actually a 5 cm sphere. A new multi-head array can burn out an 8 cm sphere, treating tumours up to 7 cm in diameter. Percutaneous radiofrequency ablation PRF is as good as cryosurgery for initial success and complications, but is superior in preventing metastatic spread. PRF is also used for renal tumours.

Liver metastases are very common from a variety of other cancers, and are treated with surgical resection where possible, with neo-adjuvant chemotherapy.

Cryotherapy can be performed on unresectable masses, with an average freezing time of 18 minutes.

NATUROPATHIC CARE OF LIVER & GALLBLADDER CANCER

Targets of therapy: mTOR inhibition, viruses, epidermal growth factor receptor EGFR, NFkB, angiogenesis.

*ALPHA LIPOIC ACID – is an important antioxidant for liver cell membranes. Combines well with vitamins C, E, selenium, grapeseed OPCs, and other antioxidants.

*ASTRAGALUS – Controls viruses such as EBV and HVC. An essential component of *Shih Chuan Da Bu Wan*.

BERBERINE – antimicrobial alkaloid found in Barberry, Oregon Grape root, Coptis and Scute. Cytostatic to cancer cells.

*CURCUMIN – COX-2 and MMP3 inhibitor, blocks growth and invasion. mTOR

& NFkB inhibitor.

GABA – Gamma-amino-butyric acid inhibits cholangiocarcinoma.

GLUTATHIONE – is the central anti-oxidant in liver detoxification and metabolism. Give intravenously, or use oral precursors such as N-acetyl cysteine, milk thistle extract and selenium.

*GRAPESEED EXTRACT – OPCs modulate free radicals of oxygen and thus apoptosis. Inhibits EGF.

*GREEN TEA EGCG – Blocks the insulin-like growth factor IGF-1 receptor, inhibits MMP3, anti-angiogenic, inhibits EGFR, inhibits mTOR, and much more.

HOMEOPATHY – *Ceanothus americanus* or *virginicus, Chelidonium majus, Cholesterinum, Lycopodium.*

HOXSEY – herbal mélange supports bile flow and suppresses cancer. May be augmented with tinctures of greater celandine *Chelidonium majus*, fringe-tree *Chionanthus virginicus* and burdock root *Arctium lappa* .

*INDOLE-3-CARBINOL – regulates transcription factors, induces cell cycle arrest and apoptosis. mTOR signalling pathway inhibitor.

*MILK THISTLE – Silibinin inhibits tumour growth and detoxifies. Inhibits EGFR and related TGFß, MMPs, NFkB transcription, and IGF-1 – by increasing IGFBP-3. Modulates VEGF and cell cyclins.

**MISTLETOE –Use Iscador Qu or Helixor A for males and M type for females.

*QUERCETIN – induces apoptosis via mitochondria, controls tumorigenic stem cells, modulates hormone signals, anti-angiogenic, inhibits EGF.

*REISHI – mushroom HMWPS extract supports immune function. *Immune Assist* formula is also useful.

SELENOMETHIONINE – for liver detox and DNA repair.

UREA – reduces angiogenesis by destabilizing fibrin stroma. Maximum dose is 30 grams daily, typically Rx: 12 to 15 grams divided in 6 doses. Mix in 1 to 2 litres of water, tomato or fruit juice. to mask the bitter taste. BUN will read high on lab tests. Within 2 weeks expect weight gain, improved wellness, tumour shrinkage and improved survival prognosis.

*VITAMIN C – anti-oxidant, detox, anti-viral.

*XIAO CHAI HU TANG – Minor Bupleurum Formula can sero-convert (cure) hepatitis C virus, a cause of hepatocellular carcinoma. It has benefited stressed livers since time immemorial.

ZINC CITRATE or PICOLINATE – prevents and assists healing of gallbladder cancer.

An American FABNO once recommended for cholangio-carcinoma:
- Curcumin – to repair liver fibrosis.
- Melatonin
- Vitamin D
- GABA – up to 3 grams
- Sho Saiko i.e. Honso 09 – 1 packet 2 to 3 times daily.

CANCER of the PANCREAS

Causative factors are unclear, but there is a correlation with exposure to environmental pollutants such as poly-chlorinated biphenyls PCBs, used in transformers and fluorescent lighting ballast resistors, and common organo-chlorine solvents and pesticides.

Abnormal micro-RNA is found, promoting proto-oncogene expression, while inhibiting tumour suppressor genes. This micro-RNA differentiates a cancer of the pancreas from pancreatitis, and is a marker for tumour aggressiveness.

Methylation of the DNA must be an issue, because intake of the methyl group donor amino acid methionine is associated with drastically reduced risk.

Carriers of BRAC-2 mutations have a six-fold increased risk of pancreatic cancer.

About 90% of cases have increased expression of EGFR. kRas mutations also occur in over 90% of cases, activating the Ras-Raf signal pathway. This can increase resistance to EGFR inhibitors.

kRas controls the PKC-iota (PKCi) oncogene, essential for growth and metastasis of pancreatic cancer. PKCi is inhibited by the arthritis drug aurothiomalate.

Pancreatic cancer cells have testosterone receptors, and aromatase enzyme to convert testosterone into estrogen.

Pancreatic cancer cells over-express COX-2 by as much as 60 times normal.

Survival after surgery is 2 times greater if the tumour is negative for calcium-binding protein S100A2.

MUC-1 is an anti-apoptotic transmembrane glycoprotein mucin expressed by pancreatic cancer cells, and involved in cell to cell and cell to extracellular matrix interactions. The amount of IgG antibodies against MUC-1 circulating in the blood is a significant predictor of survival.

Asymptomatic or sub-clinical pancreatic lesions used to be called "incidentalomas," as they were thought to be innocently benign. However, we now think they are pre-malignant, with 94% carrying a risk of transformation into an invasive malignancy.

Dietary flavonols from plant foods are linked to lower risk. These are a type of flavonoid or polyphenol. The best protectors, in order of importance, are kaempferol, quercetin and myricetin. Kaempferol is found in tea and broccoli, for example, quercetin in onions and apples, and myricetin in grapes, berries, walnuts. All fruits and vegetables are rich in a variety of flavonoids.

Adequate vitamin D intake is associated with lowered risk.

Allergy problems like asthma or hay fever are associated with lower risk of pancreatic cancer. This suggests the immune system plays some role in preventing this cancer, so it may play a role in treating it too. Immune modulation with mistletoe has produced responses in some of my patients.

Early signs are often vague, such as back pain, depression, jaundice, weight loss, anorexia, hepatomegaly (swollen liver), dark urine and light coloured stool.

Most are diagnosed at about 3 cm. in diameter, but those found when under 2 cm. have a far better prognosis.

Survival is usually less than 2 years. 5-year survival is the lowest of all cancers at about 4%.

80% of cases have spread into regional lymph nodes and 70% have liver mets at presentation.

Medical treatment is largely ineffective. Surgery can only cure in the early stages. The Whipple procedure has a 15% mortality rate, and a 10% 5 year survival rate.

The only chemo drug with any impact at all is Gemcitabine. This is reasonably mild in terms of side-effects, and can extend life by some months, though some studies show only 1 month increased lifespan. Only 5% of cases get a good response with some tumour shrinkage. About 25% of cases get some stabilization or symptomatic improvement. EGFR inhibitors may sensitize to chemo-radiation.

NATUROPATHIC CARE OF PANCREATIC CANCER

Targets of therapy: STAT-3, EGFR, NFkB, COX-2, PGE-2, IGF-1, IGFR, PPARγ, kRas, PKCi oncogene, VEGF, VEGFR, MMPs, TGF, Bcl-2, SP-1, SP-3 and SP-4 transcription factors, myeloid-derived suppressor cell MDSC, tumour-associated macrophage TAM, Akt.

AHCC – mushroom mycelia compound

*ALPHA LIPOIC ACID – 300 to 600 mg IV twice weekly or oral doses of 400 to 600 mg daily of R+ time release ALA can arrest tumour growth. Inhibits TGFß. Synergistic with low-dose Naltrexone.

BROMELAIN – inhibits Ras to reduce VEGF, PDGF and FGF, inhibiting angiogenesis.

*CAN-ARREST – controls inflammation and its growth factors, such as COX-2..

CHILIS – red chili peppers contain capsaicin which inhibits inflammation in pancreas cancer.

CHIONANTHUS – *Chionanthus. virginicus* (fringe-tree) tincture treats pancreatic inflammation.

COENZYME Q-10 – rescues mitochondria by reducing lactate. This triggers apoptosis.

*CURCUMIN – COX-2 and MMP-3 inhibitor, blocks growth and invasion. Pancreatic cancer cells can have 60 times normal COX-2.

FLAXSEED – modulates hormone growth signals, anti-androgenic.

FARE YOU – methionine from green cabbage reduces progression by acting as a methyl group donor.

FOLATE – or folic acid from green leafy vegetables donates methyl groups to silence oncogene mutations such as Ras or BRAC2.

GENISTEIN – soy genestein inhibits protein tyrosine kinases and topoisomerases.

GLA – gamma linolenic acid as from evening primrose oil is very synergistic with gemcitabine chemo. Gemcitabine alone doubles disease-free interval but has only a slight effect on survival time.

*GREEN TEA EGCG – Blocks the insulin-like growth factor IGF-1 receptor. Curbs invasion via inhibition of MMP-3. Anti-angiogenic, – decreases angiogenesis and lymphangiogenesis by inhibition of kRas protein kinases. Strongly inhibits STAT-1 DNA transcription activator. Inhibits EGFR.

HOMEOPATHY – *Carduus marianum, Cadmium sulphate, Ceanothus americanus, Hydrastis canadensis, Phosphorus, Podophyllum pelatum.*

HOXSEY – herbal tonic which can support healing.

*INDOLE-3-CARBINOL – regulates DNA transcription factor STAT-3, induces cell cycle arrest and apoptosis. Regulates hormones – pancreatic cancer cells have excess testosterone receptors and aromatase. Inhibits NFkB, Akt and MMP-9.

*JINGLI NEIXAO – TCM herbal tonic arrests growth and spread while improving overall wellness QOL.

LOW-DOSE NALTREXONE – LDN is synergistic with R+ALA. Cannot be mixed with narcotics such as morphine.

*MILK THISTLE – Silibinin inhibits tumour growth and detoxifies. Active against NFkB and EGFR.

*MISTLETOE – Iscador or Helixor can dramatically improve quality of life, and extend life significantly.

MODIFIED CITRUS PECTIN – reduces metastasis risk, increases survival.

OLEANDER – *Nerium oleander* leaves contain oleandrin, a fat-soluble cardiac glycoside. Oleander is an evergreen shrub related to dogbane, laurel and *Apocynum*. Oleandrin selectively injures pancreatic cancer cells and induces autophagic death by silencing the mTOR pathway. Akt phosphorylation is inhibited, and P13 kinase as well as MAPK signalling pathways are disrupted. Oleandrin also inhibits NFkB.

*QUERCETIN – induces apoptosis via mitochondria, controls tumorigenic stem cells, modulates hormone signals, reduces ICRA, inhibits kRas, aromatase inhibitor.

*REISHI – *Ganoderma* mushroom extract strongly inhibits NFkB.

SCUTELLARIA – baicalein controls inflammation.

SELENOMETHIONINE – repairs mutations in DNA repair gene BRAC-2.

SOY GENESTEIN – modulates androgen receptors.

TAHEEBO – tea of Pau d'Arco bark can occasionally produce dramatic responses.

VITAMIN A – and carotene provitamin A support immune function and regulate stem cells.

VITAMIN B COMPLEX –supports CoQ-10 to normalize energy production.

VITAMIN C – high oral or intravenous doses support survival by depletion of glutathione in the cancer cells.

*VITAMIN D3 – regulates differentiation to control stem cells responsible for metastasis and treatment resistance. Improves survival of Whipple surgical procedure.

Emerging therapies:

HIFU – High-intensity focused ultrasound is being used by the Chinese to reduce pain and tumour size.

MUC1 – an anti-apoptotic transmembrane mucin glycoprotein associated with a poorer prognosis.

RASFONIN – from the fungus *Trichurus terrophius* inhibits mutant Ras to promote apoptosis.

TRIPHALA – 3-Dosha Ayurvedic herb formula.

EXAMPLES OF SUCCESSFUL NATUROPATHIC PROTOCOLS FOR PANCREATIC CANCER

A protocol which created 100% wellness and 100% arrest of growth and spread of unresectable pancreatic cancer:
- Iscador mistletoe injections
- milk thistle extract
- indole-3-carbinol
- quercetin -with bromelain.

A case of metastatic pancreatic cancer was completely controlled with:
- CanArrest
- indole-3-carbinol
- green tea EGCG with vitamin E
- co-enzyme Q-10
- R+ alpha lipoic acid
- milk thistle extract
- vitamin D3.

Another case became stable for a year on this program:
- Jingli neixao
- CanArrest
- indole-3-carbinol
- green tea EGCG with vitamin E
- modified citrus pectin
- flaxseed
- Greens First food supplement
- buffered vitamin C
- Vital Victoria 1-a-day multivitamin with minerals.

Chapter Seventeen – Integrative Care Of Skin Cancers

Cancer of the skin is very common, and will happen to one in five North Americans. 97% will be non-melanoma cancers with a high cure rate. 89% with the more dangerous melanoma type skin cancers will survive 5 years.

These are mostly preventable. Lipid peroxidation is a prominent feature of skin carcinogenesis. A low-fat diet is protective.

DNA damage from ultraviolet rays is a major causative factor. It used to be thought that the UV-B rays were causing all the skin cancer, but new research that implicates UV-A as a similar hazard.

UV-A:
- longer wavelength
- penetrates to the bone
- sunscreens do <u>not</u> block these rays
- causes mutation
- destroys vitamin D

UV-B:
- penetrates skin
- responsible for sunburns
- initiates vitamin D synthesis
- blocked by sunscreens
- not a strong carcinogen

This may explain why sunscreen use hasn't prevented much skin cancer, but has caused wide-spread vitamin D deficiency. Vitamin D protects against skin cancer by regulating the hedgehog and β-catenin pathways and stimulating the DNA repair response.

Sun and other UV damage can be repaired with Co-enzyme Q-10 and green tea EGCG, orally and topically. Mixed anti-oxidants with curcumin such as QuenchFX are powerful skin protectants working from the inside.

Skin repair cream ingredients that reverse skin degeneration and sun damage are rosehip oil, vitamin C, vitamin E, MSM, grapeseed extract, vitamin A, vitamin D3, betulinic acid, green tea extract and pomegranate extract.

The best on the market is NASOBIH.

Avoiding sun exposure has created rising rates of cancers far more dangerous than skin cancers, plus an epidemic of bone and joint problems such as chondropathies (cartilage destruction). Strict sun avoidance puts people more at risk of burning when exposed to the sun – the worst injury for aging and cancer. Furthermore, studies show diligent use of sunscreens has not halted the rising rate of skin cancers.

I believe the prudent course is gradual sun or ultraviolet exposure to develop the protective coloring we have evolved for our protection. In concert with a good plant-based diet, we can handle the stress of the ultraviolet light, and turn it to our advantage. Examples of dietary supports:

- quercetin from apples, onions, and most plants blocks tumour activator protein AP-1, a critical cause of malignant melanoma, the most dangerous skin cancer.
- curcumin -from the curry spice turmeric also blocks AP-1 and controls inflammation via NFkB.
- green tea polyphenols also block AP-1.
- pomegranate, grapes and all berries contain anthocyanidins which inhibit tumour formation.
- coloured vegetables and fruits – contain beta carotene and other carotenoids which repair the skin.

Specific nutraceutical supplements can provide an even greater level of protection. Grapeseed extract OPCs restore vitamin C to an unoxidized state in the skin, sufficient to prevent sunburn. Use internally and topically, i.e. the NASOBIH™ protocol – a "naturally accelerated system for outside beauty and inner health."

Sun sensitivity is amplified by human papilloma virus HPV infection.

High-risk pre-malignant skin lesions take up the dye toluidine blue. When in doubt, we biopsy or excise the skin lesion and let the pathologist tell us what it was.

BASAL CELL CARCINOMA

BCC arises in non-keratinized cells of the basal cell layer of the epidermis, grows slowly, rarely metastasizes, but can cause extensive local damage. The characteristic lesion is a "rodent ulcer," a rolled indurated pearly edge with a depressed central area of necrosis; other lesions are nodular and spherical. Angiogenesis can produce characteristic telangiectasias, but there may be ischemic central necrosis. Neglected lesions of the head and neck can invade the subcutis and nerves and spread to the bones and lungs. Risk of extensive spread of non-melanoma skin cancers is high for basal cell carcinoma (BCC) on the nose, morpheaform BCC on the cheek, recurrent BCC in men, any skin cancer on the neck in men, location on the helix of the ear, eyelid or temple, and any lesion increasing in size pre-operatively.

Curettage and electrodessication, cryosurgery, laser or sharp excision may be used. Radiation is occasionally used in treatment, more often in palliation. Retinoids have some utility, as do platinum-based chemotherapy agents.

SQUAMOUS CELL CARCINOMA

Squamous cell carcinoma SCC is a cancer of the keratinizing cells. It is sometimes called Bowen's disease. SCC has more potential for anaplasia, rapid growth, local invasion, and if neglected, metastasis to regional lymph nodes and distant sites than basal cell carcinoma BCC. Metastasis is more likely if the lesion is on a mucosal surface such as the lips or on an injury site such as a scar or ulcer.

Ultraviolet from sunlight is the primary risk factor, but so are chemical carcinogens, inflammation, viral transformation, and mutations.

The tumour may be very irregular, and often has a surface scale or crust. It may just look like a simple sore or inflamed spot that does not heal.

Surgery is common, and a variety of modalities are used, as for basal call carcinoma.

Radiation can be an alternative to surgery for elderly patients if lesions are on the nose, lips, canthus and eyelid.

Recombinant IL-2 improves survival in oral squamous cell carcinoma. IL-2 is synergistic with melatonin, plant sterols, PSK, astragalus, L-carnitine, taurine and vitamin C.

Plant sterols may also help eradicate human papilloma virus HPV, associated with all squamous cell cancers.

The anti-viral ointment **Aldara** – Imiquimod 5% can be effective, but not in cases of hyperkeratosis. It activates several cytokines to make an inflammation response, which in time makes an immune response against the cancer cells. The degree of inflammation must be closely monitored by the prescribing doctor to keep it at a clinically active level while keeping symptoms within a comfortable range. It will be red and sore.

Regular use of prescription non-steroidal anti-inflammatory drugs NSAIDs and aspirin reduce risk by up to 60%.

Frequent intake (> 15 times) of gluco-corticoid steroids increases risk for SCC and BCC.

MALIGNANT MELANOMA

These dark lesions are less common, but much more dangerous. The melanocyte is of neural crest origin, and produces the brown-black pigment melanin. They occur in the skin, perianal area, rectum, vagina, upper digestive tract, and in the eye structures – choroid, iris and ciliary body. The incidence is rising world-wide.

Damage from UV-B rays is a prominent causal factor. Ironically, sun exposure increases melanoma survival time, and melanomas from sun-exposure are less aggressive.

Dysplastic nevi are high risk for transformation to melanoma. 3 or more atypical moles presents a 4 fold increased risk of melanoma. However, ordinary moles do not need to be removed.

The characteristic lesion is asymptomatic, has irregular borders, mixed pigmentation, with possible finger-like projections. The ABCDEs of melanoma recognition are:

Asymmetry
Border irregularity

Color variegation

Diameter > 6 mm, bigger around than a pencil eraser.

Evolving – changing size, shape, color, bleeding, itching or tenderness.

Tumour activator protein AP-1 is a critical trigger of malignant melanoma.

Melanoma growth is stimulated by anterior pituitary thyrotopin-releasing hormone TRH – also called thyroid-stimulating hormone TSH. Melanoma is more common in hypothyroid cases, associated with increased production and release of TRH. Many doctors are now prescribing thyroid hormone supplements at a level which suppresses TRH/TSH. When borderline hyperthyroid, melanoma growth is inhibited.

Interleukin eight IL-8 is associated with metastasis of melanoma. COX-2 also drives metastasis in melanoma.

Melanomas produce the immuno-suppressing interleukin ten IL-10, blocking dendritic cell processing of tumour antigens.

Tyrosinase, MART-1 (melan-A antigen), VEGF121, and PAI1 mRNA expression are significantly associated with micrometastases. Tyrosinase and MART-1 expression are significantly associated with overall survival and relapse-free survival, whereas histologically proven micrometastases and Breslow thickness are associated with relapse-free survival.

Brenner's sign – a reddish rash near or distant from the melanoma lesion – indicates activity of platelet-derived endothelial growth factor PDEGF or PDGF.

60% of melanomas have Raf kinase mutations increasing angiogenesis and cell proliferation. These are highly vascular tumours, so target angiogenesis in all cases.

Normal expression of matrix metallo-proteinase MMP-8 inhibits melanoma.

Treatment is based on the estimated tumour thickness (Breslow's) and level of invasion (Clark's) plus regional lymph node involvement. Using ultrasound and digital video microscopy, the thickness can be accurately assessed.

Wide excision around the lesion is required.

Lesions over 1 millimetre thick necessitate sentinel lymph node sampling. Approximately 2 in 3 cases with positive sentinel nodes will have a local nodal reoccurrence. There is no increased risk with micro-metastases

in a sentinel node if they are under 0.1 mm diameter, but if larger, mortality risk goes up 4 to 5-fold.

8% will have a re-occurrence within 2 years. Local reoccurrence is associated with 70% mortality within 5 years.

Survival is worse if lesions are on the scalp or neck.

IGFBP-7 induces apoptosis in melanoma cells. This binding protein is secreted extracellularly, and mediates growth inhibition via the BRAF tumour suppressor gene. This gene is mutated and actively promoting rapid proliferation in about 2/3 of melanomas. IFGBP-7 expression may be silenced by epigenetic hypermethylation, and if this occurs in the presence of BRAF mutation, melanoma cells escape senescence and apoptosis, and growth is uncontrolled.

Adjuvants include radiation, interferon alpha 2B, cisplatin, vinblastine, DTIC, thiotepa, nitrosoureas, and taxanes.

Interleukin two IL-2 works with activated lymphocytes to suppress melanoma. We can support IL-2 therapy with astragalus, taurine, vitamin C, L-carnitine and PSK mushroom extract.

Recombinant vaccines and gene therapy are under investigation.

Uveal melanoma and liver mets can be treated with chemo-embolization. Cytotoxic drugs are infused with granulocyte-macrophage colony stimulating factor GM-CSF, to disrupt the tumour blood supply. GM-CSF induces antigen-processing dendritic immune cells and improves absorption of tumour antigens.

Polarized CD4 helper cells and effector Th-17 T-cells – associated with auto-immunity – can cure melanoma.

TROY is a biomarker and potential target of therapy, co-expressed with TNF-receptor-associated factor 6.

Betulinic acid is a derivative of betulin, isolated from the bark of Betula alba, the common white birch. This compound is found in several plants, including the medicinal Chaga mushroom. Betulinic acid has anti-inflammatory, anti-HIV and antineoplastic activities. Betulinic acid induces apoptosis through induction of changes in mitochondrial membrane potential, production of reactive oxygen species, and opening of mitochondrial permeability transition pores, resulting in the release of mitochondrial apogenic factors, activation of caspases, and DNA fragmentation. Highly cytotoxic against melanoma cells.

Sample protocols for melanoma:

My esteemed colleague Jacob Schor, ND, FABNO treats melanoma with betulinic acid from Chaga mushrooms, feverfew parthenolides, vitamin C, vitamin K3, boswellia, curcumin, quercetin, resveratrol, melatonin, vitamin D and broccoli sprouts for sulforaphanes. He titrates TSH levels to under 1.0 and serum vitamin D to over 70 ng/ml.

Another American FABNO uses these same agents and adds beta-glucans, calendula, MCP and omega 3s.

NATUROPATHIC CARE OF SKIN CANCERS

Targets of therapy: EGFR, CD-44, MAPK kinases, PDGF, NFkB, COX-2, AP-1 protein activation, HPV, RAF kinase, IL-8 inhibition, IL-2 promotion, angiogenesis, hypermethylation, IGFBP-7, HSP-90.

ANDROGRAPHITES – *Andrographites paniculata* extracts increase IL-2 activity.

*ANTI-OXIDANTS – are particularly needed by the skin. Use a face cream of rosehip oil, green tea extract, vitamin C, MSM, alpha lipoic acid, grapeseed extract and vitamin E to heal injury and prevent degeneration.

ASTRAGALUS – reduces metastasis of melanoma.

*BROMELAIN – modulates cell adhesion molecule CD-44 to arrest progression and metastasis. Inhibits kRas mutations.

CHAGA – Chaga mushrooms provide betulinic acid, anti-inflammatory, pro-apoptotic, and cytotoxic to melanoma.

*CO-ENZYME Q-10 – reduces risk of melanoma metastasis by 8 fold.

*CURCUMIN – Blocks activation of AP-1 protein. Inhibits NFkB and inflammatory growth factor COX-2. Reduces invasiveness and angiogenesis.

ESCHAROTICS – Escharotics as used by Hoxsey and Bastyr are useful alternatives, although they can be painful. I have created a formula based on podophyllin resin I call *Wart Death*, which removes warts and other skin lesions.

GINGER – inhibits skin growth promoter epidermal ornithine decarboxylase EOD.

**GRAPESEED EXTRACT – OPCs in grapeseed are able to control COX-2 growth factor created by inflammation. This can be supported by curcumin and omega 3 oils.

**GREEN TEA EGCG – reduces UV damage and inflammation. Creams with green tea extract are exceptional for healing skin lesions and radiation burns. Orally it is a major cancer remedy in high dose concentrates. . Blocks activation of AP-1 protein.

HOMEOPATHY – Arsenicum bromatum, Arsenicum iodatum, Carcinosum, Conium maculatum, Lycopodium claviceps, Thuja occidentalis.

HOXSEY – herbal tincture can give great support. Hoxsey tonic can be augmented with Jason Winter's red clover adjuncts – chaparral and gotu kola. I like to add homeopathic remedies such as *Carcinosum* nosode.

LOW DOSE NALTREXONE – inhibits melanoma.

*MELATONIN –regulates biological cycles, including IL-2 levels.

*MILK THISTLE – Modulates EGFR and related TGFα, MMP's, NFkB transcription, IGF-1 (while increasing IGFBP3); modulates VEGF and cell cyclins. Inhibits skin cancer growth by inhibiting EGF-induced mitogen activated protein kinase MAPK and related ERK1/2 signalling pathway.

MISTLETOE – Iscador or Helixor P injectable mistletoe lectins from pine trees are specific for skin cancers.

**MODIFIED CITRUS PECTIN – inhibits metastasis and growth. Mandatory for melanoma cases.

PLANT STEROLS – IL-2 is greatly enhanced by plant sterols and sterolins such as Vitazan *Ultra-Immune*.

*POMEGRANATE – anthocyanidins and tannins in pomegranate fruit and juice inhibit tumorigenesis, and modulate UV-mediated phosphorylation of mitogen-activated protein kinases MAPK and activation of nuclear factor kappa B NFkB.

*QUERCETIN – Blocks activation of AP-1 protein. Quercetin is particularly active against melanomas.

REISHI –Hot water extracts from the mushroom *Ganoderma lucidum* inhibit NFkB and modulate interleukins. Mushroom and other plant beta-glucans can also be used.

VACCINES – Vaccinations against smallpox (Vaccinia) and tuberculosis (BCG) are protective against melanoma. BCG can be injected right into melanoma nodules. This may give pause to the homeopaths to consider miasmatic and constitutional remedies.

Naturopathic Oncology

*VITAMIN A – retinol palmitate, pro-vitamin A carotenes, and other mixed carotenoids reduce risk, repair skin and slow cancers. Apply topically every evening. Long-term use of oral retinol vitamin A over 3,000 IU daily interacts unfavourably with vitamin D, affecting bone health and other tissues and processes.

*VITAMIN D 3 – regulates differentiation and cellular growth. Associated with improved survival.

VITAMIN E – an antioxidant to use with green tea. EGCG polyphenol concentrate

FABNO and Naturopathic Dermatologist Professor Traub reports reliable clearance of basal and squamous cell cancers with *Aldara*, which is 5% Imiquimod. It is applied daily for about 6 weeks, but dosing is monitored closely by the physician, as the degree of immune reaction and subsequent inflammation must be kept at a tolerable but active state to effect a cure. Reoccurrence is rare.

Non-melanoma skin cancer may also respond to *Curaderm* with BEC5. The active principle is derived from an eggplant relative from Australia called "Devil's Apple." The solasodine rhamnosyl glycosides bind selectively to cancer cells and induce apoptosis. It is covered by an occlusive dressing. It can sting and itch at the tumour borders. Responses may take up to 5 weeks.

Chapter Eighteen – Integrative Care Of Brain Cancers

Cancer of the central nervous system is becoming more prevalent in the elderly and in children.

Unequivocal risk factors are exposure to ionizing radiation and immuno-suppression.

Chlorine in water increases risk by the formation of trihalomethanes.

Astrocytomas are linked to pesticide ingestion.

CNS tumours develop vasculature without the normal blood-brain barrier, allowing in toxins and proteins which cause edema. Thus even small lesions can compress adjacent vital structures within the closed vessel of the cranium.

Brain tumours are not malignant in the sense that they may spread to other tissues, but high grade lesions are dangerous and spread within the brain. Gliomas are particularly invasive.

A metastatic cell must then adhere to endothelial cells lining the blood vessels in the target organ. Insulin-like growth factors I and II are chemoattractants for metastases. The cell will stop and attach where it "smells" this chemical. These are high when the diet is rich in sugars and simple carbohydrates. The metastatic cells attach to the blood vessel walls in the brain via integrin cellular adhesion molecules.

Metastases must then extravasate, or leave the blood vessel through the basement membrane of the endothelium lining to enter the new tissue. Metastases only grow significantly if they can stimulate angiogenesis or new blood vessel growth into their new home. Brain tumours tend to nest in peri-vascular niches, dependent on angiogenic factors. It is suspected that immune cells and stem cells are essential recruits to complete this process.

Diffuse tumours are inoperable.

5-year survival is about 32% overall.

GLIOMAS

Gliomas encompass ependymomas, oligodendrogliomas and astrocytomas. They tend to be resistant to radiotherapy and other pro-apoptotic therapies. They do respond to pro-autophagy drugs such as Temozolomide, which can double survival time.

Glial cells lack a normal blood-brain barrier. As tight junctions in the microvasculature break down, there is the characteristic vasogenic edema around these tumours. Grapeseed extract oligomeric proanthocyanidins and boswellia help resolve this edema and restore the BBB integrity.

GLIOBLASTOMA

Glioblastomas inactivate apoptotic pathways, and are more susceptible to induction of autophagy. Autophagy is a process of protein recycling with extensive degradation of Golgi apparatus, poly-ribosomes endoplasmic reticulum, and finally destruction of the nucleus.

Inactivation of mTOR can induce autophagy. This is how the drug Temozolomide acts. mTOR inhibitors are supported by P13K and Akt inhibitors, namely protein tyrosine kinase inhibitors.

Glioblastomas contain "stem-cell-like" glioma cells which produce 10 to 20 times normal amount of VEGF under normal oxygen levels as well as when hypoxic. The stem-cell like cells sequester into peri-vascular niches. It is thought that anti-angiogenics are a useful therapeutic target against this phenomenon. Green tea EGCG is good in this regard.

Glioblastoma multiforme has MET oncogene amplification of the Erb-B3 pathway.

Glioblastomas are dependent on NFkB activation. Think reishi extract!

A new treatment that appears promising is laser interstitial thermal therapy LITT. This is something like radiofrequency ablation, but with laser light as the heating agent. LITT uses an MRI-guided light probe to inflict thermo coagulation on glioblastomas.

Another new therapy is an electrical field device that disrupts critical tumor cell processes. Electrodes are attached to the scalp. The Novo-TTF-100A has demonstrated increased survival time.

Targets of therapy in glioblastoma: autophagy, NFkB, mTOR, VEGF, PTKs.

SIGNS & SYMPTOMS

Symptoms arise from raised intracranial pressure, focal signs from edema and ischemia, and hydrocephalus from blocked CSF flow. The traditional Chinese TCM doctors call this a "dampness of the marrow with phlegm obstructing the channels."

- Headache is common, can be severe, persistent and is typically crescendo in presentation – relentlessly getting worse.
- Vomiting, especially on awakening, with or without nausea
- Neck and back pain at night or early in the day, usually worse laying down and improved when standing upright.
- Seizures are quite common with focal sensory and motor signs.
- Behavioural and personality changes.

Corticosteroids such as Dexamethasone are very useful as palliatives as they reduce the edema and swelling dramatically within 24 to 48 hours. This is somewhat less helpful in tumours that have metastasized to the brain from elsewhere, which are less oedematous and tend to grow as firm spheres. Corticosteroids should be taken according to a circadian rhythm – none in the evening, low dose at noon to early afternoon, and high doses in the morning. Support the patient with valerian root for sleep, glycine and GABA for anxiety, and adaptogens for adrenal gland function.

MRI and stereotactic 3 dimensional guided needle biopsy techniques have improved diagnosis and treatment.

Despite surgery and good medical care half of all cases will be fatal within one year. Only 20% are cured.

Post-surgical radiation may improve survival time. Radiation is an excellent palliative treatment. Gamma knife technology and related precision radiation techniques improve long-term survival with brain mets. To heal the damage from radiation to the nervous system inhibit IL-6 and TNFα – for example with omega 3 oils and nettles.

Temozolomide significantly adds to the survival benefit of radiation, reducing tumour bulk and aggressiveness and extending life, but cannot cure the disease and prevent reoccurrence. The patient most likely to benefit from Temozolomide has a methylated promoter for the gene encoding 0-6-methylguanidine-DNA methyltransferase.

Glial cells are radio-therapy resistant if they carry the gene to express Delta-EGFR. This can be overcome with an Akt inhibitor – such as curcumin with bromelain or CanArrest – as the Akt/mTOR pathway mediates radio-resistance.

Chemotherapy may include the carmustine nitrosourea BCNU, or the combination of PCV: procarbazine, CCNU and vincristine.

Meningiomas are estrogen dependent, so hormone therapies are used as adjuncts to surgery. Quercetin is particularly indicated, as it binds to type II estrogen receptors which are amplified in these tumours. Meningiomas tend to also express abundant receptors for testosterone, progesterone, COX-1, COX-2 and LOX-5.

Tamoxifen can stabilize gliomas. Doses used are high, i.e. 120 mg twice daily.

MENINGIOMAS

Meningiomas arise in arachnoidal cap cells of the meninges, the tough fibrous wrapping around the brain and spinal cord. They are slow growing. Surgery can be curative. Radio surgery may also be possible, with gamma knife or stereotactic radiation technologies. Hydroxyurea is a common chemotherapy. It induces apoptosis in meningioma cells by inhibition of ribonucleotide reductase enzyme, and is an efficient radio-sensitizer.

NATUROPATHIC CARE OF BRAIN CANCERS

Targets of therapy: **NFkB**, EGFR, PDGFR, **mTOR-Akt-P13K**, topoisomerase inhibition. Anti-angiogenics will inhibit cancer stem cells, which grow in peri-vascular niches. In nerve sheath tumours target IGF-1 and mTOR signalling. In glioblastoma target autophagy, VEGF, mTOR, PTKs and NFkB.

*ALKYLGLYCEROLS – from shark liver oil inhibit glioma growth and invasion by 50%.

ARTEMESININ – artemether and artemisinin rob iron to make severe oxidative stress for cancer cells.

BASIC NUTRITION – The brain uses more oxygen than any other tissue, is very fatty, and so is susceptible to lipid peroxidation and always requires anti-oxidant protection such as vitamin E and grapeseed extract. It uses so much oxygen to burn a lot of sugar, so it also requires energy cofactors such as Coenzyme Q-10, the B-vitamin complex, magnesium, and acetyl-L-carnitine. The fats needed for normal function and healing include the omega 3 oils EPA and DHA. The essential fatty acid GLA as found in evening primrose oil should not be given if blood sugars are high, including when on Dexamethasone steroids. GLA in these conditions promotes arachidonic acid, which makes inflammation, which brings growth factors and swelling. Reduce dietary arachidonic acid such as grains and grain-fed animal foods.

BERBERINE – assists or replaces BCNU chemotherapy. Topoisomerase inhibitor found in *Berberis*, *Hydrastis* and *Coptis*

BILBERRY– Delphinidins inhibit EGFR kinases and VEGFR in gliomas, including glioblastoma multiforme.

*BOSWELLIA – reduces edema in and around brain tumours, almost as well as the steroid drug Dexamethasone. It does so by inhibiting leukotriene 4 produced via the lipoxygenase LOX pathway. Boswellia can be combined with the drug to reduce the steroid dose, often to the point of replacing the drug. Boswellia can also be used to reduce swelling fast in neurological emergencies. It is a topoisomerase inhibitor cytotoxic to gliomas.

*CANARREST – for curcumin, boswellia and quercetin, plus absorption support. Suppresses VEGF and COX-2.

*CURCUMIN –reduces cerebral edema and promote autophagy in gliomas. Helps overcome radio-resistance mediated by the Akt / mTOR pathway. Inhibits platelet-derived growth factor receptor PDGFR.

DETOX – from fat-soluble pesticides is warranted when history suggests high exposure. I use homeopathic and botanical medicine, along with a defined diet; elimination diet, brown rice diet or modified fast. Foods to increase include beets, cilantro leaf, fish, walnuts, almonds, and of course, pure water.

*GENESTEIN – soy isoflavone genestein stops gliomas by increasing apoptosis, G2/M cell cycle arrest, topoisomerase I inhibition, and protein tyrosine kinase PTK inhibition

GLA – gamma linolenic acid dissolves gliomas on contact when placed in the surgical cavity, but cannot be taken orally when blood sugars are high, as when on corticosteroid drugs. Under high blood sugar conditions the omega 6 oil is directed to make pro-inflammatory arachidonic acid AA and becomes pro-oxidant.

**GRAPESEED EXTRACT – proanthocyanidins are excellent for restoring the integrity of the blood-brain-barrier, and are an effective cerebral anti-oxidant. Delphinidins in bilberry and grapeseed extracts inhibit the key glioma growth factor EGFR kinases, as well as VEGFR.

**GREEN TEA EGCG – anti-angiogenic, removes perivascular niches that brain cancers grow in, supported by growth factors from vascular endothelial cells and local stem cells. Topoisomerase inhibitor. Inhibits mTOR signalling pathway, IGF-1, and platelet-derived growth factor receptor PDGFR.

HOMEOPATHY – *Apis mellifica, Baryta carbonicum, Baryta iodatum, Calcarea phosphoricum, Conium maculatum, Plumbum iodatum, Ruta graveolens.*

HOXSEY – herbal tincture has on occasion produced dramatic responses. The red clover isoflavones modulate estrogen receptors – like Tamoxifen, which is active against gliomas.

LUTEOLIN – flavonoid which down-regulates growth factors and easily enters the brain.

MELATONIN – to regulate the pineal gland, to extend life.

*MILK THISTLE – extract inhibits EGF and NFkB.

MISTLETOE – Iscador and Helixor mistletoe extract are NOT generally recommended for tumours inside the skull – it will cause swelling around the tumour, which will increase intra-cranial pressure. This can be managed with boswellia in high doses and adjunct homeopathic *Viscum album* 30 C and *Apis mellifica* 30X, but only under close supervision by a very experienced physician. Use *Iscador P* from pine trees for peripheral nerve cancers.

OMEGA 3 OILS – 2,000 mg eicosapentaenoic acid EPA and 1,000 mg dihexanoic acid DHA will reduce PGE-2 and increase PGE-3 to control inflammation.

*QUERCETIN – is particularly active against meningiomas, as it is an aromatase inhibitor, stopping local production of estrogen.

*REISHI – Mushroom extract controls the key growth factor NFkB.

RESVERATROL – inhibits angiogenesis and tumour growth in gliomas. Angiogenesis inhibition also targets malignant bone marrow-derived stem cells.

SCUTELLARIA – Topoisomerase inhibitor and anti-inflammatory.

*SHARK LIVER OIL – alkylglycerols inhibit invasion and growth of gliomas by 50%.

STRAMONIUM – agglutinin lectin in Jimson weed *Datura stramonium* induces irreversible differentiation in astrocytic gliomas.

TARGETED VACCINES – such as chickenpox vaccine from herpes varicella zoster HVZ, to create a cytotoxic CD8+ T-cell clone response and interferon alpha INFα in peripheral nerves and the brain or spinal cord.

TCM HERBS – Survival of brain cancer cases in China are reported to be increased by 4 to 5 times when traditional Chinese medicine (TCM) is integrated with the medical oncology care! Formulas to consider:

Ping Xiao Pian, Jingli Neixao, Liu Wei Di Huang Wan. Liu Wei Di Huang Wan or Rehmannia Six formula is a classic to restore kidney yin to control yang and up-rushing wind. The patients who will benefit will have thin, smooth, shiny red tongues. Restoring the kidney nourishes the root of all health – the connection with the vital essences and the ancestors – the DNA. Zhen Gan Xi Feng Tang classic formula may be added to the program if the yang energy is agitated, creating wind i.e. seizures.

UKRAIN – Ukrain injectables can cause swelling around the tumour, which will increase intra-cranial pressure. NOT RECOMMENDED.

VITAMIN C – intravenous doses create hydrogen peroxide H_2O_2 in neuroblastoma cells, causing apoptosis.

VITAMIN E – an excellent antioxidant for high oxygen tissues. Promotes autophagy as well as apoptosis

A protocol for a meningioma, prescribed by a FABNO at Cancer Treatment Centers of America:
- Curcumin – 3-6 grams daily
- Boswellia – 1,000 mg three times daily
- Quercetin – 2 caps twice daily
- Vitamin C – 5 grams IV – use anti-oxidant doses, not pro-oxidant doses.
- Luti-Max – luteolin flavonoid lozenges four times daily.

Chapter Nineteen – Integrative Care Of Lymphoma & Leukemia

Cancer of the immune and blood cells tend to occur in the very young and the elderly. Fortunately the cure rates with conventional allopathic oncology is reasonably good. Unfortunately the treatments are very harsh, and carry a significant risk of provoking other cancers. Naturopathic co-care or complementary medicine has a clear role in moderating the harm, and increasing the proportion who can be cured.

IL-6 is a major growth factor for haematological malignancies. It is strongly inhibited by beta carotene.

HODGKINS DISEASE

Hodgkin's Disease HD is a cancer associated with chronic inflammation of the lymphoid tissue. Diagnosis is often by needle biopsy of lymph nodes. Risk of HD increases 4-fold with exposure to formaldehyde.

HD appears to correlate with an altered immune response to the Epstein-Barr virus of infectious mononucleosis, or surgery to lymphoid tissue such as tonsillectomy or appendectomy. Occurrence spikes in February and March. Defects in cell-mediated immunity involving the T-cells are common, resulting in serious infectious complications.

Cancers associated with the Epstein-Barr virus EBV:

- Hodgkin's disease
- Burkitt's lymphoma
- B-cell lymphoma
- Nasal NK/T-cell lymphomas
- some gastric cancers

Serum EBV DNA is monitored by RTQ-PCR assay – real-time quantitative polymerase chain reaction.

Early signs include painless swollen lymph nodes, but they may become tender on consuming alcohol. There is a moderate to marked neutrophilic leukocytosis and thrombocytosis, elevated serum fibrinogen, zinc and copper, anemia, and pruritus (itchiness). The lungs, liver, spleen and bone marrow are often involved. Later signs may include anorexia, weight loss, fatigue and high fever with drenching sweats.

Aggressive Hodgkin's lymphomas show elevated CDK9 / Cyclin T1 complex of proteins. Hodgkin's lymphoma also overproduces a carbohydrate-binding lectin galectin one – Gal-1, which B-cell lymphomas do not produce.

Survival is shorter if there are an increased number of tumour-associated CD68+ macrophages, so more aggressive therapies are indicated for this subset of patients.

Radiation can be curative in 90% of stage I to IIA cases. Prognosis is poorer if bulky lesions advance into the mediastinal lymph nodes or are found below the diaphragm. In stage III and IV the treatment of choice is chemotherapy with ABVD – adriamycin, bleomycin, vinblastine, and dacarbazine; or MOPP- mechlorethamine, vincristine, prednisone and procarbazine; or BEACOPP combination. Overall survival is about 85% at 5 years.

A 3 year remission often predicts a cure.

NON-HODGKINS LYMPHOMA

Lymphomas are lymphoid proliferative diseases progressing from genomic instability to chromosomal translocations involving immunoglobulin genes, cyclins, constitutive activation of NFkB and deregulation of p53 pathway and downstream, its CDK inhibitor p21.

NHL lymphomas may arise from many causes, including the hepatitis-C, Herpes-6 and EBV viruses, and the bacteria Helicobacter pylori.

There is an 80% increased risk if you were given antibiotics over 10 times during childhood.

Auto-immune disorders like rheumatoid arthritis increase risk, as does high NSAID use. Use of glucocorticoid steroids like cortisone over 15 times in the course of treatment of a chronic inflammatory disease like RA increases risk of NHL by 268 times!

Risk is increased with contamination by PCBs and furans.

Ocular adnexal MALT lymphoma is linked to infection with the avian parasite *Chlamydophila psittaci.*

Diagnosis is usually by excisional biopsy of an enlarged lymph node. The condition is usually found when already well advanced by spread through the bloodstream.

B-cell malignancies include non-Hodgkin's lymphoma, multiple myeloma, and chronic lymphocytic leukemia.

B-cell lymphomas constitutively express Bcl-6 proto-oncogene, which stifles the p53 pathway, reducing apoptosis. B-cell lymphomas up-regulate sonic hedgehog SHH signalling proteins, activating the ABC-G2 p-glycoprotein efflux pump. Counter this aberration with quercetin.

B-cell lymphomas also produce the immuno-suppressing interleukin ten IL-10, blocking dendritic cell processing of tumour antigens.

B-cell lymphomas are linked to exposure to organo-chlorine solvents and pesticides. Detox in an infrared sauna.

Mantle cell lymphomas over-express cyclin D1 and anti-apoptotic Bcl-2. MCL is aggressive, responds poorly to chemotherapy, and has a relatively short survival expectancy.

Follicular lymphomas tend to be somewhat more indolent, with a median survival of 10 to 15 years from diagnosis. These represent about 25% of lymphomas. The typical patient presents at over 30 years of age with stage 3 to 4 disease, having had a slow-growing asymptomatic lymphadenopathy for several years. Treatment usually gets a good response, but it is invariably followed by reoccurrence, and progressively

the remission period gets shorter, so the diseases is considered medically incurable. \
Adverse risk features of follicular lymphoma:

- over 4 positive nodes
- increased LDH
- age over 60 years
- Hemoglobin less than 120 g/l
- Stage 3 to 4 disease

Over 90% of follicular lymphomas over-express Bcl-2, because the gene is deregulated by translocation.

Burkitt's lymphoma (EBV) over-expresses MYC.

Lymphoma cells can have IGF-1 receptors.

Overall 5-year survival is about 58%.

Medical treatment may include radiation, alkylating CHOP protocol chemotherapy, purine analogues, stem cell transplants, monoclonal antibodies, and Bcl-2 antisense oligonucleotide therapy.

The radioactive antibody compound Bexxar has shown high remission and response rates in low grade advanced stage NHL, with a single dose. Minimal side-effects are seen including moderately low blood counts and flu-like symptoms.

Cutaneous T-cell lymphomas such as mycoides fungoides are treated with PUVA psoralen + ultraviolet light regime, as used for psoriasis. This can produce remissions, but risks skin damage in 1 in 3 cases, and increases risk of triggering secondary cancers.

Chemotherapy will not always follow rapidly after diagnosis, as is common for most cancers. Oncologists and haematologists reserve chemo for cases experiencing "B list symptoms":

Criteria for Starting Chemotherapy in Lymphoma:
- Cytopenias
- Symptomatic lymphadenopathy
- Early satiety
- Hepato-splenomegaly causing visible abdominal bloating
- Constitutional symptoms such as drenching night sweats
- Obstructive uropathy or other organ compromise
- Effusions
- High LDH
- Rapid progression

INTEGRATIVE CARE OF LYMPHOMAS

CHOP + R protocol is reasonably effective for even advanced cases of follicular lymphoma. CHOP or CHOP+R can increase survival time in a meaningful way. The drugs are cyclophosphamide, doxorubicin, vincristine, prednisone, and rituximab.

Rituximab or Rituxan is only used if there are B-cells which are CD-20+; the antibody attaches to this marker to selectively deplete these cells.

With CHOP or CHOP+R you should give:

- Shih Chuan Da Bu Wan 12 pellets twice daily (or Astragalus Combination 3 capsules twice daily).
- Vitamin. A – 10,000 IU twice daily
- Omega 3 marine oils – 3 to 4 caps daily.
- 1-a-day multivitamin + minerals for B-complex and magnesium, etc.
- Co-enzyme Q-10 – 100 mg twice daily
- melatonin – 3 mg at bedtime only – 8pm to 12 midnight and <u>only until the chemo is completed</u>.

With Rituximab maintenance therapy or with CHOP+R use beta glucans to improve responses. This mushroom polysaccharide will even create responses to Rituximab in patients previously unresponsive. An excellent source of beta glucans is *Agaricus blazei* mushroom extract. Rituximab maintenance therapy alone is usually quite helpful. Just four doses can double the event-free survival in follicular lymphoma.

Ginger root extract 2 capsules tid / prn is cheaper than the drug metoclopramide, and much more consistently effective for the nausea and vomiting.

Do not use curcumin during this chemotherapy, as it will alter the liver detox pathways for a number of these drugs.

Some lymphoma patients will require blood-thinning drugs. Heparin is more costly than Coumadin (Warfarin), but it is far safer in lymphoma patients. There are less clots, less haemorrhages, and no deaths with low molecular weight heparin.

Chemo is intrinsically pro-oxidant, and that is how it kills cancer cells. Judicious use of moderate doses of selected antioxidants can give a benefit by reducing aldehydes – which would otherwise arrest cell cycle progression and reduce cancer cells entering the checkpoint for the "apoptosis" tumour death and recycling program. This is known as the Conklin hypothesis. The net effect can be improved tumour destruction while sparing healthy cells. The best anti-oxidants are grapeseed extract and melatonin. Vitamins C, E, and beta-carotene are more risky. Do not give them on chemo days.

If neurotoxicity crops up give R+alpha-lipoic acid 150 to 300 mg three times daily at meals. Vitamin B12 shots are also very helpful.

Fare You – Vitamin U formula 4 pills three times daily for mucositis or gut irritation. It is a form of methionine from cabbage.

3 weeks after the last chemo dose give lots of antioxidants, do some detox, and move onto the next phase of care:

NATUROPATHIC LYMPHOMA CARE:

Targets of therapy – **STAT-3**, ERK and **NFkB**, COX-2, Bcl-2, B-cell, IGF-1, T-cell and HD.

*ALPHA LIPOIC ACID – R+ ALA increases apoptosis via mitochondrial rescue.

*CAN-ARREST – for curcumin, quercetin, bromelain to control inflammation and its growth factors.

CAT'S CLAW – *Una de Gato* vine alkaloids have shown in vitro activity against lymphoma cells.

*CO-ENZYME Q-10 – Co Q-10 repairs mitochondrial dysfunction in lymphoma stem cells.

DEVIL'S CLAW ROOT – *Harpagophytum procumbens* may regress follicular lymphoma, by COX-2 inhibition.

EPA – Eicosapentaenoic omega 3 oil from seals or fish is an important modulator of cytokines.

*GRAPESEED EXTRACT – OPCs are complementary to resveratrol, quercetin and grape juice.

**GREEN TEA EGCG – EGCG concentrate does it all.

HOMEOPATHICS – *Baryta carb, Baryta iodatum,* and *Phytolacca.* Hodgkin's lymphoma is based in a Luetic miasm.

HOXSEY – herbal tonic recommended by Dr. Patrick Donovan, ND for lymphomas.

**INDOLE-3-CARBINOL – I3C inhibits the key growth factor STAT-3.

**JINGLI NEIXAO – TCM herb formula

MELATONIN – NOT RECOMMENDED! It reduces apoptosis in malignant lymphocytes, while dramatically increasing oxidative stress of ROS in healthy cells. Use only short-term during chemotherapy, as a pro-oxidative agent.

MISTLETOE – injectable mistletoe lectins at one time were controversial for lymphoma, but there are published controlled studies, and I strongly recommend it. Use Iscador or Helixor type P.

MULTIVITAMIN – Vital Victoria 1-a-day multivitamin with minerals

NALTREXONE – Low dose naltrexone therapy for Hodgkin's disease and NHL. The patient cannot be on opiates for pain control.

*OMEGA 3 OIL- Marine omega 3 oils in large doses are showing responses. EPA and DHA are the active fats.

PLANT STEROLS – Plant sterols and sterolins are not recommended for lymphomas except where the Epstein-Barr virus EBV is involved.

*POMEGRANATE – Ellagic acid, quercetin, and anthocyanidins are active against lymphoma.

QUERCETIN – inhibits lymphocyte tyrosine kinases. Inhibits p-glycoprotein efflux pump in B-cell lymphomas.

**REISHI – *Ganoderma lucidum* mushroom polysaccharides are potent immune modulators and regulators of nuclear transcription factor NFkB. Avoid immune stimulants such as *Echinacea* in lymphoma. Choose only immuno-modulators or re-balancers of the immune function.

VACCINES – Lymphomas are highly immunogenic, and will respond to targeted vaccine therapy.

VITAMIN E – works with green tea EGCG.

VITAMIN C – anti-viral and immune balancer.

*VITAMIN D3 – Dr. Thorpe, PhD, of Kripps Pharmacy in Vancouver, has long

used high dose vitamin D therapy with success in lymphoma.

MULTIPLE MYELOMA

This lymphoma is characterized by diffuse destruction of bone including lytic "punched-out" lesions in the cranium and other bones.

NFkB is involved in creating these lytic bone lesions. NFkB activation is the primary trigger of multiple myeloma. NFkB increases multiple myeloma cell survival and increases treatment resistance, so target this aggressively. PTEn regulates P13K/Akt pathway, which regulates NFkB.

5-year survival rates are only about 30%.

Doxorubicin and thalidomide are used, but this combination has a high risk of causing deep vein thrombosis. Thalidomide alone will give a response in many relapsed cases, 67% see no progression for 3 months, 43% last a median of 6 months, but most eventually progress by 18 months. Side-effects include some sedation, skin rash, constipation, neuropathy and neutropenia. Most can't tolerate the top-end dose of 600 mg. Adding dexamethasone to the thalidomide doubles the response rate. Some regimes include melphalan with the prednisone and thalidomide. Overall, thalidomide extends time to progression, but not overall survival, and is very toxic.

A new thalidomide analog Lenalidomide (Revlimid) shows increased potency with less toxicity. Combined with dexamethasone it gives good response rates with impressive long-term remissions and survival.

Another regime uses vincristine, oral dexamethasone and pegylated liposomal doxorubicin.

Doxorubicin plus Bortezomib is very active against myeloma, even refractory cases. Bortezomib or *Velcade* is a proteasome inhibitor used for relapsed multiple myeloma and mantle cell lymphoma. Do not mix with Velcade with quercetin or green tea extract, which reduce efficacy. Velcade has a positive synergy with curcumin.

Arsenic trioxide is making a come-back as a therapy for myeloma

Autologous stem cell transplantation may be considered for non-responders.

Vitamin D deficiency tends to occur as multiple myeloma progresses, and is linked to poorer prognosis.

Rising CRP and creatinine also correlate with poorer outcomes.

INTEGRATIVE CARE OF MULTIPLE MYELOMA

Targets: **P13K/Akt**, HSP90, PTEN, proteasome inhibition; **NFkB** is the primary element in the pathogenesis of multiple myeloma.

*ALPHA LIPOIC ACID – R+ALA to reduce marrow fibrosis via inhibition of platelet derived growth factor PDGF. Also inhibits NFkB.

BORON – hardens bones, to inhibit the growth and spread of cancer in the bones.

BROMELAIN – Proteolytics such as bromelain enzyme increase remission times and reduce mortality by 50 to 60%, by reducing TNF receptors and B2 microglobulin.

CO-ENZYME Q-10 – CoQ-10 repairs mitochondrial dysfunction in myeloma stem cells.

*CURCUMIN – inhibits NFkB and inflammation. Positively enhances efficacy of Velcade.

DHA – omega 3 oil which regulates myeloma cell growth, and is an anti-inflammatory.

GRAPESEED OPCs- grapeseed extract proanthocyanidins robustly inhibit NFkB.

*GREEN TEA EGCG – EGCG inhibits NFkB and mTOR. Anti-angiogenic – marrow always shows increased vascular density in myeloma. <u>NOT OK WITH VELCADE</u>!

HOMEOPATHICS – multiple myeloma is based in a Luetic miasm.

*INDOLE-3-CARBINOL – I3C inhibits NFkB and mTOR.

*MCHA CALCIUM – microcrystalline hydroxyapatite calcium complex hardens and protects bones from lysis, reducing bone pain.

MELATONIN – antioxidant, biorhythm regulator, inhibits NFkB.

MILK THISTLE – Silibinin extract inhibits NFkB, and silymarin inhibits EGFR.

MISTLETOE – Use Helixor type A.

NAC – N-acetyl cysteine inhibits NFkB.

QUERCETIN – inhibits NFkB. <u>NOT OK WITH VELCADE</u>!

*REISHI – *Ganoderma lucidum* mushroom hot water extracts is the greatest inhibitor of NFkB.

RESVERATROL – inhibits NFkB.

RETINOIDS – synergistic with vitamin D3.

SELENOMETHIONINE – inhibits NFkB.

VITAMIN C – hardens bone, inhibits NFkB.

VITAMIN D3 – associated with improved survival.

VITAMIN K2 – Menaquinone hardens bone while inhibiting the cancer.

ZINC – zinc citrate helps immune competence and inhibits NFkB.

A sample protocol which has given a good response:

- milk thistle silymarin
- reishi mushroom extract
- green tea EGCG concentrate
- vitamin E
- co-enzyme Q-10
- R+ alpha lipoic acid
- MCHA calcium
- omega 3 oil
- grapeseed OPC extract
- Can-Arrest

I have even had a very positive response with just the first four items in this list.

MYELODYSPLATIC SYNDROME

The myelodysplastic syndromes MDS are a spectrum of clonal hematopoietic stem cell disorders that are associated with distinct cytogenetic abnormalities, and persistent peripheral cytopenias. In MDS, which is thought to be a cancer akin to leukemia, blood cells are derived from a malignant multi-potent progenitor cell that results in a hyper proliferative bone marrow and ineffective haematopoiesis. Ineffective haematopoiesis can sometimes develop into leukemia.

The first United States epidemiologic data reported an incidence of approximately 3.6 per 100,000 people, or over 10,000 new diagnoses yearly in the USA.

Neutropenia is common, and 65% of cases will die of infection. Thrombocytopenia is also common, and results in petechiae, gingival bleeding, retinal haemorrhage and other bleeding disorders. The platelets develop abnormal morphologies and aggregation defects.

Iron overload increases risk of death. A serum ferritin greater than 1,000 mcg /L is diagnostic. Most cases are due to blood transfusion related hemachromatosis. Iron can be chelated by IV medicines, or an oral chelator Deferasirox. Artemisinin can burn off the iron in a blaze of endo-peroxides.

Immunosuppressive drugs have had some limited success. Interleukins IL-3, IL-6 and IL-11 induce platelet production or thrombopoiesis.

The first drug to be shown to prolong survival is Azacitidine or *Vidaza*. Chemotherapy with cytarabine may be used in about 40% of cases.

Hydroxyurea is a common chemotherapy, which induces apoptosis by inhibition of ribonucleotide reductase enzyme. Prevent liver and kidney and bone marrow toxicity with Shih Chuan Da Bu Wan or Astragalus Combination, co-enzyme Q-10, and milk thistle extract.

The only curative treatment is bone marrow transplantation, but only a few qualify and find a suitable donor.

NATUROPATHIC CARE FOR MYELODYSPLASIA

Targets: Anti-angiogenics, demethylation, Src family kinase inhibitors, farnesyl transferase inhibitors and differentiation agents are thought to be helpful, and are being developed as therapies for MDS. Chelates iron.

*ALKYLGLYCEROLS – shark liver oil alkylglycerols help regulate the bone marrow and angiogenesis.

*ARTEMESININ – chelates away iron. Support by avoiding red meat; take black tea at meals, lactoferrin, DHA.

BURDOCK ROOT – *Arctium lappa* is an alterative or tonic, recommended by Bill Mitchell, ND

CAN-ARREST – for curcumin, boswellia, quercetin and bromelain.

ELLAGIC ACID – as found in pomegranate, berries and fruits, to regulate MAPK and NFkB.

*EPA – Eicosapentaenoic acid is an omega 3 fat which controls inflammation in the

marrow.

GENESTEIN – from soy, regulates growth.

GRAPESEED – for anthocyanidins and proanthocyanidins, also found in bilberry.

*GREEN TEA EGCG – concentrate is strongly anti-angiogenic, regulates stem cells.

*MELATONIN – regulates differentiation.

REISHI – mushroom extract controls NFkB.

RESVERATROL – inhibits VEGF and NFkB.

*VITAMIN D3 – regulates cell differentiation.

LEUKEMIA

Leukemia is a cancer of the white blood or immune cells. The problem is often mutation of the stem or progenitor cells in the bone marrow.

Greave's Hypothesis: reduced antigenic challenge during early post-natal development may contribute to an increased risk of childhood leukemia. In other words let kids get dirty, and play with pets.

Acute leukemias are marked by rapid proliferation and disordered differentiation, with accumulation of large numbers of immature blast cells in the blood and bone marrow. Untreated, this can be fatal in a few weeks to a few months.

A number of insults to the foetus during pregnancy increase risk for leukemia, including radiation, organo-chlorine pesticide and solvent exposure, and infections such as influenza, pneumonia, chlamydia, human papilloma virus HPV or genital herpes HSV-II.

Iron supplements by the mother during pregnancy reduces risk of acute lymphocytic leukemia in the child.

Overall survival is about 42.5% at 5 years. Children tend to fare much better than adults over age 40. Treatment is arduous, and full recovery can take several years.

Methadone binds to opoid receptors on myeloid and lymphoblastic cells, activates mitochondrial pathways, caspase activation, and down-regulates the anti-apoptotic protein Bcl-xl. *In vitro* this kills even multi-drug resistant leukemia cells. This suggests a possible role for low dose Naltrexone LDN.

A serious and potentially fatal complication of leukemia treatment by allogeneic hematopoietic stem cell transplantation is **graft-versus-host disease GVHD**, where the new immune cells attack the recipient. This can occur in close to half of cases. GVHD onset and severity is associated with increased serum levels of interleukin IL-7 and circulating CD-19 B-cells. Some help is seen with Rituximab and Bortezomib. Consider proteasome regulators such as green tea EGCG. Omega 3 marine oils also manage GVHD. My esteemed collague Dr. Eric Yarnell has suggested *Centella asiatica* or gotu kola.

Some authorities say **avoid megadoses of vitamin C** in all leukemias, as it can paradoxically increase malignant cell proliferation.

ACUTE LYMPHOBLASTIC LEUKEMIA

Acute lymphoblastic or lymphocytic leukemia ALL is the most common childhood leukemia. Causes include maternal deficiency in folate, maternal exposure to agricultural chemicals during pregnancy; and paternal exposure in the workplace to paints, solvents, degreasers and chemical cleansers. Toxic chemicals in food and the environment which are high risk for childhood leukemias include hydrocarbons such as benzene, perchloroethylene, off-gassing solvents, and pesticides – such as from food, pet products, home garden and agricultural applications. Environmental toxins which are likely a risk are dioxans, furans, tobacco smoke, 1, 3 butadiene, benz(a)pyrene, and many other volatile organic compounds.

Rates of ALL spike after influenza epidemics. This suggests a targeted vaccine strategy.

NFkB is a prominent driver of growth in ALL.

Greave's hypothesis revisited: Children have a 50 % lower risk of ALL if they regularly attend daycare in the first few months of life, as exposure to childhood infections is protective if it occurs before expanded mutant B-cell clones can develop.

Acute leukemias present with symptoms associated with altered bone marrow production of red blood cells, white blood cells and platelets: fatigue, malaise, anorexia, bruising, low-grade fevers, anemia, and immunodeficiency.

ALL has a complete remission rate of 90% in children treated with the combination chemotherapy vincristine, prednisone and asparaginase. Remission maintenance with methotrexate and mercaptopurine gives 55 to 70% long term survival. Also used are melphalan, chlorambucil, topoisomerase inhibitors, anthracyclines and etoposide. Within 5 years 14% of kids relapse, of which 1/3 are new secondary cancers induced by anti-leukemia therapies.

Adults with acute lymphocytic leukemia are treated with vincristine, prednisone, daunorubicin, methotrexate, cyclophosphamide, cytosine arabinoside, 6-thioguanine and 6-mercaptopurine, and possibly asparaginase.

High risk cases receive radiation therapy as well as intensive chemotherapy.

Acute adult T-cell leukemia and HTLV-1 infected cells respond to the carotenoids fucoxanthin and its 2X stronger metabolite fucoxanthinol, which induce apoptosis by activation of caspases 3, 8 and 9, and cell cycle arrest at G1. Beta carotene and astaxanthin are not effective.

Response rates are 60 – 80% for adults, but the duration of remissions are considerably shorter, usually under two years.

The acute leukemias ALL, AML and APL (pro-myelocytic), AMcL (monocytic) have increased numbers of insulin receptors. This also applies to CML, but not CLL and the lymphomas.

ACUTE MYELOCYTIC LEUKEMIA

Acute myelocytic or myelomonocytic leukemia AML is the most common adult form of acute leukemia, and is the type most often seen to result from exposure to radiation or chemotherapy.

15% of AML cases are known to express AML1-ETO fusion protein which prevents recruitment of critical co-activators, silencing E protein transcription factors, preventing activation of certain tumour suppressor genes.

A viral like-illness with fatigue and malaise may be followed by pain in the long bones, ribs and sternum. Unlike ALL, AML has little peripheral lymph node involvement. There are occasionally skin lesions. Blast cells may cause leukostasis syndrome, and the blast crisis phase can be fatal. The leukemic cells secrete platelet-derived growth factors which cause the fibroblasts to turn the bone marrow spaces fibrotic.

AML is initially treated with combinations of cytarabine, etoposide, mitoxantrone, daunorubicin, thioguanine and all-trans-retinoic acid. Beware cell lysis syndrome with hyperuricemia and hyperuricuria. Chemo is commonly reinforced with autologous or allogeneic bone marrow transplantation. Bone marrow transplants are less helpful in AML than other leukemias.

Hyperglycaemia increases mortality risk 40%, so close monitoring of blood sugar is recommended. There are increased numbers of insulin receptors on these cells.

Watch the hygiene and immune competence of the oral and the peri-rectal areas.

I do not use the mitochondrial rescue protocol with leukemias and lymphomas.

A sample protocol which has worked very well is:

- Indole-3-carbinol
- Green tea EGCG + vitamin E
- CanArrest – curcumin, boswellia, quercetin and bromelain
- Reishi mushroom extract
- Milk thistle extract

My American colleagues suggest:

- Vitamin A – preferably in the form of ATRA, to induce myelomonocytic differentiation.
- Vitamin D –as 1, 25 dihydroxy vitamin D3 – calcitriol, the activated form, again for differentiation.
- Quercetin – which has high affinity for type II estrogen receptors.
- Resveratrol – to suppress multi-drug resistance by inhibition of Cyp1B1.
- *Cephalotaxus spp.* – Plum yew bark is a natural source of taxanes.

Secondary remedies include:

- Anti-Cancerlin tablets
- Holy basil
- Boswellia
- Curcumin
- Barberry

- Yunnan Bai Yao
- Grapeseed extract oligomeric proanthocyanidins OPCs
- Lycopodium

Feverfew parthenolides are said to specifically kill AML and CML progenitor and stem cells, and do so better than the chemo drug ara-C (Cytarabine). This idea needs further clinical development. Standardized feverfew extracts used for migraine headaches, given in large doses, have not shown any responses in my patient population. Apparently it should work by activation of p53 and NFkB by free radicals of oxygen ROS. Perhaps feverfew will synergize with other oxidative therapies.

CHRONIC MYELOCYTIC LEUKEMIA

CML is associated with an abnormal Philadelphia Ph chromosome, and is characterized by myeloid hyperplasia. There is an increased granulocyte-macrophage stem cell pool, leading to distinct self-renewing myeloid colonies with raised nuclear beta-catenin signalling. This is a constant source of blasts – the new immature leukemic cells. This myeloid blast signalling can be moderated by enforced expression of axin. It is also driven by differentiation arrest, genomic instability, epigenetic phenomena, telomere shortening, and non-random chromosomal abnormalities. Current therapies targets the blasts, not the source. Inhibit the beta-catenin blast phase trigger!
Therapeutic targets:

- Tyrosine kinase inhibition – curcumin, EGCG, milk thistle, reishi extract
- Differentiation – vitamin A, vitamin D, quercetin, boswellia
- Beta-catenin inhibition – vitamin A, omega 3 DHA, indole-3-carbinol
- P13k / Akt / mTOR inhibitors – curcumin, green tea EGCG

Thus a basic CML protocol might be:

- green tea EGCG
- CanArrest with curcumin, boswellia, quercetin and bromelain
- Reishi extract
- vitamin D3
- beta carotene.

The TCM formula Dang Gui Lu Hui is recommended in CML.
Chronic leukemias tend to show up on routine blood tests as thrombocytosis, with elevated lactic acid dehydrogenase and elevated uric acid. The lymphocytosis is typically over 5,000 per cubic millimetre.
The disease is generally indolent, but 3 to 10% are at risk of transformation into Richter's syndrome with an aggressive lymphoma, night sweats, weight loss, abdominal pain and lymphadenopathy. CML may also exhibit hepatomegaly, and will usually involve splenomegaly with abdominal bloating and early satiety.

CML is treated with hydroxyurea and bisulphan, although they do not stop the progression of the disease. Remission periods in the chronic phase can be prolonged with alpha-interferon.

Gleevec (Imatinib mesylate) is an expensive new selective inhibitor of tyrosine kinase BCR-ABL which can restore normal blood counts in interferon-resistant CML. Children may receive allogeneic bone marrow transplantation; adults up to age 55 may find a donor, but mortality with transplants of these stem cells is about 20%.

CHRONIC LYMPHOCYTIC LEUKEMIA

The most common adult chronic leukemia, especially for men. There may be fatigue, shortness of breath or bleeding problems. The blood tests show lymphocytosis over 5,000 per cubic millimetre.

Smudge cells on the blood test are actually a good sign. These are fragile B-cells with little vimentin cytoskeleton protein. If they disappear, the prognosis is worse.

The disease is generally indolent, but 3 to 10% are at risk of transformation into the aggressive lymphoma of Richter's syndrome, marked by night sweats, weight loss, abdominal pain, and lymphadenopathy.

CLL may be treated with chlorambucil and prednisone. Fludarabine with rituximab is also used; response is less if the cell type is ZAP70+ and CD38+.30% of CLL cases have a 6 to 18 nucleotide sequence insertion in the promoter region of the anti-apoptotic gene MCL-1, which is in the Bcl-2 protein family. These individuals are at high risk of disease progression and resistance to chemotherapy.

CLL is inhibited by green tea EGCG.

HAIRY CELL LEUKEMIA

Hairy cell leukemia HCL is a rare, chronic and indolent lymphocytic leukemia. It arises from mutations in pluripotent stem cells.

HCL patients are generally low in glutathione peroxidase, catalase and super-oxide dismutase SOD activity in their red blood cells.

HCL is treated with alpha-interferon or 2-chloro-deoxyadenosine.

NATUROPATHIC LEUKEMIA SUPPORT

Targets of therapy: NFkB, differentiation inducers, stem cell regulators, proteasome inhibitors, beta-catenin inhibitors, demethylation, insulin, and CD-44 cell adhesion molecule.

Never use melatonin or high-dose vitamin C , which can stimulate these disseminated cancers

ACUPUNCTURE – in acute leukemia Bl-18, BL- 23, GB-39.

ATRA – All-trans retinoic acid has survival benefit in APL.

ANTI-CANCERLIN formula is used in leukemias.

377

AVEMAR – induces apoptosis in leukemia cells.

ASTRAGALUS & LIGUSTRICUM are supportive in leukemias, as are the herbs corydalis, iris versicolor, arctium lappa, eleutherococcus, cornus, ginseng, milletia, polygonatum, psoralea and ganoderma.

BARBERRY – berberine inhibits leukemic stem cells.

BOSWELLIA – for leukemias.

*BROMELAIN – modulates CD44 cell adhesion molecules to reduce progression and destroy leukemic stem cells.

CAT'S CLAW – Una de Gato alkaloids have shown in vitro activity against leukemia cells.

*CO-ENZYME Q-10- repairs mitochondrial dysfunction in stem cells.

CORIOLUS – Coriolus versicolor mushroom extracts inhibit leukemia.

*CURCUMIN – synergizes with vitamin D, is directly cytotoxic, promotes apoptosis, and suppresses activation of transcription factors AP-1 and NF-kappa B in chronic myeloid leukemia CML and CLL. Synegistic with green tea EGCG.

DIET – All leukemias except CLL show increased numbers of insulin receptors, so we prescribe a low glycemic diet.

FARE YOU – Vitamin U green cabbage extract heals mucositis, the primary dose-limiting side-effect in leukemia care. All leukemia patients develop painful mucositis. Half will get to stage 4 toxicity out of 4, which prevents all intake of food or liquids, may cause bleeding, and requires use of morphine for the pain. It is due to a wicked combination of high-dose chemo plus cortisone, antifungals, strong antibiotics and the anti-rejection drug cyclosporine given after bone-marrow transplant. This is preventable and treatable with timely use of Fare You -vitamin U pills, a form of methionine extracted from green cabbage.

FEVERFEW – Feverfew chrysanthemum extract standardized for parthenolides which inhibit AML stem cells. In vitro it is a better killer of leukemic stem cells than arabinase-C chemo. It is progenitor and stem cell specific, via increased reactive oxygen species, activation of p53 and nuclear factor kappa-B. Suggested dose is 20 mg tid.

*GANODERMA – The immune modulating Reishi mushroom Ganoderma lucidum mixes well with other mushrooms such as maitake, shitake and cordyceps. AHCC mushroom extract is not recommended.

GINSENG – is synergistic with vitamin C against leukemia cells.

GLA – evening primrose oil reduces the pro-inflammatory prostaglandin PGE-2 which increases apoptosis in AML and CLL.

**GRAPESEED – grapeseed extract oligomeric proanthocyanidins OPCs inhibit progression, strongly increase apoptosis via activation of JNK protein.

*GREEN TEA EGCG – inhibits CLL. Proteasome regulator. Give 2,000 mg EGCG twice daily for CLL. Synergistic with curcumin.

HOLY BASIL – increases apoptosis in leukemia cells.

HOMEOPATHY – leukemia viruses may be defeated with the Heel brand homeopathics *Engystol* and also *Echinacea Compositum.* Use by injection twice weekly for 2 weeks and as oral tablets twice daily for 3 weeks. *Lycopodium* is useful in AML. Look at *Ceanothus americanus.*

INDIRUBIN – from the botanicals Indigofera tinctoria or Isatis tinctoria or Qing dai used in Dang Gui Long Hui Wan – an effective TCM formula for chronic myelocytic leukemia CML. The active principle appears to be indirubin in the or Isatis tinctoria, which is immune stimulating and inhibits DNA synthesis specifically in immature leukemic cells in the bone marrow. Synthetic indirubin is used at oral doses of 150-200 mg Indirubin inhibits cyclin dependent kinases and glycogen synthase kinase 3 involved in G1 cell cycle phase.

*INDOLE-3-CARBINOL – Inhibits STAT-3 and beta-catenin,

MISTLETOE – Use Helixor P for CLL, and Helixor A for other leukemias. Iscador P may also be used.

NALTREXONE – 3 mg hs for CLL (patient cannot be on opiates)

NOTOGINSENG – Panax pseudoginseng is anti-leukemic. Rx: Yunnan Bai yao

*OMEGA 3 OIL – DHA inhibits beta-catenin and thus inhibits blast production and the blast crisis phase switch.

*QUERCETIN – inhibits leukemia cell proliferation. It binds growth factor receptors such as type II estrogen receptors in leukemia cells. It arrests leukemia cells in G1-S interphase

RESVERATROL – Strongly increases apoptosis.

SHIH CHUAN – Shih Chuan Da Bu Wan or Shiquan is an astragalus-based herbal formula proven to boost chemotherapy effectiveness while strongly protecting blood cells and organs.

STEROLS & STEROLINS – plant fats used as immune modulators.

*VITAMIN A – enhances bisulphan activity against CML, at 50,000 I.U. daily. Beta-catenin inhibitor.

VITAMIN B12 and folate – support normal blood cell formation. I give them as a high dose intramuscular injection on a weekly to monthly basis.

*VITAMIN D3 – at 16,000 I.U. three times weekly can put chronic myelomonocytic leukemia CML in remission.

VITAMIN E – can assist with oxidative stress when tumour load is high, such as during a blast crisis.

VITAMIN K2 – induces apoptosis in APL myelogenous leukemia.

Chapter Twenty – Integrative Care Of Urinary Tract Cancers

KIDNEY CANCER

5 year survival is about 62%. for kidney cancer, also called renal cell cancer RCC. Tumours under 3.0 cm in diameter do not tend to metastasize.

Clear cell RCC is associated with loss of functional von Hippel-Lindau VHL tumour suppressor gene. VHL normally promotes transcription of E-cadherin cell adhesion molecule. Loss of VHL results in loss of E-cadherin, with subsequent development of aggressively growing and spreading cancer.

RCC over-expresses hypoxia-inducible factor one HIF-1. HIF-1 is particularly potent in making VEGF, PDGF, and TGFa when there is a mutation or hypermethylation of the tumour suppressor gene von Hippel-Lindau VHL.

HIF-1 down-regulates MYC oncogene, which stimulates cells to make mitochondria. RCC over-expresses tyrosine kinases.

RCC tumours are immunogenic, so consider vaccines, mistletoe, and related immune therapies.

High risk patients may seek inhaled interleukin IL-2 therapy, or interferon alpha INFa, but cytokine therapies have low responses rates, minimal improvement in survival, significant toxicity, and give a median survival of just 12-15 months.

MRI-guided radiofrequency ablation can also be useful.

Monitor hematuria and urinary nuclear matrix protein twenty-two NMP-22. Onco-foetal RNA-binding protein IMP-3 is a biomarker for high risk of post-operative metastasis.

The NCCN kidney cancer guidelines use a scoring system developed at Memorial Sloan-Kettering to help predict survival in all renal cell cancer patients. The predictive items are:

- lactate dehydrogenase level of more than 1.5 times the upper limit of normal;
- hemoglobin level lower than normal;
- corrected serum calcium level of more than 10 mg/dL;
- interval of less than 1 year from original diagnosis to the start of systemic therapy;
- Karnofsky performance score of 70 or less; and
- 2 or more sites of organ metastasis.

Patients with none of these risk factors have a median survival of 30 months. Patients with 1 or 2 risk factors have a median survival of 14 months. The prognosis for patients with 3 or more of the following items is defined as poor, and such patients have a median survival of 5 months.

Targeted therapies in use and include Sutent (tyrosine kinase), Avastin(angiogenesis), Sorafenib (serine/threonine and receptor tyrosine kinase) , Torisel or temsirolimus (mTOR), Everolimus (mTOR), and in development – Axitinib (tyrosine kinase) and Pazopanib (angiogenesis).

Renal cell carcinoma can be treated by immune therapies such as interleukin IL-2 and interferon INF♦ .

INTEGRATIVE CARE OF RENAL CANCER

Targets of therapy: Raf kinase, VEGFR, HIF-1, tumour antigens, EGFR, PDGFR, mTOR, receptor tyrosine kinases, serine/threonine kinases, mitochondrial rescue, Akt (protein kinase B), P13K, PTEN support, VHL gene.

*APHA LIPOIC ACID – R+ ALA for bio-energetic regulation.

BARBERRY – Barberry or *Berberis vulgaris* is a kidney tonic, antimicrobial and astringent.

*CO-ENZYME Q-10 – Co-enzyme Q-10 activate mitochondria to restore apoptosis, the off-switch for bad cells.

*CURCUMIN – Curcumin from turmeric root squelches inflammation, including COX-2 growth factor. A powerful inhibitor of the Akt/ mTOR signalling pathway.

*GREEN TEA EGCG – EGCG does it all, particularly active against PDGFR, VEGFR, Akt and mTOR.

*INDOLE-3-CARBINOL – from cabbage inhibits mTOR, Akt regulator.

*MILK THISTLE – Milk thistle extract inhibits EGFR and PDGFR.

MISTLETOE – Iscador or Helixor mistletoe lectins. These tumours are highly immune-responsive. Use Iscador Qu or Helixor A for males and M type for females.

*MITOCHONDRIAL RESCUE – R+ alpha lipoic acid, thiamine, L-carnitine, D-ribose, CoQ-10 , omega 3 oils.

*NIACINAMIDE – form of vitamin B3 reduces hypoxia.

QUERCETIN – inhibits angiogenesis, EGFR.

BLADDER CANCER

Cancers of the urinary bladder are linked to tobacco use, and other exposures to toxic chemicals.

Low estrogen exposure, such as early menopause, increases risk – possibly via increased rates of urinary tract infections and hormone related bladder dysfunction.

Bladder urothelial cancer *in situ* has a 50% risk of transforming into an invasive cancer within 5 years. Bladder cancer 5-year survival is about 82%.

Bladder cancer often involves HER-2 expression, involving epidermal growth factor.

Elevated survivin, an apoptosis inhibitor, is a sign of a worse prognosis.

Elevated B7-H3 protein is associated with more aggressive behaviour of kidney and bladder carcinomas. This is a cell-surface ligand which binds to receptors on immune regulating lymphocytes.

Signs and symptoms of bladder cancer may include the following:

- gross or microscopic hematuria;
- irritative symptoms of dysuria, frequency, urge incontinence, and/or urgency;
- obstructive symptoms such as intermittent or decreased force of urinary stream, straining while urinating, or feeling of incomplete voiding; and
- signs and symptoms of metastases or advanced disease, which may include abdominal, bone, flank, or pelvic pain; anorexia, cachexia, or pallor; lower-extremity edema; renal failure; suprapubic palpable mass; and/or respiratory symptoms such as cough, shortness of breath, or haemoptysis.

Lymph node dissection may be extended up to the iliac bifurcation, which is appropriate.

BCG is a tuberculosis vaccine which activates the host's immune response, and is as effective as chemo for transitional cell carcinoma TCC in early stages Ta, Tis, T1. 55% can obtain a 10 year progression-free survival. Therapy begins with a 6X weekly intravesicular instillation, then 3X weekly for 3 months, then 3X weekly at 6 months and every 6 months for 2 to 3 years.

There is benefit in combining hyperthermia with intravesicular (put up into the bladder with a catheter) BCG or chemo such as mitomycin C or Doxorubicin. Interferon gamma IFN or chemo are used primarily in non-responders to BCG.

Photodynamic therapy PDT uses light to activate intravesicular hexaminolevulinate or its lipophilic ester 5-ALA.

Advanced cases can have the bladder surgically removed and a new bladder made from their own bowel.

A new screening and monitoring test is urinary telomerase by TRAP assay – telomeric repeat amplification protocol. Also under investigation is the urinary measurement of matrix metalloproteinases MMP-2 and MMP-9 as markers of neoplastic activity.

Ca-125 tumour marker can be useful to rule-out bladder cancer reoccurrence.

INTEGRATIVE CARE OF BLADDER CANCER

Targets of Therapy: HER-2, EGFR, survivin, tumour antigens, MMPs.

*CAROTENES – Carotenoids lutein, zeanthin and lycopene inhibit bladder cancer growth.

GLA – gammal linolenic acid from evening primrose or borage oils inhibits TCC.

*GREEN TEA EGCG – highly active via several mechanisms.

HOMEOPATHICS – *Terebintha*

*MILK THISTLE – milk thistle extract inhibits EGFR.

MISTLETOE – Iscador or Helixor mistletoe lectins are as effective as BCG, but have less risks. Use Iscador Qu or Helixor A for males and M type for females.

*MSM – methylsulfonylmethane – is an excellent urinary tract anti-inflammatory.

SULFORAPHANE – An isothiocyanate from cruciferous vegetables. Especially high in raw broccoli and broccoli sprouts.

TCM HERBS – Chinese herbal formulae of special interest are Jingli Neixao, Ping Xiao Pian, and Anticancerlin

*VITAMIN C – oral vitamin C acidifies the bladder, directly cytotoxic to bladder cancer cells.

Chapter Twenty-One – Nasopharyngeal, Head And Neck Cancer, Thyroid Cancer And Sarcomas

HEAD and NECK CANCER

Nasopharyngeal, head and neck cancers:

The primary autocrine growth factor in head and neck cancer is transforming growth factor alpha TGFa and therefore ultimately epidermal growth factor receptor EGFR. Mutations in the MET oncogene also amplify the Erb-B3 pathway in these cancers.

Head and neck cancers also tend to over-express vascular endothelial growth factor receptor VEGFR.

Squamous cell carcinoma of the head and neck is triggered by a complex of hyaluronan glycosaminoglycan of the extracellular matrix with the cell receptor CD44 and the signal activator LARG – leukemia-associated rho-GEF. The complex binds to epidermal growth factor receptors, setting off the tumour promoter ras pathway. The complex also alters the protein filamin in the cell cytoskeleton, allowing cell shape changes permissive of cell migration and metastasis. We can disrupt this complex with bromelain enzyme!

There is a link between squamous cell cancers and the human papilloma virus HPV, particularly the oncogenic types 16, and sometimes type 18. Blood serum can be monitored for EBV viral DNA using real-time quantitative polymerase chain reaction test. This virus is now accepted as the cause of squamous cell carcinoma of the cervix, and there is a vaccine against it called Gardasil.

Smoking is also a major trigger of these cancers.

For squamous cell carcinomas E-cadherin over-expression means a higher risk of reoccurrence or metastasis.

Squamous cell carcinomas of the head and neck have increased activity in the P13K/ Akt / mTOR pathway.

Laser surgery is possible in select cases, and is preferable to the knife.

Chemo with cisplatin only increases disease-free interval, not overall survival, and is associated with a lot of harm.

Radiation therapy is generally helpful, for loco-regional control and improved survival. Mucositis is common, as is loss of saliva production. Laryngeal and swallowing issues are common, and there can be severe late fibrosis. It is essential to have dental problems rectified before radiation, as oral tissue healing is poor afterwards, and gets worse over the years.

Zinc is useful to suppress these cancers, but is particularly helpful during radiation therapy. Zinc improves immune cell function and thymus gland maturation of T-cells, and assists wound healing and normal tissue repair, preventing and treating dermatitis and mucositis. I prescribe 30 mg zinc citrate three times daily, with a meal.

Cetuximab is a monoclonal antibody inhibitor of epidermal growth factor receptor EGFR. It improves outcomes as an adjunct to radiation therapy. Nimotuzumab is a new EGFR inhibitor with milder skin toxicities.

INTEGRATIVE CARE of HEAD and NECK CANCERS

Targets: EGFR, TGFa, TGFβ-1, NFkB, COX-2, VEGFR, p53 mutations, Ras-kinases, E-cadherin. Target EBV or HPV with anti-virals and immune modulators.

*ALPHA LIPOIC ACID – R+ ALA inhibits TGF.

BOSWELLIA – in the anti-inflammatory formulae such as Can-Arrest and Lotus Wan.

BROMELAIN – a proteolytic enzyme from pineapple stems which targets CD44 tumour cell receptor and hyaluronan. This cuts off formation of a complex with LARG (leukemia oncoprotein-associated rhoGEF) which would otherwise stimulate metastasis by stimulating the RhoA pathway to alter cell cytoskeleton protein filamin, and would also increase tumour growth by binding to EGFR to activate the ras pathway. Modulation of ras proteins slows progression.

*GREEN TEA EGCG – EGCG inhibits VEGFR, and does many other useful tasks.

*HOMEOPATHICS – use antivirals such as *Engystol* and *Thuja occidentalis*. *Causticum* for trouble swallowing after radiation therapy.

*INDOLE-3-CARBINOL – controls SP-1 and STAT-3 transcription activators.

*MILK THISTLE – milk thistle extract inhibits EGFR.

MISTLETOE – Iscador or Helixor P type mistletoe lectins are potent immune modulators and anti-virals. Iscador P is particularly indicated for naso-pharyngeal tumours. For tongue or oral cancers consider Iscador Qu or Helixor A for males and M type for females.

*PLANT STEROLS & STEROLINS – modulate the immune response against human papilloma virus HPV.

*REISHI – Ganoderma mushroom extract regulates NFkB and immune function.

TCM HERBS – Liu Wei Di Huang Wan, Lotus Wan, Shih Chuan Da Bu Wan, Jingli Neixao, Anticancerlin.

*VITAMIN A: For squamous cell carcinomas, always use in high doses. Anti-viral, re-differentiator and cell growth regulator. Helps heal radiation injury to immune and stem cells.

*VITAMIN C – anti-viral.

*ZINC – zinc citrate is anti-viral, supports immune function; always use during radiation therapy.

SAMPLE NATUROPATHIC PROTOCOL FOR HEAD & NECK CANCER

A protocol which completely removed a recurrent adenocarcinoma on the tongue, possibly of salivary gland origin. It had originally had been treated with surgery and radiation, but reoccurred and spread, for which the only medical option was to surgically

remove the entire tongue! This horror was avoided by taking:
- Jingli neixao
- vitamin C to bowel tolerance
- Can-Arrest
- green tea EGCG with vitamin E
- grapeseed extract
- reishi mushroom extract
- modified citrus pectin
- #42's and Fare You were used as needed.

THYROID CANCER

Cancers of the thyroid gland are becoming more common. There may be a link to estrogen stimulation, as well as radioactive isotope or X-ray exposure.

There is frequently mutant *Ras* expression, and PPARγ-1 expression, a fusion oncogene formed by chromosomal translocation. DNA hypomethylation and histone de-acetylation contribute to epigenetic deregulation.

Mitogen-activated protein kinase MAPK intracellular signalling causes resistance to apoptosis, increased growth and increased angiogenesis. Tumours are highly vascular.

10 year age and gender-adjusted survival can be 98%. Only anaplastic thyroid cancer has a very poor prognosis.

70% are papillary tumours. Papillary carcinoma of the thyroid is associated with hypothyroidism. There is 10% chance of spread to bones or lungs. Synthroid is often prescribed high enough to create subclinical hyperthyroidism, removing pituitary TSH as a growth factor.

10% of cases are medullary carcinoma, which arise from calcitonin secreting C-cells. Tumours can produce ACTH and histaminases, and are associated with other concurrent endocrine tumours. Lymphatic spread is usually to the neck and mediastinum. Metastases to the liver, lung and bone tend to grow slowly. Monitor CEA and calcitonin.

5 to 10% of cases are follicular carcinoma, with a risk of spread to the brain, bones, lungs and soft tissues.

1 to 3% of cases are anaplastic thyroid cancers, which are very aggressive. Invasion of local tissues and structures can be rapidly lethal. It will also try to spread to the lungs, liver, brain and bones.

Surgery is often combined with radiation. Usually a large dose of radioactive iodine is used to ablate these tumours and their metastases. To prevent xerostomia or dry mouth, flush the iodine out of the salivary glands by sipping dilute lemon juice or real lemonade during the administration of the therapy, and for some hours after.

Chemotherapy is not usually of use in thyroid cancers.

INTEGRATIVE CARE of THYROID CANCER

Targets of therapy: NFkB, protein tyrosine kinase PTK, angiogenesis, TSH, Ras, PPARγ, DNA methylation and acetylation.

*ALKYLGLYCEROLS – from shark liver oil, inhibits PTKs and angiogenesis.

*GREEN TEA EGCG – inhibits angiogenesis and PTKs.

*MILK THISTLE – extract inhibits angiogenesis and PTKs.

MISTLETOE – Iscador Qu or Helixor A for males, type M for females.

*OMEGA 3 OIL – Marine omega 3 oils inhibit thyroid cancer.

*POMEGRANATE – anthocyanidins inhibit PTKs and angiogenesis.

*QUERCETIN – inhibits VEGF.

*REISHI – mushroom extract inhibits PTKs

RESVERATROL – inhibits PTKs.

VITAMIN A – retinol palmitate

SARCOMAS

Sarcomas are connective tissue cancers, developing in soft tissue and bone.

Fibromatosis produces desmoids, a low-grade and locally invasive fibrosarcoma.

The sarcoma or connective tissue components may be mixed with carcinomatous elements, as in a mixed Mullerian tumour. The carcinomatous elements are the drivers of metastasis.

Chemo for the carcinoma elements is Carboplatin with Taxol. About 50% respond, but there is no change in survival time.

Where sarcomatous elements dominate, the chemo may include Doxorubicin, Ifosfamide and Cisplatin.

Despite chemo, presence of mets gives a prognosis of under a year survival.

There is a very significantly increased risk of clots in sarcoma patients. Fibroblasts have altered C-Myc gene expression.

Sarcomas have over-activity in the P13K / Akt /mTOR signalling pathway.

Soft-tissue sarcomas such as leiomyosarcoma and rhabdomyosarcoma may respond to topoisomerase-II inhibitors from the oleander plant.

NATUROPATHIC SARCOMA CARE

Targets of therapy: VEGF, EGFR, PDGFR, IGF-1, proteasome regulation, protein kinase C/B, Bcl-2, Raf kinase, mTOR topoisomerase-II, INR.

*ARTEMESININ – extracts of *Artemesia spp.* use iron built up in cancer cells to kill with ROS.

*CURCUMIN – bcl-2 regulator, protein kinase inhibitor, mTOR inhibitor, proteasome regulator; blocks APN protein, reducing tumour blood flow and invasiveness.

*GREEN TEA EGCG: proteasome inhibitor, protein kinase regulator, VEGF inhibitor, PDGFR inhibitor, etc.

HOMEOPATHY – Hekla lava, Symphytum officinalis.

INDOLE-3-CARBINOL – regulates mTOR signalling pathway.

*MILK THISTLE: – EGFR and PDGFR inhibitor.

MISTLETOE – Iscador or Helixor type P, or type M for osteo-muscular sarcomas.

*MITOCHONDRIAL RESCUE – R+ alpha lipoic acid, thiamine, L-carnitine,

D-ribose, Co-enzyme Q-10 and marine omega 3 oils.

OLEANDRIN – cardiac glycosides or cardenolides from *Nerium oleander* leaves, stems and twigs act as a topoisomerase- II inhibitor on soft-tissue sarcomas. Dr. DR uses injectable *Anvirzel* oleandrin, 0.8 ml/m2/day, by IM route. There may be mild pain at the injection site, fatigue, nausea or dyspnoea.

*REISHI – Reishi mushroom extract is synergistic with green tea EGCG.

*VITAMIN D3 – inhibits fibrosarcoma proliferation, increases apoptosis and fibroblast C-Myc expression.

VITAMIN K – PDGFR inhibitor.

EXAMPLES OF SARCOMA PROTOCOLS THAT WORK

A protocol which arrested a case of leiomyosarcoma with lung metastases:
- Green tea EGCG with vitamin E
- Grapeseed extract
- CoQ-10
- Indole-3-carbinol
- Quercetin with bromelain

Note that the tumour was growing fast until this treatment started, stopped progressing until the patient went on a reduced dose, at which point it began to grow slowly.

A protocol which stabilized a late-stage sarcoma:
- Jingli neixao
- Can-Arrest – for curcumin
- vitamin C to bowel tolerance
- R+ alpha lipoic acid
- co-enzyme Q-10
- benfotiamine B1
- intermittent DCA.

A protocol that regressed a nerve sheath sarcoma:
- Iscador P
- CanArrest
- Green tea EGCG + vitamin E
- Grapeseed extract
- Milk thistle extract
- Reishi mushroom extract

A high-grade histiocytoma in the lungs has been reported to have been controlled and gradually reduced to scar tissue by:
- Omega 3 oil – 7 gm EPA and 8 gm DHA – 13/15 gm as fish oil supplements
- Olive and canola oil – provided 2 gm
- Diet emphasizing reduced intake of omega 6 fats from grains, meats and vegetable oils.

Chapter Twenty-Two – Naturopathic Medicine For Cancer Morbidity & Mortality

Naturopathic Medical Care for Complications of Cancer

There are many excellent natural medicines for some of the most difficult issues that arise in the long-term management of cancer. You do not have to wait until you have failed the expensive drug treatment to try some of the truly remarkable treasures of Nature. The following are medical problems which your naturopathic physician can help you with:

ANEMIA – is common in many chronic diseases. We use iron citrate, folate, B12, and Shiquan to keep hemoglobin in the 11-12 range. Alkylglycerols are helpful to the marrow. Look at some of the Asian mushrooms. Transfusions are needed if hemoglobin falls below 90, and allopaths may use Erythropoietin, a marrow stimulating hormone from the kidney (Procrit or Epigen) injected once weekly. See the heading under radiation and chemo toxicities for more details.

ASCITES – may develop from portal hypertension – pressure in the vein from the bowels to the liver – caused by liver metastases as in colon or breast cancer. Ascites may also develop from cancer in the peritoneal membranes of the pelvis – as in ovarian, breast or GI adenocarcinomas, and occasionally from malignant lymphomas in the abdomen. The patient may report swelling of the abdomen and/or dyspnoea. Look for shifting abdominal dullness, and a palpable fluid wave. Therapeutic paracentesis – drainage of the fluid by needle, with suction – can provoke severe protein loss. This can worsen ascites, and damage the kidneys. We prescribe 5 servings of protein daily and monitor serum albumin. Dream Protein whey supplements are often needed.

Consider homeopathic *Apocynum* or *Apis mellifica.*

BLEEDING – Tumours erode into blood vessels, angiogenesis can form weak and leaky vessels, necrotic areas can erode and bleed, and clotting can be severely disturbed by a variety of mechanisms. Yunnan Baiyao is an excellent treatment for a hemorrhagic tendency. I use the capsule form. Consider also spotted cranesbill herb *Geranium maculatum* and Shepherd's purse *Capsella bursa-pastoris,* which I use in tincture form. Homeopathics such as *Phosphorus* can be added as adjuncts. To stabilize coagulation when the patient is on prescribed blood thinners, take vitamin K1 – 100 mcg., always at the same time of day, and well away from the blood thinning drugs. Vitamin K1 does not build up in the system like K2 does. The diet must be tightly controlled to restrict food sources of K1, such as green leafy vegetables. Acupuncture SP-1 and LV-1 and apply a silver ma-grain.

BLOOD CLOTS – Cancer increases risk of clots in the veins about 7-fold overall. Lymphomas and leukemias increase risk up to 28-fold. The highest risk appears to be about 3 months after diagnosis, at about 58 times normal. Presence of metastases increase risk about 20-fold. Risk is also much higher if the body mass index BMI is high, as in obese patients. Prostate cancer is notorious for promoting blood clots, as are hormonal therapies such as Tamoxifen. Watch for petechiae, ecchymosis (bruising) and deep vein thrombosis. The *Met* oncogene creates a hypercoagulable state via altered blood clotting inhibitors, increased fibrin. Fibrin in turn stimulates inflammation, releasing growth factors and angiogenesis. Excess fibrin may be followed later by a failure of clotting factors and thus a hemorrhagic state. Cancers often make pro-coagulants such as cytokines, i.e. IL-6, activators of clotting factors IX & X, increase platelet reactivity and cause venous stasis by local anatomical change. Natural control of coagulation may include *Gingko biloba* leaf, fish oils, **seal oil omega 3**, sea cucumber extract, green tea, green leafy vegetables, horse chestnut *Aesculus hippocastanum*, red clover blossom *Trifolium repens* and compression stockings. Omega 3 marine oils will thin the blood and reduce risk of clots. Bromelain and similar protein-digesting enzymes such as serratiopeptidase and Wobenzyme will reduce the inflammation while gradually and safely dissolving a clot. Homeopaths may advise Sanum *Mucokehl.* TCM herbs of interest include salvia, sporangium, pangolin, frankincense, carthamus, myrrh, curcuma, ligusticum, persica, red peony and Panax pseudo-ginseng.

      BONE METASTASES – Bone scans are the best method to screen for bony mets. Many cancers go into the bones – for example 70 to 80% of breast cancer mets and about 70% of prostate cancer mets. Cancer in the bones causes a lot of pain, usually described as gnawing, often worse at night. It may wake the person up from sleep. Pain may become sharp with weight-bearing, relieved by rest. It can cause sudden pathological fractures and skeletal collapse. Harden the bone to prevent growth and spread of tumours, and to aid pain relief. I prescribe **MCHA calcium**, properly called "microcrystalline hydroxyapatite ossein complex." MCHA calcium will actually increase bone mass and bone density, as it contains intact bone growth factors. This hardens the bone to arrest spread, growth and pain. I formulate it with magnesium citrate, vitamin C, vitamin D3, and sometimes boron. This biological calcium with vitamin D3 is compatible with bisphosphonate drugs like Pamidronate, and Fossamax and Didrocal. Vitamin C up to 1 level tablespoonful daily also hardens bone. The mineral strontium at 600 mg daily hardens bone, but may increase risk of stroke by 30%. Take soy isoflavones at 100 to 150 mg daily, vitamin D3 at 2,000 I.U. or more daily. Other Naturopathic options include vitamin K, horsetail fern *Equisetum arvense*, comfrey leaf *Symphytum officinalis*, common boneset *Eupatorium perfoliatum,* and homeopathic remedies such as *Hekla lava, Phosphorus, Silicea,* and *Carcinosum.* Inhibiting matrix metalloproteinases will slow bone breakdown – for example **green tea EGCG** polyphenols, resveratrol, **curcumin**. Monitor bone turnover with:

- urinary N-telopeptide – excess is over 100 nMol/nMol creatinine
- bone-specific serum alkaline phosphatase – excess risk if over 146 IU/L
- bone scans

      The most common medical therapy is a single high dose shot of external beam radiation. Radiation is often given as a large single palliative dose. About 70% of cases experience good pain relief in the next 5 to 20 weeks. Some will relapse. Cryoablation gives results within 1 to 2 weeks, with 54% obtaining total relief and 85% getting partial relief.

NFkB helps establish osteolytic bone mets – its nuclear localization increases bone expression of granulocyte-macrophage colony stimulating factor GMCSF, increased osteoclast activation, accelerating bone destruction. NFkB is inhibited by **reishi** mushroom extract, indole-3-carbinol, green tea EGCG, quercetin, and pomegranate.

Bone mets are treated according to where they came from, i.e. from the breast, prostate, kidney, bronchus or thyroid gland. They retain that biology, and are not a completely new "bone cancer."

CACHEXIA – is a metabolic rate increase mediated by cytokines and marked by increased glucose production, increased fat burning and protein breakdown. 80% of cancer cases are malnourished, and 40% die of malnutrition. Weight loss is a cardinal sign of cancer, and must be monitored and managed aggressively. Loss of over 20% lean body mass is critically dangerous; increase carbohydrates & protein intake. The omega 3 oil eicosapentaenoic EPA works like magic! I especially like marine omega 3 oil capsules with meals, such as fish or seal oils. Consider also melatonin, L-glutamine, and the bitter melon *Momordica charantia.* The drug hydrazine sulphate can be helpful to block gluconeogenesis, but requires an MD prescription, and requires many stringent dietary restrictions. Maintain adequate protein, calories, and exercise. Cachexia is not caused by poor appetite, but stimulating appetite with reishi extract and royal jelly with ginseng helps the patient get back to eating heartily. Dilute hydrochloric acid HCl, cannabis THC or vitamin B1 thiamine can also be helpful for appetite.

HYPERCALCEMIA – can result from bone mets, vitamin D metabolites made by tumours, excess intake of vitamin D, increased prostaglandin PGE-2, dehydration, and very rarely from tumour production of parathyroid hormone releasing protein PTH-RP. Symptoms may be weakness, fatigue, irritability, depression, nausea, vomiting, abdominal pain and reversible coma. Stop any supplemental vitamin D. Hydrate. Medical attention may be necessary.

LYMPHEDEMA – is a swelling caused by obstruction or loss of the lymphatic drainage. Lymph channels anywhere can be blocked by tumours, as well as by cutting or post-surgical and post-radiation scarring. Lymph is a fluid that leaks out of cells, percolates through tiny spaces, eventually being collected in small ducts, flowing through lymph nodes filled with immune cells monitoring the cellular debris floating by. Eventually it all flows into the thoracic duct in the chest to rejoin the bloodstream. Lymphedema is an accumulation of fluid and protein. This protein acts as a colloid or gel matrix, holding fluid by osmosis.

Lymphedema is most common in an arm after mastectomy, surgery to remove a cancerous breast, and particularly if the lymph nodes of the armpit have been disturbed. Radiation seals the deal. There may be arm swelling, pain, immobility, and tenderness. Even small injuries can precipitate inflammation in the lymph vessels (lymphangitis) and deep tissue infection (cellulitis).

The best therapy I know is the beautiful marigold flower ***Calendula officinalis.*** **Ferlow Brothers** makes a fine organic cream to rub into congested and painful areas. Calendula can be taken as a tincture, and the flower makes a very pleasant tea as well.

Strong Xiao Xin Tan capsules are a TCM herb formula which moves the lymph system.

A Juzo **compression sleeve** can help, as can pneumatic pumps or manual drainage massage. Registered massage therapists with advanced training in lymphology should be treating all cases.

Naturopathic physicians may utilize German complex homeopathics such as *Lymphomyosot* from Heel and botanical/homeopathics such as *Lymphdiaral* from Pascoe Pharmacies. Fresh *Ceanothus spp.* "red root" removes waste from the lymphatic system.

American trained naturopathic physicians use high dose protease (protein dissolving) and lipase (fat dissolving) enzymes.

PAIN – The best defence against pain is to control the growth of the tumour/s or remove the cancer!

Assess pain on a scale from 1 to 10, or with kids use a visual scale such as happy vs. sad faces. Ask if the pain level is "acceptable."

There are potent natural anti-inflammatories that are as effective as synthetic drugs, and safer. Anti-inflammatory herbs can reduce the need for dose–escalation of opioids such as morphine, preventing the constipation and stupor those heavy drugs bring. Reducing inflammation has the beneficial side-effect of slowing tumour growth.

However, analgesics of great strength are not so readily found in the natural pharmacy. We can use willow bark, devil's claw root, cayenne, and many other herbs. Frankly, they are better used in musculoskeletal pain situations. Much has been written about the need for humane and aggressive use of drug cocktails with potentially addictive drugs such as heroin in end-stage disease. Certainly we need to do all we can to ease suffering, and fear of drug addiction is not a sensible reason to refuse opiates for a person in their last days. We have a very reliable herbal therapy for the constipation caused by opiates such as morphine. If the bowels back up pain can increase dramatically, increasing need for the drugs, and conversely the drug needs are lowered when the bowels are functioning well.

I have often been able to help people die in comfort with no drugs whatsoever. Fortunately the mind is sometimes mightier than matter. Mind-body interventions that relieve pain include meditation, prayer, guided imagery, relaxation exercise, hypnosis, cognitive restructuring, biofeedback, and emotional freedom technique.

Acupuncture is very helpful for moderate cancer pain. Acupuncture is best when prescribed within the context of authentic TCM. Commonly used pain-relieving points are LI-4, BL-60, ST-36, SP-4, GB-20, GB-43, PC-6 and LV-3. Think of KI-7 for bone pain. TENS, massage, injections and heat can be more effective if applied to nerves at acupuncture points.

Detoxification relieves pain – detox with raw food, fresh juices and liver tonifying herbs such as burdock, dandelion root, milk thistle, Xiao Chai Hu Tang, or Herbotox. Detoxification must be gently scaled to the vitality of the patient.

Coffee enemas are actually helpful for pain in a toxic cancer patient. Coffee enemas were listed in the Merck Manual until 1977, for a variety of conditions. About 4 to 6 ounces of cooled fresh-brewed coffee are placed in the rectal canal and retained as long as is comfortable. Caffeine and other constituents move up the haemorrhoidal veins to the portal vein and on into the liver, increasing the bile outflow. Overuse can cause deficiencies of vitamins A and E, loss of the electrolyte mineral sodium, and dehydration.

Boswellic acid from frankincense gum Boswellia serrata or B. carteri is a powerful anti-inflammatory plant extract. It has also been shown to induce differentiation, induce apoptosis, and inhibit tumour cells. PhytoFlex from Selekta is a potent professional product using boswellic acid and other plants extracts for pain and inflammation. I use it freely.

Cox-2 cyclooxygenase inhibitors – such as cold-water fish omega 3 fatty acids, feverfew *Tanacetum parthenium*, *Scutellaria baicalensis*, rosemary, propolis, curcumin, and grapeseed extract oligomeric proanthocyanidins -help in reducing doses of narcotics, relieving side-effects of constipation, drowsiness, stupor, and confusion.

Most people respond well to Nikken magnetic and far-infrared technologies. My personal favourite is the Back-Flex pad, which takes my pain away after just a few minutes in contact with any sore spot.

Art therapy, relaxation techniques, counselling, prayer, psychotherapy, positive affirmations, visualization, guided imagery, and meditation are associated with reduced pain, improved sleep, and improved quality of life. Every effort should be made to encourage the patient to approach every life-threatening illness as a challenge which brings gifts and meaning. I often recommend reading *Love, Medicine & Miracles* by Bernie Siegel, MD

Homeopathics for pain include *Euphorbium* or *Phosphoricum acidum* 6 to 30 CH, every 2 hours. Secondary remedies: *Apis mellifica, Arnica Montana, Arsenicum album, Carbo vegetalis, Carcinosum, Colocynthis, Conium maculatum, Hydrastis canadensis.*

Cannabinoids such as marijuana or related prescription medicines such as *Marinol* and *Sativex* reduce neuropathic pain, significantly reduce muscle spasticity, and increase sleep. I have also seen patients have a much better appetite, and it is absolutely outstanding for nausea. Vaporizing the herb is a lot healthier than smoking. Oral ingestion does produce a different response, and is less seldom favoured. Cannabis may cause dizziness and impaired memory. It is a very benign psychoactive drug, if used responsibly. A medical license can be prescribed which allows limited cultivation and possession rights.

Tumours will crush organs, compress nerves, block up vessels and tubes and pressurize cavities. This is the time to move in the big guns and use high dose radiation, for example about 400 rads per dose, for 3 doses, or Prednisone (cortisone) steroids to shrink or "debulk" aggressive cancer.

PLEURAL EFFUSION – Accumulation of fluid in the lung bases and the space around the lung can make breathing difficult. If it is tapped off, there is a lot of albumin protein lost in the fluid, which should be rapidly replaced with whey supplements. I have found the homeopathic remedies *Apocynum canadensis* and *Apis mellifica* to be very useful for lung effusions.

THROMBOCYTOPENIA – low platelets can result from **myelo**suppression in bone marrow by radiotherapy or chemotherapy, from marrow replacement with tumour, or from intravascular coagulation. Lack of platelets to make a clot can lead to serious haemorrhages, often intracranial. Your doctor may prescribe a transfusion of platelets if the count falls below 20. Yunnan Baiyao *Panax pseudo-ginseng* 1 - 2 capsules three to four times daily is a reliable and fast therapy which I have seen out-perform synthetic drugs. The pineal gland hormone melatonin helps regulate the production of platelets, with efficacy comparable to Neupogen, and it's a lot safer. Consider also shark liver oil alkylglycerols, and maitake mushroom extracts. High-dose vitamin C can help recovery. It is thought that eating fresh raw pineapple may help increase the platelet count. Avoid aspirin ASA and Advil (ibuprofen), *Ginkgo biloba*, and other blood thinners. Keep vitamin E dosed under 600 IU daily. Report to your physician any signs of bleeding such as bruising, red spots on skin, bloody urine or black, tarry stools.

WHITE BLOOD CELLS – See LEUKOPENIA

CANCER EMERGENCIES

The management of advanced cancers requires vigilance for morbidity which can rapidly turn to mortality. Cancer patients die prematurely of haemorrhage, obstructions, infection, malnutrition and organ failures. Pathological fractures, ascites, bleeding and seizures can be the first sign of advanced disease. Skilled naturopathic physicians can treat some of these issues, and be alert to refer others for definitive medical care.

BOWEL OBSTRUCTION – may occur below the ileum with colorectal tumours, lymphomas, or peritoneal metastases from ovarian adenocarcinoma. Obstruction above the ileum may occur with esophageal, gastric, pancreatic, hepatocellular and biliary tumours. Watch for early satiety, cramping abdominal pains, constipation and nausea. Vomiting may follow, becoming feculent. Signs include a distended tympanic abdomen, high-pitched and frequent bowel sounds. Later bowel sounds may be absent. Dehydration can occur from vomiting and from sequestration of fluid in the distended bowel loop – "third spacing."

COMPRESSION INJURY – Tumours will crush organs, compress nerves, block up vessels and tubes and pressurize cavities. There is a time for high dose radiation about 400 rads per dose for 3 doses or for Prednisone (cortisone) steroids to shrink or "debulk" aggressive cancer.

DEPRESSION – Mood disorders, anxiety and cognitive dysfunction are linked to elevated IL-6. I prescribe marine omega 3 oils, CanArrest and green tea EGCG to regulate IL-6, and acetyl-L-carnitine to fuel mentation.

DISSEMINATED INTRAVASCULAR COAGULATION DIC – is a decline in fibrinogen and clotting factors leading to a hemorrhagic diathesis (bleeding). Neoplastic cells can release thromboplastin-like material, especially acute promyelocytic leukemia and prostate adenocarcinoma.

DYSPNEA – Homeopathics *Arsenicum album*, also called *Metal album*, and *Apocynum canadensis*, tincture of Old Man's Beard *Usnea barbata*, rhododendron leaf as in Hsiao Keh Chuan.

HAEMORRHAGE – Tumours erode into blood vessels, angiogenesis can form weak and leaky vessels, necrotic areas can erode and bleed, and clotting can be severely disturbed by a variety of mechanisms. Yunnan Baiyao is an excellent treatment for a hemorrhagic tendency. I use the capsule form. Consider also spotted cranesbill herb *Geranium maculatum* and Shepherd's purse *Capsella bursa-pastoris,* which I use in tincture form. Homeopathics such as *Phosphorus* can be added as adjuncts. To stabilize coagulation when the patient is on prescribed blood thinners, take vitamin K1 – 100 mcg., always at the same time of day, and well away from the blood thinning drugs. Vitamin K1 does not build up in the system like K2 does. The diet must be tightly controlled to restrict food sources of K1, such as green leafy vegetables. Acupuncture SP-1 and LV-1 and apply a silver ma-grain.

INTRACRANIAL PRESSURE – may rise from brain and meningeal tumours to provoke symptoms such as headaches. Nausea and visual changes are also common, followed by personality changes, lethargy, and coma. Signs your doctor can see include papilledema at the back of the eyeball, focal neurological deficits, seizures and possibly neck rigidity and pain. A dilated and fixed pupil indicates brainstem tentorial herniation, which will often progress to death by crushing the breathing centers in the brain. We use **Boswellia** aggressively, and it is complementary to Dexamethasone steroids.

LEUKOSTASIS – is a syndrome where extreme levels of circulating leukemic blast cells, i.e. over $100,000/mm3$, cause multiple infarcts and haemorrhages in the lungs and brain.

PARANEOPLASTIC SYNDROMES – 3 out of 4 cancer patients will experience a remote effect of the tumour.

1 in 5 has symptoms from tumour antigens and uncontrolled hormone output.

- **Carcinoid syndrome** occurs in gastro-intestinal GI tumours, particularly with small intestinal cancer. May cause endocardial fibrosis or bronchospastic pulmonary disease, diarrhea, abdominal cramps, malabsorption, flushing due to serotonin excess. Monitor the urinary serotonin metabolite 5-HIAA. The most common type secretes serotonin, which provokes diarrhea. Some pancreas tumours release vasoactive intestinal peptide VIP, provoking watery diarrhea. Gastrinoma carcinoids provoke stomach ulcers, insulinoma carcinoids provoke excess insulin production, and glucagonoma carcinoids provoke diabetes mellitus.
- Multiple **endocrine** adenomatosis syndrome (MEA) can provoke galactorrhea (milk secretion) and gynecomastia (breast swelling). Tumours may produce parathyroid hormone PTH, adrenocorticotrophic hormone ACTH, thyroid stimulating hormone TSH, or melanocyte stimulating hormone MSH.
- **Cutaneous** (skin) manifestations could include purpura, flushing, erythema, phlebitis, urticaria, bullae, hyperpigmentation, pruritis, erythema nodosum, and shingles.
- **Neural** (nerve) manifestations can be neuropathy, neuromyopathy, myopathy, myasthenia, progressive leukoencephalopathy, and seizures.
- **Blood cell production** may shift from aplasia to erythrocythemia from ectopic erythropoietin, a hormone normally put out by the kidney to trigger the bone marrow to make red blood cells. Haemolysis may exacerbate anemia.

Hyperviscosity – thickening of the blood – from globulin proteins or their clumping by cryoprecipitation may complicate syndromes of coagulation and fibrinolysis.

- **Kidney function** can be compromised by ectopic antidiuretic hormone (ADH) produced by small cell lung cancer. Circulating immune complexes can inflame the kidneys, causing nephrotic syndrome.
- **Rheumatic arthritis** is associated with lymphomas and ovarian cancer.
- **Amyloid** starchy deposits can occur in any organ.
- **Endocarditis** is associated with adenocarcinomas.
- **Arterial embolism** triggers infarctions which can be fatal.
- **Fever** can exacerbate fatigue and malaise. Fever control will improve patient activity and vitality. However, a slight fever can also signal good immune activity.
- **Hypercalcaemia** can occur in squamous cell lung cancer, and very rarely also from tumour production of parathyroid hormone releasing protein (PTH-RP).

PERICARDIAL TAMPONADE – is a fluid build-up in the pericardial sac to the point of limiting the filling of the heart in diastole with right-sided heart failure and diminished cardiac output. The patient will be anxious with oppressive chest discomfort, dyspnoea, orthopnea, weakness, cough and dysphagia. There may be distended jugular veins with inspiratory swelling, faint heart sounds, tachycardia, weak arterial pulses, hypotension and pulsus paradoxus. There may be hepatomegaly and peripheral edema. A chest x-ray may show cardiomegaly with a "sac-like" appearance, as well as pleural effusion. Treatment is the same as for ascites – whey protein, Wu Ling San, *Apocynum* and *Apis* homeopathics, Iscador mistletoe.

SPINAL CORD CMPRESSION – can develop insidiously with muscle weakness, sensory disturbances, changes in bowel and bladder function, paresis. Paraplegia or quadriplegia can follow in as little as 12 to 24 hours.

SUPERIOR VENA CAVA SYNDROME – is a compression of the vein returning blood from the head and thorax to the heart. Tumours in the mediastinum, next to the heart, are the culprit. These may include primary lymphomas or metastases to the mediastinal lymph nodes from lung or breast cancer. The earliest warning sign is facial edema, which can spread to the neck and upper extremities. Later cyanosis can appear, and there may be venous distension visible on the chest.

TUMOUR LYSIS SYNDROME – is a toxic overload of the kidneys due to aggressive treatment resulting in rapid necrosis. Most commonly seen in acute leukemias and lymphomas. The metabolic load of rising potassium, phosphate, and uric acid, and falling calcium, results in acidosis and azotemia. A shift of any of these blood factors of over 25% relative to pre-treatment values is diagnostic. Watch for cardiac arrhythmias, arthritis, weakness, lethargy, tachypnea, or coma with deep Kussmaul respirations. Test serum creatinine. Monitor serum lactate dehydrogenase enzyme LDH as a marker of necrosis. Medical care involves rehydration, uric acid lowering drugs such as Allopurinol, management of renal failure, and other complex medical intervention. Support the kidneys with Co-enzyme Q-10, R+alpha lipoic acid, and goat whey minerals. Give sodium bicarbonate sufficient to raise the urine pH to over 5.0. Botanicals to consider are Pipsissewa, also known as Prince's pine – *Chimaphila umbellata,* Cleavers herb – *Gallium aparense*, stinging nettle – *Urtica urens* and parsley – *Petroselinum sativum.*

END-OF-LIFE ISSUES

"The question is not, Will I die? but Will I die healed? The real question relates to the Quality of Life, not to the reality of death" Dr. Jean-Charles Crombez

Patients tend to want both honesty and hope when facing terminal cancer, the stage where death seems inevitable. Well, it always was inevitable, but now an expert is making a prognosis. Gnosis is just "Knowing," as in knowledge, but the pro means the knowledge is before it happens. Doctors who play at fortune-telling use statistical probability to estimate the likely course of events. Unlikely events do happen, even if only rarely. The only certainty is that physical life ends in death. When it will come seems at times to be as much at the whim of the mind and the spirit as of the physical frame.

The reality is that the following, among many other diagnostic factors, give a very poor prognosis:

- Lymphopenia – low white blood cell counts indicate a lack of a robust immune response to the tumour.
- Elevated LDH – indicates tumour necrosis, associated with inflammation and toxicity
- Low albumin protein – a marker of oxidative stress in the liver and low protein intake
- Liver metastases – risk ratio 2.5
- Lung metastases – risk ratio 2.4
- Cachexia – tissue wasting, particularly if over 20% loss of body mass, or weight loss over 10 kg in the last 6 months.

Prognostic indicators of the end of life are persistent problems with –

- low Karnofsky performance status – ambulatory ability, self-care activities, etc. The Victoria Hospice uses the Palliative Performance Scale version 2 – PPSv2 which grades in 10% increments.. See below.
- anorexia – oral intake, dysphagia to solids or liquids
- dyspnoea at rest
- low total white blood cell count, particularly lymphocytes.
- altered cognition – confusion, delirium, stupor, somnolence.
- edema
- diarrhea
- nausea and vomiting
- pain which becomes intractable. The relief of pain and reduction of narcotics can help move a terminal patient into the death phase.

Anorexia induces ketosis, the build up of acidic ketones in the blood. This can create mild euphoria, analgesia and over-sense of well-being. Any food intake can interrupt this defensive mechanism.

Determining the terminal stage of cancer and the active process of dying is an art and a science demanding all the skills and experience of a physician. In communicating such news we try to engage, listen and empathize with the patient or their guardian. It is best to be sure what the patient is needing or asking before attempting to answer it.

Making a prognosis of when someone will die is simply a guess, even for a physician. No-one can see the future, so we tend to speak about average life expectancies, based on similar cases. The patient should clearly understand the gravity of the situation. However, they should also have a little hope because some must always do better than the average. There may be various forms of healing still possible, including the experience that there has been time enough to see life through in a meaningful way. As Dr. Ronna Jevne says, "Hope is not about everything turning out OK. It is about being OK with how things turn out."

<u>Palliative Performance Scale version two</u> – PPSv2 – as used by the Victoria Hospice

PPS level	Ambulation	Activity & evidence of disease	Self-care	Intake	Conscious level
100%	Full	Normal activity & work No evidence of disease	Full	Normal	Full
90%	Full	Normal activity & work Some evidence of disease	Full	Normal	Full
80%	Full	Normal activity *with* effort Some evidence of disease	Full	Normal or reduced	Full
70%	Reduced	Unable to do normal work/job Significant disease	Full	Normal or reduced	Full
60%	Reduced	Unable to do hobbies/house work; significant disease	Occasional assistance needed	Normal or reduced	Full or confusion
50%	Mainly sits or lays down	Unable to do any work Extensive disease	Considerable assistance needed	Normal or reduced	Full or drowsy +/- confusion
40%	Mainly in bed	Unable to do most activity Extensive disease	Mainly with assistance	Normal or reduced	Full or drowsy +/- confusion
30%	Totally bed bound	Unable to do any activity Extensive disease	Total care	Normal or reduced	Full or drowsy +/- confusion
20%	Totally bed bound	Unable to do any activity Extensive disease	Total care	Minimal to sips	Full or drowsy +/- confusion
10%	Totally bed bound	Unable to do any activity Extensive disease	Total care	Mouth care only	Drowsy or coma +/- confusion
0%	Death	-	-	-	-

Physiological changes the family should be aware could occur in the last hours of life include:

- Fatigue, with increasing time spent sleeping or somnolent.
- Weakness, including inability to move, swallow, speak.

- Erythema or redness where bones are prominent.
- Profound loss of appetite, with severe weight loss and wasting.
- Disinterest in fluid intake with dehydration and peripheral edema.
- Racing heart from kidney and heart dysfunction.
- Delirium with agitation, restlessness, repetitive purposeless movements, moaning and groaning.
- Abnormal breathing, gurgling, aspiration, asphyxia, agonal breaths.
- Cyanosis or blueing of the extremities and lips due to poor oxygenation.
- Pain may only be evident by grimacing or tension at the nasion and forehead.
- A period of "golden glow" may occur, with temporarily increased lucidity and strength.
- At the time of death loss of sphincter control and blood and other fluids from orifices can occur.

The ethical decision to abandon curative therapy strategies for gentler palliative comfort-oriented care is a difficult one. The guiding principles are autonomy, nonmaleficence, beneficence and justice. Prudent decisions based on informed consent, fidelity to trust, compassion, integrity and temperance result in "right and good" healing actions. Physicians would be wise to study with hospice workers and call on them for support when the case is not realistically curable. Patients will often communicate their needs and problems more effectively to a non-physician. Whether it be legal advice on living wills and advanced directives, spiritual comfort, or pain control, palliation should be multidisciplinary and patient-directed. The three top medical issues to address are dyspnoea, pain and depression

The World health Organization WHO defines quality of life as "the state in which an individual, coming from a particular culture and value system, experiences conditions of existence in accordance with his aims, expectations and standards At the same time, feelings of self-worth, self-realization and obligation to society are emphasized."

Everyone wants to forestall death. We would prefer to die as young as possible, but as late as possible. I do place living at #1 on the list of priorities. However, those who experience at least the first stages of dying, such as cardiac arrest, who are later revived, all seem to have a pleasant experience. All lose their fear of death. Death is not a failure for the patient, and it is not a failure for the health care team. It is condition we will all have. I have been honoured and amazed to share births and deaths with my loved ones and with patients. These are experiences worth having, for they define BEING. We all seem to fear having too little- including having too little life. I think the point is to fear BEING too little, and use that to motivate ourselves to engage in life with gusto. How much is enough of anything – food, sex, power, money, years of existence? If we have been consciously present in our own lives, and have participated actively in living, we should find it easy to be grateful for all we have had. No matter whom we out-live or who out-lives us, we can all say a person had a full life when they were present and understood life to be a miraculous and wondrous opportunity.

Homeopathics are very helpful in the emotional and mental transitions of palliative care, e.g. *Arsenicum album* 30C for late stage depression and anxiety. This remedy gives ease to the final moments of life. Homeopathic leaders for the pain of terminal cancer are *Euphorbium*, *Arnica montana*, and *Carbo vegetalis*. Bach flower remedies are also great assists to the spirit and mind of the dying and the grieving.

Take note that normally dying patients have no appetite and may stop oral intake, even of fluids. Artificial feeding and hydration will not affect the outcome or its timing, but can increase breathlessness, edema, ascites and nausea or vomiting. It used to be thought cruel to allow a patient to dehydrate, but it turns out this releases a lot of endorphins, and people can die without pain. Oral care regards dry mouth is still indicated for comfort.

"Palliative sedation" does not hasten death, but relieves refractory vomiting, pain, agitation and delirium. Neuroleptics, benzodiazepines and opiates are combined to bring ease to the final stage before the end of all suffering.

PART SIX – PREVENTING CANCER

Chapter Twenty-Three – Preventing Cancer

I have always maintained that BAD THINGS HAPPEN TO GOOD PEOPLE – AND SO HAVING CANCER IS NOT ALL YOUR FAULT. Sure it matters if you chose to use tobacco products, get too much sun exposure, eat junk food, and neglect physical activity. However, this only explains about half of cancers. I have seen a lot of folks who "do everything right" their whole lives and end up diagnosed with advanced cancers. No one should ever feel ashamed or blamed for developing cancer. There are toxins in our environment, food and water that the government has approved as safe for us, knowing they will injure some folks. There is a lot of radiation loose on the planet. There are genetic factors you did not choose to be born with.

We are responsible for trying to do our best with the life we are given. There are winning strategies to reduce the risk and worry of cancer. They don't work every time for every person, but at the very least, those who make the effort to have a healthy lifestyle will enter into the disease with a better reserve of health, and will stand up better to the rigors of treatment, and have a better chance of survival and recovery.

The primary cause of suffering in our culture is what Dr. Anita Tannis of the Center for Integrated Health in Vancouver calls "AFFLUENZA." This is illness provoked by the relentless pursuit of more of everything. We get so stressed by a sense of time-urgency, and a feeling we need so many things.

It is critically important to simplify our lifestyle, to restore an appreciation for taking a rest, simple food, and a calm inner life. We used to joke in the cancer research labs that the leading cause of cancer was – "mouse abuse." Well, if you are living at a "rat-race" pace, and allow the chemical corporations to adulterate your food and environment, then you are being abused, and are taking a big risk.

While you cannot avoid every genetic risk, environmental insult, and the aging process, you may be able to delay or even avoid the diseases which kill two of every three Canadian adults. Choices that can help you avoid cancer – adding protective factors, reducing risky behaviours, and seeking early detection – may also help you avoid cardiovascular disease, diabetes, hypertension and other chronic degenerative conditions. It is never too late to adopt life-affirming habits in mind and body.

Choosing to be pro-active about cancer prevention also means becoming aware of our place in the ecology of the bio-sphere and our impact on the environment. I hope that when we learn to live within the tolerances of our biology and our in-born ability to handle stress, toxins and pathogenic factors, which we will also end up walking a bit more lightly upon the Earth. The ancient Chinese Taoist belief that living in harmony with Nature was the key to health and happiness is still wise and true.

PROTECTIVE FACTORS

Protecting or restoring p53 gene functionality is the primary strategy in cancer prevention.

Protection comes in many agreeable packages; delicious foods provide us with proven cancer fighters. Increasing the amount of fruits and vegetables you eat to over five servings daily adds protective ingredients such as antioxidants and bioflavonoids, resveratrol, limonene, lycopene and polyphenols to your diet. A cancer- preventative diet includes two to three servings of fruit, four to six servings of vegetables and more than seven servings of other plant foods such as whole cereal grains, beans, peas, roots and tubers daily. All the colors of the rainbow should be represented in the variety of foods you eat, but especially good cancer-fighting foods include blueberries, grapes, cherries, apples, tomatoes, celery, yams, squash, cilantro, ginger, almonds, lemons, onions, garlic, beets, broccoli and kale.

Green vegetables and green drinks such as barley grass juice and wheat grass juice are sources of that "magical" capturer of all sun energy on this planet, chlorophyll. This green substance inhibits the leading trigger of skin cancers, lipid peroxidation. Green vegetables are also powerful detoxifiers of the blood Plant fats such as sterols and sterolins, found in all fruits and vegetables, are being studied as immune modulators that may benefit cancer patients.

Folic acid (also known as **folate** if bound to a mineral) found in green leafy vegetables is a significant regulator of cell development. The long-running Nurse's Health Study showed folate to work well as a preventative factor against colorectal cancer. Both folate and vitamin B12 put methyl groups into DNA to silence overactive genes. A multivitamin with B-complex vitamins such as folate or a greens powder supplement should be included in a cancer-prevention diet, especially if you eat under five servings of vegetables daily. There is a controversy at present regarding a possible increase in colorectal cancer from polyps being stimulated by high folic acid intake.

The cabbage family of vegetables gives us **indole-3-carbinol**, which reduces the activity of potentially harmful hormones such as estrogen. Excess estrogen exposure is the primary cause of breast cancer, and sex hormones are also thought to contribute to prostate, colorectal and other common cancers. Broccoli, cauliflower, Brussels sprouts, cabbage, kale and bok choy also provide **isothiocyanates** which do two amazing things. They detoxify and protect the body from carcinogens by powerfully inducing Phase 2 detoxification. Isothiocyanates also directly kill cancer cells by inducing apoptosis that has been blocked by bcl-2 protein. Other detoxifying glucosinolates in the *Brassica* (cabbage and mustard family) include sulforaphanes and cyanohydroxybutene.

Seeds and plants contain **lignans**, which friendly bacteria in our gut turn into weak phytoestrogens. These bind to estrogen receptors on cells and block the signal to grow. Soy is rich in lignans. Flaxseed lignans are also anti-estrogenic enough to be thought to play a role in preventing and treating hormone dependent cancers. Flaxseed lignans also increase liver output of sex-hormone binding globular proteins SHBGs which further inactivate excess hormones. I take psyllium and flaxseed daily as part of my "daily detox" regime.

403

Psyllium husks are converted by bacteria in the colon to short-chain fatty acids such as butyrates which regulate the abnormal DNA in cancer cells. **Flaxseed**, hemp, nuts, seeds, seafood, fish and fish oils are excellent sources of omega 3 fats which reduce arachidonic acid and prostaglandin PGE-2, associated with inflammation. Inflammation gives rise to a host of growth stimulators which can accelerate cancer.

The delicious onion family, including leeks, chives, and **garlic** contain allyl sulphide, a fat-soluble chemoprotectant, detoxifier and anti-mutagen.

Calcium and vitamin D reduce the risk of colorectal cancer. The best form of calcium for prevention may be calcium-D-glucarate, which some researchers believe may be the most bio-available. It is found in citrus fruit, cruciferous vegetables (cabbage family again) and apples. It inhibits beta-glucuronidase, an enzyme involved in metastasis in hormone-dependent cancers.

Vitamin D levels in Canadians are decreasing as more people avoid risk of sunburn from the ultraviolet radiation in sun exposure. Vitamin D is a very good regulator of growth, helping to slow the growth and spread of cancers. The Canadian Cancer Society recently noted that science shows up to 60% reduced risk of some cancers with adequate vitamin D levels, and that higher intakes are not toxic, as previously believed. They suggest a supplement of 1,000 IU daily, but I prescribe 2,000 IU daily in the winter months, and my American colleagues are using massive doses in cancer cases.

Some research has suggested that the mineral **selenium**, taken in moderate doses, reduces risk of many cancers by acting as an antioxidant supporting DNA surveillance and repair enzymes. In one study, reported in the Journal of the American Medical Association in 1996, doses of only 200 micrograms a day appeared to reduce skin cancer risk by half. Studies also suggest selenium works very well with vitamin E to prevent cancer of the prostate. The vast SELECT study – Selenium and Vitamin E Cancer Prevention Trial, run by the National Cancer Institute and launched in 2001, involves over 400 institutions in the United States, Puerto Rico and Canada. One of them is the British Columbia Cancer Agency BCCA. The results from this study should give us a greater understanding of how selenium works to fight cancer. We do know that areas of the world with low selenium (and calcium) in soils are seeing higher rates of cancer, and that selenium can regulate the BRAC and other DNA repair genes.

Green tea is rich in polyphenols, which appear to be able to suppress the growth of many cancers. The polyphenols in green tea inhibit cancer first by checking formation of new blood vessels into tumours and second by stopping spread into other tissues. A protective or preventative amount of tea is about 5 or more cups daily (2 to 10), and it would take well over 40 cups daily to treat a tumour. In clinical applications, therefore, it is used as a polyphenol extract in capsule form in addition to being enjoyed as a beverage. I prescribe 2,100 mg of 95% EGCG routinely, which represents far more tea than one could drink without fatal injury to the kidneys. High dose EGCG, like any anti-oxidant, can be pro-oxidant in high doses, leading to oxidative stress on the kidneys and liver. Fortunately a small daily dose of vitamin E solves this problem.

Curry is a variable mix of Asian spices, but always includes turmeric root. Turmeric contains **curcumin**, which strongly quenches inflammation. Curcumin modulates detoxification by speeding up Phase 2 detoxification while slowing Phase 1. This prevents the build-up of toxic intermediates, which could cause a "healing crisis."

Omega 3 oils are generally low in the diet relative to omega 6 oils, an imbalance which leads to increased inflammation responses. Ancestral diets were much higher in omega 3's from nuts, seeds, grass-fed meat, fish and seafood. The modern diet is now much higher in pro-inflammatory omega 6 fats from corn silage fed meats, corn products including corn oil, all grains and cereals. Restoring the 3:6 ratio reduces risk of all degenerative diseases.

Mono-unsaturated oleic acid in olive oil is protective, as is the whole **Mediterranean diet**. Several world cultures found a healthy set of plant foods to maintain health and vigour. Take your pick, and get back to sensible eating.

Supplements, while not proven to prolong life, can compensate for common deficiencies in the Canadian diet. Remember that illness and cancer therapies can create metabolic and absorption issues leading to gross nutritional deficiencies. Consider supplementing a varied, whole foods organic diet with:

- multivitamins containing basic antioxidants, B-complex with 50 mg daily for B1, B3, B5, B6; 50 mcg B12; folate 1 mg; biotin 1 mg.
- minerals including selenium up to 400 mcg, iodine up to 350 mcg, and chromium up to 400 mcg.
- vitamin C up to 3,000 mg.
- grape seed extract antioxidants 100 to 300 mg
- calcium 500 to 1,500 mg with magnesium citrate up to 500 mg.
- vitamin D3 1,000 to 2,000 IU
- fish oil, seal or plant-based omega 3 fats 1,000 to 3,000 mg.
- flaxseed and/or psyllium fibre 1 to 2 Tbsp – 15 to 30 ml.
- probiotic bacteria 1 to 3 capsules
- green drinks such as chlorella, spirulina, or barley grass 1 tsp to 1 Tbsp – 5 to 15 ml.
- indole-3-carbinol 200 to 400 mg

If you are an elderly person taking a **statin** drug such as Lipitor for cholesterol, you have 25% lower risk of getting cancer

SUGAR FEEDS CANCER

Modern diets, high in processed foods, deliver fibre-reduced foods that release a lot of sugars into the blood very fast.) These foods are considered to have a high- glycemic index if they charge up the blood sugar faster than 60 percent when compared to eating pure glucose. After a meal the glucose goes into the blood, and the pancreas responds by releasing insulin, a pump that moves sugars, fats and proteins into cells where they can be used.

The liver responds by releasing insulin-like growth factors IGF-1 and IGF-2 to make cells double. IGF-1 & 2 are major stimulators of growth for many cancers, and as cancers get older and build more IGF receptors they grow faster, metastasizing throughout the body. IGF-1 and insulin associated with estrogen metabolism, and so this is very important in hormone-dependent cancers as well as those of the gastro-intestinal tract. There is evidence that a high-glycemic meal can accelerate the growth of liver metastases from colorectal cancer by up to eight-fold for up to three hours.

High-glycemic meals can include ordinary foods such as bananas and watermelon, soft breads, potatoes, parsnips, corn, beets, or cooked carrots. It is the total sugar balance which is vital, and cancer patients definitely need to carefully regulate their blood sugar. The absolute worst sugar is *high fructose corn sugar* which is widely used in soft drinks and candy. It can trigger persistent insulin problems at very low rates of consumption.

There is no excuse for the sugary "energy foods" promoted to cancer patients for "energy" during chemo and throughout oncological treatment. This dietary mismanagement has accelerated the demise of many patients.

The ideal low- glycemic sweets for cancer patients are fruits such as blueberries, strawberries, grapes, and pears.

Sugar substitutes such as Stevia and blue agave syrup are recommended. Aspartame and cyclamates are not recommended. Splenda is OK.

The most effective action one can take to live longer is to reduce caloric intake. A weight gain of over five kilograms in adulthood is enough to measurably increase risk of several of the leading causes of death such as heart disease, high blood pressure, diabetes, and cancer. Remember that storage or depot fat, created from an excess intake of sugars and fats, can generate high levels of estrogens in the body. This is due to aromatase enzymes converting testosterone into estrogen. Obesity is almost as hard on the system as tobacco.

AVOIDING CARCINOGENIC TOXINS

Xenohormones or **xenobiotics** are chemicals which may have a beneficial use in agriculture or industry, but when they enter the human body they act like hormones, hormone disruptors or growth factors. They are unintentional hormones, synthetic chemical mimics of vital biological molecules. Environmental Protection Agency EPA studies showed cancer-causing dioxin, styrene, and other xenohormones in 100% of fat samples taken from human bodies in the USA.

Xenohormones are found in non-organic fruits and vegetables, animal feeds, and due to agricultural runoff, get into our water supply. Red meat animals are particularly good at concentrating the pesticides and herbicides in their feed. Eating red meat may increase your risk of cancer due to its saturated fat content, toxins produced during grilling, and pro-inflammatory omega 6 fats in corn silage feedlot animals. This is why I insist on very clean grass fed meats, or else vegetarian meat replacement.

Vegetarian diets give a survival advantage for cancer. An excellent vegetarian source of protein, soy may also be a leading protective factor. While the research is not yet conclusive, soy isoflavones have been shown in some studies to reduce risk of breast and other cancers by inhibiting formation of estrogen in fat, blocking the enzyme aromatase, inhibiting estrogen receptors, turning hormones into inactive forms, and through various antioxidant mechanisms. Blood levels of estrogen may be reduced by moderate intakes of soy foods such as soy milk, miso and tofu.

Endocrine disruptors such as **dioxins** attach to our estrogen receptors. Dioxins are formed during the manufacture of polyvinyl chloride PVC plastics. Dioxins are also formed during incineration of waste and burning fuels such as wood, coal and oil. Over 95 percent of exposure comes from eating commercial animal fats – milk and dairy foods, eggs, and beef. Dioxins are high in farmed salmon and are found in many other fish. Green tea EGCG suppresses transformation of the aryl hydrocarbon receptor, protecting against xenobiotic carcinogens such as dioxins.

Polychlorinated biphenyls PCBs are persistent organic pollutant, now banned, that was used as electrical transformer cooling oil. It has contaminated the entire world food-chain. For example, farmed salmon are loaded with it. PCBs are hormone mimics. Other toxic environmental xenohormones we are all tainted with include dieldrin, heptachlor, kepone, mirex and toxaphene.

Bisphenol A is a common ingredient in many plastics, including those in reusable water bottles and resins lining some food cans and dental sealants. BPA can change the course of foetal development in a way that increases the risk of breast cancer.

The industrial insecticide **methychlor** is also a potent estrogen mimic which can trigger cancer.

So is the famous insecticide **DDT**, which is still in our bodies despite being banned decades ago.

Parabens are powerful estrogen mimics. Parabens are preservatives used in cosmetics, shampoos, sunscreens, toothpastes, baby wipes, and many skin lotions and creams. They accumulate in fat, such as breast tissue. Far infrared saunas help to neutralize and remove them. Chemically, they are very similar to phthalates.

Phthalates are toxic plasticizers – they make soft and flexible plastic products possible. This can include PVC intravenous bags and tubing, blood transfusion storage bags, children's toys and bottle nipples, vinyl flooring, personal care products such as detergents, soap, shampoo, deodorants, fragrances, hair spray, nail polish, and plastic food bags, plastic wrap we put food in. The phthalates will disperse into air and fats. Think about this when you unwrap some fatty meat or cheese in kitchen wrap. Do not even think about putting any of these plastics in a microwave. Phthalates are able to disrupt reproductive hormones, including male hormone cycles.

According to the Environmental Protection Agency EPA, 60 percent of herbicides, 90 percent of fungicides and 30 percent of insecticides are known to be carcinogenic. Alarmingly, pesticide residues have been detected in 50 percent to 95 percent of U.S. foods. They are linked to lymphoma, leukemia, and other cancers. The worst case scenario is exposure during foetal development.

Organophosphates are pesticides widely used on food and in homes against mosquitoes, roaches and termites.

The fruits and vegetables recently found to be very contaminated with pesticide residues include strawberries, bell peppers, spinach, cherries, peaches, cantaloupe, celery, apples, apricots, green beans, grapes and cucumbers. Commercial grade foods need to be thoroughly washed to remove these residues. Use pure Castile soap and scrub thoroughly. You also may need to disinfect the food, particularly if you are immune-suppressed due to chemotherapy, radiation therapy, steroid drugs and other stressors.. Soak briefly with cool water treated with food grade hydrogen peroxide or unscented Clorox regular bleach. Non-organic commercial-grade fruits and vegetables still have a net health benefit. I still prefer organic grown, for safety and nutritional content, and still wash organic produce.

Nitrate fertilizers are used throughout the world to boost food production. They not only accelerate plant growth, they are able to increase the growth rate of tumours. Cancers are "nitrogen sinks," a biological term for a high user of protein. Foods that are raised with soil composting and other biological measures of feeding less concentrated nitrogen compounds do not accelerate cancer growth. Drinking water must be purified of nitrates.

Inorganic phosphates from fertilizer, soda drinks and red meats are linked to risk of lung cancer in animals.

Despite claims that organic foods are a rip-off, I feel they have great value. They are non-toxic and they tend to have much higher nutrient content. I recommend organic fruits, vegetables, beans, seeds and nuts and other organic food are staples in your diet. I insist you need to eat "organic" animal foods. Milk and cheese from organic-fed cows are increasingly available, as are free-range eggs and poultry, grass-fed red meats, and wild fish.

To avoid these chemical hazards and carcinogenic **chlorine**, it is best to choose purified water to drink. The Canadian cancer Society estimates chlorination of our water is responsible for 1 to 2% of our cancers. We certainly want to disinfect water from pathogenic bacteria. Water borne diseases are a real risk, and many would die if we stopped treating water. However, once clean, which in Canadian standards means disinfected, water can be filtered to remove chlorine before consumption.

Water is a source of many toxins that enter human tissues. The sun evaporates the oceans and lakes into clouds, that fall back to earth as rain. Many chemical compounds boil up from land and water and rain down again. Well water should be tested for carcinogenic levels of arsenic. **Purify your water.** A simple, cheap Brita type water filter will remove 99% of the chlorine. I personally will only use reverse osmosis water that is oxygenated and remineralized in a Nikken Optimizer, or tap water run through a Nikken brand "Pi-Mag" water treatment system, including the Aqua-Pour. Pi-mag water is the best for detoxification. I will also drink ozonated and filtered artesian spring water.

Molds and fungi produce potent **mycotoxins** which are a significant worldwide cause of cancer, especially liver cancer. Poor food storage can allow mould to contaminate foods such as wheat, corn and peanuts. If there is any visible trace of mould on any food, please throw it out, it is ruined. Molds also grow in homes, causing great harm to occupants.

The fungicide **vinclozolin** causes changes to male mice born for as many as four subsequent generations after the initial exposure. This is reminiscent of the multigenerational disaster when **diethylstilbestrol** DES was given to women, and ended up causing cancer in their children! DES was also used to fatten up cattle.

Ellagic acid as found in berries, grapes and pomegranate, help us to eliminate carcinogens from fungal toxins. They also help resist harm from nitrosamine and polycyclic aromatic hydrocarbons, as found smoked meats, grilled or barbecued foods..

Perfluorooctanoic acid PFOA, found in grease- and water-resistant coatings like Teflon and Gore-Tex, is a likely carcinogen, yet we wear it and cook with it.

Organic solvents and volatile organic chemicals VOCs are major indoor as well as outdoor air pollutants. Glues, resins, plastics, caulking, paints and fabrics all vent off a noxious chemical cloud. The highest risk substances are 1,3-butadiene, formaldehyde, acetaldehyde, benzene, chloroform, naphthalene, acetaldehyde and dioxins. We are exposed at work, in our cars, and in our homes. It is not easy to clean up our environments, but there are air systems that reduce harm, alternative products like low-VOC paints, and ways to get these out of our bodies such as with therapeutic saunas.

We absorb toxins through our skin and lungs, including during a shower or bath, from soaps, hair products and toiletries, fragrances and cosmetics. There are literally hundreds of thousands of unpronounceable and undesirable chemicals in your daily environment that need to be moved out and replaced by "green" products.

If it is not biodegradable, it is probably degrading you. If it hurts the environment, it can hurt you. I prefer soaps, toothpastes, shampoos and related products from Ferlow Brothers Botanicals www.ferlowbotanicals.com

Chemicals that are best kept out of your home are in over 75,000 home insecticides, cleaners, glues, paints, etc.

They upset the ecology in our bodies, our homes, and then on out into the land and water, to inevitably recycle back onto our dinner plate or onto our skin. Many green solutions are at hand, cheap and easy. I recommend you see the books *Household Solutions 1- with Substitutions* and *Household Solutions 2 with Kitchen Secrets* by Reena Nerbas. These gems are loaded with green alternatives to chemicals in your home, and beyond. For books and other resources see her website www.householdsolutions.org

Another excellent resource is *The CancerSmart Consumer Guide- How to eliminate toxins from your home and garden products and how to make healthy choices for your family and the environment*, from the Labour Environmental Alliance Society, Vancouver, B.C., www.leas.ca

Using safer products in our homes and on our bodies will take some strain off the detoxification mechanisms in the liver. The liver has to get rid of a lot of non-nutritive substances in the food and water, as well as in any drugs we take. If the liver gets bogged down in the early phase of detoxifying a carcinogen, it is caught with even more toxic oxidized carcinogens. Fortunately herbs and foods such as turmeric and raspberries can rebalance detoxification, binding the oxidized chemicals to carriers that then take them out of the body. A supervised program of detoxification is recommended once or twice a year to minimize build-up of hazardous chemicals.

Heavy metals like lead, mercury, aluminum, cadmium and arsenic are able to cause cancer. Think of testing and detoxifying heavy metal load particularly in leukemia, lymphoma and multiple myeloma and sarcoma. If you have well-water, have it checked. Avoid "silver" mercury amalgam dental fillings. Do not eat the big predator fish such as swordfish and tuna that accumulate these metals.

Nitrates and **nitrites** keep cured meats such as hot dog wieners and fresh-looking, but are carcinogens linked to stomach cancer. Nitrates are found in produce grown with chemical fertilizers.

Salt in excess from pickled and preserved foods, such as cured meats, can also trigger stomach cancer.

Ferrocyanide is an anti-caking agent used in road salt all over Canada. It is also a corrosion inhibitor. Unfortunately it can break down into highly carcinogenic hydrogen cyanide gas in the presence of strong sunlight and acidic water. Cancer rates are higher in areas where road salt is applied.

Considerable gains in health come from simply not doing some foolish things, such as using **tobacco** products. Tobacco smoke delivers tars, benzene, cadmium, cyanide, formaldehyde and polycyclic aromatic hydrocarbons – quite a toxic cloud! Chewing tobacco is little better. 30% of all cancer risks are eliminated if you kick the tobacco habit. In Finland a successful program to curb smoking produced a reduction in lung cancer deaths proportional to the numbers who quit.

We cannot completely avoid these chemicals – they are too numerous, too widely used, and too persistent. They are ubiquitous (everywhere). Even people eating only organic food and wearing hemp and doing all the right things still test positive for toxins of concern. It is worthwhile to **detoxify** what we can with far-infrared saunas, milk thistle herb, flaxseed and psyllium fibre, and supplement R+ alpha lipoic acid.

ELECTROMAGNETIC POLLUTION

Microwave radiation from cell phones is capable of causing brain cancers in young people with heavy exposure for several years.

Common household and office devices can give off very dangerous levels of high-frequency voltage transients HFVT, and these signals also reverberate through the entire wiring of a building. HFVTs occur when AC is converted to DC in transformers and switch-mode power supplies. This includes dimmer switches, halogen lamps, compact fluorescent lights, and power adaptors for laptop computers, MP3 players, telephones, and other electronics. HFVTs can increase risk of melanoma, thyroid, uterine and other cancers by about 3 fold, or about 26% in one year!

Please do not sleep within a meter of any plug-in device. Use magnetic and other geopathic or *Feng shui* amendments to create a sanctuary from the power grid.

MANAGE STRESS

Research shows that the management of stress is critical to maintaining good immune function. Grief and other major life stressors can play a role in triggering cancer, and the stress of fighting cancer itself can be gruelling. The stress hormone adrenaline – epinephrine from the adrenal glands – is able to block cancer cells from dying. Throughout the *Bad* gene, it blocks apoptosis or *the cancer off-switch,* making the little stinkers immortal. Ironically, if you relax, cancer cells die.

Activities which defuse stress, regulate autonomic balance and increase

parasympathetic tone:
- diaphragmatic breathing is the most potent solution
- yoga
- meditation
- hypnosis
- biofeedback
- progressive muscle relaxation exercises
- exercise

One of the most interesting phenomena in predicting cancer risk is the role of three factors: skipping breakfast, eating between meals, and irregular hours of sleep. These little behaviours seem to measurably increase cancer risk. While the specific mechanisms at work aren't yet known, it may be because these factors characterize a chaotic lifestyle. Chaos is stressful both physically and mentally.

Maintaining a positive outlook and tapping into social support systems can improve quality of life and potentially assist survival. Prayer and meditation are currently being studied as adjunct or complementary cancer therapies. Hospice and palliative care units for terminally ill patients offer meditation, Touch for Health healing, chaplain services and other spiritual solace. Finding meaning is the ultimate human creative endeavour. Through music, art, or journaling therapies, for example, a person can explore his or her reasons for wanting to live. Finding a way to approach life with zest and positive purpose is associated with some remarkable cancer recoveries.

Sloth, on the other hand, appears to be a deadly sin. In one observational study, the death rate from cancer for older men who walked more than two miles daily was half that of those who walked less than a mile each day. Exercise helps regulate blood sugar, moves the bowels, and improves immune functions such as the activity of cancer-eating natural killer NK cells. Exercise regulates the adrenal stress hormones.

At the end of your day, you go to sleep to rest and repair. One of the most important antioxidants and hormone and cell-growth regulators is melatonin, made in the pineal gland in the brain. Between 10 pm and 1 am, melatonin is produced in the pineal gland if the person is at rest in a dark place. Any light or disturbance can disrupt this critical defensive molecule. Early studies suggest that disturbed sleep, as experienced by shift workers, may increase risk of cancer, probably by throwing off the melatonin cycle. Jet-lag is a syndrome associated with melatonin disruption by rapid transportation to a place with a markedly different light-dark period. You may need an entire month of sleeping from 10 pm to 6 am in a completely darkened bedroom to restore a natural melatonin rhythm. Even a nightlight, bathroom light or the refrigerator light can disrupt the production of melatonin. It's no wonder melatonin disturbance is a widespread problem.

One of the most consistently helpful supports for sleep if the Nikken sleep system. The mattress is magnetized, the comforter has far-infrared reflectors, and pillow is also therapeutic. It is part of their "Certified Wellness Home" line of products, including the air and water filtration systems I use in my home and clinic.

Using **alcohol** as a self-medication for stress is most unwise from a mental health perspective, but alcohol is also a potent carcinogen. Excess intake is linked to breast and many other cancers. Good folate intake helps counteract some of the carcinogenicity of alcohol.

EARLY DETECTION

The best diet, supplements, surroundings, and psychology cannot prevent all cancers. There are insidious threats like the radiation still circulating from Chernobyl, and from DDT used in the 1950's and 1960's. The final step in a healthy lifestyle must be wise use of early screening tests to detect cancer while it can still be cured. Breast exams and prostate exams, PSA blood tests, and PAP smears are examples of reliable methods that may save lives.

The earlier a cancer is detected the better the chance of a cure. Most of the recent gains in reducing cancer deaths come from better screening, rather than significant changes in therapy.

C.A.U.T.I.O.N. – Cancer Society 7 Cardinal Warning Signs of Cancer

> **C** hange in bowel or bladder habits
> **A** sore that does not heal
> **U** nusual bleeding or discharge
> **T** hickening or extension of a lump
> **I** ndigestion or difficulty swallowing
> **O** bvious change in a wart or mole
> **N** agging cough or hoarseness

Investigate these, sudden weight loss, or any disturbing health change. It may be alarming, but get an early diagnosis.

Improvements in technologies for staging and evaluating cancers have also improved the focus and efficacy of treatments. Genetic screening helps alert doctors to who needs frequent screening tests, or would benefit from certain treatments.

Recently there has been an advisory that monthly breast self-examinations by women are not as reliable at finding cancers as an examination by a skilled nurse or physician. Well, I agree with that, but do not agree that women should not be encouraged to examine themselves! I have had a huge number of women come in with breast cancer they found themselves! Please, let's all do our part – self-care and professional care are not mutually exclusive. Integrate!

Mammograms have been a controversy for decades. They do detect cancers, and are a net benefit in women over age 50. However, the radiation is a concern. Most abnormalities found on screening mammography turn out to be benign when followed up with a diagnostic mammogram, ultrasound, needle biopsy and other more precise investigations. This means a lot of women get scared out of their wits for a few weeks over nothing, in order that a few cancer cases may be found and lives saved.

The PAP smear screening for cervical cancer is likely to be replaced by human papilloma virus HPV testing.

Since colon cancer often results in microscopic blood in the stool, screening for fecal occult (hidden) blood will pick up many early cases. Test annually after age 50.

Prostate cancer screening involves a digital rectal exam DRE and a PSA blood test. Again, age 50 is a good time to start, unless family history suggests an earlier screening.

An annual exam by a physician is no guarantee of safety from hidden disease. It is important to report any concern to your primary care provider, and let them examine, test or refer as they see fit. There is no gain in denial, stoicism, fear or macho toughness. Cancer can be beaten, but cures happen most often in early stage cancers!

I have seen many patients with cancer despite a very commendable lifestyle. I can guarantee them benefit from the good basic health, fitness and habits they bring to the start of the cancer journey. The better the constitution and vitality, the quicker the recovery.

Parts of this chapter were originally published in *Alive* magazine, the "Canadian Journal of Health & Nutrition," April 2005, No. 270, p. 48-53. The full article with scientific references is posted on my website www.drneilmckinney.ca

Selected Scientific References – INTEGRATIVE ONCOLOGY

APPENDIX A – SCIENTIFIC ARTICLES
- Alkylglycerols
- Alpha lipoic acid
- Anti-oxidants & nutraceuticals in chemotherapy
- Artemisinin
- Ashwagandha (Withania)
- Avemar
- Boswellia
- Breast cancer
- Butyrate
- Chinese medicine (TCM) herbs & acupuncture
- Co-enzyme Q-10
- Curcumin & inflammation
- Diet & general integrative oncology (miscellany)
- Ginger
- Grape seed extract & resveratrol
- Green tea EGCG & polyphenols
- Indole-3-carbinol
- Low-dose Naltrexone
- Melatonin
- Milk thistle
- Mistletoe lectins
- Mitochondria
- Modified citrus pectin
- Mushrooms (Reishi, button mushrooms, etc.)
- Omega 3 oils
- Phytoestrogens and Soy
- Pomegranate & ellagic acid
- Prevention
- Quercetin
- Radiation
- Stem cells & immune cells
- Sugar, insulin & IGF
- Surgery
- Vitamin C
- Vitamin D
- Vitamin K

APPENDIX B – BIBLIOGRAPHY

APPENDIX C – RECOMMENDED RESOURCES

APPENDIX A- SCIENTIFIC ARTICLES

ALKYLGLYCEROLS

Effect of High Doses of Shark Liver Oil Supplementation on T cell Polarization and Peripheral Blood Polymorphonuclear Cell Function, Lewkowicz, Banasik, Głowacka, et al., **Pol. Merkur. Lekarski.** 2005; 18 (108): 686-692.

The Assessment of the Effectiveness of the Shark Liver Oil in Recurrent Aphthous Stomatitis Treatment: Clinical and Immunological Studies, Gurańska, Lewkowicz, Urbaniak, et al., **Pol. Merkur. Lekarski.** 2001; 11 (63): 233-238

ALPHA LIPOIC ACID

Increased ROS Generation and p53 Activation in Alpha Lipoic Acid-induced Apoptosis of Hepatoma Cells, Simbula, Columbano, Ledda, et al., **Apoptosis** 2007; 12 (1): 113-123.
Uptake, Recycling, and Antioxidant Actions of Alpha-lipoic acid in Endothelial Cells, Jones, Li, Qu, et al., **Free Radic. Biol. Med.** 2002; 33 (1): 83-93.

Alpha-Lipoic Acid Inhibits TNF-alpha Induced NF-kappa B Activation Through Blocking of MEKK1-MKK4-IKK Signalling Cascades, Lee, Lee, Kim, et al., **Int. Immunopharmacol.** 2008; 8 (2): 362-370.

Reactive Oxygen Species Mediate Caspase Activation and Apoptosis Induced by Alpha Lipoic Acid in Human Lung Epithelial Cancer Cells Through Bcl-2 Down-regulation, Moungiaroen, Nimmannit, Callery, et al., **J. Pharmacolo. Exp.** 2006; 319 (3): 1062-1069.

R-lipoic Acid Inhibits Mammalian Pyruvate Dehydrogenase Kinase, Korotchkina, Sidhu,& Patel, **Free Radic. Res.** 2004; 38 (10): 1083-1092.

Alpha Lipoic Acid Induces Apoptosis in Human Colon Cancer Cells by Increasing Mitochondrial Respiration with a Concomitant O2* Generation, Wenzel, Nickel & Daniel, **Apoptosis** 2005; 10 (2): 359-368.

Reactive Oxygen Species Mediate Caspase Activation and Apoptosis Induced by Lipoic Acid in Human Lung Epithelial Cells Through Bcl-2 Down-regulation, Moungjaroen, Nimmannit, Callery, et al., **J. Pharmacol. Exp. Ther.** 2006; 319 (3): 1062-1069. Epub. 2006 Sept. 21.

Differential Activity of Lipoic Acid Enantiomers in Cell Culture, Smith, Thiagaraj,

Seaver & Parker, **J. Herb Pharmacother.** 2005; 5 (3): 43-54.

Selective Inactivation of Alpha-ketoglutarate Dehydrogenase and Pyruvate Dehydrogenase: Reaction of Lipoic Acid with 4-hydroxy-2-nonenal, Humphries & Szweda, **Biochemistry** 1998; 37 (45): 15835-15841.

Interaction of Alpha-lipoic Acid Enantiomers and Homologues with the Enzyme Components of the Mammalian Pyruvate Dehydrogenase Complex, Löffelhardt, Bonaventura, Locher , et al., **Biochem. Pharmacol.** 1995; 50 (5): 637-646.

The Long-term Survival of a Patient with Pancreatic Cancer with Metastases to the Liver after Treatment with the Intravenous Alpha-Lipoic Acid/Low-dose Naltrexone Protocol, Berkson, Rubin & Berkson, **Integr. Cancer Ther.** 2006; 5 (1): 83-89.

Effective Treatment of Oxaliplatin-induced Cumulative Poly-neuropathy with Alpha-Lipoic Acid, Gedlicka, Scheithauer, Schull & Kornek, **J. Clin. Oncol.** 2002; 20 (5): 3359-3361.

Effects of Alpha Lipoic Acid on Transforming Growth Factor beta 1-p38 Mitogen-activated Protein Kinase-Fibronectin Pathway in Diabetic Nephropathy, Lee, Kang, Ryu, et al., **Metabolism** 2009; 58 (5): 616-623.

ANTI-OXIDANTS & NUTRACEUTICALS IN CHEMOTHERAPY

Dietary Antioxidants During Cancer Chemotherapy: Impact on Chemotherapeutic Effectiveness and Development of Side-effects, Conklin, **Nutr. Can.** 2000; 37 (1): 1-18.

Impact of Antioxidant Supplementation on Chemotherapeutic Efficacy: a Systematic Review of the Evidence from Randomized Controlled Trials, Block, Koch, Mead, et al., **Cancer Treat. Rev.** 2007; 33 (5): 407-418.

Antioxidants and Other Nutrients Do Not Interfere with Chemotherapy or Radiation Therapy and Can Increase Kill and Increase Survival, Part 2. Simone, Simone, Simone & Simone, **Altern. Ther. Health Med**. 2007; 13 (2): 40-47

Chemotherapy-associated Oxidative Stress, Conklin, **Integr. Cancer Ther.** 2004; 3 (4): 294-299.

High Doses of Multiple Antioxidant Vitamins: Essential Ingredients in Improving the Efficacy of Standard Cancer Therapy, Prasad, Kumar,et al, **J. Amer. Coll. Nutr.,** 1999; 18: 13-25.

Supplements During Chemotherapy, McKinney, **Alive** - Canadian Journal of Health & Nutrition, April 2004; 258: 36.

To Combine or Not to Combine: Natural Health products and Chemotherapy?, Lemmo, **Townsend Letter** Aug.-Sept. 2006; #277/78: 76-77.

Reduction of Paclitaxel-induced Peripheral Neuropathy with Glutamine, Vahdat, Papadopoulos, Lange, et al, **Clin. Cancer Res.** 2001; 7 (5): 1192-1197.

Glutamine Protects Against Doxorubicin-induced Cardiotoxicity, Cao, Kennedy & Klimberg, **J. Surg. Res.** 1999; 85 (1) 178-182.

Prevention of Chemotherapy and Radiation Toxicity with Glutamine, Savarese, Savy, Vahdat, et al., **Cancer Treat. Rev**. 2003; 29 (6): 501-513

Baseline Nutritional Status is Predictive of Response to Treatment and Survival in Patients Treated by Definitive Chemo-radiotherapy for a Locally Advanced Esophageal Cancer, Di Fiore, Lecleire, Pop, et al., **Am. J. Gastroenterol.** 2007; 102 (11): 2557-63. Epub 2006 Aug 4.

Antioxidants and Cancer Therapy; Their Actions and Interactions with Oncologic Therapies, Lamson & Brignall **Alt. Med. Rev.** 1999; Vol. 4 No.5: 304-329.

Antioxidants and Cancer Therapy II – Quick reference Guide, Lamson & Brignall, **Alt. Med. Rev.** 2000; Vol. 5 No. 2: 152-163.

Antioxidants and Cancer III – Quercetin, Lamson & Brignall, **Alt. Med. Rev.** 2000; Vol. 5 No. 6: 196-208.

Orthomolecular Oncology Review: Ascorbic Acid & Cancer 25 Years Later, Gonzalez, Riordan, et al, **Integr. Cancer Ther.** 2005; 4 (1): 32-44.

Antioxidants and Cancer Therapy **Integr. Cancer Ther.** Special Edition 2004; 3 (4): 277-383.
- *Multiple Dietary Antioxidants Enhance the Efficacy of Standard and Experimental Cancer Therapies & Decrease Their Toxicity,* Prasad.: 310-321.
- *Chemotherapy-Associated Oxidative Stress: Impact on Chemotherapeutic Effectiveness,* Conklin: 294-300.
- *Dietary Antioxidants & Human Cancer,* Borek: 333-341.
- *Antioxidants & Cancer Therapy: Furthering the Debate,* Block: 342-348.

The Use of Vitamin C and Other Antioxidants with Chemotherapy and Radiotherapy in Cancer Treatment, Gunn, Hoffer & Stoute **J. Orthomolec. Med.** Special Issue 2004; Vol. 19 No.4: 194-255.

- *Editorial: The Use of Vitamin C and Other Antioxidants with Chemotherapy and Radiotherapy in Cancer Treatment,* Hoffer & Gunn: 195-197.
- *The Use of Vitamin C with Chemotherapy in Cancer Treatment: An Annotated Bibliography:* Stoute: 198-245.
- *The Use of Antioxidants with Chemotherapy & Radiotherapy in Cancer Treatment: A Review,* Gunn: 246-255.

All-trans Retinoic Acid Potentiates Tamoter-induced Cell Death Mediated by Jun N-terminal Kinase in Breast Cancer Cells, Wang and Weider, **Oncogene** 2004; 23 (2): 426-433.

Retinoic Acid Enhances the Cytotoxic Effects of Gemcitabine and Cisplatin in Pancreatic Adenocarcinoma Cells, Pettersson, Colston & Dalgleish, **Pancreas** 2001; 23 (3): 273-279.

Drug Resistance Against Gemcitabine and Topotecan Mediated by Constituitive HSP70 Overexpression in vitro: *Implication of Quercetin as Sensitiser in Chemotherapy,* Sliutz, Karlseder, Temfer, et al., **Br. J. Cancer** 1996; 74 (2): 172-177.

Molecular Pathways in the Chemosensitization of Cisplatin by Quercetin in Human Head and Neck Cancer, Sharma, Sen & Singh, **Cancer Biol. Ther.** 2005; 4 (9): 949-955.

Antioxidant Levels Tied to Treatment Toxicities in ALL, Kelly, et. al. **Paediat. Blood Cancer** 2005; 44: 1-8.

Low Antioxidant Vitamin Intakes are Associated with Increases in Adverse Effects of Chemotherapy in Children with Acute Lymphoblastic Leukemia, Kennedy, et al., **J. Clin. Nutr.** 2004; 79 (6): 1029-1036.

Antioxidant Status Decreases in Children with Acute Lymphoblastic Leukemia During the First Six Months of Chemotherapy Treatment, Tapani, Nissinen, et al., **Br. J. Nutr.** 2004; 92: 665-669.

Antioxidants and Other Nutrients Do Not Interfere with Chemotherapy or Radiation Therapy and Can Increase Kill and Increase Survival, Part 1, Simone, et al., **Altern Ther. Health Med.** 2007; 13: 22-28.

Chemotherapy Alone vs. Chemotherapy Plus High-dose Multiple Antioxidants in Patients with Advanced Non-Small Cell Lung Cancer, Pathak, et al., **J. Am. Coll. Nutr.** 2005; 24 (1): 16-21.

Adjuvant Immunotherapy with Oral Tegafur/Uracil Plus PSK in Patients with Stage II or III Colorectal Cancer: A Randomized Controlled Study, Ohwadea, et al., **Br. J.**

Cancer 2004; 90 (%): 1003-1010

Vitamin E May Protect Against Chemotherapy-induced Neuropathy, Argyriou, et al, **Neurology** 2005; 64: 26-31.

Tocopherol-associated Protein-1 Accelerates Apoptosis Induced by Alpha-Tocopherol Succinate in Mesothelioma Cells, Neuzil, Dong, Wang & Zingg, **Biochem. Biophys. Res. Commun.** 2006; 343 (4): 1113-1117.

A Randomized Controlled trial Evaluating the Efficacy and Safety of Vitamin E Supplementation for Protection Against Cisplatin-induced Peripheral Neuropathy: Final Results, Argiyriou, Chroni, Koutras, et al, **Support. Care Cancer** 2006; 14 (11): 1134-1140.

Vitamin E Neuroprotection for Cisplatin Neuropathy: A Randomized, Placebo-controlled Trial, Pace, Giannarelli, Galiè, et al., **Neurology** 2010; 74 (9): 762-766.

Antioxidants Against Cancer, Moss, 2000, Equinox Press.
Augmented Efficacy of Tamoxifen in Rat Breast Tumorigenesis when Gavaged along with Riboflavin, Niacin and CoQ-10: Effects on Lipid Peroxidation and Antioxidants in Mitochondria, Perumal, Shanti & Sachdanandam, **Chem. Biol. Interact.** 2005; 152 (1): 49-58.

Supplementation with Antioxidant Micronutrients and Chemotherapy-induced Toxicity in Cancer Patients Treated with Cisplatin-based Chemotherapy: A Randomized, Double-blind, Placebo-controlled Study, Weijl, Elsendoorn, Lentjes, et al., **Eur. J. Cancer**, 2004; 40: 1713-1723.

Selenium as an Element in the Treatment of Ovarian Cancer in Women Receiving Chemotherapy, Selja, & Talerceyk, **Gynec. Oncol.** 2004; 93: 320-327.

Selenium (Se) Deficiency in Women with Ovarian Cancer Undergoing Chemotherapy and the Influence of Supplementation with this Micro-element on Biochemical Parameters, Sieja, **Pharmazie** 1998; 53 (7): 473-476.

The Protective Role of Selenium on the Toxicity of Cisplatin-contained Chemotherapy Regimen in Cancer Patients, Hu, Chen, Zhang, et al., **Biol. Trace Elem. Res.** 1997; 56 (3): 331-341.

Apoptosis Induced by Selenomethionine and Methionine is Superoxide Mediated and p53 dependent in Human Prostate Cancer Cells, Zhao, Domann & Zhong, **Mol. Cancer Ther.** 2006; 5 (12): 3275-3284.

A Pilot Study on the Relation Between Cisplatin Neuropathy and Vitamin E, Bove,

Picardo, Maresca, et al., **J. Exp. Clin. Cancer Res.** 2001; 20: 277-280.

Neuroprotective Effect of Vitamin E Supplementation in Patients treated with Cisplatin Chemotherapy, Pace, Savarese, Picardo, et al., **J. Clin. Oncol.** 2003; 21:927-931.

Neuroprotective Effect of Reduced Glutathione on Oxiplatin-based Chemotherapy in Advanced Colorectal Cancer: A Randomized Double-blind Placebo-controlled Trial, Cascinu, et al., **J. Clin. Oncol. 2002; 20 (16): 3478-3483.**

High Curative Resection Rate with Weekly Cisplatin, 5-Fluorouracil, Epidoxorubicin, 6S-Leukovorin, Glutathione & Filgastrimin Patients with Locally Advanced, Unresectable Gastric Cancer: A Report from the Italian Group Study of Digestive Tract Cancer, Cascinu, **Br. J. Cancer** 2004; 90 (8): 1521-1525.

Glutathione Reduces the Toxicity and Improves Quality of Life of Women Diagnosed with Ovarian Cancer: Results of a Double-blind Randomized Trial. Smyth, Bowman, Perren, et al., **Ann. Oncol.** 1997; 8 (6): 569-573.

Dose Intensification of Platinum Compounds with Glutathione Protection as Induction Chemotherapy for Advanced Ovarian Carcinoma, Bohm, et al., **Oncology** 1999; 57 (2): 115-120.

The Use of Antioxidants with First-Line Chemotherapy in Two Cases of Ovarian Cancer, Drisko, Chapman & Hunter, **J. Am. Coll. Nutr.** 2003; 22 (2): 118-123.

Coenzyme Q-10 for Prevention of Anthracycline-induced Cardiotoxicity, Conklin, **Integr. Canc. Ther.,** 2005; 4 (2): 110-130.

Protective Effect of Coenzyme Q-10 in Cardiotoxicity Induced by Adriamycin, Okuma, Furuta & Ota, **Gan To Kagaku Ryoho** 1984; 11 (3): 502-508.

The Use of Antioxidants with First-line Chemotherapy in Two Cases of Ovarian Cancer, Drisko, Chapman & Hunter, **J. Am Coll Nutr** 2003; 22 (2): 118-123.

Use of Antioxidant Supplements During Breast Cancer Treatment: A Comprehensive Review, Greenlee, Hershman & Jacobson, **Breast Cancer Res Treat** 2008 Oct. 7, (epub ahead of print – PMID 18839308)
Methylseleninic acid [selenium] Synergizes with Tamoxifen to Induce Caspase-mediated Apoptosis in Breast Cancer Cells, Li, et al., **Mol. Cancer Ther.** 2008; 7 (9): 3056-3063.

Ascorbic Acid and Adriamycin Toxicity, Shimpko, et al., **Am. J. Clin. Nutr.** 1991; 54 (Suppl. 6): 1298S-1301S.

Impact of Antioxidant Supplementation on Chemotherapeutic Efficacy: A Systematic Review of the Evidence from Randomized Controlled Trials, Block, Koch, Mead, et al., **Cancer Treat. Rev.** 2007; 33 (5): 407–418.

Silibinin Sensitizes Human Prostate Carcinoma DU145 Cells to Cisplatin- and Carboplatin-induced Growth Inhibition and Apoptotic Death, Dhanalakshmi, Agarwal, Glode & Agarwal, **Int. J. Cancer** 2003; 106 (5): 699-705.

Anti-proliferative Effect of Silybin on Gynaecological Malignancies: Synergism with Cisplatin and Doxorubicin, Scambia, De Vincenzo, Ranelletti, et al., **Eur. J. Cancer** Part A 1996; 32: 877-882.

Silibinin Restores Paclitaxel Sensitivity to Paclitaxel-resistant Human Ovarian Carcinoma Cells, **Anticancer Res.** 2008; 28 (2A): 1119-1127.

Drug Resistance Against Gemcitabine and Topotecan Mediated by Constitutive hsp70 Over-expression in vitro: Implication of Quercetin as Sensitiser in Chemotherapy, Sliutz, Karlseder, Tempfer, et al., **Br. J. Cancer** 1996 ; 74 (2): 172-177.

Quercetin Potentiates the Effect of Adriamycin in a Multidrug-resistant MCF-7 Human Breast Cancer Cell Line: P-glycoprotein as a Possible Target, Scambia, Ranelletti, Panic, et al., **Cancer Chemother. Pharmacol.** 1994; 34 (6): 459-464.

The Synergistic Reversal Effect of Multi-drug Resistance by Quercetin and Hyperthermia in Doxorubicin-resistant Human Myelogenous Leukemia Cells, Shen, Zhang, Wu & Zhu, **Int, J. Hyperthermia** 2008; 24 (2): 151-159.

Effects of Quercetin on the Cell Growth and the Intra-cellular Accumulation and Retention of Adriamycin, Asaum, Matsuzaki, Kawasak, et al., **Anticancer Res.** 2000; 20 (4): 2477-2483.

The Synergistic Reversal Effect of Multidrug Resistance by Quercetin and Hyperthermia in Doxorubicin-Resistant Human Myelogenous Leukemia Cells, Shen, Zhang, Wu & Zhu, **Int. J. Hyperthermia** 2008 ;24 (2): 151-159.

Synergistic Anti-cancer Effects of Grapeseed Extract and Conventional Cytotoxic Agent Doxorubicin Against Human Breast Carcinoma Cells, Sharma, Tyagi, Singh, et al., **Breast Cancer Res. Treat.** 2004; 85 (1): 1-12.

Amelioration of Doxorubicin-induced Myocardial Oxidative Stress and Immunosuppression by Grapeseed Extract Proanthocyanidins in Tumour-bearing Mice, Zhang, Wang, Song, et al., **J. Pharm. Pharmacol.** 2005; 57 (8): 1043-1052.

Five Years Survival in Metastatic Non-small Cell Lung Cancer Patients Treated with Chemotherapy Alone or Chemotherapy and Melatonin: A Randomized Trial, Lissoni,

Chilelli, Villa, et al., **J. Pineal Res.** 2003; 35 (1): 12-15.

Melatonin, a Promising Role in Taxane-related Neuropathy, Nahleh, Pruemer, Lafollette & Sweany, **Clin. Med. Insights Oncol**. 2010; 4: 35-41.

Melatonin and Doxorubicin Synergistically Induce Cell Apoptosis in Human Hepatoma Cell Lines, Fan, Sun, Wei et al., **World J Gastroenterol.** 2010; 16 (12): 1473-1481.

Protective Effect of Melatonin on Oxaliplatin-induced Apoptosis Through Sustained Mcl-1 Expression and Anti-oxidant Action in Renal Carcinoma Caki Cells, Um & Kwon, **J. Pineal Res.** 2010 Jul 2. [Epub ahead of print] <http://www.ncbi.nlm.nih.gov/pubmed/20626587?dopt=Abstract>

Bio-modulation of Cancer Chemotherapy for Metastatic Colorectal Cancer: A Randomized Study of Weekly Low-dose Irinotecan Alone versus Irinotecan Plus the Oncostatic Pineal Hormone Melatonin in Metastatic Colorectal Cancer Patients Progressing on 5-fluorouracil-containing Combinations, **Cerea, Vaghi, Ardizzoia, et al., Anticancer Res.** 2003; 23 (2C): 1951-1954.

Oxidant-Antioxidant Status in Relation to Survival Among Breast Cancer Patients, Saintot, Mathieu-Daude, Astre, et al., **Int. J. Cancer** 2002; 97 (5): 574-579.

A Phase II Study of Chemo-neuroimmunotherapy with Platinum, Subcutaneous Low-dose Interleukin-2 and the Pineal Neurohormone Melatonin (P.I.M.) as a Second-line Therapy in Metastatic Melanoma Patients Progressing on Dacarbazine Plus Interferon-alpha, Lissoni, Vaghi, Ardizzoia, et al., **In Vivo.** 2002; 16 (2): 93-96.

Decreased Toxicity and Increased Efficacy of Cancer Chemotherapy Using the Pineal Hormone Melatonin in Metastatic Solid Tumour Patients with Poor Clinical Status, Lissoni, Barni, Mandalà, et al., **Eur. J. Cancer** 1999; 35 (12): 1688-1692

Use of Herbs and Supplements by Chemotherapy Patients Attending an Integrative Cancer Clinic, Block, Gyllenhaal, Koch, et al., Presented at annual meeting of the **Society for Integrative Oncology,** San Francisco CA, Nov. 21 2007.

A Pilot Study on the Effect of Acetyl-l-Carnitine in Paclitaxel and Cisplatin-induced Peripheral Neuropathy, Maestri, De Pasquale Ceratti, Cdari et al., **Tumori** 2005; 91 (2): 135-138.

Potential Role of Levo-Carnitine Supplementation for the Treatment of Chemotherapy-induced Fatigue in Non-anaemic Cancer Patients, Graziano, Bisonni, Catalano, et al., **Br. J. Cancer** 2002; 86 (12): 1854-1857.

Prevention by L-carnitine of Interleukin-2 Related Cardio-toxicity During Cancer Chemotherapy, Lissoni, Galli, Tancini & Barni, **Tumori** 1993; 79 (3): 202-204.

Acetyl-l-carnitine Prevents and Reduces Paclitaxel-induced Painful Peripheral Neuropathy, Flatters, Xiao & Bennett, **Neurosci. Lett.** 2006; 397 (3): 219-223.

Reversal of Doxorubicin-induced Cardiac Metabolic Damage by L-Carnitine, Sayed-Ahmed, Shaarawy, Shouman & Osman, **Pharmacol Res.** 1999; 39 (4): 289-295

Oral Glutamine is Effective for Preventing Oxaliplatin-induced Neuropathy in Colorectal Cancer Patients, Wang Lin, Lin et al., **Oncologist** 2007; 12 (3): 312-319.

Oral Glutamine Reduces the Duration and Severity of Stomatitis after Cytotoxic Cancer Chemotherapy, Anderson, Schroeder & Skubitz, **Cancer** 1998; 83 (7): 1433-1439.

Glutamine Supplementation in Cancer Patients, Yoshida, Kaibara, Ishibashi & Shirouzu, Nutrition 2001; 17 (9): 766-768.

Clinical Use of Glutamine Supplementation, Wernerman, **J. Nutr.** 2008; 138 (10): 2040S-2044S.

The Effect of Glutamine Supplementation on Hematopoietic Stem Cell Transplant Outcome in Children: A Case-control Study, Kuskonmaz, Yalcin, Kucukbayrak, et al., **Pediatr. Transplant.** 2008; 12 (1): 47-51.

Glutamine Supplementation in Cancer Patients Receiving Bone Marrow Transplantation and High-dose Chemotherapy, Ziegler, **J. Nutr.** 2001; 131 (9 Supplement): 2578S-2584S; discussion 2590S.

Nutrition Support for Bone Marrow Transplant Patients, Murray & Pindoria, **Cochrane Database Syst. Rev.** 2008; (4): CD002920.

Effects of Oral Glutamine Supplementation on Children with Solid Tumours Receiving Chemotherapy, Okur, Ezgu, Tumer, et al., **Pediatr. Hematol. Oncol.** 2006; 23 (4): 277-285.

Exogenous Glutamine: the Clinical Evidence, Bongers, Griffiths & McArdle, **Crit. Care Med.** 2007; 35 (9 Supplement): 545S-552S.

Bolus Oral Glutamine Protects Rats Against CPT-11-induced Diarrhea and Differentially Activates Cytoprotective Mechanisms in Host Intestine But Not Tumour, Xue, Sawyer, Field, et al., **J. Nutr.** 2008; 138 (4): 740-746.

Prevention of Chemotherapy and Radiation Toxicity with Glutamine, Savarese, Savy,

Vahdat, et al., **Cancer Treat. Rev.** 2003: 29 (6): 501-513.

Oral Glutamine for the Prevention of Chemotherapy-induced Peripheral Neuropathy, Amara, **Ann. Pharmacother.** 2008; 42 (10): 1481-1485.

Oral Glutamine Ameliorates Chemotherapy-induced Changes of Intestinal Permeability and Does Not Interfere with the Antitumor Effect of Chemotherapy in Patients with Breast Cancer: A Prospective Randomized Trial, Li, Yu, Liu, et al., **Tumori,** 2006; 92 (5): 396-401.

Oleic Acid, the Main Monounsaturated Fatty Acid of Olive Oil, Suppresses Her-2/ neu (erbB-2) Expression and Synergistically Enhances the Growth Inhibitory Effects of Trastuzumab (Herceptin) in Breast Cancer Cells with Her-2/neu Oncogene Amplification, Menendez, Vellon, Colomer & Lupu, **Ann. Oncol.** 2005; 16 (3): 359-371.

Clinical Corner: Herb-drug Interactions in Cancer Chemotherapy: Theoretical Concerns Regarding Drug Metabolizing Enzymes, Block & Gyllenhaal, **Integr. Cancer Ther.** 2002; 1 (1): 83-89.

Treatment with Antioxidant and Other Nutrients in Combination with Chemotherapy and Irradiation in Patients with Small-cell Lung Cancer, Jaakkola , Lähteenmäki , Laakso, et al., **Anticancer Res.** 1992; 12 (3): 599-606.

Neuroprotective Effect of Reduced Glutathione on Cisplatin-based Chemotherapy in Advanced Gastric Cancer: A Randomized Double-blind Placebo Controlled Trial, Cascinu, Cordella, Del Ferro E, et al., **J. Clin. Oncol.** 1995; 1: 26-32.

Glutathione Improves the Therapeutic Index of Cisplatin and Quality of Life for Patients with Ovarian Cancer, Smyth, Bowman, Perren, et al., **Proc. ASCO** 1995; 14: 761.

Anti-tumour Activity of Gemcitabine and Oxaliplatin is Augmented by Thymoquinone in Pancreatic Cancer, Banerjee, Kaseb, Wang, et al., **Cancer Res.** 2009; 69 (13): 5575-5583.

Weekly Cisplatin and Glutathione in Relapsed Ovarian Carcinoma, Colombo, Bini, Miceli, et al., **Int. J. Gynecol. Cancer** 1995; 5: 81-86.

ARTEMESININ

Clinical Pharmacology of Artemisinin-based Combination Therapies, German & Aweeka, **Clin. Pharmacokinet.** 2008; 47 (2): 91-102.

Artemesinin and the Anti-malarial Endoperoxides: from Herbal Remedy to Targeted Chemotherapy, Meshnick, Taylor & Kamchonwongpaisan, **Microbiol. Rev.** 1996; 60 (2): 301-315.

Pharmacokinetics and Pharmacodynamics of Endoperoxide Antimalarials, Gautam, Anirudh, Ahmed, et al., **Curr. Drug Metab.** 2009; 10 (3): 289-306.

Artemisinin Blocks Prostate Cancer Growth and Cell Cycle Progression by Disrupting Sp1 Interactions with the Cyclin-dependent Kinase-4 (CDK4) Promoter and Inhibiting CDK4 Gene Expression, Willoughby, Sundar, Cheung, et al., **J. Biol. Chem.** 2009; 284 (4): 2203-2213.

The Anti-malarial Artesunate is Also Active Against Cancer, Efferth, Dunstan, Sauerberry et al., **Int. J. Oncol.** 2001; 18: 767-773.

Experimental Therapy of Hepatoma with Artemisinin and Its Derivatives: In vitro and In vivo Activity, Chemosensitization ,and Mechanisms of Action, Hou, Wang, Zhang & Wang, **Clin. Cancer Res.** 2008; 14 (17): 5519-5530.

ASHWAGANDHA

Antitumor and Radiosensitizing Effects of Withania somnifera (Ashwagandha) on a Transplantable Mouse Tumour, Sarcoma -180. Devi & Solomon **Ind. J. Exp. Biol. July** 1993; 31 (7): 607-611.

In vivo Growth Inhibitory Effect of Withania somnifera *(Ashwagandha) on a Transplantable Mouse Tumour Sarcoma-180,* Devi, Sharada, Solomon, et al., **Ind. J. Exp. Biol.** 1992; 30: 169-172.

Withania somnifera dunal: Potential Plant Source of a Promising Drug for Chemotherapy and Radiosensitization, Devi, **Ind. J. Exp. Biol.** 1996; 34 (10): 927-932.

In vivo growth Inhibitory and Radiosensitizing Effects of Withaferin A on Mouse Erlich Ascites Carcinoma in vivo, Devi, Sharada & Solomon, **Acat. Oncol.** 1996; 35: 95-100.

Modulation of TCA Cycle Enzymes and Electron Transport Chain Systems (by Withania) In Experimental Lung Cancer, Senhilnathan, Padmavathi, Magesh & Sakthisekaran, **Life Sci.** 2006; 78 (9): 1010-1014.

Immunoprotection by Botanical Drugs in Cancer Chemotherapy, Diwanay, Chitre & Patwardhan, **J. Ethnopharmacol.** 2004; 90 (1): 49-55

The Protective Effect of a Purified Extract of Withania somnifera Against

Doxorubicin-induced Cardiac Toxicity in Rats, Hamza, Amin & Daoud, **Cell Biol. Toxicol.** 2008; 24 (1): 63-73.

AVEMAR

Fermented Wheat Germ Extract (Avemar) in the Treatment of Cancer and Autoimmune Diseases, Boros, Nichelatti & Shoenfeld, **Ann. N.Y. Acad. Sci.** 2005; 1051: 529-542.

Antimetastatic Effect of Avemar in High-risk Melanoma Patients, Demidov, Manzjuk, Kharkevitch, et. al., **18th UICC International Cancer Congress**, 2002; P868 - Oslo, Norway.

Adjuvant Fermented Wheat Germ Extract (Avemar) Nutraceutical Improves Survival of High-risk Melanoma Patients: A Randomized, Pilot, Phase II Clinicnal Study with a 7-year Follow-up, Demidov, Manzuik, Kharkevitch, et al., **Cancer Biother. Radiopharm.** 2008; 23 (4): 477-482.

A Medical Nutriment Has Supportive Value in the Treament of Colorectal Cancer, Jakab, Schoenfeld, Balogh, et al., **Br. J. Cancer** 2003; 89 (3): 465-469.

BOSWELLIA

Boswellic Acids and Malignant Glioma: Induction of Apoptosis but No Modulation of Drug Sensitivity, Glaser, Winters, Groscurth, et. al., **Br. J. Cancer** 1998; 80 (5-6): 756-765.

Boswellic Acids Inhibit Glioma Growth: A New Treatment Option?, Winking, Sarikaya, et. al., **J. Neurooncol** 2000; 46: 97-103.

Boswellic Acids in the Palliative Therapy of Children with Progressive or Relapsed Brain Tumours, Janssen, Bode, Breu, et. al., **Klin. Paediatr.** 2000; 212: 189-195.

Response of Radio-Chemotherapy-associated Cerebral Edema to a Phytotherapeutic Agent H15, Streffer, Bitzer, Schabet, et al., **Neurology** 2001; 56: 1219-1221.

Boswellic Acid Acetate Induces Differentiation and Apoptosis in Leukemia Cell Lines, Jing, Nakato, et al., **Leuk. Res.** 1999; 23: 43-50.

Boswellic Acids: Novel, Specific, Non-redox Inhibitors of 5-lipoxygenase, Safayhi, Mack, Sabieraj, et al., **J. Pharmacol. Exp. Ther.** 1992; 261 (3): 1143-1146

BUTYRATE

Sodium Butyrate Inhibits Cell Growth and Stimulates P21 Protein in Human Colonic Adenocarcimoma Cells Independently of p53 Status, Kobayashi, Tan & Fleming, **Nutr. & Cancer** 2003; 46 (2): 202-211.

Butyrate Induces Glutathione S-Transferase in Human Colon Cells and Protects from Genetic Damage by 4-Hydroxy-2-Nonenal, Ebert, et al., **Nutr. & Cancer** 2001; 41 (1): 156-164.

Topical Butyrate for Acute Radiation Proctitis: Randomised, Cross-over Trial, Vernia, Fracasso, Casale, et al., **Lancet** 2000; 356 (9237): 1232-1235.

BREAST CANCER

Survival Impact of Integrative Cancer Care in Advanced Metastatic Breast Cancer, Block, Gyllenhaal, Tripathy, et al., **Breast J.** 2009; 154: 357-366.

Apparent Partial Remission of Breast Cancer in "High-Risk" Patients Supplemented with Nutritional Antioxidants, Essential fatty acids and Coenzyme Q-10, Lockwood, Moesgaard, Hanioka, et. al., **Mol. Aspects. Med.** 1994; Suppl. 15: 231-240.

Progress on Therapy of Breast Cancer with Vitamin Q-10 and the Regression of Metastases, Lockwood, Moesgaard, Yamamoto & Folkers, **Biochem. Biophys. Res. Commun.** 1995; 212 (1): 172-177.

The Israeli Breast Cancer Anomaly, Westin & Richter, **Annals N.Y. Acad. Sci.** 1989; 609: 269-279.

Alteration of the Effects of Cancer Therapy Agents on Breast Cancer Cells by the Herbal Medicine Black Cohosh, Rockwewll, Liu & Higgins, **Breast Cancer Res. Treat.** 2005; 90: 233-239.

Fibroblasts Isolated from Common Sites of Breast Cancer Metastasis Enhance Cancer Cell Growth Rates and Invasiveness in an Interleukin-6-Dependent Manner, Studebaker, Storci, Werbeck, et al., **Cancer Res.** 2008; 68 (21): 9087-9095.

Psychologic Intervention Improves Survival for Breast Cancer Patients: A Randomized Clinical Trial, Andersen, Yang, Farrar, et al., **Cancer** 2008; 113:3450-3458.

Perspectives on the Soy-Breast Cancer Relation, Messina & Wu, **Am. J. Clin. Nutr.** 2009; 895: 1673S-1679S.

Co-enzyme Q-10, Riboflavin and Niacin Supplementation on Alteration of DNA Repair Enzyme and DNA Methylation in Breast Cancer Patients Undergoing Tamoxifen Therapy, Premkumar, Yuvaraj & Sachdanandam, **Br. J. Nutr.** 2008; 1006: 1179-1182.

Cytotoxic Effects of Ultra-diluted Remedies on Breast Cancer Cells, Frenkel, Mishra,

Sen, et al., **Int. J. Oncol.** 2010; 36: 395-403.

PARP Inhibitors and the Treatment of Breast Cancer: Beyond BRCA1/2?, Frizzell & Kraus **Breast Cancer Res.** 2009; 11: 111.

CHINESE MEDICINE (TCM) HERBS & ACUPUNCTURE

Traditional Chinese Medicine In Cancer Symposium, Vanc. Gen. Hosp. Sept. 21, 2003

Astragalus-based Chinese Herbs and Platinum-based Chemotherapy for Advanced Non-small-cell Lung Cancer: Meta-analysis of Randomized Trials, McCulloch, See, Shu, et al., **J. Clin. Oncol.** 2006; 24 (3): 419-430.

Astragalus-containing Chinese Herbal Combinations for Advanced Non-Small Cell Lung Cancer:A Meta-analysis of 65 Clinical Trials Enrolling 4751 Patients, Dugoua, Wu, Seeley, et al., **Lung Cancer: Targets and Therapy** Dove Medical Press, 2010; 1: 1–16.

A Phase II Study of an Herbal Decoction That Includes Astragali Radix for Cancer-Associated Anorexia in Patients With Advanced Cancer, Lee & Lee, **Integr. Cancer Ther.** 2010; 9 (1): 24–31.

Traditional Chinese Medicine Astragalus Reverses Predominance of Th2 Cytokines and Their Up-stream Transcript Factors in Lung Cancer Patients, Wei, Sun, Xiao, et al., **Oncol. Rep.** 2003; 10 (5): 1507-1512

Shi-Quan-Da-Bu-Tang (Ten Significant Tonic Decoction), SQT. A Potent Chinese Biological Response Modifier in Cancer Immunotherapy, Potentiation and Detoxification of Anticancer Drugs, Zee-Cheng, **Methods Find Exp Clin Pharmacol.** 1992; 14 (9): 725-736

Immunotherapy with Chinese Medicinal Herbs. I. Immune Restoration of Local Xenogeneic Graft-versus-host Reaction in Cancer Patients by Fractionated Astragalus membranaceus in vitro, Chu, Wong & Mavligit, **J. Clin. Lab. Immunol.** 1988; (3): 119-123.

A Phase II Study of an Herbal Decoction That Includes Astragali Radix for Cancer-Associated Anorexia in Patients with Advanced Cancer, Lee & Lee, **Integr. Cancer Ther.** 2010; 9 (1): 24-31.

Chinese Medical Herbs for Chemotherapy Side-effects on Colorectal Cancer Patients, Taixiang, Munro & Guanjian, **Cochrane Database Syst. Rev.** 2005; (1): CD004540.

Cohort Study on the Effect of a Combined Treatment of Traditional Chinese Medicine and Western Medicine on the Relapse and Metastasis of 222 Patients with Stage II and III Colorectal Cancer After Radical Operation, Yang, Ge, Wu, et al., **Chin. J. Integr. Med.** 2008; 144: 251-256.

Clinical Observation on Treatment of Colonic Cancer with Combined Treatment of Chemotherapy and Chinese Herbal Medicine, Zhou, Shan & You, **Chin. J. Integr. Med.** 2009; 152: 107-111.

Immune System Effects of Echinacea, Ginseng and Astragalus: A Review, Block & Mead,**Integr. Cancer Ther.** 2003; 2 (3): 247-267.

Chinese Medicinal Herbs Reverse Macrophage Suppression Induced by Urological Tumours, Rittenhouse, Lui & Lau, **J. Urol.** 1991; 146 (2): 486-490.

Integrating Chinese & Conventional Medicine in Colorectal Cancer Treatment, Lahans, **Integr. Cancer Ther.** 2007; 6 (1): 89-94.

Chinese Herbal Medicine and Chemotherapy in the Treatment of Hepatocellular Carcinoma: A Meta-analysis of Randomized Controlled Trials, Shu, McCulloch, Xiao, et al., **Integr. Cancer Ther.** 2005; 4 (3): 219-229.

Chinese Herbal Medicine for Cancer Pain, Xu, Lao, Ge, et al., **Integr. Cancer Ther.** 2007; 6 (3): 208-234.

Cancer Chemo-preventative and Therapeutic Activities of Red Ginseng, Xiaoguang, Hongyan, Xiaohong, et al., **J. Ethnopharmacol.** 1998; 60 (1): 71-78.

The Effects of P6 Acupressure in the Prophylaxis of Chemotherapy-Related Nausea and Vomiting in Breast Cancer Patients, Molassiotis, Helin, Dabbour, et al., **Complement. Ther. Med.** 2007; 15 (1): 3-12.

Acupuncture: Role in Comprehensive Cancer Care – A Primer for the Oncologist and Review of the Literature, Cohen, Menter & Hale, **Integr. Cancer Ther.** 2005; 4 (2): 131-143.

The Management of Cancer Related Fatigue After Chemotherapy with Acupuncture and Acupressure: A Randomized Controlled Trial, Molassiotis, Sylt & Diggins, **Complement. Ther. Med.** 2007; 154: 228-237.

Acupuncture to Alleviate Chemotherapy-induced Nausea and Vomiting in Paediatric Oncology – A Randomized Multicenter Cossover Pilot Trial, Gottschling, Reindl, Meyer, et al., **Klin. Paediatr.** 2008; 220 (6): 365-370.

Acupuncture Versus Venlafaxine for the Management of Vasomotor Symptoms in Patients with Hormone Receptor-Positive Breast Cancer: A Randomized Controlled Trial, Walker, Rodrigues, Kohn, et al., **J. Clin. Oncol.** 2009; Epub ahead of print

Naturopathic Oncology

PMID: 20038728.

Acupuncture in the Rehabilitation of Women After Breast Cancer Surgery- A Case Series, Alem & Gurgel, **Acup. Med.** 2008; 262: 86-93.

Monitoring of Neuromuscular Blockade at the P6 Acupuncture Point Reduces the Incidence of Post-operative Nausea and Vomiting, Arnberger, Stadelmann, Alischer, et al., **Anesthesiology** 2007; 107 (6): 903-908.

Acupuncture for the Treatment of Vasomotor Symptoms in Breast Cancer Patients Receiving Hormone Suppression Treatment, Walker, et al., **Int. J. Rad. Oncol. – Biol. – Phys.** 2008; Abstract No. 228. Volume 72, Number 1.

Clinical Observations on Post-operative Vomiting Treated by Auricular Acupuncture, Kim, Kim & Kim, **Am. J. Chin. Med.** 2003; 31 (3): 475-480.

Clinical Uses of P6 Acupuncture Anti-emesis, Dundee & McMillan, **Acupunct. Electrother. Res.** 1990; 15 (3-4): 211-215.

Acupuncture for Nausea and Vomiting: An Update of Clinical and Experimental Studies, Streitberger, Ezzo & Schneider, **Auton. Neurosci.** 2006; 129(1-2): 107-117.

Effect of Acupressure on Nausea and Vomiting Induced by Chemotherapy in Cancer Patients, Gardani, Cerrone, Biella, et al., **Minerva Med.** 2006; 97 (5): 391-394.

Electroacupuncture for Refractory Acute Emesis Caused by Chemotherapy, Choo, Kong, Lim, et al., **J. Altern. Complement. Med.** 2006; 12 (10): 963-969.

Acupuncture-point Stimulation for Chemotherapy-Induced Nausea or Vomiting, Ezzo, Richardson, Vickers, et al., **Cochrane Database Syst. Rev.** 2006; (2): CD002285.

Effects of Electro-acupuncture on T-cell Subpopulations, NK Activity, Humoral Immunity and Leukocyte Count in Patients Undergoing Chemotherapy, Ye, Liu, Wang & Xu, **J. Trad. Chin. Med.** 2007; 271: 19-21.

Acupuncture for the Treatment of Hot Flashes in Breast Cancer Patients, a Randomized, Controlled Trial, Hervik & Mjaland, **Breast Cancer Res. Treat.** 2009; 1162: 311-316.

Acupuncture as Palliative Therapy for Physical Symptoms and Quality of Life for Advanced Cancer Patients, Dean-Clower, Doherty-Gilman, Keshaviah, et al., **Integr. Cancer Ther.** 2010; 9 (2): 158-167.

CO-ENZYME Q-10

Coenzyme Q-10 Plasma Levels Predict Melanoma Metastasis, Rusciani, et al, **J. Am. Acad. Dermatology**, 2006; 54: 234-241.

Coenzyme Q Differentially Modulates Phospholipid Hydroperoxide Glutathione Peroxidase Gene Expression and Free Radicals Production in Malignant and Non-malignant Prostate Cells, Quiles, Farquharson, Ramirez-Tortosa, et al., **Biofactors** 2003; 18 (1-4): 265-270.

Clinical Response of Myelodysplastic Syndromes Patients to Treatment with Coenzyme Q-10, Galili, Sechman, Cerny, et al., **Leuk Res.** 2007 J; 31 (1): 19-26.

Coenzyme q-10 for Prevention of Anthracycline-induced Cardiotoxicity, Conklin, **Integr Cancer Ther.** 2005; 4 (2): 110-130.

CoQ-10: Could It Have a Role in Cancer Management?, Hodges, Hertz, Lockwood & Lister, **BioFactors** 1999; 9: 365-370.

An Analysis of the Role of Coenzyme Q in Free Radical Generation and As an Antioxidant, Beyer, **Biochem. & Cell Biol**.1992; 70 (6): 390-403.

The Mode of Action of Lipid-soluble Antioxidants in Biological Membranes. Relationship Between the Effects of Ubiquinol and Vitamin E as Inhibitors of Lipid Peroxidation in Submitochondrial Particles, Ernster, Forsmark & Nordenbrand, **J. Nutr. Sci. & Vitamin.** 1992; Spec No: 548-551.

CURCUMIN & INFLAMMATION

Curcumin and Green Tea Polyphenols: Synergistic Anticancer Compounds, Yarnell, **Quart. Rev. Nat. Med.** 1998; Fall: 218-220.

Antioxidant and Anti-inflammatory Properties of Curcumin, Menon & Sudheer, **Adv. Exp. Med. Biol.** 2007; 595: 105-125.

Curcumin and Resveratrol Inhibit Nuclear Factor-kappaB-mediated Cytokine Expression in Adipocytes, Gonzales & Orlando, **Nutr. Metab.** (Lond). 2008; 5 (1): 17.

Regulation of COX and LOX by Curcumin, Rao, **Adv. Exp. Med. Biol.** 2007; 595: 213-226.

Induction of Apoptosis by Curcumin and its Implications for Cancer Therapy, Karunagaran, Rashmi & Kumar, **Curr. Cancer Drug Targets** 2005; 5 (2): 117-129.

Biological Effects of Curcumin and its Role in Cancer Chemoprevention and Therapy, Singh & Khar, **Anticancer Agents Med.Chem.** 2006; 6 (3): 259-270.

Chemotherapeutic Potential of Curcumin for Colorectal Cancer, Chauhan, **Curr. Pharm. Des.** 2002; 8 (19): 1695-1706.

Synergistic Inhibitory Effects of Curcumin and 5-FluoroUracil on the Growth of the Human Colon Cancer Cell Line HT-29, Du, Jiang, Xia & Zhong, **Chemotherapy** 2006;52 (1): 23-28.

Curcumin Inhibits Human Colon Cancer cell Growth by Suppressing Gene Expression of Epidermal Growth Factor Receptor Through Reducing the Activity of the Transcription Factor Egr-1, Chen, Xu & Johnson, **Oncogene** 2005; Sept. 19, Epub.

Molecular Targets of Curcumin, Lin, **Adv. Exp. Med. Biol.** 2007; 595: 227-243.

Curcumin, an Anti-oxidant and Anti-tumour Promoter, Induces Apoptosis in Human Leukemia Cells, Kuo, Huang & Lin, **Biochem Biophys Acta** 1996; 131 (7): 95-100.

The Chemopreventive Agent Curcumin is a Potent Radiosensitizer of Human Cervical Tumour Cells via Increased Reactive Oxygen Species Production and Overactivation of the Mitogen-activated Protein Kinase Pathway, Javvadi, Segan, Tuttle & Koumenis, **Mol Pharmacol.** 2008 May; 73 (5): 1491-501.

Curcumin, a Dietary Component, has Anti-cancer, Chemo-sensitization, and Radio-sensitization Effects by Down-regulating the MDM2 Oncogene Through the P13K/mTOR/ETS2 Pathway, Zhang, Hill, Wang & Zhang, **Cancer Res.** 2007; 67 (5): 1988-1996.

Cellular Foundation of Curcumin-induced Apoptosis in Follicular Lymphoma Cell Lines, Skommer, Wlodkowic & Pelkonen, **Exp. Hematol.** 2006; 34 (4): 463-474.

Curcumin Inhibits Human Colon Cancer Cell Growth by Suppressing Gene Expression of Epidermal Growth Factor Receptor Through Reducing the Activity of the Transcription Factor Egr-1, Chen, Xu & Johnson, **Oncogene** 2006; 25: 278-287.

Therapeutic Potential of Curcumin in Human Prostate Cancer-1. Curcumin Induces Apoptosis in Both Androgen-dependent and Androgen-independent Prostate Cancer Cells, Dorai, Gehani & Katz, **Prost. Cancer Prost. Dis.** 2000; 3: 84-93.

Dietary Curcumin Inhibits Chemotherapy-induced Apoptosis in Models of Human Breast Cancer, Somasundaram, Edmund, Moore, et al., **Cancer Res.** 2002; 62 (13): 3868-3875.
Can a Common Spice be Used to Treat Cancer?, Witter, **Oncolog.** 2007; 52 (9): 4-5.

Curcumin as Chemosensitizer, Limtrakul, **Adv. Exp. Med. Biol.** 2007; 595: 269-300.

Curcumin Inhibits Prosurvival Pathways in Chronic Lymphocytic Leukemia B Cells and May Overcome Their Stromal Protection in Combination with EGCG, Ghosh, Kay, Secreto & Shanafelt, **Clin. Cancer Res.** 2009; 15 (4): 1250-1258.

Elimination of Colon Cancer Stem-like Cells by the Combination of Curcumin and FOLFOX, Yu, Kanwar, Patel, et al., **Transl. Oncol.** 2009; 2 (4): 321-328.

Dietary Curcumin Inhibits Chemotherapy-induced Apoptosis in Models of Human Breast Cancer, Somasundaram, Edmund, Moore, et al., **Cancer Res.** 2002; 62 (13): 3868-3875.

Modulation of Function of Three Drug Transporters, P-Glycoprotein (ABCB1), Mitoxantrone Resistance Protein (ABCG2) and Multi-drug Resistance Protein 1 (ABCC1) by Tetrahydrocurcumin, a Major Metabolite of Curcumin, Limtrakul, Chearwae, Shukia, et al., **Mol. Cell Biochem.** 2007; 296 (1-2): 85-95.

Aspirin, COX-2 Inhibitors Effective as Adjuvant Therapy in Stage III Colon Cancer, Fuchs, **Amer. Soc. Clin. Onc.**, AGM May 16, 2005; Abstract 3530, as reported by Schuster, Medscape Medical News, May 2005; article 504976.

Helicobacter Infection, Chronic Inflammation and the Development of Malignancy, Crowe, **Curr. Opin. Gastroenterol.** 2005; 21 (1): 32-38.

Nutritional and Botanical Modulation of the Inflammatory Cascade – Eicosanoids, Cyclooxygenases and Lipoxygenases – As an Adjunct in Cancer Therapy, Wallace, **Integr. Cancer Ther**. 2002; 1 (1): 7-37.

Inflammation, COX-2 Inhibitors, & Cancer, Block, **Integr. Cancer Ther.** 2005; 4 (1): 3-4.

Inflammation and Cancer: An Ancient Link with Novel Potentials, Perwez Hussain & Harris, **Int. J. Cancer** 2007; 121 (11): 2373-2380.

NF-kappaB: A Stress-regulated Switch for Cell Survival, Piva, Belardo & Santoro, **Antioxid. Redox Signal.** 2006; 8 (3-4): 478-486.

Cancer Cachexia and Targeting Chronic Inflammation: A Unified Approach to Cancer Treatment and Palliative/Supportive Care, MacDonald, **J. Support. Oncol.** 2007; 5 (4): 157-162.

Inflammation and Cancer, Coussens & Werb, **Nature** 2002; 420 (6917): 860-867.

Significance and Relationship Between Infiltrating Inflammatory Cell and Tumour Angiogenesis in Hepatocellular Carcinoma Tissues, Peng, Deng, Yang, et al., **World J Gastroenterol.** 2005; 11 (41): 6521-6524.

Inflammatory Cell Infiltration of Tumours: Jekyll or Hyde, Talmadge, Donkor, & Scholar, **Cancer Metastasis Rev.** 2007; 26 (3-4): 373- 400.

Bioavailability of Curcumin: Problems and Promises, Anaand, Kunnumakkara, Newman, et al., **Molec. Pharm.** 2007; 4 (6): 807-818.

Phase II Trial of Curcumin in Patients with Advanced Pancreatic Cancer, Dhillon, Aggarwal, Newman, et al., **Clin. Cancer Res.** 2008; 14 (14): 4491-4499.

Inflammation and Prostate Cancer, Vasto, Carruba, Candore, et al., **Future Oncol.** 2008; 4 (5): 637-645.
Prevention and Treatment of Pancreatic Cancer by Curcumin in Combination with Omega-3 Fatty Acids, Swamy, Citineni, et al, **Nutr. Cancer** 2008; 60 Suppl. 1: 81-89.

Curcumin Inhibits Human Colon Cancer Cell Growth by Suppressing Gene Expression of Epidermal Growth Factor Receptor Through Reducing the Activity of the Transcription Factor Egr-1, Chen, Xu & Johnson, **Oncogene** 2006; 25 (2): 278-287.

Phase II Trial of Curcumin in Patients with Advanced Pancreatic Cancer, Dhillon, Aggarwal, Newman, et al., **Clin. Cancer Res.** 2008; 14 (14): 4491-4499.

Inhibitory Effect of Curcumin, a Food Spice from Turmeric, on Platelet-activating Factor and Arachidonic Acid-mediated Platelet Aggregation Through Inhibition of Thromboxane Formation and Ca2+ Signalling, Shah, Nawaz, Pertani, et al., **Biochem. Pharmacol.** 1999; 58 (7): 1167-1172.

Combination Treatment with Curcumin and Quercetin of Adenomas in Familial Adenomatous Polyposis, Cruz-Correa, Shoskes, Sanchez, et al., **Clin. Gastroenterol. Hepatol.** 2006; 4 (8): 1035-1038.

Curcumin Inhibits Proliferation, Invasion, Angiogenesis and Metastasis of Different Cancers Through Interaction with Multiple Cell Signaling Proteins, Kunnumakkara, Anand & Aggarwal, **Cancer Lett.** 2008; [Epub ahead of print].

Curcumin (Diferuloylmethane) Down-regulates Expression of Cell Proliferation and Anti-apoptotic and Metastatic Gene Products Through Suppression of I-kappaB-alpha Kinase and Akt Activation, Aggarwal, Ichikawa, Takada, et al., **Mol. Pharmacol.** 2006; 69 (1): 195-206.

Curcumin Down-regulates the Multidrug-resistance Mdr1b Gene by Inhibiting the PI3K/Akt/NF kappa B Pathway, Choi, Kim, Lim, et al., **Cancer Lett.** 2008; 259 (1): 111-118.

Amelioration of Immune Cell number Depletion and Potentiation of Depressed Detoxification System of Tumour-bearing Mice by Curcumin, Pal, Bhattacharyya, Choudhuri, et al., **Cancer Detect. Prev.** 2005; 29 (5): 470-478

Vitamin Antioxidants, Lipid Peroxidation, Tumour Stage, the Systemic Inflammatory Response and Survival in Patients with Colorectal Cancer, Leung, Crozier, Talwar, et al., **Int. J. Cancer** 2008; 12310: 2460-2464.

Evaluation of Anti-inflammatory Property of Curcumin (diferuloyl methane) in Patients with Postoperative Inflammation, Satoskar, Shah & Shenoy, **Int. J. Clin. Pharmacol. Ther. Toxicol.** 1986; 24: 651-654.

Biological Effects of Curcumin and its Role in Cancer Chemoprevention and Therapy, Singh & Khar, **Anticancer Agents Med. Chem.** 2006; 6 (3): 259-270.

Chemotherapeutic Potential of Curcumin for Colorectal Cancer, Chauhan, **Curr. Pharm. Des.** 2002; 8 (19): 1695-1706

Suppression of the Nuclear Factor-kappaB Activation Pathway by Spice-derived Phytochemicals: Reasoning for Seasoning, Aggarwal & Shishodia, **Ann. N. Y. Acad. Sci.** 2004; 1030: 434-441.

Phase I Dose Escalation Trial of Docetaxol Plus Curcumin in Patients with Advanced and Metastatic Breast Cancer, Bayet-Robert, Kwiatkowski, Leheurteur, et al., **Cancer Biol. Ther.** 2010, 9 (1): [Epub ahead of print}. PMID 19901561.

Curcumin in Combination with Bortezomib Synergistically Induced Apoptosis in Human Multiple Myeloma U266 Cells, Park, Ayyappan, Bae, et al., **Molecular Oncology** 2009 2 (4): 317-326.

Curcumin Circumvents Chemoresistance in vitro *and Potentiates the Effect of Thalidomide and Bortezomib Against Human Multiple Myeloma in Nude Mice Model,* Sung, Kunnumakkara, Sethi, et al., **Mol. Cancer Ther.** 2009; 8 (4): 959-970.

Curcumin as an Anti-cancer Agent: Review of the Gap Between Basic and Clinical Applications, Bar-Sela, Epelbaum & Schaffer, **Curr. Med. Chem.** 2010; 17 (3): 190-197(8).

Aromatase Inhibitor Letrozole in Synergy with Curcumin in the Inhibition of Xenografted Endometrial Carcinoma Growth, Liang, Hao, Wu, et al., **Int. J. Gynecol. Cancer** 2009; 19 (7): 1248-1252

Curcuma wenyujin Extract Induces Apoptosis and Inhibits Proliferation of Human Cervical Cancer Cells in Vitro and in Vivo, Lim, Ky, Ng, et al., **Integr. Cancer Ther.** 2010; 9 (1): 36-49.

Curcumin Inhibits Prosurvival Pathways in Chronic Lymphocytic Leukemia B Cells and May Overcome Their Stromal Protection in Combination with EGCG, Ghosh, Kay, Secreto & Shanafelt, **Clin. Cancer Res.** 2009; 15 (4): 1250-1258.
Elimination of Colon Cancer Stem-like Cells by the Combination of Curcumin and FOLFOX, Yu, Kanwar, Patel, et al., **Transl. Oncol.** 2009; 2 (4): 321-328.

Regression of Follicular Lymphoma with Devil's Claw: Coincidence or Causation?, Wilson, **Curr. Oncol.** 2009; 16 (4): 67-70.

DIET & GENERAL INTEGRATIVE ONCOLOGY

Natural Health Products and Cancer Treatment, Hal Gunn, Complementary Corner, Summer 2003 Vol. 4 No. 3 www.abreastinthewest.ca (BCCA policy re: natural agents)

Cancer Therapy – The Independent Consumer's Guide to Non-toxic Treatment and Prevention, Ralph Moss 1992/6 Equinox Press.

Use of Complementary / Integrative Nutritional Therapies During Cancer Treatment: Implications in Clinical Practice, Kumar et al., **Cancer Control** 2002; 9 (3): 236-243.

Complementary Therapies for Cancer-related Symptoms, Deng, Cassileth & Yeung, **J. Support Oncol.** 2004; 2: 419-429.

Complementary and Alternative Therapies for Cancer, Cassileth & Deng, **Oncologist** 2004; 9: 80-89.

Integrative Oncology: Complementary Therapies in Cancer Care, Cassileth, Heitzer & Gubili, **Cancer Chemother. Rev.** 2008; 3 (4): 204-211.

Lifestyle Changes and the 'Spontaneous' Regression of Cancer: An Initial Computer Analysis Foster, **Int. J. Biosoc. Res.**, 1988; 10 (1): 17-33.

Exercise in Prevention and Management of Cancer, Newton & Galvao, **Curr. Treat. Opt. Oncol.** 2008; 92 (3): 135-146.

Molecular Targets of Dietary Agents for Prevention and Therapy of Cancer, Aggarwal & Shishodia, **Biochem. Pharmacol.** 2006; 71: (10): 1397-1421.

Analysis of Botanicals and Dietary Supplements for Antioxidant Capacity: a Review, Prior & Cao, **J. AOAC Int.** 2000; 83 (4): 950-956.

Dietary Fat, Fibre, Vegetable, and Micronutrients are Associated with Overall Survival in Postmenopausal Women Diagnosed with Breast Cancer, McEligot, Largent, Ziogas, Peel & Anton-Culver, **Nutr. Cancer.** 2006; 55 (2): 132-140.

Dietary Influences on Survival After Ovarian Cancer, Nagle, Purdie, Webb, et al., **Int. J. Cancer** 2003; 106 (2): 264-269.

Association of Dietary Patterns with Cancer Recurrence and Survival in Patients with Stage III Colon Cancer, Meyerhardt , Niedzwiecki , Hollis, et al., **J. Amer. Med. Assoc.** 2007; 298 (7):754 -764.

Greater Survival After Breast Cancer in Physically Active Women with High Vegetable-Fruit Intake Regardless of Obesity, Pierce, Stefanick, Flatt, et al., **J. Clin. Oncol.** 2007; 25 (17): 2345-2351.

Influence of a Diet Very High in Vegetables, Fruit and Fibre and Low in Fat on Prognosis Following Treatment for Breast Cancer, **J. Amer. Med. Assoc.** 2007; 298 (3): 289-298.

Baseline Nutritional Status is Predictive of Response to Treatment and Survival in Patients treated by Definitive Chemo-Radiotherapy for a Locally Advanced Esophageal Cancer, Di Fiore, Lecleire, Pop, et al., **Am. J. Gastroenterol.** 2007; 102 (11): 2557-2563.

Is Voluntary Vitamin and Mineral Supplementation Associated with Better Outcome in Non-Small Cell Lung Cancer Patients? Results from the Mayo Clinic Lung Cancer Cohort. Jatoi, Williams, Nichols, et al., **Lung Cancer.** 2005; 49 (1): 77-84.

Survival Impact of Integrative Cancer Care in Advanced Metastatic Breast Cancer, Block, Gyllenhaal, Tripathy, et al., in press, **The Breast Journal** 2009; 15 (4).

Survival Impact of Integrative Care in Advanced Prostate Cancer, Block, Gyllenhaal, Chodak, et al., **Proc. Am. Soc. Clin. Oncol**. 2003; 22: abstract 1746.

Mind-body Therapies for the Management of Pain, Astin, **Clin. J. Pain** 2004; 20 (1): 27-32.

Pilot Crossover Trial of Reiki vs. Rest for Treating Cancer-related Fatigue, Tsang, Carlson & Olson, **Integr. Cancer Ther.** 2007; 6 (1): 25-35.

The Hoxsey Treatment: Cancer Quackery or Effective Physiological Adjuvant?, Brinker, **J. Naturopathic Med.** 1996; 6(1): 9-23.

Broad in vitro *Efficacy of Plant-derived Betulinic Acid Against Cell Lines Derived from the Most Prevalent Human Cancer Types,* Kessler, Mullauer, dee Roo & Medema, **Cancer Lett.** 2007; 251 (1): 132-145

437

Naturopathic Oncology

Complementary & Alternative Medicine, Larson, **Trustee Mag.** 2006, Sept.

Survival Impact of Integrative Care in Advanced Prostate Cancer, Block, Gyllenhaal, Chodak et al., **Proc. Am Soc. Clin. Oncol.** 2003; 22: abstract 1746.

Survival Impact of Integrative Cancer Care in Advanced Metastatic Breast Cancer, Block, Gyllenhaal, Tripathy et al., **The Breast Journal.** 2008; in press.

Genetic Program Linking Cancer to Hemostasis Identified, Boccaccio, et al., **Nature** 2005; 434: 396-400.

Metastasis: A Therapeutic Target for Cancer, Steeg & Theodorescu, **Nat. Clin. Pract. Oncol.** 2008; 5 (4): 206-219.

Effect of Gamma-Linolenic Acid on the Transcritional Activity of the Her-2/neu (erbB-2) Oncogene, Menendez, Vellon, Colomer & Lupu, **J. Natl. Cancer Inst.** 2005; 97 (2): 1611-1615.

Therapeutic Applications of Whey Protein, Marshall, **Altern. Med. Rev.** 2004; 9 (2): 136-156.
Herb-Drug Interactions in Oncology: Focus on Mechanisms of Induction, Meijerman, Bejnen and Schellens, **Oncologist** 2006; 11: 742-752.

L-Glutamine Use in the Treatment and Prevention Mucositis and Cachexia: A Naturopathic Perspective, Noé, **Integr. Cancer Ther.** 2009; 8 (4): 409-415.

Energy-modulating Vitamins – A New Combinatorial Therapy Prevents Cancer Cachexia in Rat Mammary Carcinoma, Perumai, Shanthi & Sachdanandam, **Br. J. Nutr.** 2005; 93(6): 901-909.

P13 Kinase /Akt Pathway as a Therapeutic Target in Multiple Myeloma, Harvey & Lonial, **Future Oncol.** 2007; 3(6): 639-647.

Starvation-dependent Differential Stress Resistance Protects Normal but Not Cancer Cells Against High-dose Chemotherapy, Raffaghello, Lee, Sadfie, et al., **Proc Natl Acad Sci USA** 2008; 105 (24): 8215-8220.

Adherence to Mediterranean Diet and Health Status: Meta-analysis, Sofe, Cesari, Abbate, et al., **BMJ** 2008; 337: a1344.

Early Hormonal Data from a Multicentre Phase II Trial Using Transdermal Oestrogen Patches as a First-line Hormonal Therapy in Patients with Locally Advanced or Metastatic Prostate Cancer, Langley, Godsland, Kynastn, et al., **BJU Int** 2008; 102 (4): 442-445.

Starvation-dependent Differential Stress Resistance Protects Normal but Not Cancer Cells Against High-dose Chemotherapy, Raffaghello, Lee, Sadfie, et al., **Proc Natl Acad Sci USA** 2008; 105 (24): 8215-8220.

Dietary Alpha-, Beta-, Gamma- and Delta-Tocopherols in Lung Cancer Risk, Mahabir, Schendel, Dong, et al., **Int. J. Cancer** 2008; 123: 1173-1180.

Allergic Pulmonary Inflammation Promotes the Recruitment of Circulating Tumour Cells to the Lung, Taranova, Maldonado, Vachon, et al., **Cancer Res.** 2008; 68 (20): 8582-8589.

Interaction of Warfarin with Drugs, Natural Substances, and Foods, Greenblatt & von Moltke, **J. Clin. Pharmacol.** 2005; 45 (2): 127-132.

Intensive Lifestyle Changes May Affect the Progression of Prostate Cancer, Ornish, Weidner, Fair, et al., **J Urol**. 2005; 174 (3): 1065-1069.

High Casein-Lactalbumin Diet Accelerates Blood Coagulation in Rats, Chan, Lou & Hargrove, **J. Nutr.** 1993; 123 (6): 1010-1016.

Dairy Products, Calcium, and Vitamin D and Risk of Prostate Cancer, Chan & Giovannucci, **Epidemiol. Rev.** 2001; 23 (1): 87-92.

Dairy Products and Breast Cancer: the IGF-I, Estrogen, and bGH Hypothesis, Outwater, Nicholson & Barnard, **Med. Hypotheses** 1997; 48 (6): 453-461.

Prospective Study of Grapefruit Intake and Risk of Breast Cancer in Postmenopausal Women: the Multi-ethnic Cohort Study, Monroe, Murphy, Kolonel & Pike, **Br. J. Cancer** 2007; 697 (3): 440-445.

Does Grapefruit Juice Increase the Bioavailability of Orally Administered Sex Steroids? Fingerová, Oborná, Petrová, et al., **Ceska Gynekol.** 2003; 68 (2): 117-121.

Gamma-linolenic Acid Therapy of Human Glioma- A Review of in vitro, in vivo, and Clinical Studies, Das, **Med. Sci. Monit.** 2007; 13 (7): RA119-131.

Gamma Linolenic Acid: An Antiinflammatory Omega-6 Fatty Acid, Kapoor & Huang, **Curr. Pharm. Biotechnol.** 2006; 7(6): 531-534.

Non-linear Dynamics for Clinicians: Chaos Theory, Fractals, and Complexity at the Bedside, Goldberger, **Lancet** 1996; 347: 1312–1314.

Megadose Vitamins in Bladder Cancer: A Double-blind Clinical Trial, Lamm, Riggs, Shriver et al., **J. Urol.** 1994; 151 (1): 21-26

Health Implications of Mediterranean Diets in Light of Contemporary Knowledge: Meat, Wine, Fats, and Oils, Kushi, Lenart & Willett, **Am. J. Clin. Nutr**. 1995; 61 (6Suppl): 1416S-1427S.

Adherence to the Mediterranean Diet Attenuates Inflammation and Coagulation Process in Healthy Adults: The ATTICA Study, Chrysohoou, Panagiotakos, Pitsavos, et al., **J. Am. Coll. Cardiol**. 2004; 44 (1): 152-158.

Fibrinogen: A Novel Predictor of Responsiveness in Metastatic Melanoma Patients Treated with Bio-chemotherapy: IMI (Italian Melanoma Inter-group) Trial, Guida, Ravaioli, Sileni, et al., **J. Transl. Med**. 2003; 1 (1): 13.

Analysis of Botanicals and Dietary Supplements for Antioxidant Capacity: A Review, Prior, Cao, Prior & Cao, **J. AOAC Int**. 2000; 83 (4): 950-956.

Seronea repens (Permixon, Saw Palmetto)Inhibits the 5-alpha-reductase Activity of Human Prostate Cancer Cell Lines Without Interfering with PSA Expression, Habib, Ross, Ho, et al., **Int. J. Cancer** 2005; 114 (2); 190-194.

Efficacy of Homeopathic Therapy in Cancer Treatment, Milazzo, Russell & Ernst, **Eur. J. Cancer**, 2006; 42 : 282-289.

Series of Case Reports: Clinical Evaluation of a Complex Homeopathic Injection Therapy in the Management of Pain in Patients After Breast Cancer Treatment, Orellana, Ruiz de Viñaspre & Kaszkin-Bettag, **Altern. Ther. Health Med**. 2010; 16 (1): 54-59.

Ultra-diluted Remedies on Breast Cancer Cells, Frenkel, Mishra, Sen, et al., **Int. J. Oncol**. 2010; 36 (2): 395-403. PMID: 20043074

Pancreatic Proteolytic Enzyme Therapy Compared With Gemcitabine-Based Chemotherapy for the Treatment of Pancreatic Cancer, Chabot, Tsai, Fine, et al., **J. Clin. Oncol**. 2009 Aug 17. [Epub ahead of print] PMID 19687327.

Berberine and Berberine-containing Plants as Antineoplastic Agents, Tang, Feng, Wang, et al., **J. Ethnopharmacol**. 2009; 128: 5-17.

Gamma Tocopherol Traps Mutagenic Electrophiles such as NOx and Complements Alpha Tocopherol: Physiological Implications, Christen, Woodall, Shigenaga, et al., **Proc. Natl. Acad. Sci. USA** 1997; 94: 3217–3222.

GINGER

Ginger for Chemotherapy-related Nausea in Cancer Patients: A URCC CCOP Randomized, Double-blind, Placebo-controlled Clinical Trial of 644 Cancer Patients,

Ryan, Heckler, Dakhil et al., **J. Clin. Oncol.** 2009: 27: 15s, (suppl; abstr 9511 - 2009 ASCO Annual Meeting).

Phase II Trial of Encapsulated Ginger as a Treatment for Chemotherapy-induced Nausea and Vomiting, Zick, Ruffin, Lee et al., **Support Care Cancer** 2009; 17 (5): 563-572.

A Phase II/III Randomized, Placebo-Controlled, Double-Blind Clinical Trial of Ginger (Zingiber officinale) for Nausea Caused by Chemotherapy for Cancer: A Currently Accruing URCC CCOP Cancer Control Study, Hickok, Roscoe, Morrow & Ryan, **Support Cancer Ther.** 2007; 4 (4): 247-250.

Protein and Ginger for the Treatment of Chemotherapy-induced Delayed Nausea, Levine, Gillis, Koch et al., **J. Altern. Complement. Med.** 2008; 14 (5): 545-551.

Antiemetic Effect of Ginger in Gynecologic Oncology Patients Receiving Cisplatin. Manusirivithaya, Sripramote, Tangjitgamol et al., **Int. J. Gynecol. Cancer** 2004; 14 (6): 1063-1069.

GRAPESEED EXTRACT & RESVERATROL

Oligomeric Proanthocyanidin Complexes: History, Structure & Phytopharmaceutical Applications, A. M. Fine. **Alt. Med Rev**. 2000; Vol. 5, No. 2: 144-151.

Cellular Protection with Proanthocyanidins Derived from Grape Seeds, Bagchi, Bagchi & Stohs, et al, **Ann. N. Y. Acad. Sci**. 2002; 957: 260-270.
Oligomeric Proanthocyanidins (OPCs) – Monograph, **Alt. Med. Rev**. 2003; Vol. 8, No.4: 442-450.
Chemoprevention of Colorectal Cancer by Grapeseed Proanthocyanidin is Accompanied by a Decrease in Proliferation and Increase in Apoptosis, Nomoto, Iigo, Hamada, et al. **Nutr. & Cancer**. 2004; Vol. 49, No. 1: 81-89.

Alcohol and Polyphenolic Grape Extract Inhibit Platelet Adhesion in Flowing Blood, de Lange, Scholman, Kraaijenhagen, et al., **Eur. J. Clin. Invest.** 2004; 4 (12): 818-824.

Red Wine and Red Wine Polyphenolic Compounds But Not Alcohol Inhibit ADP-induced Platelet Aggregation, de Lange, van Golden, Scholman, et al., **Eur. J. Intern. Med.** 2003; 14 (6): 361-366.

Grape Seed and Skin Extracts Inhibit Platelet Function and Release of Reactive Oxygen Intermediates, Vitseva, Varghese, Chakrabarti, et al., **J. Cardiovasc. Pharmacol.** 2005; 46 (4): 445-451.

Proanthocyanidin from Grape Seeds Enhances Anti-tumour Effect of Doxorubicin Both in vitro & in vivo, Zhang, Bai, Wu, et al, **Pharmazie**, 2005; 60: 533-538.

Grape Seed Proanthocyanidin Extract Induced Mitochondria-associated Apoptosis in Human Acute Myeloid Leukaemia 14.3D10 Cells, Hong & Qin, **Chin. Med. J.** 2006; 119 (5): 417-421.

Grapeseed Extract Induces Apoptotic Death of Human Prostate Carcinoma DU145 Cells Via Caspases Activation Accompanied by Dissipation of Mitochondrial membrane Potential and Cytochrome C Release, Agarwal, Singh & Agarwal, **Carcinogenesis** 2002; 23 (11): 1869-1876.

Suppression of Estrogen Biosynthesis by Procyanidin Dimers in Red Wine and Grape Seeds, Eng, Ye, Williams, et al., **Cancer Res**. 2003; 63 (23): 8516-8522.

Grapeseed Extract is an Aromatase Inhibitor and a Suppressor of Aromatase Expression, Kijima, Phung, Hur, et al., **Cancer Res.** 2006; 66 (11): 5960-5967.

Grapeseed Extract Inhibits Advanced Human Prostate Cancer Growth and Angiogenesis and Upregulates Insulin-like Growth Factor Binding Protein 3, Singh, Tyagi, Dhanalakshmi, et al., **Int. J. Cancer** 2004; 108 (5): 733-740.

Grape Seed Extract Induces Anoikis and Caspase-mediated Apoptosis in Human Prostate Carcinoma LNCaP Cells: Possible Role of Ataxia Telangiectasis Mutated-p53 Activation, Kaur, Agarwal & Agarwal, **Mol. Cancer Ther.** 2006; 5 (5): 1265-1274.

Grape Seed Proanthocyanidin Extract Induced Mitochondria-associated Apoptosis in Human Acute Myeloid Leukaemia 14.3D10 cells, Hu & Qin, **Chin. Med. J.** 2006; 119 (5): 417-421.

Proanthocyanidins from Grape Seeds Inhibit Expression of Matrix Metalloproteinases in Human Prostate Carcinoma Cells, Which is Associated with the Inhibition of Activation of MAPK and NF kappa B, Vayalil, **Carcinogenesis** 2004; 25 (6): 987-985.

Anti-angiogenic Efficacy of Grape Seed Extract in Endothelial Cells, Agarwal, Singh, Dhanalakshmi & Agarwal, **Oncol. Rep.** 2004; 11 (3): 681-685.

Grape Seed Extract Inhibits Advanced Human Prostate Tumour Growth and Angiogenesis and Upregulates Insulin-like Growth Factor Binding Protein-3, Singh, Tyagi, Dhanalakshmi,et al., **Int. J. Cancer** 2004; 108 (5): 733-740.

Anti-cancer Activity of Grape and Grape Skin Extracts Alone and Combined with Green Tea Infusions, Morré & Morré, **Cancer Lett.** 2006; 238 (2): 202-209.

Grape Seed Extract Induces Apoptotic Death of Human Prostate Carcinoma DU145 Cells Via Caspases Activation Accompanied by Dissipation of Mitochondrial Membrane Potential and Cytochrome C Release, Agarwal, Singh & Agarwal, **Carcinogenesis** 2002; 23 (11): 1869-1876.

Inhibition of NF-kappaB Pathway in Grape Seed Extract-induced Apoptotic Death of Human Prostate Carcinoma DU145 Cells, Dhanalakshmi, Agarwal & Agarwal, **Int. J. Oncol.** 2003; 23 (3): 721-727.

Grape Seed Extract Inhibits EGF-induced and Constituitively Active Mitogenic Signallng but Activated JNK in Human Prostate Carcinoma DU145 Cells:Possible Role in Antiproliferation and Apoptosis, Tyagi, Agarwal & Agarwal, **Oncogene** 2003; 22 (9): 1302-1316.

Matrix Metalloproteinases in Cancer Metastasis: Molecular Targets for Prostate Cancer Prevention by Green Tea Polyphenols and Grape Seed Proanthocyanidins, Katiyar, **Endocr. Metabol. Immune Disord. Drug Targets,** 2006; 6 (1): 17-24.

Grape Seed Extract Inhibits EGF-induced and Constitutively Active Mitogenic Signaling But Activates JNK in Human Prostate Carcinoma DU145 Cells: Possible Role in Anti-proliferation and Apoptosis, Tyagi, Agarwal & Agarwal, **Oncogene** 2003; 22 (9): 1302-1316.

Grape Seed Extract Inhibits in vitro and in vivo Growth of Human Colorectal Carcinoma Cells, Kaur, Singh, Gu, et al., **Clin. Cancer Res.** 2006; 12 (20 Pt 1): 6194-6202.

Proanthocyanidin from Grape Seeds Inactivates the PI3-kinase/PKB Pathway and Induces Apoptosis in a Colon Cancer Cell Line, Engelbrecht, Mattheyse, Ellis, et al., **Cancer Lett.** 2007; 258 (1): 144-153.

Experimental Model for Treating Pulmonary Metastatic Melanoma Using Grape-seed Extract, Red wine and Ethanol, Martínez Conesa, Vicente Ortega, et al., **Clin. Transl. Oncol.** 2005; 7 (3): 115-121.

Grapeseed Extract Inhibits Angiogenesis via Suppression of the Vascular Endothelial Growth Factor Receptor Signaling Pathway, Wen, Lu, Zhang & Chen, **Cancer Prev. Res.** 2008; 1 (7): 554-561

Grapeseed Extract Inhibits VEGF Expression via Reducing HIF-1 alpha Protein Expression, Lu, Zhang, Chen & Wen, **Carcinogenesis** 2009; 30 (4): 636-644.

Free Radicals and Grape Seed Proanthocyanidin Extract: Importance in Human Health and Disease Prevention, Bagchi, Bagchi, Stohs, et al., **Toxicol.** 2000; 148

(2-3): 187-197.
Chemoprevention of Colorectal Cancer by Grape Seed Proanthocyanidin is Accompanied by a Decrease in Proliferation and Increase in Apoptosis, Nomoto, Hiroshi, Iigo, et al., **Nutr. & Cancer** 2004; 49 (1): 81-89.

Synergistic Anti-cancer Effects of Grapeseed Extract and Conventional Cytotoxic Agent Doxorubicin Against Human Breast Carcinoma Cells, Sharma, Tyagi, Singh, et al., **Breast Cancer Res. Treat.** 2004; 85 (1): 1-12.

Chemopreventative Effects of Grape Seed Proanthocyanidin Extract on Chang Liver Cells, Joshi, Kuszynski, Bagchi & Bagchi, **Toxicol.** 2000; 155: 83-90.

Dermal Wound Healing Properties of Redox-active Grape Seed Proanthocyanidins, Khanna, Venojarvi, Roy, et al., **Free Rad. Biol. Med.** 2002; 33: 1089.
Gallic Acid, an Active Constituent of Grapeseed Extract, Exhibits Anti-proliferative, Por-apoptotic and Anti-tumorigenic Effects Against Prostate Carcinoma Xenograft Growth in Nude Mice, Kaur, Velmurugan, Rajamanickam, et al., **Pharm. Res.** 2009; June 20 [Epub ahead of print] PMID: 19543955.

Molecular Mechanisms Behind the Chemopreventive Effects of Anthocyanidins, Hou, Fujii, Terahara & Yoshimoto, **Biomed. Biotechnol.** 2004; 2004 (5): 321-325.
Signal Transduction Pathways: Targets for Chemoprevention of Skin Cancer, Bode, **Lancet Oncol.** 2000; 1: 181-188.

The Cytotoxic Effects of a Novel Grape Seed Proanthocyanidin Extrct on Cultured Human Cancer Cells, Joshi, Ye, Liu, et al., **Sci. Proc. 89th Ann. Meet. Amer. Assoc. Cancer Res.** 1998, Vol. 39.

Anti-thrombotic Effect of Proanthocyanidin, a Purified Ingredient of Grape Seed, Sano, Oda, Yamashita, et al., **Thromb. Res.** 2005; 115: 115-121.

Pycnogenol as an Adjunct in the Management of Childhood Asthma, Lau, Riesen, Truong, et al., **J. Asthma** 2004; 41 (8): 825-832.

Role of Resveratrol in Prevention and Therapy of Cancer: Preclinical and Clinical Studies, Aggarwal, Bhardwaj, Aggarwal, et al., **Anticancer Res.** 2004; 24 (5A): 2783-2840.

Resveratrol-induced Apoptosis in Human Breast Cancer Cells is Mediated Primarily Through the Caspase-3-dependent Pathway, Alkhalaf, El-Mowafy, Renno, et al., **Arch. Med. Res.** 2008; 39 (2): 162-168.

Resveratrol Inhibits Proliferation, Induces Apoptosis, and Overcomes Chemo-resistance Through Down-regulation of STAT3 and Nuclear factor-kappaB-regulated

Anti-apoptotic and Cell Survival Gene Products in Human Multiple Myeloma Cells, Bhardwaj, Sethi, Vadhan-Raj, et al., **Blood** 2007; 109 (6): 2293-2302.

Resveratrol Induces the Suppression of Tumour-derived CD4+CD25+ Regulatory T Cells, Yang, Paik, Cho, et al., **Int. Immunopharmacol.** 2008; 8 (4): 542-547.

Resveratrol Induces Apoptosis and Differentiation in Acute Pro-myelocytic Leukemia (NB4) Cells, Cao, Wang, Liu, et al., **J. Asian Nat. Prod. Res.** 2005; 7 (4): 633-641.

Resveratrol: A Candidate Nutritional Substance for Prostate Cancer Prevention, Stewart, Artime & O'Brian, **J. Nutr.** 2003; 133 (7 Suppl): 2440S-2443S.

Resveratrol Inhibits Aggregation of Platelets from High-risk Cardiac Patients with Aspirin Resistance, Stef, Csiszar, Lerea, et al., **J. Cardiovasc. Pharmacol.** 2006; 48 (2): 1-5.

Anti-angiogenic Activity of Resveratrol, a Natural Compound from Medicinal Plants, Cao, Fu, Wang, et al., **J. Asian Nat. Prod. Res.** 2005; 7 (3): 205-224.

Resveratrol Acts as an Estrogen Receptor (ER) Agonist in Breast Cancer Cells Stably Transfected with ER alpha, Levenson, Gehm, Pearce, et al., **Int. J. Cancer** 2003; 104: 587-597.

The Cancer Preventative Agent Resveratrol is Converted to the Anti-cancer Agent Piceattanol by the Cytochrome P-450 Enzyme CYP1B1, Potter, Patterson, Wanogho, et al., **Br. J. Cancer** 2002; 86: 774-778.

Involvement of p21WAF1/Cip1, pRB, Bax and NF-kappaB in Induction of Growth Arrest and Apoptosis by Resveratrol in Human Lung Carcinoma A549 cells, Kim, Lee, Choi, et al., **Int. J. Oncol.** 2003; 23 (4): 1143-1149.

GREEN TEA EGCG

Green Tea Monograph, McKenna, Hughes & Jones, **Alt. Ther.** May 2000; Vol. 6, No. 3: 61-84.

Green Tea Extract and (-)-Epigallocatechin-3-gallate, the Major Tea Catechin, Exert Oxidant but Lack Antioxidant Activites, Elbling, Weiss, Teufelhofer, et al., **FASEB J.** 2005; 19 (7): 807-809.

Prospective Cohort Study of Green Tea Consumption and Colorectal Cancer Risk in Women, Yang, Shu, Li. Et al., **Cancer Epidemiol. Biomarkers Prev.** 2007; 16 (6): 1219-1223.

Green Tea (Camellia sinensis) Extract Does Not Alter Cytochrome P-450 3A4 or 2D6 Activity in Healthy Volunteers, Donovan, Chavin & Devane **Drug. Metab. Dispos.**

2004; 32: 906-908.

Efficacies of Tea Components on Doxorubicin-induced Anti-tumour Activity and Reversal of Multi-drug Resistance, Sadzuka, Sugiyama & Sonobe, **Toxicol. Letters** 2000; 114: 155-162.

Green Tea Inhibits VEGF Induction in Human Breast Cancer Cells, Sartippour, Shao, Heber, et al, **J. Nutr**. 2002; 132: 2307-2311.

The Effects of Green Tea Consumption on Incidence of Breast Cancer and Recurrence of Breast Cancer: A Systematic Review and Meta-analysis, Seely, Mills, Wu P, et al., **Integr. Cancer Ther.** 2005; 4 (2): 144-155.

Green Tea Catechins Inhibit VEGF-induced Angiogenesis in vitro *Through Suppression of VE-Cadherin Phosphorylation & Inactivation of Akt Molecule,* Tang, Nguyen & Meydani, **Int. J. Cancer** 2003; 106: 871-878.

Epigallocatechin-3-gallate Inhibits Epidermal Growth Factor Receptor Signalling Pathway. Evidence for Direct Inhibition of ERK1/2 and AKT Kinases, Sah, Balasubramanian, Eckert & Rorke, **J. Biol. Chem.** 2004; 279 (13): 12755 – 12762.

Green Tea Appears to Protect Against Breast Cancer, Wu, **Int. J. Cancer** 2003; 106: 574-579.

Green Tea Component Destroys Leukemia Cells, Kay, **Blood** Mar.2, 2004 On-line edition.

Green Tea Catechins Containing a Galloyl Group in the 3' Position Inhibit Tissue Factor-Induced Thrombin Generation, Stampfuss, Schror & Weber, **Thromb. Haemost.** 2005; 93 (6): 1200-1201.

Green Tea Epigallocatechin-3-gallate Inhibits Platelet Signalling Pathways Triggered by Both Proteolytic and Non-proteolytic Agonists, Deana, Turetta, Donella-Deana, et al., **Thromb Haemost.** 2003; 89 (5): 866-874.

Tea Polyphenols, Their Biological Effects and Potential Molecular Targets, Chen, Milacic, Chen, et al., **Histol. Histopathol.** 2008; 23 (4): 487-496.

Antioxidant Activity of Tea Polyphenols in vivo: *Evidence from Animal Studies,* Frei & Higdon, **J. Nutr.** 2003; 133 (10): 3275S-3284S.

Clinical Effects of Oral Green Tea Extracts in Four Patients with Low Grade B-cell Malignancies, Shanafelt, Lee, Call, et al., **Leuk. Res.** 2006; 30: 707-712.

Green Tea Polyphenols and Cancer Chemoprevention: Multiple Mechanisms and

Endpoints for Phase II Trials, Moyers & Kumar, **Nutr. Rev.** 2004; Vol. 62 No. 5: 204-211.

Pigments in Green Tea Leaves (Camellia sinensis) Suppress Transformation of the Aryl Hydrocarbon Receptor Induced by Dioxin, Fukada, Sakane, Yabushita, et al., **J. Agric. Food Chem.** 2004; 52 (9): 2499-2506.

Clinical Effects of Oral Green Tea Extracts in Four Patients with Low Grade B-cell Malignancies, Shanafelt, Lee, Call, et al., **Leuk. Res.** 2006; 30 (6): 707-712.
Anti-oxidants from Green Tea and Pomegranate for Chemoprevention of Prostate Cancer, Adhami and Mukhtar, **Biotechnol.** 2007; 37 (1): 52-57.
Inhibition of Aromatase Activity by Green Tea Extract Catechins and Their Endocrinological Effects of Oral Administration in Rats, Satoh, Sakamoto, Ogata, et al., **Food Chem. Toxicol.** 2002; 40 (7): 925-933.

Structure-Activity Relationships for Inhibition of Human 5-alpha-reductases by Polyphenols, Hiipkka, Zhang, Dai, et al., **Biochem. Pharmacol.** 2002; 63 (6): 1165-1176.

Selective Inhibition of Steroid 5-alpha-reductase Isozymes by Tea Epicatechin-3-gallate and Epigallocatechin-3-gallate, Liao & Hipakka, **Biochem. Biophys. Res. Commun.** 1995; 214 (3): 833-838.

The Antifolate Activity of Tea Catechins, Navarro-peran, Cabezas-Herrera, Garcia-Canovas, et al., **Cancer Res.** 2005; 65 (6): 2059-2064.

Effects of Aqueous Green Tea Extract on Activities of DNA Turn-over Enzymes n Cancerous and Non-cancerous Human Gastric and Colon Tissues, Ergruder, Namusui, Sozener, et al., **Altern. Ther. Health Med.** 2008; 14 (3): 30-33.

Interactions Affecting the Bioavailability of Dietary Polyphenols in vivo, Scholz & Williamson, **Int. J. Vitam. Nutr. Res.** 2007; 77 (3): 224-235.

Green Tea Extracts for the Prevention of Metachronous Colorectal Adenomas: A Pilot Study, Shimizu, Fukutomi, et al., **Cancer Epidemiol. Biomarkers Prev.** 2008; 17 (11): 3020-3025.

Essential Role of Caspases in Epigallocatechin-3-gallate-mediated Inhibition of Nuclear Factor kappa B and Induction of Apoptosis, Gupta, et al., **Oncogene** 2004; 23 (14): 2507-2522.

Epigallocatechin-3-gallate is a Potent Natural Inhibitor of Fatty Acid Synthase in Intact Cells and Selectively Induces Apoptosis in Prostate Cancer Cells, Brusselmans, De Schrijver, Heyns, et al., **Int. J. Cancer** 2003; 106 (6): 856-862.

Prostate Carcinoma and Green Tea: PSA-triggered Basement Membrane Degradation and MMP-2 Activation are Inhibited by (-) Epigallocatechin-3-gallate, Pezzato, Sartor, Dell'Aica, et al., **Int. J. Cancer** 2004; 112 (5): 787-792.

EGCG Inhibits Activation of HER3 and Expression of Cyclooxygenase-2 in Human Colon Cancer Cells, Shimizu, Deguchi , Joe, et al., **J. Exp. Ther. Oncol.** 2005; 5 (1): 69-78.

Epigallocatechin-3-gallate Inhibits Activation of HER-2/neu and Downstream Signaling Pathways in Human Head and Neck and Breast Carcinoma Cells, Masuda, Suzui, Lim & Weinstein, **Clin. Cancer Res.** 2003; 9 (9): 3486-3491.

Role of p53 and NF-kappaB in Epigallocatechin-3-gallate-induced Apoptosis of LNCaP Cells, Hastak, Gupta, Ahmad, et al., **Oncogene** 2003; 22 (31): 4851-4859.

Green Tea Constituent (-)-Epigallocatechin-3-gallate Inhibits Hep G2 Cell Proliferation and Induces Apoptosis Through p53-dependent and Fas-mediated Pathways, Kuo & Lin, **J. Biomed. Sci.** 2003;10 (2): 219-227.

Combined Effect of Green Tea and Ganoderma lucidum on Invasive Behaviour of Breast Cancer Cells, Thyagarajan, Zhu & Sliva, **Int. J. Oncol.** 2007; 30 (4): 963-969.

The Tea Polyphenol, (-)-Epigallocatechin Gallate Effects on Growth, Apoptosis, and Telomerase Activity in Cervical Cell Lines, Yokoyama, Noguchi, Nakao, et al., **Gynecol. Oncol.** 2004; 92 (1): 197-204.
EGCG Down-regulates Telomerase in Human Breast Carcinoma MCF-7 Cells, Leading to Suppression of Cell Viability and Induction of Apoptosis, Mittal, Pate, Wylie, et al., **Int. J. Oncol.** 2004; 24 (3): 703-710.

Matrix Metalloproteinases in Cancer Metastasis: Molecular Targets for Prostate Cancer Prevention by Green Tea Polyphenols and Grape Seed Proanthocyanidins, Katiyar, **Endocr. Metabol. Immune Disord. Drug Targets,** 2006; 6 (1): 17-24.

Anti-cancer Activity of Grape and Grape Skin Extracts Alone and Combined with Green Tea Infusions, Morré & Morré, **Cancer Lett.** 2006; 238 (2): 202-209.

Green Tea Polyphenol Causes Differential Oxidative Environments in Tumour versus Normal Epithelial Cells, Yamamoto, Hsu, Lewis, et al., **J. Pharmacol. Exp. Ther.** 2003; 307 (1): 230-236.

EGCG Inhibits Growth, Invasion, Angiogenesis and Metastasis of Pancreatic Cancer, Shankar, Ganapathy, Hingorani & Srivastava, **Front. Biosci.** 2008; 13: 440-452.

(-)-Epigallocatechin Gallate Inhibits Membrane-type 1 Matrix Metalloproteinase,

MT1-MMP, and Tumour Angiogenesis, Yamakawa, Asai, Uchida, et al., **Cancer Lett.** 2004; 210 (1): 47-55.

Combined Effect of Green Tea and Ganoderma lucidum *on Invasive Behaviour of Breast Cancer Cells,* Thyagarajan, Zhu & Silva, **Int. J. Oncol.** 2007; 30 (4): 963-969.

Dietary Intakes of Mushrooms and Green Tea Combine to Reduce the Risk of Breast Cancer in Chinese Women, Zhng, Huang, Xie & Holman, **Int. J. Cancer** 2009; 1246: 1404-1408.

Phase II Randomized, Placebo-Controlled Trial of Green Tea Extract in Patients with High-Risk Oral Premalignant Lesions, Tsao, Liu, Martin, et al. **Cancer Prev Res** 2009; 2 (11): 931-941.

Natural Compounds with Proteasome Inhibitory Activity for Cancer Prevention and Treatment, Yang, Landis-Piwowar, Chen, et al., **Curr. Protein Pept. Sci.** 2008; 9 (3): 227-239.

Phase II Trial of Daily, Oral Green Tea Extract in Patients with Asymptomatic, Rai Stage 0-II Chronic Lymphocytic Leukemia (CLL), Shanafelt, Call, Zent, et al., **J. Clin. Oncol.** 2010; 28: 7s, (suppl; abstr 6522).

INDOLE-3-CARBINOL

Indole-3-carbinol – Monograph, **Alt. Med. Rev.** 2005; Vol. 10 No. 4: 337-342.

Molecular Targets and Anticancer Potential of Indole-3-carbinol and Its Derivatives, Aggarwal & Ichikawa, **Cell Cycle** 2005; 4 (9): 1201-1215.

Changes in Levels of Urinary Estrogen Metabolite After Oral Indole-3-carbinol Treatment in Humans, Michnovicz, Adlercreutz & Bradlow, **J. Natl. Cancer Inst.** 1997; 89 (10): 718-723.

Indole-3-carbinol and Tamoxifen Cooperate to Arrest the Cell Cycle of MCF-7 Human Breast Cancer Cells, Cover, Hsieh, Cram, et al., **Cancer Res.** 1999; 59 (6):1244-1251.

Indole-3-carbinol and Prostate Cancer, Sarkar, **J. Nutr.** 2004; 134 (12 Suppl): 3493S-3498S.

Indole-3-carbinol as a Chemopreventive and Anti-cancer Agent, Weng, Tsai, Kulp & Chen, **Cancer Lett.** 2008; 262 (2): 153-163.

Multiple Molecular Targets of Indole-3-carbinol, a Chemopreventative Anti-Estrogen in Breast Cancer, Ashtok, Chen, Garikapaty, et. al., **Eur. J. Cancer Prev.** 2002;

Suppl. 2: 86-93.

Placebo-controlled Trial of Indole-3-carbinol in the Treatment of CIN, Bell, Crowley-Nowick, Bradlow, et al., **Gynecol. Oncol.**, 2000 Aug.; 78(2): 123-129.

BRCA1 and BRCA2 as Molecular Targets for Phytochemicals Indole-3-carbinol and Genistein in Breast and Prostate Cancer Cells. Fan, Meng, Auborn, et al., **Br. J. Cancer** 2006 Feb 13; 94(3): 407-426.

Indole-3-carbinol and 3'-3'-Diindolylmethane Antiproliferative Signaling Pathways Control Cell-cycle Gene Transcription in Human Breast Cancer Cells by Regulating Promoter-Sp1 Transcription Factor Interactions, Firestone & Bjeldanes, **J. Nutr.** 2003; 133: 2448S-2455S.

Indole-3-carbinol Activates the ATM Signaling Pathway Independent of DNA Damage to Stabilize p53 and Induce G1 Arrest of Human Mammary Epithelial Cells. Brew, Aronchik, Sheen, et al., **Int. J. Cancer** 2006 Feb 15; 118(4): 857-868.

Gene Expression Profiling Revealed Survivin as a Target of 3,3'-Diindolylmethane-Induced Cell Growth Inhibition and Apoptosis in Breast Cancer Cells. Rahman, Li, Wang, et al., **Cancer Res.** 2006 May 1; 66(9): 4952-4960.

Indole-3-Carbinol (I3C) Inhibits Cyclin-dependent Kinase-2 Function in Human Breast Cancer Cells by Regulating the Size Distribution, Associated Cyclin E Forms, and Subcellular Localization of the CDK2 Protein Complex. Garcia, Brar, Nguyen, et al., **J. Biol. Chem.** 2005 Mar. 11; Vol. 280, No. 10: 8756-8764.

Synthetic Dimer of Indole-3-carbinol: Second Generation Diet Derived Anti-Cancer Agent in Hormone Sensitive Prostate Cancer. Garikapaty, Ashok, Tadi, et al., **Prostate** 2006 Apr 1; 66(5): 453-462.

Indole-3-carbinol (I3C) Induces Apoptosis in Tumorigenic but Not in Non-tumorigenic Breast Epithelial Cells, Rahman, Aranha, & Sarkar, **Nutr. Cancer** 2003; 45 (1): 101-112.

Translocation of Bax to Mitochondria Induces Apoptotic Cell Death in Indole-3-carbinol (I3C) Treated Breast Cancer Cells, Rahman, Aranha, Glazyrin, et al, **Oncogene** 2000; 19 (50): 5764-5771.

Indole-3-carbinol Enhances Ultraviolet-B-induced Apoptosis by Sensitizing Human Melanoma Cells, Kim, Jeong, Moon, et al., **Cell. Mol. Life Sci.** 2006; 63 (22): 2661-2668.

3,3'-Diindolylmethane is a Novel Mitochondrial H(+)-ATP Synthase Inhibitor That Can Induce p21(Cip1/Waf1) Expression by Induction of Oxidative Stress in Human Breast Cancer Cells, Gong, Sohn, Xue, et al., **Cancer Res.** 2006; 66 (9): 4880-4887.

450

Apoptosis-inducing Effect of Erlotinib is Potentiated by 3,3'-diindolylmethane in vitro and in vivo Using an Orthoptic Model of Pancreatic Cancer, Ali, Banerjee, Ahmad, et al., **Mol. Cancer Ther.** 2008; 7 (6): 1708-1719.

Indole-3-carbinol and Prostate Cancer, Sarkhar & Li, **J. Nutr.** 2004; 134 (12Suppl.): 3493S-3498S.

Indole-3-carbinol Inhibition of Androgen Receptor Expression and Down-regulation of Androgen Responsiveness in Human Prostate Cancer Cells, Hsu, Zhang, Dev, et al., **Carcinogenesis** 2005;

Indole-3-carbinol (I3C) Induced Cell Growth Inhibition, G1 Cell Cycle Arrest and Apoptosis in Prostate Cancer Cells, Chinni, Li, Upadhyay, et al., **Oncogene** 2001;

Akt Inactivation is a Key Event in Indole-3-carbinol-induced Apoptosis in PC-3 Cells, Chinni & Sarkhar, **Clin. Cancer Res.** 2002; 8 (4): 1228-1236.

Anti-carcinogenic and Anti-metastatic Properties of Indole-3-carbinol in Prostate Cancer, Garikpaty, et al., **Oncol. Rep.** 2005; 13 (1): 89-93.

Indole-3-carbinol Induces a G1 Cell Cycle Arrest and Inhibits Prostate-specific Antigen Production in Human LNCaP Prostate Carcinoma Cells, Zhang, Hsu, Kinseth, et al., **Cancer** 2003; 98 (11): 2511-2520.

Selective Growth Regulatory and Pro-apoptotic Effects of DIM is Mediated by AKT and NF-kappaB Pathways in Prostate Cancer Cells, Li, Chinni & Sarkhar, **Front. Biosci.** 2005; 10: 236-243.

Indole-3-carbinol Prevents PTEN Loss in Cervical Cancer in vivo, Qi, Anderson, Chen, et al., **Mol. Med.** 2005; 11 (1-12): 59-63.

BRCA1 and BRCA2 as Molecular Targets for Phytochemicals Indole-3-carbinol and Genistein in Breast and Prostate Cancer Cells, Fan, Meng, Auborn, et al., **Br. J. Cancer** 2006; 94 (3): 407-426.

Molecular Targets and Anticancer Potential of Indole-3-carbinol and its Derivatives. Aggarwal & Ichikawa, **Cell Cycle** 2005; 4 (9): 1201-1215.

Intake of Cruciferous Vegetables Modifies Bladder Cancer Survival, Tang, Zirpoli, Guru, et al., **Cancer Epidemiol. Biomarkers Prev.** 2010; 19 (7): 1806-1811.

A Novel Mechanism of Indole-3-carbinol Effects on Breast Carcinogenesis Involves Induction of Cdc25A Degradation, Wu, Feng, Jin, et al.**, Cancer Prev. Res.** 2010; 3 (7): 818-828.

<u>LOW-DOSE NALTREXONE</u>

Neuro-immunotherapy of Untreatable Metastatic Solid Tumours with Subcutaneous Low-dose Interleukin-2, Melatonin and Naltrexone: Modulation of Interleukin-2-induced Anti-tumour Immunity by Blocking the Opioid System, Lissoni, Malugani, Malysheva, et al., **Neuroendocrinol. Lett.** 2002; 23 (4): 341-344.

A New Neuro-immunotherapeutic Strategy of Subcutaneous Low-dose Interleukin-2 plus the Long-acting Opioid Antagonist Naltrexone in Metastatic Cancer Patients Progressing on Interleukin-2 Alone, Lissoni, Malugani, Bordin, et al., **Neuroendocrinol. Lett.** 2002; 23 (3): 255-258.

Opioid Growth Factor Regulates the Cell Cycle of Human Neoplasias, Zagon, Roesener, Verderame, et al., **Int. J. Oncol.** 2000; 17 (5): 1053-1061.

Methylnaltrexone Inhibits Opiate and VEGF-induced Angiogenesis: Role of Receptor Transactivation, Singleton, Lingen, Fekete, et al., **Microvasc. Res.** 2006; 72(1-2): 3-11.

Reversal of Signs and Symptoms of a B-cell Lymphoma in a Patient Using only Low-dose Naltrexone, **Integr. Cancer Ther.** 2007; 6 (3): 293-296.

The Long-term Survival of a Patient with Pancreatic Cancer with Metastases to the Liver after Treatment with the Intravenous Alpha-Lipoic Acid/Low-dose Naltrexone Protocol, Berkson, Rubin & Berkson, **Integr. Cancer Ther.** 2006; 5 (1): 83-89.

Revisiting the ALA/N (alpha lipoic acid/low dose naltrexone) Protocol for People with Metastasic and Non-Metastatic Pancreatic Cancer; A Report of 3 New Cases, Berkson, Rubin & Berkson, **Integr. Cancer Ther.** 2009; (4): 416-422.

<u>MELATONIN</u>

The Therapeutic Application of Melatonin in Supportive Care and Palliative Medicine, Mahmoud, Sarhill & Mazurczak, **Am. J. Hosp. Palliat. Care** 2005; 22: 295-309.

Aromatase Inhibitor-induced Joint Pain: Melatonin's Role, Burk, **Med. Hypoth.** 2008; doi: 10.1016/j.mehy.2008.07.040.

Melatonin – Monograph, **Alt. Med. Rev.** 2005; Vol. 10, No. 4: 326-336.

Melatonin Provokes Cell Death in Human B-Lymphoma Cells by Mitochondria-dependent Apoptotic Pathway Activation, Trubiani, Recchioni, Moroni, et al., **J. Pineal Res.** 2005; 39 (4): 425-431.

Melatonin Induces Apoptosis in Human Neuroblastoma Cancer Cells, Garcia-Santos, Antolin, Herrara, et al., **J. Pineal Res.** 2006; 41 (2): 130-135.

Increased Survival Time in Brain Glioblastoma by a Radio-neuro-endocrine Strategy with Radiotherapy Plus Melatonin Compared to Radiotherapy Alone, Lissoni, Meregalli, Nosetto, et al., **Oncology** 1996; 53: 43-46.

Five-Years Survival in Metastatic Non-Small Cell Lung Cancer Patients Treated with Chemotherapy Alone or Chemotherapy with Melatonin: A Randomized Trial, Lissoni, et al., **J. Pineal Res.** 2003; 35 (1): 12-15.

Circadian Function in Patients with Advanced Non-small-cell Lung Cancer, Levin, Daehler, Grutsch, et al., **Br. J. Cancer** 2005; 93 (11): 1202-1208.

Light at Night Co-distributes with Incident Breast But Not Lung Cancer in the Female Population of Israel, Kloog, Haim, Stevens, et al., **Chronobiol. Int.** 2008; 25 (1): 65-81.

Global Co-distribution of Light at Night (LAN) and Cancers of Prostate, Colon, and Lung in Men, Kloog , Haim, Stevens & Portnov, **Chronobiol. Int**. 2009; 26 (1): 108-125.

Randomized Study with the Pineal Hormone Melatonin versus Supportive Care Alone in Advanced Non-small-cell Lung Cancer Resistant to a First-line Chemotherapy Containing Cisplatin, Lissoni, Barni, Ardizzoia, et al., **Oncology** 1992; 49 (5): 336-339.

Neuro-immunotherapy of Untreatable Metastatic Solid Tumours with Subcutaneous Low-dose Interleukin-2, Melatonin and Naltrexone: Modulation of interleukin-2-induced Anti-tumour Immunity by Blocking the Opioid System, Lissoni, Malugani, Malysheva, et al., **Neuro. Endocrinol. Lett.** 2002; 23 (4): 341-344.

Melatonin in Human Breast Cancer Tissue: Association with Nuclear Grade and Estrogen Receptor Status, Maestroni & Conti, **Lab. Inv.**1996; 75 (4): 557-561.

Immune and Endocrine Mechanisms of Advanced Cancer-related Hypercortisolemia, Lissoni, Brivio, Fumagalli, et al., **In Vivo** 2007; 21 (4): 647-650.

Melatonin Increase as Predictor for Tumour Objective Response to Chemotherapy in Advanced Cancer Patients, Lissoni, Tancini, Barni, et al., **Tumori** 1998; 74 (3): 339-345.

Chronotherapy for Cancer, Eriguchi, Levi, Hisa, et al., **Biomed. Pharmacother.** 2003; 57 Suppl 1: 92s-95s.

Biomodulation of Cancer Chemotherapy for Metastatic Colorectal Cancer: A

Randomized Study of Weekly Low-dose Irinotecan Alone versus Irinotecan Plus the Oncostatic Pineal Hormone Melatonin in Metastatic Colorectal Cancer Patients Progressing on 5-fluorouracil-containing Combinations, Cerea, Vagh, Ardizzoia, et al., **Anticancer Res.** 2003; 23 (2C): 1951-1954.

Making Circadian Cancer Therapy Practical, Block, Block, Fox, et al., **Integr. Cancer Ther.** 2009;8(4):371-386.

Melatonin in Clinical Oncology, Bartsch, Bartsch & Karasek, **Neuro. Endocrinol. Lett.** 2002; 23 Suppl 1: 30-

Melatonin: Fifty Years of Scientific Journey from the Discovery in Bovine Pineal Gland to Delineation of Functions in Human, Chowdhury, Sengupta & Maitra, **Indian J Biochem Biophys.** 2008; 45 (5): 289-304.

The Immune-Pineal Axis: Stress as a Modulator of Pineal Gland Function, Couto-Moraes, Palermo-Neto & Markus, **Ann N Y Acad Sci.** 2009; 1153: 193-202.

A Review of the Evidence Supporting Melatonin's Role as an Antioxidant, Reiter, Melchiorri, Sewerynek, et al., **J Pineal Res.** 1995; 18 (1): 1-11.

Health Disorders of Shift Workers, Knutsson, **Occup Med** (Lond). 2003; 53 (2): 103-108.

Night-shift Work and Risk of Colorectal Cancer in the Nurses' Health Study, Schernhammer, Laden, Speizer, et al., **J. Natl. Cancer Inst.** 2003; 95 (11): 825-828.

Molecular Mechanisms of Melatonin Anticancer Effects, Hill, Frasch, Xiang, et al., **Integr. Cancer Ther.** 2009; 8 (4): 337-346.

Circadian Stage-Dependent Inhibition of Human Breast Cancer Metabolism and Growth by the Nocturnal Melatonin Signal: Consequences of its Disruption by Light at Night in Rats and Women, Blask, Dauchy, Brainard & Hanifin, **Integr. Cancer Ther.** 2009; 8 (4): 347-353.

MILK THISTLE

Toward the Definition of the Mechanism of Action of Silmarin: Activites Related to Cellular Protection from Toxic Damage Induced by Chemotherapy, Comelli, Mengs, Schneider, et al., **Integr. Cancer Ther.** 2007; 6 (2): 120-129.

Clinical Applications of Silybum marianum in Oncology, Greenlee, Abascal, Yarnell, et al, **Integr. Cancer Ther.** 2007; 6 (2): 158-165.

Milk Thistle (Silybum marianum) *is Associated with Reductions in Liver Function Tests (LFTs) in Children Undergoing Therapy for Acute Lymphoblastic Leukemia (ALL),* Ladas, Cheng, Hughes, et al., **Int. Conf. Soc. Integr. Oncol.** 2006; abstract D045.

Antiproliferative Effect of Silybin on Gynaecological Malignancies: Synergism with Cisplatin and Doxorubicin, Scambia, DeVincenzo, Ranelletti, et al., **Eur. J. Cancer** 1996; 32 A (5): 877-882.

Silybin and its Bioavailable Phospholipid Complex (IdB 1016) Potentiate in vitro and in vivo the Activity of Cisplatin, Giacomelli, Gallo, Apollonio, et al, **Life Sci.** 2002; 70 (12): 1447-1459.

Effect of Silibinin on the Growth and Progression of Primary Lung Tumours in Mice, Singh, Deep, Chittezhath, et al., **J. Natl. Cancer Inst.** 2006; 98 (12): 846-855.

Advances in the Use of Milk Thistle, Post-White, Ladas & Kelly, **Integr. Cancer Ther.** 2007; 6 (2): 104-109.

A Randomized, Controlled, Double-blind, Pilot Study of Milk Thistle for the Treatment of Hepatotoxicity in Childhood Acute Lymphoblastic Leukemia (ALL), Ladas, Kelly, et al., **Cancer** 2009; DOI: 10.1002/cncr.2472.

MISTLETOE

Differential Effects of Viscum album Extract Iscador Qu on Cell Cycle Progression and Apoptosis in Cancer Cells, Harmsma, Gromme, Ummelin, et. al., **Int. J. Oncol.** 2004; 25: 1521 – 1529.

Impact of Complementary Mistletoe Extract Treatment on Quality of Life in Breast, Ovarian and Non-Small Cell Lung Cancer Patients. A Prospective, Randomized Controlled Clinical Trial, Piao, Wang, Xie, et al. **Anticancer Res.** 2004; 34: 303-309.

Use of Iscador, an Extract of European Mistletoe (Viscum album) in Cancer Treatment: Prospective Non-randomized and Randomized Matched-pair Studies Nested Within a Cohort Study, Grossarth-Maticek, Kiene, Baumgartner & Ziegler **Alt. Ther.** 2001; Vol. 7 No. 3: 57-78.

Treatment of Advanced Pancreatic Cancer with Mistletoe: Results of a Pilot Trial Friesse, et al. 1996; **Anticancer Res.** 16 : 915-920.

Mistletoe Extract May Be Alternative Bladder Cancer Therapy, Elsaesser-Beile, et al. July 2005; **J. Urol.** 174: 176-179.

Naturopathic Oncology

Final Results of the EORTC 18871 / DKG 80-1 Randomised Phase III Trial: rIFN-alpha2b vs. rIGN-gamma vs. Iscador M vs. Observation After Surgery in Melanoma Patients with Either High-risk Primary or Regional Lymph Node Metastasis, Kleeberg, Suciu, Brocker, et al., **Eur. J. Cancer** 2004; 40: 390-402.

Safety and Efficacy of the Long-term Treatment of Primary Intermediate to High-risk Malignant Melanoma (UICC/AJCC stage II and III) with a Standardized Fermented European Mistletoe Extract: Results from a Multicenter, Comparative, Epidemiological Cohort Study in Germany and Switzerland, Augustin, Bock, Hanisch, et. al., **Arzeimittelforschung,** 2005; 55 (1):38-49.
Anti-proliferative Effect of Iscador Against Urinary Bladder Carcinoma, Urech, et al., **Anti-Cancer Res.** 2006; 26: 3049-3056.

Iscador Qu Spezial Inhibits Tube Formation, Elluru, et al, **Drug Res.,** 2006; 56: 461.

Palliative In-Patient Cancer Treatment in an Anthroposophic Hospital: II. Quality of Life During and After Stationary Treatment, and Subjective Treatment Benefits, Heusser, Braun, Burtschy et al., **Forsch Komplementarmed**, 2006; 13: parts I & II.
Iscador in Breast Cancer (I), Leroi, **Helvet Chir Acta** 1977; 44.

Iscador in Breast Cancer (II), Hellan, et. al., **Krebs und Alternativ-Medizin II**, 1990, Springer.

Iscador in Breast Cancer (III), Grossarth-Maticek, et. al., **Altern. Ther. Health Med.,** 2001; 7.

Iscador in Breast Cancer (IV), Grossarth-Maticek, et. al., **Altern. Ther. Health Med.,** 2001; 7.

Iscador in Breast Cancer (V), Bock et. al., **Drug Res**. 2004; 58.

Iscador in Cancer of Different Locations, Grossarth-Maticek, et. al., **Altern. Ther. Health Med.,** 2001; 7: 3.

Efficacy and Safety of Long-term Complementary Treatment with Standardized European Mistletoe Extract (Viscum album. L.) in Addition to the Conventional Adjuvant Oncological Therapy in Patients with Primary Non-metastatic Breast Cancer – Results of a Multicentre, Comparative, Epidemiological Cohort Study, Bock, Friedel, Hanisch et. al., **Arneim-Forsch/ Drug Res.** 2004; 54 No. 8: 456 – 466.

Anticancer Activity of a Lectin-rich Mistletoe Extract Injected Intratumorally into Human Pancreatic Cancer Xenografts, Rostock, Huber, Greiner, et al., **Anticancer Res** 2005; 25 (3B): 1969-1975.

Reducing Malignant Ascites Accumulation by Repeated Intraperitoneal Administrations of a Viscum album Extract, Bar-Sela, Goldberg, Beck, et al., **Anticancer Res.** 2006; 26 (1B): 709-713.

Quality of Life is Improved in Breast Cancer Patients by Standardized Mistletoe extract PS76A2 During Chemotherapy and Follow-up: a Randomised, Placebo-controlled, Double-Blind, Multicentre Clinical Trial, Semiglazov, Stepula, Dudov, et al., **Anticancer Res.** 2006; 26 (2B): 1519-1529.

Nitric-Oxide Involvement in the Anti-Tumour Effect of Mistletoe (Viscum album L.) Extract Iscador on Human Macrophages, Mossalayi, Alkharrat & Malvy, **Arzneimittelforschung** 2006; 56 (6A): 457-460.

Immunological Effector Mechanisms of a Standardized Mistletoe Extract On the Function of Human Monocytes and Lymphocytes in vitro, ex vivo and in vivo, Heinzerling, von Baehr, Liebenthal, et al., **J. Clin. Immunol.** 2006; 26 (4): 347-359.

Anticancer Activity of a Lectin-rich Mistletoe Extract Injected Intratumorally into Human Pancreatic Cancer Xenografts, Rostock, Huber, Greiner, et al., **Anticancer Res** 2005; 25 (3B): 1969-1975.

Prospective Controlled Cohort Studies on Long-term Therapy of Breast Cancer Patients with a Mistletoe Preparation (Iscador(r), Grossarth-Maticek & Ziegler, **Forsch Komplementarmed** 2006; 13 (5): 285-292.

Immune Modulation Using Mistletoe (Viscum album L.) Extracts Iscador, Büssing, **Arzneimittelforschung** 2006; 56 (6A): 508-515.

Anti-proliferative Effects of Mistletoe (Viscum album L.) Extract in Urinary Bladder Carcinoma Cell Lines, Urech, Buessing, Thalmann, et al., **Anticancer Res.** 2006; 26 (4B): 3049-3055.

Mistletoe for Cancer? A Systematic Review of Randomised Clinical Trials, Ernst, Schmidt & Steuer-Vogt, **Int. J. Cancer** 2003; 107 (2): 262-267.

Complementary Cancer Therapy: A Systematic Review of Prospective Clinical Trials on Anthroposophic Mistletoe Extracts, Kienle & Kiene, **Eur. J. Med. Res.** 2007; 12 (3): 103-119

Mistletoe Therapy in Oncology, Horneber, Bueschel, Huber R, et al.,**Cochrane Database Syst. Rev.** 2008; (2): CD003297.
Survival of Cancer Patients Treated with Mistletoe Extract (Iscador): A Systematic Literature Review, Ostermann, Raak & Bussing, **BMC Cancer** 2009; 9 (1): 451.

Viscum album L. Extracts in Breast and Gynaecological Cancers: A Systematic Review of Clinical and Preclinical Research, Kienle, Glockmann, Schink & Kiene, **J. Exp. Clin. Cancer Res**. 2009; 28: 79.

Systematic Evaluation of the Clinical Effects of Supportive Mistletoe Treatment within Chemo-and/or Radiotherapy Protocols and long-Term Mistletoe Application in Nonmetastatic Colorectal Carcinoma: Multicenter, Controlled, Observational Cohort Study, Friedel, Matthes, Bock & Zanker, **J. Soc. Integr. Oncol.** 2009; 7 (4): 137-145.

Influence of Viscum album L. (European Mistletoe) Extracts on Quality of Life in Cancer Patients: A Systematic Review of Controlled Clinical Studies, Kienle & Kienle, **Integr. Cancer Ther.** 2010; 9 (2): 142-157.

MITOCHONDRIA

Mitochondria and Cancer, Jurasunas, **Townsend Letter** 2006; # 277/78: 83-86, 146-148.
A Mitochondria-K+ Channel Axis is Suppressed in Cancer and its Normalization Promotes Apoptosis & Inhibits Cancer Growth, Bonnet, Archer, Allalunis-Turner, et al., **Cancer Cell** 2007; 11 (1): 37-51. PubMed ID# 17222789

Restoration of Cellular Energetic Balance with L-Carnitine in the Neuro-bioenergetic Approach for Cancer Prevention and Treatment, Hoang, Shaw, Pham & Levine, **Med. Hypotheses** 2007; 69 (2): 262-272.

Increased Carnitine-dependent Fatty Acid Uptake into Mitochondria of Human Colon Cancer Cells Induces Apoptosis, Wenzel, Nickel & Daniel, **J. Nutr.** 2005; 135 (6): 1510-1514.
Carnitine Supplementation Alleviates Cancer-Related Fatigue, Cruciani, et al., **J. Pain Sympt. Man.** 2006; 32: 551-559.

Voltage-Dependent Anion Channel (VDAC) as Mitochondrial Governator – Thinking Outside the Box, Lemasters & Holmuhamedov, **Biochem.Biophys. Acta** 2006; 1762 (2): 181-190.

Lactate: mirror and motor of tumour malignancy, Walenta & Mueller-Klieser ,**Semin Radiat Oncol.** 2004; 14 (3): 267-74.

High lactate levels predict likelihood of metastases, tumour recurrence, and restricted patient survival in human cervical cancers, Walenta, Wetterling, Lehrke, et al., **Cancer Res.** 2000; 60 (4): 916-921.

Tumour-derived lactic acid modulates dendritic cell activation and antigen expression, Gottfried, Kunz-Schughart, Ebner, et al., **Blood.** 2006; 107 (5): 2013-2021.

Lactate dehydrogenase 5 expression in operable colorectal cancer: strong association with survival and activated vascular endothelial growth factor pathway--a report of the Tumour Angiogenesis Research Group, Koukourakis, Giatromanolaki, Sivridis, et al., **J Clin Oncol.** 2006; 24 (26): 4301-4308. Epub 2006 Aug 8.

Lactate dehydrogenase 5 (LDH5) relates to up-regulated hypoxia inducible factor pathway and metastasis in colorectal cancer, Koukourakis, Giatromanolaki, Simopoulos, et al., **Clin Exp Metastasis** 2005; 22(1): 25-30.

Studies with glycolysis-deficient cells suggest that production of lactic acid is not the only cause of tumour acidity, Newell, Franchi, Pouysségur & Tannock, **Proc Natl Acad Sci U S A.** 1993; 90 (3): 1127-1131.

Early and Late Apoptosis Events in Human Transformed and Non-transformed Colonocytes are Independent of Intracellular Acidification, Wenzel & Daniel, **Cell Physiol Biochem**. 2004;14 (1-2): 65-76.

Mitochondria and cancer: Warburg addressed, Wallace, **Cold Spring Harb. Symp. Quant. Biol.** 2005; 70: 363-374.

Cu2+ Toxicity Inhibition of Mitochondrial Dehydrogenases in vitro and in vivo, Sheline & Choi, **Ann. Neurol.** 2004; 55 (5): 645-653.

Cofactors of Mitochondrial Enzymes Attenuate Copper-induced Death in vitro and in vivo, Sheline, Choi, Kim-Han, et al., **Ann Neurol.** 2002; 52 (2): 195-204.

The Biological Significance of Cancer: Mitochondria as a Cause of Cancer and the Inhibition of Glycolysis with Citrate as a Cancer Treatment, Halabe Bucay, **Med Hypotheses** 2007; 69(4): 826-828.

Cheap, Safe Drug Kills Most Cancers, Coghlan, **New Scientist** January 2007.

Effect of Thiamine Phosphates on the Activity of Regulatory Enzymes of the Pyruvate Dehydrogenase Complex, Parkhomenko, Chernysh, Cjurilova, et. al., **Ukr. Biokhim. Zh.** 1987; 59 (5): 49-54.

Bovine Heart Pyruvate Dehydrogenase Kinase Stimulation by Alpha-ketoisovalerate, Robertson, Barron & Olson, **J. Biol. Chem.** 1990; 265 (28): 16814-16820.

Co-enzyme Q-10 Improves Lactic Acidosis, Stroke-like Episodes and Epilepsy in a Patient with MELAS (Mitochondrial Myopathy, Encephalopathy, Lactic Acidosis and Stroke-like Episodes), Berbel-Gacia, Barbera-Farre, Etessam, et al., **Clin. Neuropharmacol.** 2004; 27 (4): 187-191.

Mitochondria Rescue (Possibly) Heals Cancer? McKinney, **Naturopathic Doctor**

Naturopathic Oncology

News & Review - May 2008; 4 (5): 10-11.

MODIFIED CITRUS PECTIN

Modulation of the Lung Colonization of B16-F1 Melanoma Cells by Citrus Pectin, Platt & Raz, **J. Natl. Cancer Inst.** 1992; 84 (6): 438-442.

Citrus Pectin: Characterization and Inhibitory Effect on Fibroblast Growth Factor-Receptor Interaction, Liu, Ahmad, Luo, et. al., **J. Agric. Food Chem.** 2001, 49 (6): 3051-3057.

Inhibition of Spontaneous Metastasis in a Rat Prostate Cancer Model by Oral Administration of Modified Citrus Pectin, Pienta, Naik, Akhtar, et. al, **J. Natl. Cancer Inst.** 1995; 87 (5): 348-353.

Inhibition of Human Cancer Cell Growth and Metastasis in Nude Mice by Oral Intake of Modified Citrus Pectin, Nangia-Makker, Pratima, Hogan, et al., **J. Natl. Cancer Inst.** 2002; 94 (24): 1854-1862.

Galectin-3 Induces Endothelial Cell Morphogenesis and Angiogenesis, Nangia-Makker, Honjo, Sarvis, et. al., **Am. J. Pathol.** 2000, 156 (3): 899-909.

Recognition of Galactan Components of Pectin by Galectin-3, Gunning, Bongaerts & Morris, **Fed. Amer. Soc. Exp. Biol. J.** 2008; 10.1096: fj. O8-106617.

MUSHROOMS

Anti-Aromatase Activity of Phytochemicals in White Button Mushrooms (Agaricus bisporus), Chen, Oh, Phung, et al., **Cancer Res.** 2006; 66 (24): 12026-12034.

White Button Mushroom Phytochemicals Inhibit Aromatase Activity and Breast Cancer Cell Proliferation, Grube, Eng, Kao, et al., **J. Nutr.** 2001; 131 (12): 3288-3293.

Ganodermic Acid T from Ganoderma lucidum *Mycelia induces Mitochondria Mediated Apoptosis in Lung Cancer Cells,* Tang, Liu, Zhao, et al., **Life Sci.** 2006; 80 (3): 205-211.
Ganoderic acid T from Ganoderma lucidum mycelia induces mitochondrial-medicated apoptosis in lung cancer cells, Tang, Liu, Zhao, et al., **Life Sci.** 2006; 80 (3): 205-211. Epub. 2006 Sept. 6, 2006

Enhanced induction of mitochondrial damage and apoptosis in human leukemia HL-60 cells by Ganoderma lucidum and Duchesnea chrysantha extracts, Kim, Kim, Son & Kim, **Cancer Lett.** 2007; 246 (1-2): 210-217.

Coriolus versicolor (Yunzhi) Extract Attenuates Growth of Human Leukemia Xenografts and Induces Apoptosis Through the Mitochondrial Pathway, Zhang, Soboloff, Zhu & Berger, **Mol. Pharmacol.** 2006; 16 (3): 609-616.

Ganoderma lucidum Inhibits Proliferation of Human Breast Cancer Cells by Down-regulation of Estrogen Receptor and NF-kappaB Signalling, Jiang, Slivova & Sliva, **Int. J. Oncol.** 2006; 29 (3): 695-703.

Androgen Receptor-Dependent and -Independent Mechanisms Mediate Ganoderma lucidum Activities in LNCaP Prostate Cancer Cells, Zaidman, Wasser, Nevo & Mahajna, **Int. J. Oncol.** 2007; 31 (4): 959-967.

Effects of Water-soluble Ganoderma lucidum Polysaccharides on the Immune Functions of Patients with Advanced Lung Cancer, Gao, Tang, Dai, et al., **J. Med. Food** 2005; 8 (2): 159-168.

Effects of Ganopoly (A Ganoderma lucidum Polysaccharide Extract) on the Immune Functions in Advanced-stage Cancer Patients, Gao, Zhou, Jiang, et al., **Immunol. Invest.** 2003; 32 (3): 201-215.

Combined Effect of Green Tea and Ganoderma lucidum on Invasive Behaviour of Breast Cancer Cells, Thyagarajan, Zhu & Sliva, **Int. J. Oncol.** 2007; 30 (4): 963-969.

Telomerase-associated Apoptotic Events by Mushroom Ganoderma lucidum on Pre-malignant Human Urothelial Cells, Yuen, Gohel & Au, **Nutr. Cancer** 2008; 60 (1): 109-119.

Dietary Intakes of Mushrooms and Green Tea Combine to Reduce the Risk of Breast Cancer in Chinese Women, Zhng, Huang, Xie & Holman, **Int. J. Cancer** 2009; 1246: 1404-1408.

Ganoderma lucidum (Reishi) in Cancer Treatment, Sliva, **Integr. Cancer Ther.** 2003; 2 (4): 358-364.

The Use of Mushroom Glucans and Proteoglycans in Cancer Treatment, Kidd, **Altern. Med. Rev.** 2000; 5(1): 4-27.

Anticancer Effects of Ganoderma lucidum: A Review of Scientific Evidence, Yuen & Gohel **Nutr. Cancer** 2005; 53 (1): 11-17

Natural Killer Cell Activity and Quality of Life Were Improved by Consumption of a Mushroom Extract, Agaricus blazei Murill Kyowa, in Gynecological Cancer Patients Undergoing Chemotherapy, Ahn, Kim, Chae, et al., **Int. J. Gynecol. Cancer** 2004; 14 (4): 589-594.

461

Secretion of TNF-alpha, IL-8 and Nitric Oxide by Macrophages Activated with Agaricus blazei Murill Fractions in vitro, Sorimachi, Akimoto, Ikehara, et al., **Cell Struct. Funct.** 2001; 26 (2): 103-108.

Characterization and Immuno-modulating Activities of Polysaccharide from Lentinus edodes, Zheng, Jie, Hanchuan & Moucheng, **Int. Immunopharmacol.** 2005; 5 (5): 811-820.

Effects of Ganopoly (a Ganoderma lucidum Polysaccharide Extract) on the Immune Functions in Advanced-stage Cancer Patients, Gao, Zhou, Jiang, et al., **Immunol. Invest.** 2003; 32 (3): 201-215.

Protective Effects of Ganoderma lucidum Polysaccharides Peptide on Injury of Macrophages Induced by Reactive Oxygen Species, You & Lin, **Acta Pharmacol. Sin.** 2002; 23 (9): 787-791.

The Use of Mushroom Glucans and Proteoglycans in Cancer Treatment, Kidd, **Altern. Med. Rev**. 2000; 5 (1): 4-27.

Anticancer Effects and Mechanisms of Polysaccharide-K (PSK): Implications of Cancer Immunotherapy, Fisher & Yang, **Anticancer Res.** 2002; 22 (3): 1737-1754.

A Review of Research on the Protein-bound Polysaccharide (Polysaccharopeptide, PSP) from the Mushroom Coriolus versicolor (Basidiomycetes: Polyporaceae), Ng, **Gen. Pharmacol.** 1998; 30 (1): 1-4.

*Augmentation of Various Immune Reactivities of Tumour-bearing Hosts with an Extract of Cordyceps sinensis,*Yamaguchi, Yoshida, Ren et al., **Biotherapy** 1990; 2 (3): 199-205.

Effect of Cordyceps sinensis on the Th1/Th2 Cytokines in Patients with Condylomata Acuminata, Gao, Wuu & He, **Zhong Yao Cai** 2000; 23 (7): 402-404.

The Use of Mushroom Glucans and Proteoglycans in Cancer Treatment, Kidd, **Altern. Med. Rev**. 2000; 5 (1): 4-27.

Supplements for Immune Enhancement in Hematological Malignancies, Sze & Chan, **Hematology** 2009; 313-319.

OMEGA 3 OILS

Modulation of Angiogenesis by Omega-3 Polyunsaturated Fatty Acids is Mediated by Cyclooxygenases, Szymczak, Murray & Petrovic, **Blood** 2008; 111 (7): 3514-3521.

N-3 Fatty Acids, Cancer and Cachexia: A Systematic Review of the Literature, Colomer, Moreno-Nogufeira, Garcia-Luna, et al., **Br. J. Nutr.** 2007; 975: 823-831.

Dietary Omega-3 Fatty Acids, Cyclooxygenase-2 Genetic Variation, and Aggressive Prostate Cancer Risk, Fradet, Cheng, Casey &Witte, **Clin Cancer Res.** 2009; 15 (7): 2559-2566.

Prevention and Treatment of Pancreatic Cancer by Curcumin in Combination with Omega-3 Fatty Acids, Swamy, Citineni, et al, **Nutr. Cancer** 2008; 60 Suppl. 1: 81-89.

Omega 3 Fatty Acids: Biological Activity and Effects on Human Health, La Guardia, Giammanco, Di Majo, et al., **Panminerva Med.** 2005; 47 (4): 245-257.

Effect of Eicosapentaenoic Acid, Protein and Amino Acids on Protein Synthesis and Degradation in Skeletal Muscle of Cachectic Mice, Smith, Greenberg & Tisdale, **Br. J. Cancer** 2004; 91 (2): 408-412.

Role of Omega-3 Fatty Acid Supplementation in Inflammation and Malignancy, Jho, Cole, Lee & Espat, **Integr. Cancer Ther.** 2004; (2): 98-111.

Cytotoxic Drugs Efficacy Correlates with Adipose Tissue Docosahexaenoic Acid Level in Locally Advanced Breast Carcinoma, Bougnoux, Germain, Chajes, et al., **Br. J. Cancer** 1999; 79 (11-12): 1765-1769.

Complementary Actions of Docosahexaenoic Acid and Genistein on COX-2, PGE2 and Invasiveness in MDA-MB-231 Breast Cancer Cells, Horia E, Watkins BA. **Carcinogenesis** 2007; 28 (4): 809-815.

n-3 PUFAs Modulate T-cell Activation via Protein Kinase C-alpha and -epsilon and the NF-kappaB Signaling Pathway, Denys , Hichami & Khan, **J. Lipid Res.** 2005; 46 (4): 752-758.

n-3 Fatty Acids, Inflammation, and Immunity: Relevance to Post-surgical and Critically Ill Patients, Calder, **Lipids** 2004; 39 (12): 1147-1161.

Impact of Post-operative Omega-3 Fatty Acid-supplemented Parenteral Nutrition on Clinical Outcomes and Immuno-modulations in Colorectal Cancer Patients, Liang, Wang, Ye, et al., **World J. Gastroenterol.** 2008; 14 (15): 2434-2439.

High Omega-3 Fat Intake Improves Insulin Sensitivity and Reduces CRP and IL6, But Does Not Affect Other Endocrine Axes in Healthy Older Adults, Tsitouras, Gucciardo, Salbe, et al., **Horm. Metab. Res.** 2008; 40 (3): 199-205.

Dietary Omega-3 Fatty Acids, Cyclo-oxygenase-2 Genetic Variation, and Aggressive

Prostate cancer Risk, Fradet, Cheng, Casey & Witte, **Clin, Cancer Res.** 2009; 15 (7): 2559-2566.

The Potential for Treatment with Dietary Long-chain Polyunsaturated n-3 Fatty Acids During Chemotherapy, Biondo, Brindley, Sawyer & Field, **J. Nutr. Biochem.** 2008; 1912: 787-796.

Chemoprotective and Renal Protective Effects for Docosahexaenoic Acid (DHA): Implications of CRP and Lipid Peroxides, Elmesery, et al., **Cell Div.** 2009; 4 (1): 6.

Omega-3 Fatty Acids Can Improve Radioresponse Modifying Tumour Interstitial Pressure, Blood Rheology and Membrane Peroxidability, Baronzio, Freitas, Griffini et al., **Anticancer Res.** 1994; 14 (3A): 1145-1154

Neuroblastoma Cell Death in Response to Docosahexaenoic acid: Sensitization to Chemotherapy and Arsenic-induced Oxidative Stress, Lindskog, Gleissman, Ponthan et al., **Int. J. Cancer** 2006; 118 (10): 2584-2593.

Differential Sensitization of Cancer Cells to Doxorubicin by DHA: A Role for Lipoperoxidation, Maheo, Vibet, Steghens et al., **Free Radic. Biol. Med.** 2005; 39 (6): 742-751.

Cytotoxic Drugs Efficacy Correlates with Adipose Tissue Docosahexaenoic Acid Level in Locally Advanced Breast Carcinoma, Bougnoux, Germain, Chajes et al., **Br. J. Cancer** 1999; 79 (11-12): 1765-1769.

Sensitization by Docosahexaenoic Acid (DHA) of Breast Cancer Cells to Anthracyclines Through Loss of Glutathione Peroxidase (GPx1) Response, Vibet, Goupille, Bougnoux, et al., **Free Radic. Biol. Med.** 2008; 44 (7): 1483-1491.

Phase II Study of High-dose Fish Oil Capsules for Patients with Cancer-related Cachexia, Burns, Halabi, Clamon, et al., **Cancer** 2004; 101: 370-378.

The Effect of Dietary Omega-3 Polyunsaturated Fatty Acids on T-lymphocyte Subsets of Patients with Solid Tumours, Gogos, Ginopoulos, Zoumbos, et al., **Cancer Detect. & Prev.** 1995; 19 (5): 415-417.

Effect of a Protein and Energy Dense N-3 Fatty Acid Enriched Oral Supplement on Loss of Weight and Lean Tissue in Cancer Cachexia: A Randomised Double Blind Trial, Fearon, Von Meyenfeldt, Moses, et al., **Gut** 2003; 52 (10): 1479-1486.

Modulation of Inflammation and Cytokine Production by Dietary (n-3) Fatty Acids, Blok, Katan & van der Meer, **J. Nutr.** 1996; 126 (6): 1515-1533.

Effect of Dietary Fish Oil on Development and Selected Functions of Murine Inflammatory Macrophages, Hubbard, Somers & Eriskson, **J. Leukoc. Biol.** 1991; 49: 592.

Antitumor Activity of Fish Oils Against Human Lung Cancer is Associated with Altered Formation of PGE_2 and PGE_3 and Regulation of Akt Phosphorylation, Yang, Chan, Cartwright, et al., **5th AACR Int. Conf. Frontiers Cancer Prev. Res.** 2006.

Dietary Omega-3 Polyunsaturated Fatty Acids Plus Vitamin E Restore Immunodeficiency and Prolong Survival for Severely Ill Patients with Generalized Malignancy: A Randomized Control Trial, Gogos, Ginopoulos, Salsa, et al., **Cancer** 1998; 82 (2): 395-402.

Improving Outcome of Chemotherapy of Metastatic Breast Cancer by Docosahexaenoic Acid: A Phase II Trial, Bougnoux, Hajjaji, Ferrasson, et al., **Br. J. Cancer** 2009; 101 (12): 1978–1985.

Dietary Omega-3 Fatty Acids, Cyclooxygenase-2, Genetic Variation and Aggressive Prostate Cancer Risk, Fradet, Cheng, Casey & Witte, **Clin. Cancer Res.** 2009; 157: 2559-2566.

PHYTOESTROGENS & SOY

Phytoestrogens and Antioxidants – Bits of Experimental Evidence, Mariani, **Medscape** General Medicine 01/24/2005

Phytoestrogens in Botanical Dietary Supplements: Implications for Cancer, Piersen, **Integr. Cancer Ther.**, 2003; 2 (2): 120-138.

Dietary Phytoestrogen Intake – Lignans, Isoflavones – and Breast Cancer Risk (Canada), Cotterchio, Boucher, Kreiger, et al., **Cancer Causes & Control** 2008; 193: 259-272.

Dietary Lignan Intakes in Relation to Survival Among Women with Breast Cancer: The Western New York Exposures and Breast Cancer (WEB) Study, McCann, Thmpson, Nie, et al., **Breast Cancer Res. Treat.** 2010; 122 (1): 229-235.

Phytoestrogen Content of Foods Consumed in Canada, Including Isoflavones, Lignans, and Coumestan, Thompson, Boucher, Liu, et al., **Nutri. Cancer**, 2006; 54 (2): 184-201.

Inhibitory Effect of Isoflavones on Prostate Cancer Cells and PTEN Gene, Cao, Jin & Zhou, **Biomed. Environ. Sci.** 2006; 19 (1): 35-41.

Induction of Apoptosis in Low to Moderate Grade Human Prostate Carcinoma by Red Clover-Derived Dietary Isoflavones, Jarred, Keikha, Dowling, et al., **Cancer Epidemiol. Biomarkers Prev.** 2002; 11 (12): 1689-1696.

Multi-targeted Therapy of Cancer by Genistein, Banerjee, Li, Wang & Sarkar, **Cancer Lett.** 2008; 269 (2): 226-242.

Xenoestrogens Modulate Vascular Endothelial Growth Factor Secretion in Breast Cancer Cells Through an Estrogen Receptor-dependent Mechanism, Buteau-Lozano, Velasco, Cristofari, et al., **J. Endocrinol.** 2008; 196 (2): 399-412.

Potentiation of the Effect of Erlotinib by Genistein in Pancreatic Cancer: The Role of Akt and Nuclear Factor-kappaB, E-Rayes, Ali, Ali, et al., **Cancer Res.** 2006; 66 (21): 10553-10559.

Effect of Soybean on Breast Cancer According to Receptor Status: A Case-control Study in Japan, Suzuki, Matsuo, Tsunoda, et al., **Int. J. Cancer** 2008; 123 (7): 1674-1680.

Soy Isoflavones, Estrogen Therapy, and Breast Cancer Risk: Analysis and Commentary, Messina & Wood, **Nutr. J.** 2008; 7: 17.

Genestein Inhibits p38 Map Kinase Activation, Matrix Metalloproteinase Type 2, and Cell Invasion in Human Prostate Epithelial Cells, Huang, Chen, Xu, et al., **Cancer Res.** 2005; 65 (8): 3470-3478.

Genestein Induces Cell Growth Inhibition in Prostate Cancer Through the Suppression of Telomerase Activity, Ouchi, Ishiguro, Ikeda, et al., **Int. J. Urol.** 2005; 12 (1): 73-80.

Genestein Inhibits Vitamin D Hydroxylases CYP24 and CYp27B1 Expression in Prostate Cells, Farhan, et al., **J. Steroid Biochem. Mol. Biol.** 2003; 84 (4): 423-429.

Implications of Phytoestrogen Intake for Breast Cancer, Duffy, Perez & Partridge, **CA Cancer J. Clin.** 2007; 57 (5): 260-277.

Genestein Potentiates the Growth Inhibitory Effects of 1,25-dihydroxyvitamin D(3) in DU145 Human Prostate Cancer Cells: Role of the Direct Inhibition of CYP24 Enzyme Activity, Swami, et al., **Mol. Cell Endocrinol.** 2005;

Soy-derived Isoflavones Inhibit the Growth of Adult T-cell Leukemia Cells in vitro and in vivo, Yamasaki, Fujita, Ishiyama, et al., **Cancer Sci.** 2007; 98 (11): 1740-1746.

Effects of a Flaxseed Mixture and Plant Oils Rich in Alpha-linolenic Acid on the Adenoma Formation in Multiple Intestinal Neoplasia (Min) Mice, Oikarinen, Pajari,

Salminen et al., **Br. J. Nutr.** 2005; 94 (4): 510-518.

Flaxseed Oil Reduces the Growth of Human Breast Tumors (MCF-7) at High Levels of Circulating Estrogen,
Truan, Chen & Thompson, **Mol. Nutr. Food Res**. 2010; 54: 1–8.

Flaxseed Oil–Trastuzumab Interaction in Breast Cancer, Mason, Chen & Thompson, **Food Chem Tox.** 2010;
doi:10.1016/j.fct.2010.05.052

Addressing the Soy and Breast Cancer Relationship: Review, Commentary, and Workshop Proceedings, Messina M, McCaskill-Stevens W, Lampe JW. **J. Natl. Cancer Inst.** 2006; 98 (18): 1275-1284.

Point-Counterpoint: Soy Intake for Breast Cancer Patients, Block, Constantinou, Hilakivi-Clarke et al., **Integr. Cancer Ther.** 2002; 1 (1): 90-100.

Various Doses of Soy Isoflavones Do Not Modify Mammographic Density in Postmenpausal Women, Masarinec, Verheus, Steinberg et al., **J. Nutr.** 2009; 139 (5): 981-986.

Flaxseed and its Lignans Inhibit Estradiol-induced Growth, Angiogenesis, and Secretion of Vascular Endothelial Growth Factor in Human Breast Cancer Xenografts in vivo, Bergman, Jungeström, Thompson & Dabrosin, **Clin. Cancer Res**. 2007; 13 (3): 1061-1067.

Dietary Intake of Isoflavones and Breast Cancer Risk by Estrogen and Progesterone Receptor Status, Zhang, Yang & Holman, **Breast Cancer Res. Treat.** 2009; Epub Feb. 28, 2009; DOI 10.1007/s10549-009-0354-9.

Dietary Soy Intake and Breast Cancer Risk, Enderlin, Coleman, Stewart & Hakkak, **Oncol. Nurs. Forum** 2009; 36 (5): 531-539.

Effects of Diverse Dietary Phytoestrogens on Cell Growth, Cell Cycle and Apoptosis in Estrogen-Receptor Positive Breast Cancer, Sakamoto, Horiguchi, Oguma & Kayama, **J. Nutr. Biochem.** 2009; Oct 2. [Epub ahead of print] PMID: 19800779.

Soy Food Intake and Breast Cancer Survival, Shu, Zheng, Cai, et al., **JAMA** 2009; 302: 2437-2443.

POMEGRANATE & ELLAGIC ACID

Pomegranate Extract Inhibits Androgen-independent Prostate Cancer Growth Through a Nuclear Factor Kappa-B dependent Mechanism, Rettig, et al., **Mol.**

Cancer Ther. 2008; 7 (9): 2662-2671.

In vitro Anti-proliferative, Apoptotic and Antioxidant Activities of Punicalagin, Ellagic Acid and a Total Pomegranate Tannin Extract are Enhanced in Combination with other Polyphenols as Found in Pomegranate Juice, Seeram, Adams, Henning, et al., **J. Nutr. Biochem.** 2005; 16 (6): 360-367.

Pomegranate Polyphenols Down-regulate Expression of Androgen-synthesizing Genes in Human Prostate Cancer Cells Over-expressing the Androgen Receptor, Young, Hong, Seeram & Heber, **J. Nutr. Biochem.** 2008; 19 (12): 848-855.

Ellagic Acid Induces Apoptosis Through Inhibition of Nuclear Factor Kappa B in Pancreatic Cancer Cells, Edderkaoui, Odinokova, Ohno, et al., **World J. Gastroenterol.** 2008; 14 (23): 3672-3680.
Combined Inhibition of PDGF and VEGF Receptors by Ellagic Acid, a Dietary-derived Phenolic Compound, Labrecque, Lamy, Chapus, et al., **Carcinogenesis** 2005; 26 (4): 821-826.

In vitro Anti-proliferative Activities of Ellagic Acid, Losso, Bansode, Trappey, et al., **J. Nutr. Biochem.** 2004; 15 (11): 672-678.

Support Ellagic Acid Therapy in Patients with Hormone Refractory Prostate Cancer (HRPC) on Standard Chemotherapy Using Vinorelbine and Estramustine Phosphate, Falsaperla, Morgia, Tartarone, et al., **Eur. Urol.** 2005; 47 (4): 449-454.

Berry Phytochemicals, Genomic Stability and Cancer: Evidence for Chemoprotection at Several Stages in the Carcinogenic Process, Duthie, **Mol. Nutr. Food Res.** 2007; 51 (6): 665-674.

Phase II Study of Pomegranate Juice for Men with Rising Prostate-Specific Antigen Following Surgery or Radiation for Prostate Cancer, Pantuck, Leppert, Zomorodian, et al., **Clin. Cancer Res.** 2006; 12 (13): 4018-4026.

PREVENTION

Prostate Cancer Prevention by Nutritional Means to Alleviate Metabolic Syndrome, Barnard, **Amer. J. Clin. Nutr.** 2007; 863, s. 889-893.

Chemoprevention of Human Prostate Cancer by Oral Administration of Green Tea Catechins in Volunteers with High-grade Prostate Intraepithelial Neoplasia, A Preliminary Report from a One-year Proof-of-Principle Study, Betuzzi, Brausi, Rizzi & Castagnetti, **Cancer Res.** 2006; 66 (2): 1234-1240.

Resveratrol: a Candidate Nutritional Substance for Prostate Cancer Prevention,

Stewart, Artime & O'Brian, **J. Nutr.** 2003; 133 (7 Suppl.): 2440S-2443S.

Cancer Prevention – the Easy Choices, McKinney, **Alive** - Canadian Journal of Health & Nutrition, April 2005; 270: 48-53.

How to Prevent and Treat Cancer with Natural Medicine, Murray, Birdsall, Pizzorno & Reilly, **Riverhead Books**, 2002.

Antioxidant Vitamin and Mineral Supplementation May Help Prevent Prostate Cancer Meyer, et al., **Int. J. Cancer**, 2005; 116: 182-186.

Herbicides and Non-Hodgkins Lymphoma: New Evidence from a Study of Saskatchewan Farmers, Blair, **J. Int. Cancer Inst**. 1990; 85: 544-545.

Glutathione Treatment of Hepatocellular Carcinoma, Dalhoff, et al., **Liver** 1992; 12: 341-343.

EcoCancers: Do Environmental Factors Underlie a Breast Cancer Epidemic?, Raloff, **Sci. News** 1993; 144: 10-13.

Paraben Esters: Review of Recent Studies of Endocrine Toxicity, Absorption, Esterase and Human Exposure, and Discussion of Potential Human Health Risks, Darbe & Harvey, **J. Appl. Toxicol.** 2008; 285: 561-578.

Coffee Consumption and the Risk of Oral, Pharngeal and Esophageal Cancers in Japan: The Miyagi Cohort Study, Naganuma, Kuriyama, Kakizaki, et al., **Am. J. Epidemiol.** 2008; 16812: 1425-1432.

Red Meat Intake, Doneness, Polymorphisms in Genes that Encode Carcinogen-metabolizing Enzymes, and Colorectal Cancer Risk, Cotterchio, Boucher, Manno, et al., **Cancer Epidemiol. Biomarkers & Prev.** 2008; 1711: 3098-3107.

Multi-targeted Prevention of Cancer by Sulforaphane, Clarke, Dashwood & Ho, **Cancer Lett.** 2008; 269 (2): 291-304.

<u>QUERCETIN</u>

Suppression of Insulin-like Growth Factor Signalling Pathway and Collagen Expression in Keloid-derived Fibroblasts by Quercetin: It's Therapeutic Potential Use in the Treatment and/or Prevention of Keloids, Phan, See, Tran, et al., **Br. J. Dermatol.** 2003; 148 (3): 544-552.

Differential Responses of Skin Cancer Chemoprotective Agents Silibinin, Quercetin and Epigallocatechin 3-Gallate on Mitogenic Signalling and Cell Cycle Regulators in Human Epidermoid carcinoma A431 Cells, Bhatia, Agarwal & Agarwal, **Nutr. & Cancer.** 2001; 39 (2); 292-299.

Role of Mitochondria in Quercetin-enhanced Chemotherapeutic Response in Human Non-Small Cell Lung Carcinoma H-520 Cells, Kuhar, Sen & Singh, **Anticancer Res.** 2006; 26 (2A): 1297-1303.

Inhibition of Lung Cancer Cell Growth by Quercetin Glucoronides via G2/M Arrest and Induction of Apoptosis, Yang, Hsia, Kuo, et al., **Drug Metab. Dispos.** 2006, 34 (2): 296-304.

Induction of Cell-cycle Arrest and Apoptosis in Human Breast cancer Cells by Quercetin, Choi, Kim, Lee, et al., **Int. J. Oncol.** 2001; 19 (4): 837-844.

Antioxidants and Cancer III – Quercetin, Lamson & Brignall, **Alt. Med. Rev.** 2000; Vol. 5 No. 6: 196-208.

Quercetin decreases intracellular GSH content and potentiates the apoptotic action of the antileukemic drug arsenic trioxide in human leukemia cell lines, Ramos & Aller, **Biochem Pharmacol.** 2008;75 (10):1912-1923.

Enhanced Bioavailability of Tamoxifen after Oral Administration of Tamoxifen with Quercetin in Rats, Shin, Choi & Li, **Int. J. Pharm.** 2006; 313 (1-2): 144-149.

Inhibition of P-Glycoprotein by Flavonoid Derivatives (Quercetin and Morin) in Adriamycin-Resistant Human Myelogenous Leukemia (K562/ADM) Cells, Ohtani, Koyabu, Juichi, et al., **Cancer Lett.** 2002; 177 (1): 89-93.

Effects of Quercetin on the Cell Growth and the Intracellular Accumulation and Retention of Adriamycin, Asaum, Matsuzaki, Kawasak, et al., **Anticancer Res.** 200; 20 (4): 2477-2483.

Quercetin Potentiates the Effect of Adriamycin in a Multi-Drug-Resistant MCF-7 Human Breast Cancer Cell Line: P-Glycoprotein as a Possible Target, Scambia, Ranelletti, Panici, et al., **Cancer Chemother. Pharmacol.** 1994; 34 (6): 459-464.

Suppression of Multi-Drug Resistance Via Inhibition of Heat Shock Factor by Quercetin in MDR Cells, Kim, Yeo, Lim, et al., **Exp. Mol. Med.** 1998; 30 (2): 87-92.

Synergistic Antiproliferative Activity of Quercetin and Cisplatin on Ovarian Cancer Cell Growth, Scambia, Ranelletti, Benedetti, et al., **Anticancer Drugs** 1990; 1 (1): 45-48.

Drug Resistance Against Gemcitabine and Topotecan Mediated by Constituitive HSP-

70 Over-expression in vitro: Implication of Quercetin as a Sensitiser in Chemotherapy, Sluitz, Karlseder, Temfer, et al., **Br. J. Cancer** 1996; 74 (2): 172-177.

Low-concentrations of Quercetin and Ellagic Acid Synergistically Influence Proliferation, Cytotoxicity and Apoptosis in MOLT-4 Human Leukemia Cells, Mertens-Talcott, Talcott & Percival, **J. Nutr.** 2003; 133 (8): 2669-2674.
Spontaneous mitochondrial membrane potential change during apoptotic induction by quercetin in K562 and K562/adr cells, Kothan, Dechsupa, Leger, et al., **Can. J. Physiol. Pharmacol.** 2004, 82 (12): 1084-1090.

Food-derived Polyphenols Inhibit Pancreatic Cancer Growth Through Mitochondrial Cytochrome C Release and Apoptosis, Suolinna, Buschbaum & Racker, **Cancer Res.** 1975; 35 (7): 1865-1872.

Quercetin Induces Necrosis and Apoptosis in SCC-9 Oral Cancer Cells, Haghiac & Walle, **Nutr. Cancer** 2005; 53 (2):220-231.

Selective Aromatase Inhibition for Patients with Androgen-independent Prostate Carcinoma, Smith, Kaufman, George, et al., **Cancer** 2002; 95 (9): 1864-1868.

Absorption and Disposition Kinetics of the Dietary Antioxidant Quercetin in Man, Hollman, vd Gaag, Mengelers, et al., **Free Rad Biol Med** 1996; 21 (5): 703-707.

Quercetin Potentiates the Effect of Adriamycin in a Multidrug-resistant MCF-7 Human Breast-Cancer Cell Line: P-glycoprotein as a Possible Target, Scambia, Ranelletti, Panici, et al. **Cancer Chemother. Pharmacol.** 1994; 34 (6): 459-464.

Flavonoids: a Class of Modulators with Bifunctional Interactions at Vicinal ATP- and Steroid-binding Sites on Mouse P-glycoprotein, Conseil, Baubichon-Cortay, Dayan, et al., **Proc. Nat. Acad. Sci.** 1998; 95 (17): 9831-9836.

The Synergistic Reversal Effect of Multidrug Resistance by Quercetin and Hyperthermia in Doxorubicin-Resistant Human Myelogenous Leukemia Cells, Shen, Zhang, Wu & Zhu, **Int. J. Hyperthermia** 2008 ;24 (2): 151-159.

RADIATION

Timing is Everything in Combined Antiangiogenic / Radiation Therapy, Jain, **Cancer Cell** 2004; 6: 553-563.

Effects of Zinc Supplementation on Clinical Outcomes in Patients Receiving Radiotherapy for Head and Neck Cancers: a Double-blinded Randomized Study, Lin, Que, Lin, et al., **Int. J. Radiat. Oncol. Biol. Phys.** 2008; 702: 368-373.

Curcumin – a New Radiosensitizer of Squamous Cell Carcinoma Cells, Khafif, et al., **Otolarngol. Head Neck Surg.**, 2005; 132: 317-321.

The Chemopreventative Agent Curcumin is a Potent Radiosensitizer of Human Cervical Tumour Cells via Increased ROS production and Overactivation of the MAPK Pathway, Javvadi, Segan, Tuttle, et al., **Mol. Pharmacol.** 2008 Feb. 5 Epub ahead of print, PMID# 18252805.

Effects of Rhubarb Extract on Radiation Induced Lung Toxicity Via Decreasing Transforming Growth Factor Beta-1 and Interleukin-6 in Lung Cancer Patients Treated with Radiotherapy, Yu, Liu, Cheng, et al., **Lung Cancer** 2008; 592: 219-226.

ARCON (accelerated radiotherapy with carbogen and nicotinamide): a Novel Biology-based Approach in Radiotherapy Kanders, Bussink & van der Kogel, **Lancet Oncol.** 2002; 3 (12): 728-737.

Radiosensitization by Nicotinamide in vivo: *A Greater Enhancement of Tumour Damage Compared to that of Normal Tissue,* Horsman, Chaplin & Brown, **Rad. Res.** 1987; 109: 479-489.

Mechanism of Action of the Selective Tumour Radio-Sensitizer Nicotinamide, Horsman, Brown, et al, **Int. J. Rad. Onc. Biophys.** 1988; 15: 685-690. *Nicotinamide and Other Benzamide Analogs as Agents for Overcoming Hypoxic Cell Radiation Resistance in Tumours. A Review,* Horsman, **Acta Oncol.** 1995; 34 (5): 571-587.

Do Antioxidants Interfere with Radiation Therapy for Cancer?, Moss, **Integr. Cancer Ther.** 2007, 6 (3): 281-292.

Acute Adverse Effects of Radiation Therapy and Local Recurrence in Relation to Dietary and Plasma Beta Carotene and Alpha Tocopherol in Head and Neck Cancer Patients, Meyer, Bairati, Jobin, et al., **Nutr. Cancer** 2007; 59 (1): 29-35.

Dietary Counselling Benefits Patients Undergoing Radiotherapy, Ravasco. et al., **J. Clin. Oncol.** 2005; 23: 1348-1349, 1431-1438.

Effect of Concomitant Naturopathic Therapies on Clinical Tumour Response to External Beam Radiation Therapy for Prostate Cancer (Abstract), Birdsall, Alschuler, Martin, et al., **Soc. Integr. Oncol.** Nov. 2006, Boston, Mass.

Effect of Complementary Alternative Medical (CAM) Therapy on Tumour Response in Prostate Cancer Patients Treated with Radiation Therapy, Cain, Flynn, Kelly, et al., **J. Clin. Oncol.** 2007; 25: 15585.

Potential for Combined Modality Therapy of Cyclooxygenase Inhibitors and Radiation, Saha & Choy, **Prog Exp Tumour Res.** 2003; 37: 193-209.

Long-term Use of Cellular Phones and Brain Tumours: Increased Risk Associated with Use for >=10 Years, Hardell, Carlberg, Soderqvist, et al., **Occup. Envir. Med.** 2007; 64 (9): 626-632.

Oral Vitamin A Therapy for a Patient with a Severely Symptomatic Post-Radiation Anal Ulceration, Levitsky, Hong, Jani & Ehrenpreis, **Dis Colon Rectum** 2003; 46 (5): 679- 682.

Phase I Study of Concurrent Radiotherapy with TS-1 and Vitamin A (TAR Therapy) for Head and Neck Cancer, Nakashima, Kuramoti, Yamamoto, et al., **Gan To Kagaku Ryoho** 2005; 32 (6): 803-807.

Sensitization of Cervical Cancer Cell Lines to Low-dose Radiation by Retinoic Acid Does Not Require Functional p53, Tillmanns, Kamelle, Guruswamy, et al., **Gynecol Oncol** 2005; 97 (1): 142-150.

Supplemental Vitamin A Prevents the Acute Radiation-induced Defect in Wound Healing, Levenson, Gruber, Rettura, et al., **Ann Surg** 1984; 200 (4): 494-512.

Protective Effect of Vitamin A on Acute Radiation Injury in the Small Intestine, Beyzadeoğlu, Balkan, Demiriz, et al., **Radiat. Med.** 1997; 15 (1): 1-5.

A New Electromagnetic Exposure Metric: High Frequency Voltage Transients Associated with Increased Cancer Incidence in Teachers in a California School, Milham & Morgan, **Am J Ind Med** 2008; 51 (8): 579-586.

Arachidonic Acid Metabolites Mediate the Radiation-induced Increase in Glomerular Albumin Permeability, Sharma, McCarthy, Sharma, et al., **Exp. Biol. Med.** 2006; 231: 99-106.

Enhanced Radiosensitivity of Rat Autochthonous Mammary Tumours by Dietary Docosahexaenoic Acid, Colas, Paon, Denis, et al., **Int. J. Cancer** 2004; 109 (3): 449- 454.

[Omega-3 Fatty Acid-containing Diet (Racol) Reduces Toxicity of Chemo-radiation Therapy for Patients with Esophageal Cancer], Minami, Miyata, Doki, et al., **Gan To Kagaku Ryoho** 2008; 35 (3): 437-440.

Aloe vera for Preventing Radiation-induced Skin Reactions: A Systematic Literature Review, Richardson, Smith, McIntyre, et al., **Clin. Oncol (R. Coll. Radiol).** 2005; 17 (6): 478-484.

Prevention of Chemotherapy and Radiation Toxicity with Glutamine, Savarese, Savy,

Vahdat, et al., **Cancer Treat. Rev**. 2003; 29 (6): 501-513.

Successful and Sustained Treatment of Chronic Radiation Proctitis with Antioxidant Vitamins E and C, Kennedy, Bruninga, Mutlu, et. al., **Am. J.Gastroenterol.** 2001; 96 (4): 1080-1084.

Protective effects of Berberine on Radiation-induced Lung Injury via Intercellular Adhesion Molecule-1 and Transforming Growth Factor beta-1 in Patients with Lung Cancer, Liu, Yu, Zhang, et al., **Eur. J. Cancer** 2008; 44 (16): 2425-2432.

Curcumin Sensitizes Human Colorectal Cancer Xenografts in Nude Mice to □-Radiation by Targeting Nuclear Factor-B–Regulated Gene Products, Kunnumakkara1, Diagaradjane, Guha, et al., **Clin.Cancer Res.** *2008;*14: 2128-2136. *Curcumin Induces Chemo/Radio-Sensitization in Ovarian Cancer Cells and Curcumin Nanoparticles Inhibit Ovarian Cancer Cell Growth,*Yallapu, Maher, Sundram et al., **J. Ovarian Res.** 2010; 3: 11.

Can the Therapeutic Gain of Radiotherapy Be Increased by Concurrent Administration of Asian Botanicals?, Sagar, **Integr. Cancer Ther.** 2010; 9 (1): 5-13. Dr. Lawenda's response pp. 14-15.

STEM CELLS & IMMUNE CELLS

Tumour Stem Cells: Rooting Out Resistance, Rich, et al., **Nat. Rev. Cancer** 2006; 6 (12): 904-905. Medscape article 550020

The Paradox of Response and Survival in Cancer Therapeutics, Huff, Matsui, Smith & Jones, **Blood** 2006; 107: 4321-434.

Will Cancer Stem Cell Provide New Therapeutic Targets?- Review, Behbod & Rosen, **Carcinogenesis** 2004; 26 (4): 703-711.

Cancer Stem cells: Are We Missing the Target? – Commentary, Jones, Matsui & Smith, **J. Natl. Cancer Inst.** 2004; 96 (8): 583-585.

On Mammary Stem Cells, Woodward, Chen, Behbod & Rosen, **J. Cell Sci.** 2005; 118: 3585-3594.

Cancer Stem Cells - Review, Jordan, Guzman & Noble, **NEJM** 2006; 355 (12): 1253-1261.

Bone Marrow Derived Cells & Cancer – An Opportunity for Improved Therapy, Houghton, **Nat. Clin. Pract. Oncol.** 2007; 4 (1): 2-3. Medscape article 551187

The Lymphovascular Embolus of Inflammatory Breast Cancer Expresses a Stem Cell-like Phenotype, Xiao, Ye, Yearsley, et al., **Amer. J. Pathol.** 2008; 173 (2): 561-574.

Leukaemia Stem Cells & the Evolution of Cancer Stem Cell Research, Huntley & Gilliand, **Nat. Rev. Cancer** 2005; 5: 311-321.

Human Pancreatic Cancer Stem Cells Identified, Simenone, et al., **Cancer Res.** 2007 Medscape article 551581

Targeting Breast Stem Cells with the Cancer Preventive Compounds Curcumin and Piperine, Kakarala, Brenner,
 Korkaya, et al., **Breast Cancer Res. Treat.** 2009 [Epub ahead of print] PMID: 19898931

Brain Tumour Cells Lurk in Perivascular Niches, Gilbertson, **Cancer Cell** 2007; 11: 3-5, 69-82. Medscape article 551315.

Bone Morphogenetic Proteins Inhibit the Tumorigenic Potential of Human Brain Tumour-initiating Cells, Piccirillo & Vescovi, **Nature** 2006; 444: 761-765.

Brain Tumour Stem Cells, Vescovi, Galli, and Reynolds, **Nat. Rev. Cancer** 2006; 6 (1): 425-436.

Relation of tumour associated macrophages and mast cells of tumour interstitum and angiogenesis in non-small cell lung cancer, Zou & Hu, **Zhong Nan Da Xue Xue Bao Yi Xue Ban** 2007; 32 (6):1037-1041.

Association of macrophages, mast cells and eosinophil leukocytes with angiogenesis and tumour stage in non-small cell lung carcinomas (NSCLC), Tataroğlu, Kargi, Ozka, et al., **Lung Cancer** 2004; 43 (1): 47-54.

Inflammatory cell infiltration of tumours: Jekyll or Hyde, Talmadge, Donkor & Scholar, **Cancer Metastasis Rev.** 2007; 26 (3-4): 373-400.

Human macrophages promote the motility and invasiveness of osteopontin-knockdown tumour cells, Cheng, Huo, Kuang, et al., **Cancer Res.** 2007; 67(11): 5141-5147.

Dynamics of the immune reaction to pancreatic cancer from inception to invasion, Clark, Hingorani , Mick, et al.,**Cancer Res.** 2007;67 (19): 9518-9527.

Increased expression of human macrophage metalloelastase (MMP-12) is associated with the invasion of endometrial adenocarcinoma, Yang, Dong, Zhao,et al., **Pathol Res Pract.** 2007; 203 (7): 499-505. Epub 2007 Jun 14.

Role of tumour-associated macrophages in tumour progression and invasion, Mantovani, Schioppa, Porta, et al., **Cancer Metastasis Rev.** 2006;25(3): 315-322.

Co-opting macrophage traits in cancer progression: a consequence of tumour cell fusion? Pawelek, Chakraborty, Lazova, etr al., **Contrib Microbiol.** 2006; 13: 138-155.

Macrophages: obligate partners for tumour cell migration, invasion, and metastasis, Condeelis & Pollard, **Cell** 2006;124 (2): 263-266.

Prostate Cancer: Genes, Environment, Immunity and the Use of Immunotherapy, Karan, Thrasher & Lubaroff, **Prostate Cancer Prostatic Dis.** 2008; 11 (3): 230-236.

ER Alpha Status of Disseminated Tumour Cells in Bone Marrow of Primary Breast Cancer Patients, Fehm, Krawczyk, Solomayer, et al., **Breast Cancer Res.** 2008; 0 (5): R76.

Resistance of Cancer Cells to Immune Recognition and Killing, Lipinski & Egyud, **Med. Hypoth.** 2000; 54 (3): 456-460.

Molecular Biology of Macrophage Activation: A Pathway Whereby Psychosocial Factors Can Potentially Affect Health, Adams, **Psychosomat. Med.** 1994; 56: 316-327.

Disregulation in TH1 and TH2 Subsets of CD4+ T Cells in Peripheral Blood of Colorectal Cancer Patients and Involvement in Cancer Establishment and Progression, Pellegrini, Berghella, Del Beato, et al., **Cancer Immunol. Immunother.** 1996; 42 (1): 1-8.

Th1/Th2 balance: The Hypothesis, Its Limitations, and Implications for Health and Disease, Kidd, **Altern. Med. Rev.** 2003; 8(3):223-46

Anesthesia, Surgery, and the Immune System, Kotani, **Curr. Opin. Anesthesiol.** 1993; 6: 562-568.

Effect of Major Dietary Modifications on the Immune System in Patients with Breast Cancer, Garritson, Nikaein, Peters, et al., **Cancer Practice** 1995; 3 (4): 239-246.

In vivo Effect of Ascorbic Acid on Enhancement of Human Natural Killer Cell Activity, Vojdani & Ghoneum, **Nutr. Res.**1993; 13: 753-754.

Enhancement of Human Natural Killer Cytotoxic Activity by Vitamin C in Pure and Augmented Formulations, Vojdani & Namatalla, **J. Nutr. Environ. Med.** 1997; 7 (3): 187-195.

Cancer-expanded Myeloid-derived Suppressor Cells Induce Anergy of NK Cells Through Menbrane-bound TGF-beta 1, Li, Han, Guo, et al., **J. Immunol.** 2009; 182 (1): 240-249.

Signaling Mechanism(s) of Reactive Oxygen Species in Epithelial-Mesenchymal Transition Reminiscent of Cancer Stem Cells in Tumor Progression, Wang, Li & Sarkar, **Curr. Stem Cell Res. Ther.** 2010; 5 (1): 1-7.

<u>SUGAR, INSULIN & IGF</u>

Insulin and Cancer, Boyd, **Integr. Cancer Ther.**, 2003; 2 (4): 315-329.

Insulin-like Growth Factor 1 Tied to Prostate Cancer Risk, Douglas, **Medscape** 487836 8/25/04.

Insulin-Like Growth Factor I Receptor Promotes Gastric Cancer Adachi. et al., **Gut** 2005; 54: 591-600.

Diabetes, High Glucose Levels Linked to Cancer in Korean Study, Jee, et al., **JAMA** 2005; 194-202 and editorial p. 235-236.

Diabetes Triples Risk of Liver Cancer, El-Serag, et al, **Gut**, 2005; 54: 533-539.

Elevated IGF-1 Linked to Raised Risk of Cancer in Premenopausal Women, Shi, et al, **Int. J. Cancer** 2004; 111: 418-423.

High Dietary Glycemic Load May Increase Colorectal Cancer Risk in Women, Higginbotham, et al, **J. Natl. Cancer Inst.** 2004; 96: 229-233.

High Dietary Glycemic Load and Insulin Resistance Combine to Increase Pancreatic Cancer Risk, Michaud, et al., **J. Natl. Cancer Inst.** 2002; 94: 1293-1300.

Controlling Hyperglycemia as an Adjunct to Cancer Therapy, Krone & Ely, **Integr. Cancer Ther.** 2005; 4 (1): 25-31.

Fasting insulin and outcome in early-stage breast cancer- results of a prospective cohort study, Goodwin, et al, **J. Clin. Oncol.**, 2002; 20: 42-51.

Glycemic Index, Glycemic Load and Thyroid Cancer Risk, Randi, Ferraroni, Talamini, et al., **Annals of Oncol.** 2008; 192: 380-383.

Green Tea Polyphenols Inhibit IGF-1 Signalling in Prostate Cancer Model, Mukhtar, et al., **Cancer Res.** 2004; 64: 8715-8722.

Postprandial Hyperinsulinemia Accelerates Growth of Hepatocellular Carcinoma, Kawata, et al., **Gut** 2002; 51: 100-104.

Insulin-like Growth Factor -1 Activates Gene Transcription Programs Strongly

Associated with Poor Breast Cancer Prognosis, Chreighton, Casa, Lazard, et al., **J Clin Oncol** 2008; 26 (25): 4078-4085.

Insulin, Insulin-like Growth Factors and Colon Cancer: A Review of the Evidence, Giovannucci, **J Nutr**
2001; 131 (Suppl. 11): s3109-3120.

Glycemic Index, Glycemic Load, and Cancer Risk: A Meta-analysis, Gnagnarella, Gandini, La Vecchia, & Maisonneuve, **Amer. J. Clin. Nutr.** 2008; 87 (6): 1793-1801.

Up-regulation of IGF Binding Protein-1 as an Anti-carcinogenic Strategy: Relevance to Caloric Restriction, Exercise, and Insulin Sensitivity, McCarty, **Medical Hypotheses** 1997; 48 (4): 297-308.

The Insulin-like Growth Factor System as a Treatment Target in Breast Cancer, Yee, **Sem. Oncol.** 2002; 29 (3 Suppl 11): 86-95.

Cross-talk Among Estrogen Receptor, Epidermal Growth Factor, and Insulin-like Growth Factor Signaling in Breast Cancer, Lee, Cui & Oesterreich, **Clin. Cancer Res.** 2001; 7 (12 Suppl): 4429s-4435s.
Tyrosine Kinase Signalling in Breast Cancer: Insulin-like Growth Factors and Their Receptors in Breast Cancer, Zhang & Yee, **Breast Cancer Res.** 2000; 2 (3): 170-175.

Insulin-like Growth Factors and Cancer, Furstenberger & Senn, **Lancet Oncol.** 2002; 3 (5): 298-302.

Insulin-Like Growth Factor (IGF) Family and Prostate Cancer, Gennigens, Menetrier-Caux & Droz, **Crit. Rev. Oncol. Hematol.** 2006; 58 (2): 124-145.

Activation of Estrogen Receptor-mediated Gene Transcription by IGF-I in Human Breast Cancer Cells, Lee, Weng, Jackson & Yee, **J. Endocrinol.** 1997; 152 (1): 39-47.

Vitamin D Analogue EB1089-induced Prostate Regression is Associated with Increased Gene Expression of Insulin-like Growth Factor Binding Proteins, Nickerson T. Huynh H. **J. Endocrinol.** 1999; 160 (2): 223-229.

Pharmacological Modulation of IGF Serum Concentrations as a Therapeutic Approach to Control the Growth of Malignant Breast Tumours, Singer, Hudelist, Schreiber & Kubista, **Drugs Today** (Barc). 2003; 39 (2): 115-125.

Inhibition of Insulin-like Growth Factor I Receptor Signaling by the Vitamin D Analogue EB1089 in MCF-7 Breast Cancer Cells: A Role for Insulin-like Growth Factor Binding Proteins, Rozen & Pollak, **Int. J. Oncol.** 1999; 15 (3): 589-594.

Insulin, Insulin-like Growth Factors, Insulin Resistance, and Neoplasia, Pollack **Am. J. Clin. Nutr.** 2007; 86 (3): s820-822.

Role of Sugars in Human Neutrophilic Phagocytosis, Sanchez, Reeser, Lau, et al., **Am. J. Clin. Nutr.** 1973; 26: 1180-1184.

SURGERY

Micrometastases Often Persist in Breast Cancer Patients, Slade, et al, **Int. J. Cancer** 2005; 114: 94-100.

Wounding from Biopsy and Breast Cancer Progression, Retsky, Demichelli & Hrushesky, **Lancet** 2001; 357 (9261): 1048.

Port-sites Excision for Gallbladder Cancer Incidentally Found After Laparoscpic Cholecystectomy, Guiliante, Ardito, Velone, et al., **Am. J. Surg.** 2006; 191 (1): 114-116.

Primary Tumour Removal Increases Vascular Density in Liver Metastases, **Int. J. Cancer**, 2004; 112: 554-559.

Menopausal Status Dependence of the Timing of Breast Cancer Recurrence After Surgical Removal of the Primary Tumour, Demicheli, et al, **Breast Cancer Res.,**2004; 6 (6): 689-696.

A Randomized Clinical Trial of a Brief Hypnosis Intervention to Control Side-effects in Breast Surgery Patients, Montgomery, Bovbjerg, Schnur, et al., **J. Natl. Cancer Inst.** 2007; 99 (17): 1304-1312.

Impact of Psycho-therapeutic Support for Patients with Gastro-intestinal Cancer Undergoing Surgery: 10-Year Survival Results of a Randomized Trial, Kuchler, Bestmann, Rappat, et al., **J. Clin. Oncol.** 2007; 25 (19): 2702-2708.

Needle Track Seeding Following Biopsy of Liver Lesions in the Diagnosis of Hepatocellular Carcinoma: A Systematic Review and Meta-analysis, Silva, Hegab, Hyde, et al., **Gut 2008; 57 (11): 1592-1596.**

VITAMIN C

Vitamin C Deficiency in Cancer Patients, Mayland,Bennett & Allan, **Palliat. Med.** 2005; 19: 17-20.

High-Dose Vitamin C Selectively Kills Cancer Cells, Levine, et al., **Proc. Natl. Acad. Sciences USA,** 2005; 102: 13604-13609.

Naturopathic Oncology

High-dose Vitamin C Therapy: Renewed Hope or False Promise? Assouline & Miller, **Can. Med. Assoc. J.** 2006; *174*: 956–957.

Intravenous Ascorbate as a Tumour Cytotoxic Chemotheraeutic Agent, Riordan, et al., **Med. Hypotheses** 1995; 44: 207-213.
Prolonged Survival linked to Intravenous Vitamin C Seen in Three Cancer Patients, Levine, et al, **Can. Med. Assoc. J.**, 2006; 174: 937-942.

Changes of Terminal Cancer Patients' Health-related Quality of Life After High Dose Vitamin C Administration, Yeom, Jung & Song, **J. Korean Med Sci** 2007; 22 (1): 7-11.

Intravenously Administered Vitamin C as a Cancer Therapy: Three Cases, Padayatty, Riordan, Hewitt, et al., **CMAJ** 2006; 174 (7): 937-942.

A Pilot Clinical Study of Continuous Intravenous Ascorbate in Terminal Cancer Patients, Riordan, Casciari, Gonzalez, et al., **P R Health Sci J** 2005; 24 (4): 269-276.

Innovation vs. Quality Control: An 'Unpublishable' Clinical Trial of Supplemental Ascorbate in Incurable Cancer, Cameron & Campbell, **Med Hypotheses** 1991; 36 (3): 185-189.

Reticulum Cell Sarcoma: Two Complete 'Spontaneous' Regressions, in Response to High-dose Ascorbic Acid Therapy. A Report on Subsequent Progress, Campbell, Jack & Cameron, **Oncology** 1991; 48 (6): 495-497.

Changes of Terminal Cancer Patients' Health-related Quality of Life After High Dose Vitamin C Administration, Yeom, Jung & Song, **J. Korean Med Sci** 2007; 22 (1): 7-11.

Supplemental Ascorbate in the Supportive Treatment of Cancer: Prolongation of Survival Times in Terminal Human Cancer, Cameron & Pauling, **Proc. Natl Acad Sci USA** 1976; 73 (10): 3685-3689.

Supplemental Ascorbate in the Supportive Treatment of Cancer: Reevaluation of Prolongation of Survival Tmes in Terminal Human Cancer, Cameron & Pauling, **Proc Natl Acad Sci USA** 1978; 75: 4538–4542.

Vitamin C Inhibits p53-induced Replicative Senescence Through Suppression of ROS Production and p38 MAPK Activity, Kim, Jin, Lee, et al., **Biochem Pharmacol.** 2008; 22 (5): 651-655.

Pharmacological Doses of Ascorbate Act as a Pro-oxidant and Decrease Growth of Aggressive Tumour Xenografts in Mice, Chen, Espey, Sun, et al., **Proc. Natl. Acad.**

Sci. USA 2008; 1105: 11105-11109.

Pharmacologic Ascorbic Acid Concentrations Selectively Kill Cancer Cells: Action as a Pro-drug to Deliver Hydrogen Peroxide to Tissues, Chen, Espey, Krishna, et al., **Proc. Natl. Acad. Sci. U S A** 2005; 102 (38): 13604-13609.

Vitamin C Pharmacokinetics: Implications for Oral and Intravenous Use, Padayatty, Sun, Wang, et al., **Ann. Intern. Med.** 2004; 140 (7): 533-537.

Ascorbate in Pharmacologic Concentrations Selectively Generates Ascorbate Radical and Hydrogen Peroxide in Extracellular Fluid in vivo, Chen, Espey, Sun, et al., **Proc. Natl. Acad. Sci U S A** 2007; 104 (21): 8749-8754.

Phase I Clinical Trial of I.V. Ascorbic Acid in Advanced Malignancy, Hoffer, Levine, Assouline, et al., **Ann. Oncol.** 2008; [Epub ahead of print]

Emerging Role of Ascorbic Acid in the Management of Advanced Breast Carcinoma as a Chemosensitizer, Goel, Agarwal, Mandal, et al., **Asian J. Surg.** 1999; 22: 333-336.

In vivo Effect of Ascorbic Acid on Enhancement of Human Natural Killer Cell Activity, Vojdani & Ghoneum, **Nutr. Res.**1993; 13: 753-754.

Enhancement of Human Natural Killer Cytotoxic Activity by Vitamin C in Pure and Augmented Formulations, Vojdani & Namatalla, **J. Nutr. Environ. Med.** 1997; 7 (3): 187-195.

The Orthomolecular Treatment of Cancer II. Clinical Trial of High-dose Ascorbic Acid Supplements in Advanced Human Cancer, Cameron & Campbell, **Chem. Biol. Interact.** 1974; 9: 285–315.

Mega-dose Vitamin C as Therapy for Human Cancer? Borst, **Proc Natl Acad Sci USA**; 2008; 105: E95.

Vitamin C and Cancer Revisited, Frei & Lawson, **Proc Natl Acad Sci USA** 2008;105: 11037–11038.

The Antioxidant Ascorbic Acid Mobilizes Nuclear Copper Leading to a Prooxidant Breakage of Cellular DNA: Implications for Chemotherapeutic Action Against Cancer, Ullah, Khan, Zubair, et al., **Cancer Chemother. Pharmacol.** 2010 March 6 [Epub ahead of print] PMID: 20213077.

VITAMIN D

Vitamin D and Cancer, Ali & Vaidya, **J. Cancer Res. Ther.** 2007; 3 (4): 225-230.

Naturopathic Oncology

Vitamin D Signalling Pathways in Cancer: Potential for Anti-cancer Therapeutics, Deeb, Trump & Johnson, **Nat. Rev. Cancer** 2007; 7 (9): 684-700.

Induction of Ovarian Cancer Cell Apoptosis by 1,25-dihydroxy-Vitamin D3 Through the Down-regulation of Telomerase, Jiang, Bao , Li, et al., **Biol. Chem.** 2004; 279 (51): 53213-53221.

High Vitamin D Levels Linked to Improved Lung Cancer Survival, Zhou, et al., **J. Clin. Oncol.** 2007; 25: 479-485.

Vitamin D and Calcium Supplementation Reduces Cancer Risk: Results of a Randomized Trial, Lappe, et al., **Am. J. Clin. Nutr.** 2007; 85 (6): 1586-1591.

Vitamin D Supplementation and Total Mortality: a Meta-analysis of Randomized Controlled Trials, Autier and Gandini, **Arch. Intern. Med.** 2007; 167 (16): 1730-1737. *Do Sunlight and Vitamin D Reduce the Likelihood of Colon Cancer?*, Garland & Garland, **Int. J. Epidemiol.** 2006; 35 (2): 217-220.

Circulating 25-hydroxy Vitamin D Levels and Survival in Patients with Colorectal Cancer, Ng, Meyerhardt, Wu, et al., **J Clin Oncol** 2008; 26 (18): 2937-2939.

Molecular Basis of Potential of Vitamin D to Prevent Cancer, Ingraham, Bragdon & Nohe, **Curr. Med. Res. & Opin.** 2008; 241: 139-149.

1{alpha}, 25-Dihydroxyvitamin D3 Potentiates Cisplatin Anti-tumour Activity by p73 Induction in a Squamous Cell Carcinoma Model, Ma, et al., **Mol. Cancer Ther.** 2008; 7 (9): 3047-3055

Association Between Serum 25(OH)D and Death from Prostate Cancer, Tretli, Hernes, Berg, et al., **Br. J. Cancer** 2009; 1003: 450-454.

Chemotherapy is Linked to Severe Vitamin D Deficiency in Patients with Colorectal Cancer, Fakih, Trump, Johnson, et al., **Int. J. Colorectal Dis.** 2009; 242: 219-224. *Dairy Products, Calcium, and Vitamin D and Risk of Prostate Cancer*, Chan & Giovannucci, **Epidemiol. Rev.** 2001; 23 (1): 87-92.

Vitamin D is Associated with Improved Survival in Early-stage Non-Small Cell Lung Cancer Patients, Zhou, Suk, Liu, et al., **Cancer Epidemiol. Biomarkers Prev.** 2005; 14 (10): 2303-2309.

Vitamin D Analogue EB1089-induced Prostate Regression is Associated with Increased Gene Expression of Insulin-like Growth Factor Binding Proteins, Nickerson T. Huynh H. **J. Endocrinol.** 1999; 160 (2): 223-229.

Inhibition of Insulin-like Growth Factor I Receptor Signaling by the Vitamin D Analogue EB1089 in MCF-7 Breast Cancer Cells: A Role for Insulin-like Growth Factor Binding Proteins, Rozen & Pollak, **Int. J. Oncol.** 1999; 15 (3): 589-594.

A Combined Pretreatment of 1,25-Dihydroxyvitamin D3 and Sodium Valproate Enhances the Damaging Effect of Ionizing Radiation on Prostate Cancer Cells, Gavrilov Leibovich, Ariad, Lavrenkov & Shany, **J. Steroid Biochem. Mol. Biol.** 2010 [Epub ahead of print] PMID: 20214985.

Vitamin D3 Distribution and Status in the Body, Heaney, Horst, Cullen & Armas, **J. Am. Coll. Nutr.** 2009; 28 (3): 252-256.

<u>VITAMIN K</u>

The Anticancer Effects of Vitamin K, Lamson & Plaza, **Alt. Med. Rev.** 2003; 8 (3): 303-318.

The Mechanisms of Vitamin K2- induced Apoptosis of Myeloma Cells, Tsujioka, Miura, otsuki, et al., **Haematologica** 2006, 91 (5): 613-619.

Oxidative Stress by Ascorbate (Vit C) / Menadione (K3) Association Kills K562 Human Chronic Myelogenous Leukemia Cells and Inhibits its Tumour Growth in Nude Mice, Verrax, Stockis, Tison, et al, **Biochem. Pharmacol.** 72 (6): 671-680.

Vitamin K2 Inhibits the Growth and Invasiveness of Hepatocellular Carcinoma Cells Via Protein Kinase A Activation, Otsuka, Kato, Shao, et al., **Hepatology** 2004; 40 (1): 243-251.

Phase I Trial of Menadiol Diphosphate (Vitamin K3) in Advanced Malignancy, Lim, et al., **Invest. New Drugs** 2005; 23: 235–239.

Alpha-Tocopheryl Succinate Promotes Selective Cell Death Induced by Vitamin K3 in Combination with Ascorbate, Tomasetti, Strafella, Staffolani, **Br. J. Cancer.** 2010; 102 (8):1224-34.

Cell Damage and Death by Autoschizis in Human Bladder (RT4) Carcinoma Cells Resulting from Treatment with Ascorbate and Menadione, Gilloteaux, Jamison, Loukas, et al., **Ultrastructural Pathology** 2010; 34:140–160.

<u>APPENDIX B – BIBLIOGRAPHY/SUGGESTED READING</u>

Life Over Cancer, Keith Block, MD 2009

The Paleolithic Prescription – A Program of Diet and Exercise and a Design for Living, Eaton, Shostak, and Konner, 1988.

Dietary Options for Cancer Survivors – A Guide to Research on Foods, Food Substances, Herbals and Dietary Regimens That Might Influence Cancer, Weldon, et al, American Institute for Cancer Research, 2002.

Stopping Cancer Before It Starts – The American Institute for Cancer Research's Program for Cancer Prevention, The American Institute for Cancer Research, 1999.

Naturally There's Hope – A Handbook for the Naturopathic Care of Cancer Patients, McKinney, **Trafford Press**, 2003.

Guns, Germs and Steel – the Fates of Human Societies, Jared Diamond, 1997.

Foods That Fight Cancer, Preventing Cancer by Diet, Richard Beliveau and Denis Gingras, 2007

Cooking with Foods That Fight Cancer, Richard Beliveau and Denis Gingras, 2007

The Complete Natural Medicine Guide to Breast Cancer – A Practical Manual for Understanding, Prevention and Care, Sat Dharam Kaur, ND 2003.

Natural Compounds in Cancer Therapy – Promising Non-toxic Anti-tumour Agents from Plants and Other Natural Sources, John Boik, Oregon Medical Press 2001.

An Alternative Medicine Definitive Guide to Cancer, Diamond, Cowden & Goldberg, Future Medicine Publishing, 1997.

Healing the Planet- One Patient at a Time, A Primer in Environmental Medicine, Jozef Krop, 2000.

Healing with Whole Foods - Asian Traditions and Modern Nutrition, Paul Pritchard, 2003.

Breast Cancer – Beyond Convention, edited by Tafliaferri, Cohen & Tripathy, 2002, Atria Books.

Iscador- Mistletoe preparations used in anthroposophically extended cancer treatment, Gorter, 1998, Erlag fur GanzheitsMedizin.

Iscador Mistletoe and Cancer Therapy, edited by Christine Murphy, 2001, Lantern Books.

Staying Alive Cookbook for Cancer Free Living, Sally Errey, 2004, Belissimo Books.

The Complete Cancer Cleanse, Calbom, Calbom & Mahaffey, 2003, Thomas Nelson, Inc.

Cancer as a Turning Point, Lawrence LeShan, 1994, Plume/Penguin.

You Can Fight for Your Life, Lawrence LeShan, 1977, M. Evans & Co.

Questioning Chemotherapy, Ralph Moss, 1995, Equinox Press.

Antioxidants Against Cancer, Ralph Moss, 2000, Equinox Press.

Cancer and Vitamin C, Cameron & Pauling, revised ed. 1993, Camino Books.

Healing Cancer- Complementary Vitamin & Drug Treatments, Hoffer & Pauling, 2004, CCNM Press.

Nutrition After Cancer, 2002, American Institute for Cancer Research.

Alternatives in Cancer Therapy, Pelton & Overholser, 1994, Fireside.

Comprehensive Cancer Care – Integrating Alternative, Complementary and Conventional Therapies, Gordon & Curtin, 2001, Perseus Publishing.

The Biology of Cancer, Robert A. Weinberg, 2007; Garland Science

Clinical Oncology, American Cancer Society, 2000

Cancer Medicine 7 : Holland,Frei et al., editors, 7th edition, BC Decker, 2006.

Robbins Pathologic Basis of Disease, Sixth edition, R. Cotran, V. Kumar, & T. Collins, W.B. Saunders Company

Cancer & Natural Medicine - a Textbook of Basic Science and Clinical Research, John Boik, 1996, Oregon Medical Press

Natural Compounds in Cancer Therapy – Promising Non-toxic Anti-tumour Agents from Plants and Other Natural Sources, John Boik, 2001, Oregon Medical Press.

Cancer and Natural Medicine – a Textbook of Basic Science and Clinical Research , John Boik, 1996 Oregon Medical Press.

Naturally There's Hope – A Handbook for the Naturopathic Care of Cancer Patients, McKinney, **Trafford Press**, 2003.

You Don't Have to Die, Harry Hoxsey, N.D., 1956 Milestone Books

The Cancer Industry -Unravelling the Politics, Ralph W. Moss, 1989, Paragon

A Family Guide - Coping with Chemotherapy Using Homeopathy, Laura Fenton, 2003, Health Harmony Books.

An Introduction to Integrated Healing - Participants' guide to self-care, healthful nutrition, vitamins, supplements, complementary medical therapies and healing, Center for Integrated Healing, 1998

Third Opinion: An International Directory to Alternative Therapy Centres for the Treatment and Prevention of Cancer and Other Degenerative Diseases, Second edition, J. M. Fink, 1992; Avery Publishing Group.

A Guide to Unconventional Cancer Therapies, Ontario Breast Cancer Information Exchange Project, 1994

Breast Cancer - What you should know (but may not be told) about prevention, diagnosis and treatment, Steve Austin, N.D. and Cathy Hitchcock, M.S.W., 1994, Prima Health Publishing

Breast Cancer - The Complete Guide, Third edition, Yashar Hirshaut & Peter Pressman, 2000, Bantam Books.

Breast Cancer - A Nutritional Approach, Carlton Fredericks, Ph.D., 1977, Grosset & Dunlap

Beating Cancer with Nutrition, Patrick Quillan, 1994, Nutrition times Press.

Secrets to Great Health, Jonn Matsen, N.D., 2001, Prima Publishing

The Schwarzbein Principle, Diana Schwarzbein, MD, 1999, Health Communications

A Holistic Approach to Cancer Therapy, Wolfgang Woeppel, 1995, Pascoe

Love, Medicine & Miracles - Lessons learned about self-healing from a surgeon's experience with exceptional patients, Bernie. S. Siegel, M.D., 1986, Harper & Row

Homeopathic Medical Repertory, Robin Murphy, N.D., 1993; Hahnemann Academy of North America.

The Cancer Epidemic: Shadow of the Conquest of Nature, Gotthard Booth, 1974, Edwin Mellen Press

Cancer Therapy - the Independent Consumer's Guide to Non-toxic Treatment and Prevention, Ralph Moss, Equinox Press

Healthy Fats For Life - Preventing and treating common health problems with essential fatty acids, L. Vanderhaege, K. Karst, 2003, Quarry Health Books

How to Prevent and Treat Cancer with Natural Medicine, Michael Murray, Tim Birdsall, Joseph E. Pizzorno & Paul Reilly, 2002, Riverhead Books

Cancer and Vitamin C, Ewan Cameron & Linus Pauling, 1979, Linus Pauling Institute of Science and Medicine

Cancer as a Turning Point, Lawrence LeShan, Penguin Press

Nutritional Management of Cancer Patients, Abby S. Block, Aspen Publishers

Everyone's Guide to Cancer Therapy, M. Dollinger, E. Rosebaum, & G. Cable, Andrews-McMeel Publishers

The Wheatgrass Book, Ann Wigmore, 'Doctor of Natural Laws,' 1985, Avery Publishing Group.

Healing Words – The Power of Prayer and the Practice of Medicine, Larry Dossey 1993.

Head First – The Biology of Hope, Norman Cousins, 1989.

Cancer Principles and Practices, V. DeVita, S. Hellman,& S. Rosenberg, Lipincott-Raven Publishers

Handbook of Cancer Chemotherapy, Roland T. Skeel, Lipincott.

Manual of Clinical Oncology, D. Casciato & B. Lowitz, Little Brown

Primer of Epidemiology, Gary Friedman, 1980, McGraw-Hill

Foundations of Epidemiology, A. Lilienfeld, 1976, Oxford U. Press

FDA Supplement Warnings - Misleading, Exaggerated or Unproven, Zoltan Rona, June/July 1998, Health Naturally.

Increasing and Improving Research in Complementary and Alternative Medicine, Carlo Calabrese, 2000, NIH Office of Alternative Medicine.

The Cancer Blackout - A history of denied and suppressed remedies, Maurice Natenberg, 1959, Regent House.

The Medical Mafia - How to get out of it alive and take back our health & wealth, Ghislaine Lanctot, 2002 edition, self-published.

Hard to Swallow – The Truth About Food Additives, Sargeant and Evans, 1995, Alive Books

Fight for Your Health, Byron Richards, 2006, Walter Publishing.

Cancer - A Healing Crisis - the whole-body approach to cancer therapy, Jack Tropp, 1980, Exposition Press.

The Healing of Cancer - The cures, the cover-ups and the solution now, Barry Lynes, 1989, Marcus Books.

The Tao of Medicine, Stephen Fulder, 1982, Destiny Books.

Cancer Treatment with Fu Zheng Pei Ben Principle, Pan Mingji, et al, 1992, Fujian Science & Technology Publishing House.

7-Day Detox Miracle 2nd ed.,, Bennett & Barrie , 2001; Three Rivers Press.

Living Downstream: An Ecologist Looks at Cancer and the Environment, Steingraber, 1997, published by Addison-Wesley.

Our Toxic World – A Wake-up Call - Chemicals damage your body, brain, behaviour and sex, Doris Rapp, 2004.

Toxic Deception - How the chemicals industry manipulates science, bends the law and endangers your health, Dan Fagin, Marianne Lavelle

The CancerSmart Consumer Guide- How to eliminate toxins from your home and garden products and how to make healthy choices for your family and the environment, Labour Environmental Alliance Society, Vancouver, B.C., www.leas.ca

Clinical Purification, A Complete Treatment and Reference Manual, Gina Nick, 2001, Longevity Through Prevention.

Cancer Therapy – The Independent Consumer's Guide to Non-toxic Treatment and Prevention, Ralph Moss 1992/6 Equinox Press.

<u>APPENDIX C – RESOURCES</u>

RECOMMENDED JOURNALS

- Cancer
- Nutrition & Cancer
- Journal of Clinical Oncology
- Journal of the National Cancer Institute
- Cancer Research
- Integrative Cancer Therapies
- American Journal of Clinical Nutrition
- Alternative Medicine Review
- International Journal of Cancer
- Clinical Pearls
- Anticancer Research
- Townsend Letter for Doctors & Their Patients

WEB RESOURCES

- www.oncanp.org
- www.aicr.org
- www.lifeovercancer.com
- www.cancerfacts.com
- www.nci.nih.gov
- www.cancernet.nci.nih.gov/clinpdq
- www.cancer.org American Cancer Society 1-800-ACS-2345
- www.cdc.gov.org/cancer
- www.bccancer.bc.ca
- www.y-me.org
- www.asco.org
- www.Medscape.com - oncology database
- www.inspirehealth.ca
- www.denvernaturopathic.com
- www.camresearch.net
- www.ncbi.nlm.nih.gov/**PubMed**/
- www.oncologystat.com
- www.epec.net

ACKNOWLEDGEMENTS & THANKS

I thank Terry Fox for demonstrating the courage to try to get things moving forward for today's cancer patients.

I thank Dr. John Bastyr, N.D. for his example of the pursuit of knowledge and brevity in communicating it.

I am much indebted to my colleagues at Cancer Treatment Centers of America, and members of the Oncology Association of Naturopathic Physicians for sharing their advanced knowledge of integrated cancer care.

Thank you my dear wife Lynda, for tolerating all that time looking at the back of my head while I write.

I am grateful to Pete Allen, my publisher, for his support and friendship.

With all my heart I thank my patients for sharing their lives so freely with me.

—Neil McKinney, ND
—Naturopathic Physician in Oncology

March 21, 2010

CLINIC COORDINATES

Vital Victoria Naturopathic Clinic, Ltd.
Ste. 125 – 1555 McKenzie Avenue, Victoria, BC CanadaV8N 1A4
Phone: (250) 386 -3534 Fax: (250) 386 -3500 Toll-free 1-888-722-6401
Web: www.drneilmckinney.ca Email: drneilmckinney@shaw.ca

INDEX

CPSIA information can be obtained at www.ICGtesting.com

227864LV00003B/2/P